Contraceptive Technology

Nineteenth Revised Edition

Robert A. Hatcher, MD, MPH

James Trussell, PhD

Anita L. Nelson, MD

Willard Cates Jr., MD, MPH

Felicia Stewart, MD

Deborah Kowal, MA, PA

ARDENT MEDIA, INC.
New York

ISSN 0091-9721

ISBN 978-1-59708-001-9/ISBN 1-59708-001-2 (Paperback with Single-User CD-ROM)
ISBN 978-1-59708-002-6/ISBN 1-59708-002-0 (Hardcover with Single-User CD-ROM)
ISBN 978-1-59708-003-3/ISBN 1-59708-003-9 (Single-User CD-ROM)

Credits:

Executive and Managing Editor: Deborah Kowal, MA, PA
Composition: Melissa Colbert, ATLIS Systems, Inc.
Production Coordination: Jerry Balan, ATLIS Systems, Inc.
CD-ROM Preparation: Jason Blackburn, Digital Impact Design
Indexer: WordCo Indexing Services, Inc.
Cover artist: KC Hatcher
Proofreader: Kelly Cleland, MPA, MPH

WP
630
C764
2008

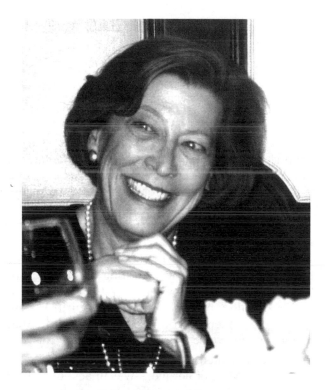

Felicia Hance Stewart

1943–2006

She made us laugh.
She made us think.
She made us care.
She made us act.
She made us proud.

"The respect colleagues accord her is tinged with the particular affection reserved for cheerful human gale forces."

—Jan Hoffman on Felicia Stewart,
The New York Times Magazine, January 10, 1993

Dedication

THE TWO FELICIAS:

Felicia Stewart

Felicia (Fifi) Guest

Felicia is an uncommon name, but we somehow managed to find two of them in our authors' group. Each woman was as uncommon as her name. Fitting too were the synonyms for 'uncommon': rare, unusual, singular, exceptional, remarkable, special. Especially special. It is to these two special colleagues, friends, and in a way, family members, that we dedicate this 19th edition.

Although the idea of dedicating the book to the two Felicia's generated much enthusiasm, the thought of writing the dedication pages left us all unwilling to volunteer to do the task. What could we possibly say that captured their intellect, humor, wise insight, spirit? We are impaired by not being able to ask them to craft the sentences and paragraphs, for they were our most poetic voices.

Felicia Stewart became an author in 1978, contributing to 11 editions, including this, her last. Most of her work was unacknowledged by a tagline under the chapter titles, because that was not how we did things back then. But she wrote the chapters that most directly addressed women's vulnerabilities and sensitivities: managing the changes that came at the end of the reproductive years, touching private parts to insert awkward barrier contraceptives, responding to the 'uh-oh' moments after unprotected intercourse, hanging in some suspense over a pregnancy test to give good news or bad, and going through the most difficult of decisions over whether to terminate a pregnancy. No one was a better advocate for women's unique health care needs; no one had a better ear for using language that was non-victim blaming and nonsexist; no one had a better sense of 'do no harm' as she advised, always, against hoping that the next prescription would change women's lives without recognizing there would be prices to pay. Even in the old days of gynecological unenlightenment, Felicia respected the symptoms that others failed to see as physiologic, such as PMS or menopausal complaints. She never oversold pharmaceutical panaceas. Read her early chapters on hormone replacement therapy... she was ever suggesting caution in weighing risks and benefits and casting healthy doubt on studies that fell short of randomized, controlled trials. "Prudent" was one of her favorite, and most heavily used, words. These things we will sorely and surely miss. Although we can find other good minds to write chapters, we cannot replace her vision, the way she always got to the marrow of a policy issue. We cannot replace the small things either, such as the way she took special note of something one of us had done well (or at least tried to) and made sure others were appreciative, or the way she could reduce life's complexities to stories of lost umbrellas or vagaries of ophthalmic diagnoses (an inside joke). However, if you are reading this dedication, turn next to Chapter 1 on Values in Family Planning. Felicia wrote the chapter from her heart, from her unerring sense of moral value, and from her front-line experiences as a caring clinician

Fifi Guest became an author on the book in 1976, writing for 11 editions. Up through the last edition, she wrote the chapter on education and counseling, roles for which she was quintessentially suited. With the simplest of words, Fifi explained the most complicated of topics. With the gentlest but most forthright of words, she rendered percipient counsel. To the book and to our group, she brought balance, unprejudicially weighing all sides of a debate. Fifi's sense of balance graced the pages of the HIV/AIDS chapter. Seldom does a family planning problem have such terrible consequences, and Fifi neither sensationalized nor medicalized the infection or its disease. She wrote about facts and statistics but never forgot matters on which relationship decisions really rest: romance and power and adolescent fantasies of people of every age. She respected that people make mistakes, and being allowed to make them was a kind of Bill of Rights, so clinicians (and friends and family) had best hold back judgment. One of her most dearly held beliefs was that "people do the best they can do at the time." Fifi never raised her voice, but she was never unheard. She was our storyteller. And she was funny as hell. (We particularly remember being seized with laughter over hearing her story involving a farmer's field in her native Alabama, impetuous youths, and a randy mule.) With passions ranging from direct patient counseling to the Atlanta Braves, from great restaurants to memorized passages of beginning and final paragraphs of great literature, Fifi shared freely her many means to *carpe* her *diem*. It is this rich, layered personality that gives her perspective, that informs her work, and that moves us still to call for her point of view.

As different as each of these Felicias were, they complemented each other perfectly. Optimists in the best sense of the word, they shared a belief in the potential of people to change, to be good, and to do good. Each had her own unique approach. Felicia Stewart worked incessantly to remodel the world, its laws, its attitudes, and even its vocabulary, urging people to fulfill their potential for good. Felicia Guest taught us how to find the good inside people and how to motivate them to act on their best instincts and qualities. Our two Felicias poured years of their creativity, caring, and enormous hearts into their work as teachers, activists, and role models. Readers of *Contraceptive Technology*, and those who have been touched in other ways by their wisdom and their souls, owe them an inestimable debt of gratitude. Let us never lose sight of their visions and values.

Preface

As many as 500,000 to one million women in the United States become pregnant while depending on birth control pills as their contraceptive. That statistic means, to me, that we have about a million challenges. We need to improve how we present information to women about their contraceptive choices and help them to choose and use contraceptives *consistently* and *correctly*.

For three decades, combined contraceptive pills, the major reversible contraceptive in the United States, have been taken 21/7, 21/7, 21/7. Pills taken this way lead to very regular withdrawal bleeding. Women who take the final hormonally active pill on Saturday morning will often say their periods came every 28 days and they came like clockwork: every Monday between 12 noon and 9 pm, for example, or every Sunday evening between 6 p.m. and 9 p.m.

This is so different than naturally occurring menses. Large studies of women's periods over their lifetime show that only 10% to 15% of cycles are exactly 28 days. To many of these women, the regularity was a contraceptive benefit from pills taken in the usual schedule. Accompanying this benefit, however, is a disadvantage—the potential to miss pills during the vulnerable first week of hormones, leading to the potential for a contraceptive failure.

Today, a number of women take pills continuously for extended periods of time. While extended use is not a completely new idea, it is a new practice for many women. Another practice is just starting: use of hormonally active pills for 24 days followed by just 4 days of taking no hormones.

Since 1990, the landscape has changed dramatically, with methods and practices that often change the flow and timing of a woman's 'monthly' menses:

- Depo-Provera injections (1992)
- Mirena, the levonorgestrel IUS (2001)
- Seasonale, the 3 month pill (2003)
- Extended use of NuvaRings (2001)
- Lybrel, the 1 year pill (2007)
- Implanon implants (2006)

Far from causing menstrual regularity, most of these methods consistently lead to irregular menses, spotting, and amenorrhea. These methods last longer, may be easier to use, and are more effective. They also have important non-contraceptive benefits. But for a woman to enjoy those advantages, they will need excellent counseling when they begin their method and at follow up visits. In the following chapters of *Contraceptive Technology*, readers will find the education and counseling tools to help women correctly use these important and effective options

I want to call attention to two other new insights that should change the way we practitioners counsel our patients. The first is the hysteroscopic approach to tubal occlusion, called Essure, which may help decrease the cumulative failure that had been associated with tubal ligation over the years. Hysteroscopic sterilization with Essure microinserts has been studied for 5 years with no pregnancies in a group of 643 women in Australia. Since 1-2% of women having laparoscopic tubal sterilization procedures become pregnant over the next 10 years, the Essure technique could prevent thousands upon thousands of pregnancies worldwide.

The second significant 'good news' concerns an old method. Evidence is increasing that condoms really work. They are reliable contraceptives if used consistently and correctly, and they are also effective at decreasing the risk of many sexually transmitted infections. A mid-2006 study of university students within a month of their first act of intercourse demonstrated that women using condoms 100% of the time were one-third as likely to test positive for HPV as women using condoms less than 5% of them. In 8 months, there were no cervical intraepithelial lesions among women always using condoms after 32 person-years of exposure while there were 14 incident lesions in 97 person-years of exposure among women who did not use condoms or used them less consistently.[1]

Between the day you read this and the next edition of *Contraceptive Technology*, consider the ways in which you can provide pills continuously, for extended periods of time (e.g., 84 days), or with shorter hormone-free intervals. Do what you can do to bring Essure into residency training programs and into physicians' offices (an operating room is *not* necessary). And encourage condom use.

Ours remains a dynamic field. We all need to work to keep up on the latest evidence-based findings. I have found family planning so exciting over the past four decades, and I am proud to be a colleague of the devoted, compassionate, and intelligent women and men who join me in this field.

Robert A. Hatcher, MD, MPH
Tiger, Georgia

[1]Winer RL, Hughes JP, Feng Q, O'Reilly S, Kiviat NB, Holmes KK, Koutsky LA. Condom use and the risk of genital human papillomavirus infection in young women. N Engl J Med. 2006 Jun 22;354(25):2645-54.

Author-Editors

Robert A. Hatcher, MD, MPH
Professor of Gynecology and Obstetrics
Emory University School of Medicine

James Trussell, PhD
Professor of Economics and Public Affairs
Director, Office of Population Research
Princeton University

Anita L. Nelson, MD
Professor, Obstetrics and Gynecology
David Geffen School of Medicine at UCLA

Medical Director, Women's Health Care Programs
Harbor-UCLA Medical Center

Willard Cates, Jr., MD, MPH
President, Research
Family Health International

Felicia H. Stewart, MD
Adjunct Professor, Department of Obstetrics, Gynecology and
    Reproductive Sciences
Co-Director, UCSF Center for Reproductive Health Research & Policy
University of California, San Francisco

Deborah Kowal, MA, PA
President and CEO, Contraceptive Technology Communications, Inc.

Adjunct Assistant Professor, Department of International Health
Rollins School of Public Health
Emory University

Chapter Authors

Marcos Arevalo, MD, MPH
Director of Biomedical Research, Institute for Reproductive Health
Assistant Professor, Department of Obstetrics and Gynecology
Georgetown University Medical Center

Susie Baldwin, MD, MPH
Women's Health Fellow
Greater Los Angeles VA Healthcare
Assistant Clinical Professor, Obstetrics and Gynecology
University of California-Los Angeles

Mark A. Barone, DVM, MS
Senior Medical Associate
EngenderHealth

Kathryn M. Curtis, PhD
Epidemiologist, Division of Reproductive Health
Centers for Disease Control and Prevention

Jacqueline E. Darroch, PhD
Senior Fellow
The Guttmacher Institute

Mary Fjerstad NP, MHS
Clinical Training Director
Planned Parenthood Consortium of Abortion Providers

Henry L. Gabelnick, PhD
Executive Director
CONRAD

Alisa B. Goldberg, MD, MPH
Assistant Professor of Obstetrics, Gynecology & Reproductive Biology
Harvard Medical School & Brigham and Women's Hospital
Director of Clinical Research and Training
Planned Parenthood League of Massachussetts

David A. Grimes, MD
Vice President of Biomedical Affairs
Family Health International
Clinical Professor, Department of Obstetrics and Gynecology
University of North Carolina School of Medicine

Felicia Guest, MPH, CHES
Director of Training, Southeast AIDS Training and Education Center
Emory University School of Medicine

Victoria H. Jennings, PhD
Professor of Obstetrics and Gynecology,
Georgetown University Medical Center

Director, Institute for Reproductive Health
Georgetown University

Kathy I. Kennedy, DrPH
Associate Clinical Professor of Preventive Medicine
University of Colorado at Denver and Health Sciences Center

Director, Regional Institute for Health and Environmental Leadership

Jeanne M. Marrazzo, MD, MPH
Associate Professor, Division of Allergy and Infectious Diseases
University of Washington

Medical Director, Seattle STD/HIV Prevention Training Center

John R. Marshall, MD
Clinical Professor of Obstetrics and Gynecology
UCLA School of Medicine

Attending Physician
Harbor/UCLA Medical Center

Anne Brawner Namnoum, MD
Atlanta Center for Reproductive Medicine

Kavita Nanda, MD, MHS
Medical Scientist, Clinical Research Department
Family Health International

Consulting Associate, Department of Obstetrics and Gynecology
Duke University Medical Center

Maureen Paul MD, MPH
Associate Clinical Professor, Department of Obstetrics, Gynecology, and
   Reproductive Services
Mt. Sinai School of Medicine

Chief Medical Officer
Planned Parenthood of New York City

Herbert B. Peterson, MD
Professor and Chairman, Department of Maternal and Child Health
School of Public Health

Professor, Department of Obstetrics and Gynecology
School of Medicine, The University of North Carolina at Chapel Hill

Michael S. Policar, MD, MPH
Associate Clinical Professor of Obstetrics, Gynecology and Reproductive
  Sciences
University of California, San Francisco

Amy E. Pollack, MD, MPH
Past President, EngenderHealth

Adjunct Assistant Professor
Mailman School of Public Health
Columbia University

Elizabeth G. Raymond, MD, MPH
Scientist
Family Health International

Jill Schwartz, MD
Clinical Research Manager, CONRAD

Assistant Professor of Obstetrics and Gynecology
Eastern Virginia Medical School

Markus J. Steiner, PhD, MSPH
Senior Epidemiologist
Family Health International

Lisa J. Thomas, MD, FACOG
Director of Reproductive Health Programs
The Susan Thompson Buffett Foundation

Paul F.A. Van Look, MD, PhD, FRCOG
Director, Department of Reproductive Health and Research
World Health Organization

Lee Warner, PhD, MPH
Senior Health Scientist, Division of Reproductive Health
Centers for Disease Control and Prevention

Reviewers

Frances Batzer, MD, MBE
Professor, Obstetrics and Gynecology
Division of Reproductive Endocrinology
Thomas Jefferson University Hospital

Eli Carter, BS
Director, Product Quality and Compliance Division
Family Health International

Laura Castleman, MD, MPH
Medical Director, Ipas
Clinician, Planned Parenthood Mid-Michigan
Adjunct Assistant Clinical Professor
University of Michigan

Soledad Diaz, MD
Member of the Board of Directors
Instituto Chileno de Medicina Reproductiva

Mary Lyn Gaffield, PhD
Technical Officer, Department of Reproductive Health and Research
World Health Organization

Marji Gold MD
Professor, Family and Social Medicine
Director, Family Planning Fellowship
The Center for Reproductive Health Education in Family Medicine
Albert Einstein College of Medicine/Montefiore Medical Center

Roy Jacobstein, MD, MPH
Clinical Director, ACQUIRE Project, EngenderHealth
Adjunct Professor, Maternal and Child Health
University of North Carolina School of Public Health

Miriam H. Labbok MD, MPH
Professor, Practice of Public Health
Director, Center for Infant and Young Child Feeding and Care
Department of Maternal and Child Health, School of Public Health
University of North Carolina-Chapel Hill

Helain Landy, MD
Professor and Chair of Obstetrics-Gynecology
Georgetown University

Monica Hau Le, MD
Women's Health Fellow
Harbor-UCLA Medical Center

E. Steve Lichtenberg MD, MPH
Assistant Professor of Clinical Obstetrics-Gynecology
Northwestern University Feinberg School of Medicine
Medical Director, Family Planning Associates Medical Group, Ltd.

Maurizio Macaluso, MD, DrPH
Senior Research Scientist and Chief, Division of Reproductive Health
Centers for Disease Control and Prevention

Cristina Muñoz, MD
Assistant Professor, Division of Women's Primary Healthcare
Department of Obstetrics and Gynecology
University of North Carolina, Chapel Hill

LeRoy E. Nelson, MS

Mark D. Nichols, MD
Professor, Obstetrics and Gynecology
Oregon Health & Science University

Nuriye Ortayli, MD, MPH
Medical Officer, Department of Reproductive Health and Research
World Health Organization

Roberto Rivera, MD
Senior Advisor
Family Health International

George F. Sawaya, MD
Associate Professor
Departments of Obstetrics, Gynecology and Reproductive Sciences
Epidemiology and Biostatistics
University of California, San Francisco

Sharon Schnare, MSN, FNP, CNM
Clinician and Consultant
South Kitsap Family Care Clinic

John J. Sciarra, MD, PhD
Thomas J. Watkins Professor and Chairman, Department of Obstetrics and
   Gynecology
Northwestern University Medical School

Donna Shoupe, MD
Professor, Obstetrics and Gynecology and Family Medicine
Keck School of Medicine
University of Southern California

Joe Leigh Simpson, MD
Professor and Chair of Obstetrics-Gynecology
Baylor College of Medicine

Matthew Stewart

Kathryn Stewart

Katherine M. Stone, MD
Consultant
Atlanta, GA

Helena von Hertzen, MD, DDS
Medical Officer
UNDP/UNFPA/WHO/World Bank Special Programme of Research,
   Development and Research Training in Human Reproduction
Department of Reproductive Health and Research
World Health Organization

Edio J. Zampaglione, MD, FACOG
Senior Director, Women's Healthcare
Medical Affairs
Organon USA, Inc.

Table of Contents

Color Photos of Pills follow page 418

Invitations and Conferences

New Media Survey

CD-ROM Information

*Managing Contraceptio*n **Information and Order Form**

Safely Sexual **Information**

Contraceptive Technology **Order Forms**

List of Tables

List of Figures

Contraceptive Technology

Values in Family Planning

Felicia H. Stewart, MD

Contraception, family planning, and reproductive health care available before 1960 would seem remarkably limited to us today. The "modern" method was the diaphragm, not legal yet in many states because of Comstock laws and, in any case, not likely to be available at all to unmarried women. The "Pill" was still a research method. The first edition of *Contraceptive Technology* was published over thirty years ago (1969) when hormonal contraceptives had only recently become commonplace. Since then, an entire generation has grown up with the potential benefits of a variety of safe and effective contraceptive methods. (See Table 1–1 for a list of modern milestones in reproductive health.) These technologies have enabled men and women to decide when and whether to become parents, a profound advance that has indelibly shaped modern life.

In these beginning pages of the 19th edition, the authors* take a moment to talk about why providing reproductive health care, researching, teaching, and writing remain so satisfying and rewarding to each of us.

Professionals in our field are familiar with its amazing scientific and medical advances, and are comfortable explaining the research evidence and science involved. Many of us, however, are less accustomed to the other important dimension of this work—its *moral* value. For most of us, this dimension is why working in reproductive health care is so compelling. When we counsel patients about birth control, help patients make decisions about an unintended pregnancy, help women plan for pregnancy and safely traverse its nine months, work to shape public policy, or contribute to reproductive health research, whether or not we are aware of it, we are engaged in a critically important and deeply moral undertaking.

---

*Felicia Guest, MPH, CHES; Deborah Kowal, MA, PA; Matthew Stewart; and Kathryn Stewart provided assistance on this chapter.

For some areas in clinical medicine, the *why* seems hardly to need a chapter. Becoming an expert on heart disease management has self-evident value, and is not controversial. The value of work as a heart disease clinician is not likely to be attacked as immoral, and heart problems are not likely to be carved out for special scrutiny as expenditures by public health services. The local town council or school board is not likely to ask the local heart specialist to testify about proposed local policies. Unfortunately, this is not true for clinicians working in the field of family planning services and reproductive health.

Table 1–1 Milestones: reproductive health in the United States

1960s
1960 Enovid, first oral contraceptive, approved[7]
1964 Lippes Loop IUD introduced
1965 Supreme Court assures access to contraception for married couples on right to privacy grounds in *Griswold* v. *Connecticut*[4]
1968 Pope Paul VI publishes *Humanae Vitae*, reaffirming opposition to all contraception except for rhythm method
1969 CDC begins abortion surveillance to document legal abortion rates and adverse events[1,2]

1970s
1970 Title X of Public Health Services Act funds public family planning services
1970 First oral contraceptive package insert written for consumers
1971 First bound edition of *Contraceptive Technology* (32 pages)
1971 CDC establishes the National Survey of Family Growth, first reliable nationl data on contraception, infertility, marriage[1]
1972 Supreme Court rules that the right to privacy includes an unmarried person's right to use contraception in *Eisenstadt* v. *Baird*[4]
1973 Supreme Court upholds abortion on right to privacy grounds in *Roe* v. *Wade*
1973 *Our Bodies, Ourselves* published by Boston Women's Health Book Collective[3]
1974 CDC launches Collaborative Review of Sterilization (CREST) study with NIH to investigate safety and efficacy of sterilization procedures in the U.S.[1,2]
1974 Dalkon Shield IUD no longer manufactured.
1976 First over-the-counter pregnancy test kit advertised in women's magazines[3]
1976 First Hyde Amendment bars use of Medicaid funds for abortion[9]

1980s
1981 First cluster of U.S. AIDS cases described[6]
1983 Toxic Shock Syndrome determined to be related to tampon characteristics
1983 CDC and FDA recommend women still using Dalkon Shields have them removed due to excess PID risk[1]

(continued)

Table 1–1 Milestones: reproductive health in the United States—*(cont'd)*

1984 Copper T 380A (ParaGard) approved by FDA

1985 HIV antibody screening test becomes available[6]

1982 Cancer and Steroid Hormones (CASH) initial study concludes that oral contraceptives do not cause cancer and actually decrease risk for certain kinds of cancer

1986 CDC begins surveillance of maternal mortality

1988 Oral contraceptives with more than 50 mcg of estrogen withdrawn due to association with rare but fatal thromboembolism[8]

1988 Title X "gag rule" prohibits nondirective pregnancy options counseling and referral[9]

1990s

1990 Norplant approved

1991 Meta-analysis of estrogen replacement therapy shows increase in breast cancer rate for long-term users[1]

1991 CDC recommends hepatitis vaccine for infants[1]

1992 Depo Provera approved[7]

1992 Abortion access in steady decline. No abortion provider in 84% of U.S. counties

1993 Female condom approved

1993 *Chlamydia trachomatis* identified by CDC and Office of Population Affairs as leading cause of infertility among women[1]

1993 President Clinton revokes 1988 "gag rule"[9]

1994 CDC publishes recommendations for prevention of perinatal HIV transmission

1995 National Institute of Justice and CDC cosponsor National Violence Against Women survey[1]

1997 CDC releases first annual report of pregnancy success rates for U.S. fertility clinics

1998 Emergency contraception approved[7]

1999 World population tops 6 billion[3]

2000s

2000 First major international microbicide conference

2000 FDA approves first U.S. rapid HIV diagnostic test kit[6]

2000 FDA approves mifepristone for abortion in early pregnancy[10]

2000 CDC CREST study reports tubal sterilization not associated with menstrual problems

2001 Scientific review panel confirms condoms are effective against HIV/AIDS[6]

2002 NuvaRing vaginal ring and Ortho Evra patch introduced

2002 Women's CARE study concludes that oral contraceptive users are not more likely than other women to develop breast cancer between 35 and 64[1]

Timeline compiled from web sites for CDC Divisions of Women's Health[1] and Reproductive Health[2], the National Institutes of Health[3], the New York Times[4], U.S. Agency for International Development[5], the Food and Drug Administration[6], WebMD[7], the Public Broadcasting System[8], Planned Parenthood of NorthEast Pennsylvania[9], and the National Abortion Federation[10]

It is not only abortion that is under attack. Emergency contraception, IUDs, and OCs are challenged by arguments based on questionable evidence. Failure to provide insurance coverage for contraception is *prima facie* evidence of the second-class status of women in this country. In the face of these challenges to individual freedoms, we need to rededicate ourselves to the goal that a woman does have the right to control her own fertility and that she needs access to information, services and psychological support for her decisions. And we need to remember that fertility control improves pregnancy outcomes.

As scientists, clinicians, and educators, we may not be accustomed to talking about values. For many of us, however, the moral importance of our work is its most compelling appeal, and it helps sustain us in the face of political challenges that are increasingly trumping science. As we work with colleagues and policymakers, we need to convey not only the science of reproductive health, but also why it is of vital importance in people's lives. If we fail to do so, we are abdicating the moral high ground to those who oppose efforts to provide reproductive health care.

When we perform our work in clinics, hospitals, laboratories, and offices, we are engaged in a critically important and *deeply moral* undertaking. Reproductive health care enables individuals and couples to make and implement some of the most important decisions that shape their lives, and thus in turn shape society.

Today, we are still faced with an environment in which actions and decisions are "compromised by discriminatory practices and policies:"[1]

1. National public health statistics hide disgraceful or even shocking disparities in health status for disadvantaged communities. For example, minorities are more likely than whites to be diagnosed with late-stage breast cancer. The risk of dying from pregnancy or delivery is three to four times higher for black women than for white women.

2. Women are disproportionately stuck at the low end of the job scale where benefits—including health coverage—are less likely.

3. More than half of U.S. women report ever having been physically assaulted. Those who need assurance of protection find the mechanisms are scant.

4. Women have been shortchanged in funding and insurance coverage for essential reproductive health care services that only women need: cervical cancer screening, routine exams, and contraceptives.

5. To this day, illnesses that primarily affect women are less well understood than those that affect men because of the research gap in women's health.

6. Preventive care lives under the 'poverty line.' For example, funding for Title X, the program that provides reproductive health and family planning care to low-income men and women, is adequate to provide care for only half the people who need it.

7. Women find their status as moral agents who have the capacity, right, and responsibility to make their own reproductive decisions[2] is being challenged.

8. Within some of our national health agencies, ideology has distorted scientific evidence and the disseminated information has gone against the recommendations of mainstream prevention experts on a wide range of public health issues. Men and women need evidence-based education in order to make sound reproductive decisions ranging from whether to use condoms (which are effective in reducing the risk of STIs) to being able to obtain emergency contraceptives.

9. There still exist in America unwanted babies, some of whom grow up to be unwanted children. Family planning services should receive the support they need[3]—in funding, policy, research, and community cooperation—to help every child be a wanted child.

Reproductive health care reflects a deep commitment to parenthood and children. Our work helps ensure that every pregnancy is intended and as safe as possible, and that children are born when their parents are best able to provide the love and support they need to thrive. Reproductive health care makes an essential contribution to the human infrastructure we count on for our society to thrive. Our participation in strengthening individuals, families, and the community provides each of us—including those who write this book—with a foundation for our own unique moral code, which brings meaning to our lives.

REFERENCES

1. Hwang AC, Shields WC, Stewart FH. Ten priorities in women's health. Contraception 2004;70:265–268.
2. Colloquium of Theologians. An open letter to religious leaders on abortion as a moral decision. Religious Institute on Sexual Morality, Justice, and Healing, 2005.
3. Alan Guttmacher Institute. Women and societies benefit when childbearing is planned. Issues in brief. Maternal health. The Alan Guttmacher Institute, 2002.

The Menstrual Cycle

Robert A. Hatcher, MD, MPH
Anne Brawner Namnoum, MD

- Normal ovulatory cycles require the integration of hormones and peptides from the hypothalamus, pituitary gland, and ovaries. When a woman's cycles are irregular, it is usually due to differences in the length of the follicular phase of the cycle.

- The perfect 28-day cycle is the most common pattern, but it occurred in only 12.4% of more than 30,000 cycles recorded by 650 women.[1]

- Hormonal contraceptives have many desirable effects on the cyclic symptoms women experience during their menstrual cycles.

A thorough understanding of the menstrual cycle is fundamental to the discussion of contraception. The ovaries are the source of oocytes (eggs) as well as the hormones that regulate female reproduction. In contrast to the male reproductive system where large numbers of gametes are produced continuously, in women only one gamete is released each month from the time of menarche to the time of menopause. During each monthly interval, or menstrual cycle, a series of events occurs that culminates in ovulation and the preparation of the endometrium for implantation of an embryo. The corpus luteum begins to atrophy 9 to 11 days after ovulation if pregnancy does not occur. Shortly thereafter the process of oocyte maturation and endometrial preparation begins anew. Under complex regulation by the hypothalamus, the pituitary gland, and the ovaries, cyclic changes in gonadotropins and steroid hormones induce the development of a dominant follicle, resulting in ovulation and corpus luteum formation.[2] Responding to the cyclic changes in ovarian steroids, the endometrium prepares for implantation should fertilization occur. If pregnancy does not occur, the endometrium sloughs, resulting in menstrual bleeding.

Most women have cycles lasting from 24 to 35 days. Only 0.5% of cycles are shorter than 21 days and 0.9% of cycles are longer than 35 days. At least 20% of women experience irregular cycles.[3] The normal ovulatory menstrual cycle can be divided into four functional phases: follicular (pre-ovulatory), ovulatory, luteal, and menstrual.

MENSTRUAL CYCLE REGULATION
HYPOTHALAMUS AND ANTERIOR PITUITARY

Gonadotropin-releasing hormone (GnRH), a neurohormone synthesized in the hypothalamus, travels via the portal circulation to the anterior pituitary gland. GnRH is secreted in a pulsatile fashion every 60 to 90 minutes, stimulating cells in the anterior pituitary (gonadotropes) to produce follicle-stimulating hormone (FSH) and luteinizing hormone (LH).[4,5] FSH and LH are secreted in a pulsatile manner in response to GnRH pulses. The pulse frequency varies, depending on the phase of the menstrual cycle. FSH plays a dominant role in the promotion of ovarian follicular growth by causing the granulosa cells that line each follicle to proliferate and produce estrogen. LH stimulates androgen production in theca cells adjacent to the granulosa cells. These androgens are the substrates for estrogen production. LH also promotes ovulation and final oocyte maturation and converts estrogen-secreting granulosa cells to progesterone-secreting cells after ovulation.

STEROID PRODUCTION IN THE OVARIES

Together, theca cells and granulosa cells synthesize steroid hormones. According to the two-cell, two-gonadatrophin theory, at the beginning of an ovulatory cycle the outer theca cells can only be stimulated by luteinizing hormone (LH) and the inner granulosa cells can only be stimulated by follicle stimulating hormone (FSH). Theca cells respond to LH by producing the androgens testosterone and androstenedione. These androgens diffuse from the theca cells across the basement membrane of the follicle into granulosa cells, where they are converted to estrogens by the enzyme aromatase. Theca cells have little intrinsic aromatase activity, and granulosa cells are relatively deficient in the enzymes necessary to synthesize androgens; thus the two cell types depend on each other to produce estrogen in the developing follicle. Androgens are critical to follicular development because they are the precursors of estrogens, but if androgens exist in excess amounts, they induce follicular atresia. At low levels, androgens in granulosa cells have two effects: they are the substrate for conversion into estrogen, and they stimulate aromatase activity. Androgen production therefore must be delicately balanced to allow for normal ovarian function.

Moderate levels of estrogen produced by the follicles act on both the hypothalamus and the anterior pituitary to inhibit FSH and LH secretion in a classic negative feedback effect.[6] Progesterone and androgens have a negative feedback effect as well, but theirs is not as prominent as that of estrogen. Paradoxically, higher levels of estrogen have a positive feedback effect on gonadotropin secretion during the middle of a cycle, which initiates the preovulatory surge of LH and FSH.[3] When levels of estradiol in the range of 200 to 300 picograms/milliliter (ml) are present for 2 to 3 days, a gonadotropin surge is elicited. Low levels of progesterone produced before ovulation amplify this positive estrogen feedback effect. The pituitary is the major site of such estradiol action, but there may be a hypothalamic site of action as well. This positive feedback effect of estrogen is critical for ovulation and regular menstrual cycles.

PEPTIDE HORMONES IN THE OVARIES

A variety of peptide hormones produced in the ovary help modulate follicular development and steroid production. One of the more important of these substances is inhibin, a protein composed of alpha and beta subunits. Synthesized in granulosa and theca cells, inhibin suppresses FSH secretion.[7] Activin, composed of two of the beta subunits of inhibin, has the opposite effect and enhances FSH secretion. Ovarian follicular fluid contains more inhibin than activin, thus inhibin from the dominant follicle has a negative feedback effect on FSH secretion. Inhibin and activin also act directly within the ovary to regulate androgen and estrogen production. A third peptide, follistatin, also suppresses FSH, probably by binding activin.

Insulin and insulin-like growth factors also seem to play a significant role as regulators within the ovary. Insulin-like growth factor 1 (IGF-1) stimulates cell division and growth in many tissues. The ovary is now known to be a site of IGF-1 production and action. IGF-1 has been shown to amplify LH-stimulated androgen production in theca cells and to amplify FSH action in granulosa cells. It may also serve to communicate messages between granulosa cells and theca cells.

Oocyte maturation inhibitor (OMI), a peptide hormone present in follicular fluid, prevents final maturation of the oocyte until the time of ovulation. OMI suppression ends within hours following the midcycle LH surge just prior to ovulation.

ENDOMETRIUM

The endometrium responds to the cyclic changes in ovarian steroids. Estrogen increases the thickness of the endometrium by increasing the number and size of endometrial cells. Estrogen also stimulates the formation of progesterone receptors on endometrial cells and increases the blood flow (via spiral arterioles) to the endometrium. Progesterone causes the proliferated endometrium to differentiate and secrete proteins that are important in the survival and implantation of an early embryo if pregnancy occurs. Progesterone and exogenous progestins also decrease the proliferative effects of estrogens on the endometrium by causing down-regulation of estrogen receptors. Withdrawal of estrogen and progesterone results in the orderly and controlled sloughing of the functional zone of the endometrium. This monthly shedding of the lining of the uterus occurs from 400 to 500 times during a woman's reproductive years.[8]

CERVIX

The cervix and cervical mucus also change in response to estrogen and progesterone. The cervical mucus facilitates selective sperm penetration from the vagina to the fallopian tube during the periovulatory period; at other times, the mucus prevents microorganisms and sperm from entering the uterine cavity. When estradiol levels increase during the mid to late follicular phase, the cervical mucus becomes clear, thin, more profuse, and extrudes from the cervical os into the vagina. The cervix itself swells and softens, and the cervical os dilates. After ovulation, progesterone causes the cervix to become more firm, the cervical os to close, and the cervical mucus to become scant, thick, and turbid. Progesterone and exogenous progestins produce a contraceptive effect by causing a thick cervical mucus that sperm cannot penetrate.

THE INTEGRATED CYCLE
FOLLICULAR PHASE

Pulsatile GnRH release by the hypothalamus results in pulses of FSH and LH. FSH stimulates the proliferation of granulosa cells, which produce estradiol from androgen precursors synthesized in theca cells.[3] In the first half of the follicular phase (days 1 to 5), many follicles are "recruited" and begin to grow. The increasing local estradiol levels induce more FSH receptors on the largest follicle, thus producing greater amounts of estradiol. Estradiol and inhibin begin to provide negative feedback on FSH secretion by the anterior pituitary. (See Figures 2–1 and 2–2.)

During days 5 to 7 of the cycle, one of the recruited follicles becomes "dominant," producing the most estradiol, the largest number of granulosa cells and developing the most FSH receptors.[2] As FSH levels decline, the dominant follicle survives while the non-dominant follicles undergo atresia. After day 7, the dominant follicle is selected. The dominant follicle continues to mature and produce high levels of estradiol in the latter half of the follicular phase.[9] The length of the follicular phase is variable from individual to individual, but usually ranges from 10 to 17 days.

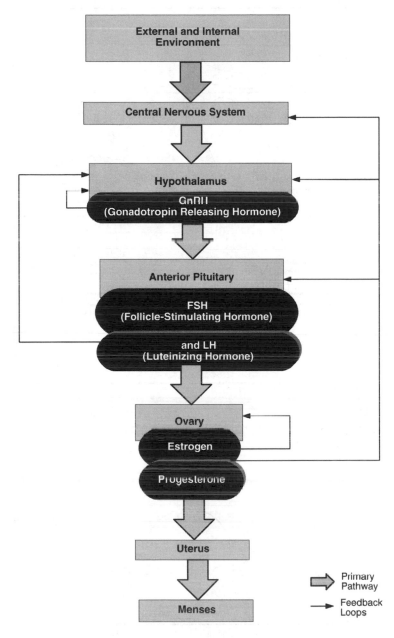

Primary hormone pathways ( ) in the reproductive system are
modulated by both negative and positive feedback loops (→).
Prostaglandins, secreted by the ovary and by uterine endometrial
cells, also play a role in ovulation, and may modulate hypothalamic
function as well.

Figure 2–1 Regulation of the menstrual cycle

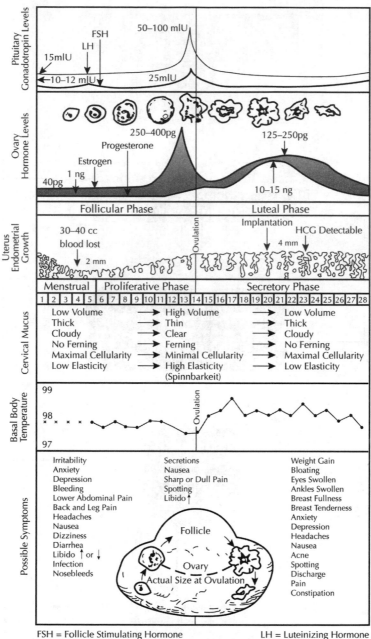

Figure 2–2 **Menstrual cycle events: hormone levels, ovarian, and endometrial patterns and cyclic temperature and cervical mucus changes**

Very late in the follicular phase LH activity stimulates stromal tissue causing a rise in androgen levels: a 15% increase in androstenedione and a 20% increase in testosterone. Libido can be stimulated by androgens, and a peak in sexual behavior initiated by women occurs in the ovulatory phase of the cycle. The mid-cycle rise in androgens may therefore increase sexual activity at the time most likely to lead to a pregnancy.

OVULATORY PHASE

Once the estradiol level has exceeded a critical level for 2 to 3 days, a positive feedback occurs in the pituitary, resulting in a surge of LH and FSH.[10] The estradiol level reaches its peak about 24 hours before ovulation. The LH surge leads to resumption of meiosis in the dominant oocyte, luteinization of granulosa cells, and resultant progesterone production. Prostaglandins, proteolytic enzymes, and the contraction of smooth muscle cells within the follicle result in a break down of the follicular wall. The oocyte and follicular fluid exude about 32 to 44 hours after the onset of the LH surge and 10 to 12 hours after the LH peak. The onset of the LH surge appears to be the most reliable indicator of impending ovulation, and ovulation predictor kits detect this increasing surge of LH.

LUTEAL PHASE

Following the rupture of the follicle, the granulosa and theca cells take up steroids and lutein pigment to give the corpus luteum ("yellow body") a yellow appearance. The hallmark of the luteal phase is the shift from the estrogen-dominated follicular phase to one of progesterone dominance. Progesterone suppresses new follicular growth and causes secretory changes in the endometrium.[11] Peak progesterone production occurs 7 to 8 days after the LH surge, at the approximate time of implantation if fertilization has occurred. The length of the luteal phase tends to be more constant than the follicular phase, approximately 14 days unless pregnancy occurs.

Because progesterone causes an elevation in basal body temperature, daily measurement of basal body temperature can be used to determine whether or not ovulation has occurred. (See Chapter 16 on Fertility Awareness.) Basal body temperatures cannot be used to predict ovulation, as the temperature rise does not occur until after ovulation, but can confirm that ovulation has occurred.

MENSTRUAL PHASE

If a woman does not become pregnant, the corpus luteum rapidly declines 9 to 11 days after ovulation, resulting in a decline of progesterone and estrogen levels.[3] The withdrawal of these hormones initially shrinks endometrial height, decreases blood flow, and begins vasodilation followed by rhythmic vasoconstriction of the spiral arterioles. Ischemia and stasis are followed by interstitial hemorrhage and tissue disorganization, resulting in menstrual flow.[12]

The normal amount of blood lost during a normal menstrual period is 20 to 80 ml. Seventy percent of the blood will slough by the second day, and 90% by the third day.[8] The average duration of the menstrual phase is 4 to 6 days.

Thrombin-platelet plugs limit blood loss, and rising estrogen levels of the new cycle induce clot formation and regrowth of the endometrium. Delayed, asynchronous, or incomplete shedding of the endometrium, as might occur in anovulatory cycles, can be associated with heavier and longer bleeding.

FERTILIZATION AND IMPLANTATION

A woman is most likely to conceive if fresh sperm are present in the upper reproductive tract when ovulation occurs. The oocyte retains potential for fertilization for 12 to 24 hours, and sperm usually remain viable in the reproductive tract for 72 hours. The extreme intervals at which women have achieved pregnancy after a single act of coitus are 6 days prior to and 3 days after ovulation.[13] The several days prior to ovulation are thus the most fertile cycle days, or the days that conception is most likely to occur. (See Chapter 25 on Impaired Fertility.) After ovulation and during the very early follicular phase, the likelihood of pregnancy is much lower. If a woman has very regular cycles and is monitoring her cycle closely, it may be feasible to use periodic abstinence during the fertile period as a means of contraception. (See Chapter 16 on Fertility Awareness.)

IMPLANTATION

During intercourse, the man deposits into the woman's vagina as many as 300 million spermatozoa suspended in seminal fluid. Because cervical mucus does not mix with semen, the sperm have to pass into the mucus, but this occurs within minutes. Under optimal conditions (in the pre-ovulatory period), the number of sperm that enter the mucus within the first few minutes is often sufficient to accomplish fertilization. Within 30 minutes, several hundred thousand sperm can be found in the cervical canal, and this number remains stable for approximately 24 hours. Because cervical mucus allows easier passage of normal sperm, the sperm population improves over that present in the ejaculate. Sperm pass through the fallopian tubes fairly rapidly, but spermatozoa in the cervical crypts can supply sperm to the upper reproductive tract for several days.

Following extrusion of the oocyte and cumulus complex at the time of ovulation, the oocyte is swept into the lumen of the tube by the fimbria within minutes to hours. Fertilization occurs in the ampullary region of the fallopian tube, and the early embryo is then transported to the uterine cavity within 2 to 3 days. Implantation begins approximately 6 to 7 days after fertilization, when the embryo is at the blastocyst stage.

ANOVULATION

Because normal ovulatory cycles require the integration of hormones and signals from the hypothalamus, pituitary gland, and ovaries, problems at any of these sites may result in anovulation. Inadequate GnRH secretion by the hypothalamus inhibits normal FSH and LH production and results in anovulation. Problems such as weight loss, extensive exercise, stress, depression and anorexia nervosa can interfere with GnRH secretion. Hyperprolactinemia may also result in ovulatory dysfunction or anovulation.

Alterations in the critically balanced factors in the ovary may also lead to anovulation. Excessive concentration of androgens in ovarian follicles may inhibit the emergence of a dominant follicle and result in follicular atresia. As in individuals with polycystic ovarian syndrome, hyperinsulinemia may contribute to the excessive androgen production in the ovaries.

THE MENSTRUAL CYCLE AND AGING

Menstrual cycle length varies as a woman ages. Cycles tend to be longer when a woman is under age 20 and over age 40. It may be several years after menarche before regular, ovulatory cycles are achieved. Several years prior to menopause, menstrual cycles tend to lengthen and anovulatory cycles become more frequent again.[14]

HORMONAL CONTRACEPTIVE EFFECTS

Hormonal contraceptives prevent fertilization in part by disrupting the menstrual cycle. Combined oral contraceptives contain both estrogen and progestin. Progestin-only contraceptives include Depo-Provera injections, Norplant implants, progestin-only pills (minipills), and intra-uterine devices (IUDs) such as the Progestasert System and the Levonorgestrel Intrauterine System. Estrogens and progestins act upon many different organ systems and produce a broad range of effects.[3] Among the most important noncontraceptive benefits of pills are their beneficial effects on the cyclic symptoms women may experience as a result of their menstrual cycles.

Estrogenic Effects

- Ovulation is inhibited because estrogen suppresses FSH and LH, thus preventing the pituitary gland from releasing ovary-stimulating hormones.
- The endometrial secretions and cellular structure are altered.
- Altered local levels of prostaglandins contribute to the degeneration of the corpus luteum.

Progestational Effects

- Ovulation is inhibited by suppression of the midcycle peak of LH and FSH.
- Thickened cervical mucus decreases sperm penetration.
- The activity of the cilia in the fallopian tubes is reduced.
- The endometrium becomes atrophic and impairs implantation.

REFERENCES

1. Vollman RF, the menstrual cycle, In: Friedman E, ed. Major problems in obstetrics and gynecology, W.B. Saunders Co., Philadelphia, 1977.
2. Henderson KM. Gonadotrophic regulation of ovarian activity. Br Med Bull 1979; 35:161.
3. Speroff L, Glass RH, Kase G. Clinical gynecologic endocrinology and infertility. 6th edition. Baltimore MD: Lippincott Williams & Wilkins, 1999.
4. Filicori M, Santoro N, Merriam GR, Crowley WF Jr. Characterization of the physiological pattern of episodic gonadotropin secretion throughout the human menstrual cycle. J Clin Endocrinol Metab 1986;62:1136.
5. Reame N, Sauder SE, Kelch RP, Marshall JC. Pulsatile gonadotropin secretion during the human menstrual cycle: evidence for altered frequency of gonadotropin-releasing hormone secretion. J Clin Endocrinol Metab 1984;59:384.
6. Kase NG, Speroff L. The ovary. In: Bondy P, Rosenberg L (eds). Metabolic control and disease. 8th edition. Philadelphia PA: WB Saunders, 1980.
7. Bicsak TA, Tucker EM, Cappel S, Vaughan J, Rivier J, Vale W, Hseuh AJW. Hormonal regulation of granulosa cell inhibin biosynthesis. Endocrinology 1986;119:2711.
8. Swartz DP, Butler W. Normal and abnormal uterine bleeding. In: Thompson JD, Rock JA (eds). TeLindeÕs operative gynecology. 7th edition. Philadelphia PA: J.B. Lippincott, 1992.
9. Clark JR, Dierschke DJ, Wolf RC. Hormonal regulation of ovarian folliculogenesis in rhesus monkey. III. Atresia on the preovulatory follicle induced by exogenous steroids and subsequent follicular development. Biol Reprod 1981;25:332.
10. Hoff, JD, Quigley ME, Yen SSC. Hormonal dynamics at midcycle: a reevaluation. J Clin Endocrinol Metab 1983;57:792.
11. Kase NG, Weingold AB, Gershenson DM. Principles and practice of clinical gynecology. 2nd edition. New York: Churchill Livingstone, 1990.

12. Sixma JJ, Cristiens GCML, Haspels AS. The sequence of hemostasis events in the endometrium during normal menstruation. In: Diczfalusy E, Fraser IS, Webb WTG (eds). WHO symposium on steroid contraception and endometrial bleeding. London: Pittman Press Ltd, 1980.

13. France JT, Graham FM, Gosling L, Hair P, Knox BS. Characteristics of natural conception cycles occurring in a prospective study of sex preselection: fertility awareness symptoms, hormone levels, sperm survival, and pregnancy outcome. Int J Fertil 37:244, 1992.

14. Gosden RG. Follicular status at menopause. Human Reprod 1987;2:617.

Choosing a Contraceptive: Efficacy, Safety, and Personal Considerations

James Trussell, PhD

- Correct and consistent use of most contraceptive methods results in a low risk of pregnancy.

- The simultaneous use of methods dramatically lowers the risk of pregnancy.

- Emergency contraception provides a last chance to prevent pregnancy after unprotected intercourse or when the extent of contraceptive protection is unclear.

- Most contraceptives pose little risk to most users' health, although personal risk factors should influence personal choice.

- Half of all pregnancies are unintended (3.1 million each year); more than four in ten unintended pregnancies end in an induced abortion and half result from contraceptive failure. One-third of all births are unintended (1.4 million each year).

Choosing a method of contraception is an important decision. A method that is not effective for an individual can lead to an unintended pregnancy. A method that is not safe for the user can create unfortunate medical consequences. A method that does not fit the individual's personal lifestyle is not likely to be used correctly or consistently. Individuals themselves must make the decision about the contraceptive method they use, taking into consideration the feelings and attitudes of their partners. The best method of contraception for an individual or couple is one that is safe and that will actually be used correctly and consistently.

Because most people will use a variety of contraceptive methods throughout their lives, they should be knowledgeable about various contraceptive methods. The patient's choice of a contraceptive method depends on several major factors: efficacy, safety, cost, noncontraceptive benefits, and personal considerations. Through counseling, you can help your patient choose the most suitable contraceptive method. You also can influence the user's motivation and ability to use the method correctly.[1] Encourage clients to educate themselves about the various methods available. Direct clients toward available literature.

Information on levels and trends in contraceptive use in the United States is based on the National Surveys of Family Growth (NSFG), periodic surveys conducted by the National Center for Health Statistics in which women ages 15 to 44 are interviewed about topics related to childbearing, family planning, and maternal and child health. Among the 61.6 million women of reproductive age (ages 15 to 44) in 2002, about 62% (38.1 million) were using some method of contraception, according to the 2002 NSFG. Among the 38% (23.5 million) who were not currently using a method, only about one-fifth were at risk of pregnancy. The remaining four-fifths were not at risk because they had been sterilized for noncontraceptive reasons, were sterile, were trying to become pregnant, were pregnant, were interviewed within 2 months after the completion of a pregnancy, or were not having intercourse during the 3 months prior to the survey.[2]

Almost 90% of the women at risk of an unintended pregnancy were using a contraceptive method, but 10.7% of all women at risk of unintended pregnancy were not using any contraceptive method. Today, the most popular contraceptive methods are oral contraceptive pills (11.6 million), female sterilization (10.3 million), male condoms (6.8 million), and male sterilization (3.5 million). See Table 3–1 for information on contraceptive method use by age of woman.

Use of the male condom and withdrawal is higher than indicated in Table 3–1, because some women are protected by dual methods. In the 2002 NSFG, women were asked to report all contraceptive methods used in the current month for any reason (for protection against either pregnancy or STIs). When more than one method was reported, only the most effective method is coded as the current method. When the data in Table 3–1 are recoded to capture all use of the male condom, the fraction using male condoms among all women at risk rises by 33%, from 16.0% to 21.2%. Increases are greatest among women ages 15 to 19 (a 67% increase, from 22.1% to 36.8%) and among women ages 20 to 24 (a 56% increase, from 20.2% to 31.5%). When the data in Table 3–1 are recoded to capture all use of withdrawal, the fraction using withdrawal among all women at risk rises by 117%, from 3.6% to 7.8%. Increases are greatest among women ages 15 to 19 (a 486% increase, from 2.1% to 12.3%) and among women ages 20 to 24 (a 131% increase, from 4.5% to 10.4%).[2]

Table 3–1 Percent and number of women at risk[a] and percent at risk currently using various methods, from the 2002 National Survey of Family Growth

Contraceptive method	Percent Using among Women at Risk[a]						
	15–44	15–19	20–24	25–29	30–34	35–39	40–44
Oral contraceptive pill	27.2	43.5	46.1	33.7	28.6	16.8	10.0
Female sterilization	24.1	0.0	3.2	13.5	24.9	37.2	45.8
Condom	16.0	22.1	20.2	18.4	15.5	14.1	10.5
No method	10.7	18.0	12.1	10.5	9.2	9.8	8.8
Male sterilization	8.2	0.0	0.7	3.7	8.4	12.8	16.8
Depo-Provera	4.8	11.4	8.8	5.8	3.8	1.8	1.5
Withdrawal	3.6	2.1	4.5	6.9	3.4	3.1	1.3
Intrauterine device (IUD)	1.9	0.2	1.6	3.3	2.8	1.3	1.0
Fertility awareness-based methods	1.3	0.0	1.1	0.9	1.5	1.8	2.0
Calendar rhythm	1.0	0.0	1.1	0.4	1.2	1.4	1.5
Implant, combined injectable or Patch	1.2	1.0	1.3	2.2	1.2	0.7	0.3
Other methods[b]	0.6	1.0	0.1	0.4	0.1	0.4	1.2
Diaphragm	0.3	0.0	0.1	0.4	0.2	0.0	0.5
Spermicides	0.3	0.5	0.1	0.1	0.4	0.3	0.3
Number of Women in Cohort, Percent and Number at Risk[a]							
Number (millions) of Women	61.6	9.8	9.8	9.2	10.3	10.9	11.5
Percent at Risk[1] 69.4	38.4	69.2	76.0	76.2	78.6	75.9	
Number (millions) at Risk[1]	42.7	3.8	6.8	7.0	7.8	8.5	8.7

Source: Mosher et al. (2004).

Notes:

[a] At risk = those who *either* are current contraceptive users *or* are nonusers who have had sex in the past three months and are not trying to become pregnant, are not pregnant, or were not interviewed within two months after the completion of a pregnancy and are not sterile. Percentages may not add to 100 due to rounding.

[2] Other methods = cervical cap, sponge, and female condom.

The mix of methods shown in Table 3–1, including the 10.7% of women at risk who do not use any method, resulted in a staggering 3.1 million unintended pregnancies in 2001, the latest year for which data are available.[3] Nearly half (48%) of unintended pregnancies result from contraceptive failure.[3] Nearly half (49%) of the 6.4 million pregnancies and one-third (34% or 1.4 million) of the 4.0 million births were unintended.[3] Every night in the United States, about 9.7 million couples at risk of unintended pregnancy have intercourse; among these, about 31,000 experience a condom break or slip, and over 1 million are not protected against pregnancy at all (see Table 3–1 and Chapter 27 on Contraceptive Efficacy).[2,4]

EFFICACY: "WILL IT WORK?"

"Is the condom really effective?"
"Which would be the most effective method for me?"
"Why did one magazine say diaphragms are 94% effective and another say they're 84% effective?"
"Can you still get pregnant if you take your pills every day on schedule?"

"Will it work?" is the question usually asked first and most frequently about any method of contraception.[5] Although this question cannot be answered with certainty for any particular couple, clinicians and counselors can try to help patients understand something of the difficulty of quantifying efficacy.

It is useful to distinguish between measures of contraceptive effectiveness and measures of the risk of pregnancy during contraceptive use. Many persons, including clinicians and clients, prefer positive rather than negative statements; instead of the negative statement that 20% of women using a method become accidentally pregnant during their first year of use, they prefer the alternative positive statement that the method is 80% effective. However, it does not follow that the method is 80% effective, because it is not true that 100% of these women would have become pregnant if they had not been using contraception. If 90% of these method users would have become pregnant had they used no method, then the use of the method reduced the number of accidental pregnancies from 90% to 20%, a reduction of 78%. In this sense, the method could be said to be 78% effective at reducing pregnancy in the first year. But if only 60% of these women would have become pregnant if they did not use contraception, then the method would be only 67% effective. Because no study can ascertain the proportion of women who would have become pregnant had they not used the contraceptive method under investigation, it is simply not possible to measure effectiveness directly. Therefore, we focus attention entirely on pregnancy rates or probabilities of pregnancy during contraceptive use, which are directly measurable. However, we continue to use the term effectiveness in its loose everyday sense of how well a method works throughout this book, and we use the terms effectiveness and efficacy interchangeably. We also provide estimates of the proportion of women who would become pregnant if they did not use contraception, so that the reader may calculate rough effectiveness rates if they are needed.

THE RISK OF PREGNANCY DURING TYPICAL AND PERFECT USE

Four pieces of information about contraceptive efficacy would help couples to make an informed decision when choosing a contraceptive method:

- Pregnancy rates during *typical use* show how effective the different methods are during actual use (including inconsistent or incorrect use).

- Pregnancy rates during *perfect use* show how effective methods can be, where perfect use is defined as following the directions for use.

- Pregnancy rates during *imperfect use* show how ineffective methods will be if they are used incorrectly or inconsistently. Pregnancy rates can be computed separately for different categories of imperfect use to reveal which types of imperfect use are most risky.[6]

- The percentage of *perfect users* or percentage of months during which a method is used perfectly reveals how hard it is to use a method correctly and consistently.

The difference between pregnancy rates during *imperfect use* and pregnancy rates during *perfect use* reveals how forgiving of *imperfect use* a method is. The difference between pregnancy rates during *typical use* and pregnancy rates during *perfect use* reveals the consequences of *imperfect use*; this difference depends both on how unforgiving of *imperfect use* a method is and on how hard it is to use that method perfectly. Only the first two pieces of information are currently available. Our current understanding of the literature on contraceptive efficacy is summarized in Table 3–2.[7,8]

Typical Use

In the second column of Table 3–2, we provide estimates of the probabilities of pregnancy during the first year of typical use of each method in the United States. This information is shown graphically in Figure 3–1 in a way that clients may find more useful.[9] For most methods, these estimates were derived from the experience of women in the 1995 NSFG, so that the information pertains to nationally representative samples of users.[10] For the other methods, we based the estimates on evidence from surveys and clinical investigations. See Chapter 27 on Contraceptive Effi-

Table 3–2 Percentage of women experiencing an unintended pregnancy during the first year of typical use and the first year of perfect use of contraception, and the percentage continuing use at the end of the first year. United States.

Method (1)	% of Women Experiencing an Unintended Pregnancy within the First Year of Use		% of Women Continuing Use at One Year[3]
	Typical Use[1] (2)	Perfect Use[2] (3)	(4)
No method[4]	85	85	
Spermicides[5]	29	18	42
Withdrawal	27	4	43
Fertility awareness-based methods	25		51
Standard Days method[6]		5	
TwoDay method[6]		4	
Ovulation method[6]		3	
Sponge			
Parous women	32	20	46
Nulliparous women	16	9	57
Diaphragm[7]	16	6	57
Condom[8]			
Female (Reality)	21	5	49
Male	15	2	53
Combined pill and progestin-only pill	8	0.3	68
Evra patch	8	0.3	68
NuvaRing	8	0.3	68
Depo-Provera	3	0.3	56
IUD			
ParaGard (copper T)	0.8	0.6	78
Mirena (LNG-IUS)	0.2	0.2	80
Implanon	0.05	0.05	84
Female sterilization	0.5	0.5	100
Male sterilization	0.15	0.10	100

Emergency Contraceptive Pills: Treatment initiated within 72 hours after unprotected intercourse reduced the risk of pregnancy by at least 75%.[9]

Lactational Amenorrhea Method: LAM is a highly effective, *temporary* method of conception.[10]

Source: See Chapter 27.
(continued)

Notes:

[1] Among *typical* couples who initiate use of a method (not necessarily for the first time), the percentage who experience an accidental pregnancy during the first year if they do not stop use for any other reason. Estimates of the probability of pregnancy during the first year of typical use for spermicides, withdrawal, fertility awareness-based methods, the diaphragm, the male condom, the oral contraceptive pill, and Depo-Provera are taken from the 1995 National Survey of Family Growth corrected for underreporting of abortion; see the text for the derivation of estimates for the other methods.

[2] Among couples who initiate use of a method (not necessarily for the first time) and who use it *perfectly* (both consistently and correctly), the percentage who experience an accidental pregnancy during the first year if they do not stop use for any other reason. See the text for the derivation of the estimate for each method.

[3] Among couples attempting to avoid pregnancy, the percentage who continue to use a method for 1 year.

[4] The percentages becoming pregnant in columns (2) and (3) are based on data from populations where contraception is not used and from women who cease using contraception in order to become pregnant. Among such populations, about 89% become pregnant within 1 year. This estimate was lowered slightly (to 85%) to represent the percentage who would become pregnant within 1 year among women now relying on reversible methods of contraception if they abandoned contraception altogether.

[5] Foams, creams, gels, vaginal suppositories, and vaginal film.

[6] The Ovulation and TwoDay methods are based on evaluation of cervical mucus. The Standard Days method avoids intercourse on cycle days 8 through 19.

[7] With spermicidal cream or jelly.

[8] Without spermicides.

[9] The treatment schedule is one dose within 120 hours after unprotected intercourse, and a second dose 12 hours after the first dose. Both doses of Plan B can be taken at the same time. Plan B (1 dose is 1 white pill) is the only dedicated product specifically marketed for emergency contraception. The Food and Drug Administration has in addition declared the following 22 brands of oral contraceptives to be safe and effective for emergency contraception: Ogestrel or Ovral (1 dose is 2 white pills), Levlen or Nordette (1 dose is 4 light-orange pills), Cryselle, Levora, Low-Ogestrel, Lo/Ovral, or Quasence (1 dose is 4 white pills), Tri-Levlen or Triphasil (1 dose is 4 yellow pills), Jolessa, Portia, Seasonale, or Trivora (1 dose is 4 pink pills), Seasonique (1 dose is 4 light-blue-green pills), Empresse (one dose is 4 orange pills), Alesse, Lessina, or Levlite, (1 dose is 5 pink pills), Aviane (one dose is 5 orange pills), and Lutera (one dose is 5 white pills).

[10] However, to maintain effective protection against pregnancy, another method of contraception must be used as soon as menstruation resumes, the frequency or duration of breastfeeds is reduced, bottle feeds are introduced, or the baby reaches 6 months of age.

cacy for more complete explanations and for tables summarizing the efficacy literature for each method.

Pregnancy rates during typical use reflect how effective methods are for the average person who does not always use methods correctly or consistently. Typical use does not imply that a contraceptive method was always used. In the NSFG and in most clinical trials, a woman is 'using' a contraceptive method if she considers herself to be using that method. So typical use of the condom could include actually using a condom only occasionally, and a woman could report that she is 'using' the pill even though her supplies ran out several months ago. In short, 'use'—which is identical to 'typical use'—is a very elastic concept that depends entirely on an individual woman's perception.

Perfect Use

In the third column of Table 3–2, we provide our best guess of the probabilities of *method* failure (pregnancy) during the first year of perfect

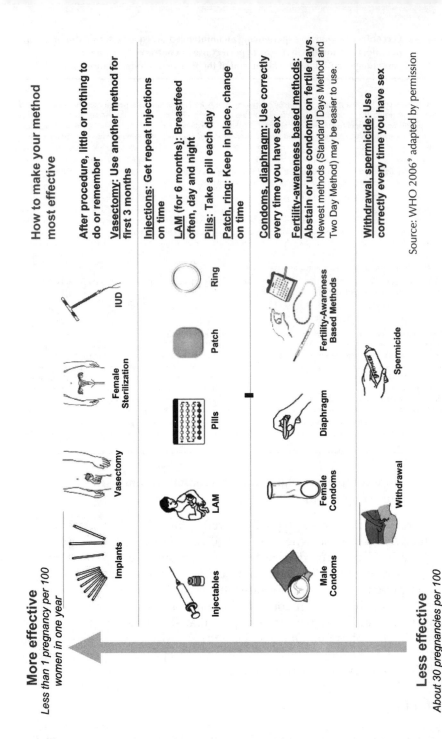

More effective
Less than 1 pregnancy per 100 women in one year

Implants   Vasectomy   Female Sterilization   IUD

Injectables   LAM   Pills   Patch   Ring

Male Condoms   Female Condoms   Diaphragm   Fertility-Awareness Based Methods

Withdrawal   Spermicide

Less effective
About 30 pregnancies per 100 women in one year

How to make your method most effective

After procedure, little or nothing to do or remember
<u>Vasectomy</u>: Use another method for first 3 months

<u>Injections</u>: Get repeat injections on time
<u>LAM</u> (for 6 months): Breastfeed often, day and night
<u>Pills</u>: Take a pill each day
<u>Patch, ring</u>: Keep in place, change on time

<u>Condoms, diaphragm</u>: Use correctly every time you have sex

<u>Fertility-awareness based methods</u>: Abstain or use condoms on fertile days. Newest methods (Standard Days Method and Two Day Method) may be easier to use.

<u>Withdrawal, spermicide</u>: Use correctly every time you have sex

Source: WHO 2006[9] adapted by permission

Figure 3–1 Comparing typical effectiveness of contraceptive methods

use. A method is used perfectly when it is used consistently according to a specified set of rules. For many methods, perfect use requires adherence at every act of intercourse. Virtually all method failure rates reported in the literature have been calculated incorrectly and are too low (see the discussion of methodological pitfalls below). Hence, we cannot empirically justify our estimates except those for the ovulation method (a fertility awareness-based method),[6] the diaphragm,[11] the sponge,[11] the male condom,[12-14] the female condom,[15] spermicides,[16] and methods for which there are extensive clinical trials with very low pregnancy rates. (See Chapter 27 on Contraceptive Efficacy.) Even the estimates for the ovulation method, female condom, diaphragm, spermicides, and sponge are based on only one or two studies. Our hope is that our understanding of efficacy during perfect use for these and other methods will be enhanced by additional studies.

Continuation

The fourth column of Table 3–2 displays the first-year probabilities of continuing use. They are based on the same sources used to derive the estimates in the second column (typical use). (See Chapter 27 on *Contraceptive Efficacy.)

Comparison with Pregnancy Rates Among Women Using Isotretinoin (Accutane)

It is interesting to compare these estimates with pregnancy rates observed among women using isotretinoin, which is effective in treating severe acne but is also teratogenic. To minimize pregnancies among women undergoing treatment, the manufacturer and the U.S. Food and Drug Administration (FDA) implemented a pregnancy prevention program. Among 76,149 women who reported using contraception, 268 became pregnant, yielding a rate of 3.6 per 1,000 20-week courses of therapy;[17] this rate, if constant for a year, would be equivalent to an annual probability of pregnancy of 0.9%. The estimated annual probabilities of pregnancy were 0.8%, 2.1%, and 2.6% among women who reported using oral contraceptives, diaphragms, and condoms, respectively. Thus, women using diaphragms achieved lower rates of pregnancy than we estimate would occur during perfect use, and those using condoms and oral contraceptives experienced about the same pregnancy rates that would be expected during perfect use. Pregnancy rates for women using any of these three methods, however, were substantially below rates generally observed during typical use; this finding would appear to indicate that users' understanding of the teratogenic risks of isotretinoin substantially enhanced correct and consistent use. It is also possible that women in this study had lower than average fecundity (because acne is a marker for excess androgen production associated with anovulation[18]), that they lowered their coital frequency during treatment, or that they under-reported their number of pregnancies (and abortions).

SIMULTANEOUS USE OF METHODS

Using two methods at once dramatically lowers the risk of unintended pregnancy, provided they are used consistently. If one of the methods is a condom or vaginal barrier, protection from disease transmission is an added benefit. For example, the probabilities of pregnancy during the first year of perfect use of male condoms and spermicides are estimated to be 2% and 18%, respectively, in Table 3–2. It is reasonable to assume that during perfect use the contraceptive mechanisms of condoms and spermicides operate independently, since lack of independence during typical use would most likely be due to imperfect use (either use both methods or not use either). The annual probability of pregnancy during simultaneous perfect use of condoms and spermicides would be 0.2%, about the same as that achieved by the combined pill (0.3%) and LNG-IUS (0.1%) during perfect use.[19]

EFFICACY OVER TIME

We confine attention to the first-year probabilities of pregnancy solely because probabilities for longer durations are generally not available. There are three main points to remember about the effectiveness of contraceptive methods over time. First, the risk of pregnancy during either perfect or typical use of a method should remain constant over time *for an individual woman* with a specific partner, providing that her underlying fecundity and frequency of intercourse do not change (although it is possible that the risk for a woman could decline during typical use of certain methods because she learns to use her method correctly and consistently). Second, in contrast, the risk of pregnancy during typical use of a method will decline over time *for a group of users*, primarily because those users prone to fail do so early, leaving a pool of more diligent contraceptive users, those who are relatively infertile, or those who have lower coital frequency. This decline will be far less pronounced among users of those methods with little or no scope for imperfect use. The risk of pregnancy during perfect use for a group of users should decline as well, but this decline will not be as pronounced as that during typical use, because only the relatively more fecund and those with higher coital frequency are selected out early. For these reasons, the probability of becoming pregnant for a group of users during the first year of use of a contraceptive method will be higher than the probability of becoming pregnant during the second year of use. Third, probabilities of pregnancy cumulate over time. Suppose that 15%, 12%, and 8% of women using a method experience a contraceptive failure during years 1, 2, and 3, respectively. The probability of not becoming pregnant *within* 3 years is calculated by multiplying the probabilities of not becoming pregnant for *each* of the 3 years: 0.85 times 0.88 times 0.92, which equals 0.69. Thus, the percentage becoming pregnant within 3 years is 31% (= 100% − 69%).

The lesson here is that the differences among probabilities of pregnancy for various methods will increase over time. For example, suppose that each year the typical proportion of women becoming pregnant while taking the pill is 8% and while using the diaphragm is 16%. Within 5 years, 34% of pill users and 58% of diaphragm users will become pregnant.

CONTRACEPTIVE FAILURES IN A LIFETIME

Data from the 1995 NSFG have been used to estimate age-specific contraceptive failure rates to produce a total lifetime contraceptive failure rate: the number of contraceptive failures that the typical woman would experience in a lifetime if she used reversible methods of contraception continuously (except for the time spent pregnant after a contraceptive failure) from exact age 15 to exact age 45. This estimate is based on the standard synthetic-cohort assumption: that the typical woman uses at each age the same mix of methods observed at each age in the NSFG and experiences the same rate of contraceptive failure observed at that age. The typical woman who uses reversible methods of contraception continuously from age 15 to age 45 would experience 1.8 contraceptive failures. If we consider both reversible methods and sterilization, the typical woman would experience only 1.3 contraceptive failures from age 15 to age 45.[20]

FACTORS THAT INFLUENCE REPORTED EFFICACY

Our understanding of the efficacy of contraceptive methods is entirely dependent on results published in the literature and is influenced by three primary factors (1) the inherent efficacy of the method when used correctly and consistently (perfect use) and the technical attributes of the method that facilitate or interfere with proper use, (2) characteristics of the user, and (3) the quality of published evidence.

Inherent Method Efficacy

For some methods, such as sterilization, implants, levonorgestrel and the copper T IUDs, the inherent efficacy is so high, and proper and consistent use is so nearly guaranteed, that extremely low pregnancy rates are found in all studies, and the range of reported pregnancy rates is quite narrow. For other methods such as the pill and injectable, inherent efficacy is high, but there is still room for potential misuse (forgetting to take pills or failure to return on time for injections), so that the second factor can contribute to a wider range of reported probabilities of pregnancy. In general, the studies of sterilization, injectable, implant, pill, patch, ring, and IUD use have been competently executed and analyzed. Studies of fertility awareness-based methods, spermicides, and the barrier methods display a wide range of reported probabilities of pregnancy because the potential for misuse is high, the inherent efficacy is relatively low, and the competence of the investigators is mixed.

User Characteristics

Characteristics of the users can affect the pregnancy rate for any method under investigation, but the impact will be greatest when the pregnancy rates during typical use are high, either because the method has low inherent efficacy or because it is hard to use consistently or correctly.

Imperfect use. The most important user characteristic is imperfect use of the method. The importance of perfect use is demonstrated in the few studies where the requisite information on quality of use was collected. For example, in a World Health Organization (WHO) study of the ovulation method, the proportion of women becoming pregnant among those who used the method perfectly during the first year was 3.1%, whereas the corresponding proportion failing during a year of imperfect use was 86.4%.[6] In a large clinical trial of the cervical cap conducted in Los Angeles, among the 5% of the sample who used the method perfectly, the fraction failing during the first year was 6.1%. Among the remaining 95% of the sample who at least on one occasion used the cap imperfectly, the first-year probability of pregnancy was nearly twice as high (11.9%).[21]

Frequency of intercourse. Among those who use a method consistently and correctly (perfect users), the most important user characteristic that determines the risk of pregnancy is frequency of intercourse. For example, in a study in which users were randomly assigned to either the diaphragm or the sponge, diaphragm users who had intercourse 4 or more times a week became pregnant in the first year twice as frequently as those who had intercourse fewer than 4 times a week.[22] In that clinical trial, among women who used the diaphragm at every act of intercourse, only 3.4% of those who had intercourse fewer than 3 times a week became pregnant in the first year, compared with 9.7% of those who had intercourse 3 or more times per week.[11]

Age. A woman's biological capacity to conceive and bear a child declines with age. This decline is likely to be pronounced among those who are routinely exposed to STIs such as chlamydia and gonorrhea. Among those not exposed, the decline is likely to be moderate until a woman reaches her late thirties.[23] Although many investigators have found that contraceptive failure rates decline with age,[24-27] this effect almost surely overstates the pure age effect because age in many studies primarily captures the effect of coital frequency, which declines both with age and with marital duration.[28] User characteristics such as race and income seem to be less important determinants of contraceptive failure.

Regular cycles. Women with regular cycles were 7.2 times as likely as were women with irregular cycles (one or more cycles < 17 days or > 43 days) to become pregnant while using the Reality female condom.[29]

Quality of Published Evidence

The errors committed by investigators range from simple arithmetical mistakes to improper design, execution or analysis of studies to outright fraud.[7]

Fraud. One well-documented instance of fraud involved the Dalkon Shield. In a two-page article published in the *American Journal of Obstetrics and Gynecology*, a first-year probability of pregnancy of 1.1% was presented and the claim made that "only the combined type of oral contraceptive offers slightly greater protection."[30] It was not revealed by the researcher that some women had been instructed to use spermicides as an adjunctive method to reduce the risk of pregnancy, nor that he was part-owner of the Dalkon Corporation. Furthermore, he never subsequently revealed (except to the A.H. Robins Company, which bought the Shield from the Dalkon Corporation but did not reveal this information either) that as the original trial matured, the first-year probability of pregnancy more than doubled.[31]

What gets published. The incentives to conduct research on contraceptive failure vary widely from method to method. Many studies of the pill and IUD exist because companies wishing to market them must conduct clinical trials to demonstrate their efficacy. In contrast, few studies of withdrawal exist because there is no financial reward for investigating this method. Moreover, researchers face differing incentives to report unfavorable results. The vasectomy literature is filled with short articles by clinicians who have performed 500 or 1,000 or 1,500 vasectomies. When they report pregnancies (curiously, pregnancy is seldom mentioned in discussions of vasectomy "failures," which focus on the continued presence of sperm in the ejaculate), their pregnancy rates are invariably low. Surgeons with high pregnancy rates simply do not write articles calling attention to their poor surgical skills. Likewise, drug companies do not commonly publicize their failures. Even if investigators prepared reports describing failures, journal editors would not be likely to publish them.

Analytical pitfalls. Several analytical pitfalls can snare investigators. Three of the most common are: (1) use of a misleading measure of contraceptive failure called the Pearl index, (2) the incorrect calculation of method failure rates; and (3) failure to follow up subjects in a trial. Other, more technical, errors that have biased reported results are discussed elsewhere.[7,32,33]

Pearl index. The Pearl index is obtained by dividing the number of unintended pregnancies by the number of years of exposure to the risk of unintended pregnancy contributed by all women in the study. This measure can be misleading when one wishes to compare pregnancy rates obtained from studies with different average amounts of exposure. The likelihood of pregnancy declines over time because those most likely to become pregnant do so at earlier durations of contraceptive use and exit from observation. Those still using contraception after long durations are unlikely to become pregnant, so that an investigator could (wittingly or unwittingly) drive the reported pregnancy rate toward zero by running the trial "forever." Two investigators using the NSFG could obtain Pearl-index pregnancy rates of 7.5 and 4.4 per 100 woman-years of exposure for the condom.[34] One (who got 4.4) allowed each woman to contribute a maximum of 5 years of exposure while the other (who got 7.5) allowed each woman to contribute only 1 year. Which investigator is incorrect? Neither. The two rates are simply not comparable. Life-table measures of contraceptive failure are easy to interpret and control for the distorting effects of varying durations of use. Another problem occurs when deciding which pregnancies to count. Most studies count only the pregnancies observed and reported by the women. If, on the other hand, a pregnancy test were administered every month, the number of pregnancies (and hence the pregnancy rate) would increase because early fetal losses not observed by the woman would be added to the number of observed pregnancies. Such routine pregnancy testing in the more recent contraceptive trials has resulted in higher pregnancy rates than would otherwise have been obtained and makes the results not comparable to those from other trials.

Incorrect calculation of method failure rates. Unfortunately, nearly all investigators who have attempted to calculate "method" and "user" failure rates have done so incorrectly. Investigators routinely separate the unintended pregnancies into two groups. By convention, pregnancies that occur during a month in which a method was used improperly are classified as user failures (even though, logically, a pregnancy might be due to failure of the method, if it was used correctly on some occasions and incorrectly on others), and all other pregnancies are classified as method failures. But investigators do not separate the exposure (the denominator in the calculation of failure rates) into these two groups.

For example, suppose that 2 method failures and 8 user failures occur during 100 woman-years of exposure to the risk of pregnancy. Then the common calculation is that the user failure rate is 8% and the method failure rate is 2%; the sum of the two is the overall failure rate of 10%. By definition, however, method failures can occur only during perfect use and user failures cannot occur during perfect use. If there are 50 years of perfect use and 50 years of imperfect use in the total of 100 years of exposure, then the method failure rate would be 4% and the user failure rate would be 16%. The difference between the two rates (here 12%) provides a measure of how forgiving of imperfect use the method is. However, since investigators do not generally inquire about perfect use except when a pregnancy occurs, the proper calculations cannot be performed.

Loss-to-follow-up. The standard assumption made at the time of analysis is that women who are lost-to-follow-up (LFU) experience unintended pregnancy at the same rate as those who are observed. This assumption is probably innocuous when the proportion LFU is small. But in many studies the proportion LFU may be 20% or higher, so that what really happens to these women could drastically affect the estimate of the proportion becoming pregnant. Our strong suspicion is that women LFU are more likely to experience a contraceptive failure than are those who remain in the trial. For example, one study found that the pregnancy rate for calendar rhythm rose from 9.4 to 14.4 per 100 woman-years of exposure as a result of resolution of cases LFU.[35]

GOALS FOR COMMUNICATING ABOUT EFFICACY

Keep these thoughts in mind when counseling about contraceptive efficacy:

1. **What matters most is correct and consistent use.** For example, an 8% probability of pregnancy during the first year for typical use of the pill will not protect the careless user. The 16% probability of pregnancy during the first year of typical diaphragm use need not discourage a careful and disciplined woman who has infrequent intercourse from using a diaphragm.

2. **Methods that protect a person for a long time and do not require daily or coital adherence** (sterilization, implants, IUDs, and long-acting injections) **tend to be associated with lower pregnancy rates,** primarily because they allow little scope for user error.

3. **Abstinence is always available as an option, as is withdrawal.**

4. **Emergency contraception provides a last chance to prevent pregnancy after unprotected intercourse.** Emergency contraceptive pills (ECPs) are an especially important second method

for those relying on condoms, in cases of breakage or slippage, those who do not actually use their ongoing method for whatever reason, and those who are forced to have unprotected intercourse. Even more effective than ECPs is the insertion of a copper IUD.

5. **Using two methods at once dramatically lowers the risk of unintended pregnancy,** provided they are used consistently. If one of the methods is a condom, protection from disease transmission is an added benefit.

6. **Make sure your staff provides consistent and correct information.** One study of the information provided by family planning staff indicated that providers tended to give the lowest reported probabilities of pregnancy for pills and IUDs, typical-use probabilities of pregnancy for diaphragms and spermicides, and higher than typical-use probabilities of pregnancy for condoms.[36] Thus, family planning providers may extensively bias their patient education in favor of methods they provide most frequently. Condoms and withdrawal get an undeserved low efficacy score within many family planning clinics and offices. You can avoid unintentional bias by deciding carefully what pregnancy rates your clinic or staff members are going to use.

7. **Technology fails people just as people fail technology.** Patients are sometimes told that unintended pregnancies are their own fault because they did not use their method correctly or carefully. Contraceptive methods are imperfect and can fail even the most diligent user.

S AFETY: "WILL IT HURT ME?"

"I smoke. Won't the pill give me a heart attack?"
"Could the IUD puncture my womb?"
"Will I be able to get pregnant after stopping my method?"

In general, contraceptives pose few serious health risks to users. Moreover, the use of contraceptive methods is generally far safer than pregnancy. Unintended pregnancies unnecessarily place women at risk. Women in many developing countries will experience an even greater advantage in using contraceptive methods than those in the developed world because pregnancy-related mortality is higher. Nonetheless, use of some contraceptive methods may entail potential risks:

- Use of the method may lead to serious outcomes such as pain, hospitalization, surgery, medical side effects, infections, loss of reproductive capacity, or, in rare cases, death.

- Contraceptive failure (pregnancy) is associated with risk: a woman must assess the likelihood of contraceptive failure and the dangers that a pregnancy would pose.

- Future fertility may be influenced by choice of a contraceptive method.

Major Health Risks

When it comes to the most serious outcome of all—death—the absolute level of risk is extraordinarily low for most women. Table 3–3 puts into perspective some of the mortality risks of everyday life in the United States.[37-45] Other major health risks from contraceptive use are not only uncommon, but they are also most likely to occur in women who have underlying medical conditions.

Cardiovascular Disease

The combined pill (and presumably the patch and ring as well) has been associated with an increased risk of myocardial infarction (MI) and stroke. Smoking definitely increases the risk of MI, especially in women over age 35. However, nonsmoking, normotensive, nondiabetic women of any age who use combined OCs are not at increased risk for MI. The risk of stroke in nonsmoking women under age 35 is not increased by use of OCs with less than 50 μg estrogen.[46] The risk of venous thromboembolism is increased by combined OC use, but the absolute risk is quite low among women who use OCs with less than 50 μg estrogen, ranging from 9 events per 100,000 woman-years of exposure among those aged 20–24 to 18 events per 100,000 woman-years of exposure among those aged 40 44.[46]

Cancer

The combined pill (and presumably the patch and ring as well) protects users against cancers of the endometrium and ovary.[46] Use of combined OCs is associated with an increased risk of cancers of the cervix and liver, an increased risk of breast cancer in young women, and a decreased risk of colorectal cancer. However, there is great uncertainty regarding the causal link, if any, between combined OC use and liver and colorectal cancer,[46] and recent evidence suggests no association between current or former combined OC use and breast cancer.[47] Regardless, the net effect of combined pill use on cancer is negligible.[46]

Persistent infection with certain types of HPV is the most important cause of cervical cancer (see Chapter 21 on Reproductive Tract Infections). However, the incidence of cervical cancer is increased in women using oral contraceptives, particularly long-term users, among women

Table 3–3 Voluntary risks in perspective

Activity	Risk of Death	Source
Risk per year		
While skydiving	1 in 1,000	Laudan (1994)[37]
From an accident	1 in 2,900	
From an automobile accident	1 in 5,000	
From a fall	1 in 20,000	
From a fire	1 in 50,000	
From riding your bicycle	1 in 130,000	
In an airplane crash	1 in 250,000	
From being struck by lightning	1 in 2,000,000	
Risk per year for women preventing pregnancy		
Using combined oral contraceptives (and presumably the patch and ring as well)		Schwingl et al. (1999)[38]
Nonsmoker		
Aged 15–34	1 in 1,667,000	
Aged 35–44	1 in 33,300	
Smoker		
Aged 15–34	1 in 57,800	
Aged 35–44	1 in 5,200	
Undergoing tubal sterilization	1 in 66,700	Escobedo et al. (1989)[39]
Risk per year from using tampons	1 in 5,734,000	Hajjeh et al. (1999);[40] U.S Census Bureau (2003)[41]
Risk from pregnancy	1 in 8,700	Berg et al. (2003)[42]
Risk from spontaneous abortion	1 in 142,900	Saraiya et al. (1999)[43]
Risk from legal induced abortion		
Mifepristone/misoprostol	1 in 162,500	Summers (2006)[44]
Surgical	1 in 142,900	Bartlett et al. (2004)[45]
≤ 8 weeks	1 in 1,000,000	
9–10 weeks	1 in 500,000	
11–12 weeks	1 in 250,000	
13–15 weeks	1 in 58,800	
16–20 weeks	1 in 29,400	
≥ 21 weeks	1 in 11,200	

who test positive for HPV; this risk increases as duration of use increases.[48] Results from limited data also suggest a slight increase in the risk of cervical cancer among women who use injectable contraceptives for five years or longer.

Analysis of pooled data from 54 epidemiologic studies conducted in 25 countries found that women face a slightly increased risk (about 25%

higher) of having breast cancer diagnosed while they are using combined oral contraceptives. Cancers diagnosed in these women are less advanced clinically than those diagnosed in women of the same age who have never used combined pills.[49] The increased risk is apparent soon after combined pill use begins but does not increase with duration of use, declines after use ceases, and does not persist beyond ten years after exposure ceases. These patterns are not typical for a carcinogenic agent but would be consistent with promotion of already existing tumors or with earlier diagnosis of breast cancer in women who have used the combined pill. A more recent study in the United Sates found that among women aged 35–64, current or former combined OC use is not associated with an increased risk of diagnosis of breast cancer.[47]

SIDE EFFECTS

Often, the minor side effects of contraceptive methods, in addition to the more serious complications, influence whether an individual selects a certain method. "What physical changes will I undergo?" "Will I be annoyed by spotting, cramping, or the sensation or messiness of using a given method?" Do not dismiss the important role that side effects play when an individual must repeatedly assess whether to continue using a method or whether to use it consistently.

Side effects can be hormonally, chemically, or mechanically induced. Headaches, nausea, dizziness and breast tenderness can be side effects of hormonal methods. Menstrual changes such as spotting and decreased or increased bleeding can be caused by hormonal methods and IUDs. Physical sensations such as decreased penile sensitivity, pressure on pelvic walls, or uterine cramping may be caused by mechanical methods. Other chemically-induced side effects include allergic reactions to latex or copper.

With the great majority of these side effects, instruction and patient education can help users accept and understand what is happening. The appearance of side effects that are not serious is not a medical reason to preclude use of a method.

GOALS FOR COMMUNICATING ABOUT SAFETY

1. **Try to educate the patient about misconceptions.** People who are afraid do not respond well to rational persuasions. Many patients hold certain opinions about contraceptive methods—that the pill is very dangerous even to healthy, non-smoking young women or that injectables lead to permanent sterility. If you see that you are getting nowhere, stop. Help

each client select a method that can be used correctly and consistently without fear.

2. **Make sure that you and your staff know all about the major side effects** of contraceptive methods, such as the relation between combined pill use and blood clots or reproductive cancers. Give accurate information.

3. **Tell patients what they need to know** even if they do not ask. Patients do not always ask the questions they need answered.

4. **Compare risks of using contraception with pregnancy risks.** In general, the risks of pregnancy, abortion, and delivery are far greater than those of using a contraceptive method.

5. **Help patients make contraceptive method choices that will protect them from both pregnancy and STIs.** Safety concerns often overlap with worries about infections. With the exception of abstinence, currently available methods (male and female condoms) that protect against infection are not those that provide greatest protection against pregnancy. Conversely, the most highly effective methods of contraception provide *no* protection against infection. Therefore, highly effective protection against both risks requires use of two methods. Even "abstinence" has different rules for protection against pregnancy and protection against infection: oral and anal intercourse can result in STI transmission but not in pregnancy.

6. **Teach patients the danger signals** of the method they select. If a danger signal does appear, the informed user can quickly seek help.

NONCONTRACEPTIVE BENEFITS

Although the noncontraceptive benefits provided by certain methods are not generally the major determinant for selecting a contraceptive method, they certainly can help patients decide among suitable methods. (See Table 3–4.) Awareness that a method of contraception has major noncontraceptive benefits (cancer prevention, protection of future fertility or diminished menstrual cycle symptoms) may also increase the likelihood of continuing to use that method. Make it a practice to tell your patients about the noncontraceptive benefits of the various methods. If patients have additional reasons for using the contraceptive method, their motivation to use it correctly and consistently will probably be improved.

Table 3–4 Major methods of contraception and some related safety concerns, side effects, and noncontraceptive benefits

Method	Dangers	Side Effects	Noncontraceptive Benefits
Combined hormonal contraception (pill, and presumably Evra patch, and NuvaRing.)	Cardiovascular complications (stroke, heart attack, blood clots, high blood pressure), depression, hepatic adenomas, increased risk of cervical and possibly liver cancers, earlier development of breast cancer in young women	Nausea, headaches, dizziness, spotting, weight gain, breast tenderness, chloasma	Decreases dysmenorrhea, menorrhagia, anemia and cyclic mood problems (PMS); protects against ectopic pregnancy, symptomatic PID, and ovarian, endometrial, and possibly colorectal cancer; reduces acne
Progestin-only pill	May avoid some dangers of combined hormonal contraceptives	Less nausea than with combined pills	Lactation not disturbed
IUD	Infection post insertion, uterine perforation, anemia	Menstrual cramping, spotting, increased bleeding with non-progestin-releasing IUDs	Mirena decreases menstrual blood loss and menorrhagia and can provide progestin for hormone replacement therapy
Male condom	Anaphylactic reaction to latex	Decreased sensation, allergy to latex	Protects against STIs, including HIV; delays premature ejaculation
Female condom	None known	Aesthetically unappealing and awkward to use for some	Protects against STIs
Implanon	Infection at implant site; may avoid some dangers of combined hormonal contraceptives	Headache, acne, menstrual changes, weight gain, depression, emotional lability	Lactation not disturbed; decreases dysmenorrhea
Depo-Provera	Depression, allergic reactions, pathologic weight gain, bone loss; may avoid some dangers of combined hormonal contraceptives	Menstrual changes, weight gain, headache, adverse effects on lipids	Lactation not disturbed; reduces risk of seizures; may protect against ovarian and endometrial cancers

(continued)

Table 3–4 Major methods of contraception and some related safety concerns, side effects, and noncontraceptive benefits—(cont'd)

Method	Dangers	Side Effects	Noncontraceptive Benefits
Sterilization	Infection; possible anesthetic or surgical complications; if pregnancy occurs after tubal sterilization, high risk that it will be ectopic	Pain at surgical site, psychological reactions, subsequent regret that the procedure was performed	Tubal sterilization reduces risk of ovarian cancer and may protect against PID
Abstinence	None known		Prevents STIs, including HIV, if anal and oral intercourse are avoided as well
Diaphragm, Sponge	Vaginal and urinary tract infections, toxic shock syndrome; possible increase in susceptibility to HIV/AIDS acquisition if exposed to positive partner	Pelvic discomfort, vaginal irritation, vaginal discharge if left in too long, allergy	
Spermicides	Vaginal and urinary tract infections; possible increase in susceptibility to HIV/AIDS acquisition if exposed to positive partner	Vaginal irritation, allergy	
Lactational Amenorrhea Method (LAM)			Provides excellent nutrition for infants under 6 months old

CONTRACEPTIVE TECHNOLOGY

Reducing the user's risk of STIs may weigh as heavily as preventing pregnancy. Any sexually active person who may be at risk of acquiring STIs should consider condoms (see Chapter 21 on Reproductive Tract Infections). Because condoms reduce the risk of STIs that cause PID and thus lead to infertility, they protect future fertility.

Fertility awareness methods educate women about their menstrual physiology. This knowledge can also help couples achieve a planned pregnancy.

Mirena (LNG-IUS) markedly reduces menstrual blood loss (thereby reducing anemia) and has a low ectopic pregnancy rate; it can be used to treat menorrhagia and to provide progestin in hormone replacement therapy.[50]

Combined oral contraceptives protect against ectopic pregnancy, symptomatic PID, and ovarian, endometrial and colorectal cancer, and may improve bone health in women with normal estrogen levels. High-dose pills, but not low-dose pills, protect against functional ovarian cysts. High-dose pills protect against benign breast disease, and low-dose pills may also offer protection. Some combined oral contraceptives protect against acne, a key concern among youth. The combined pill reduces dysmennorhea, menorrhagia, and anemia, and is effective in treating dysfunction uterine bleeding. All these benefits presumably accrue to users of the Evra patch and NuvaRing.[46]

PERSONAL CONSIDERATIONS

The best method of contraception for patients is one that will be in harmony with their wishes, fears, preferences, and lifestyle; a method that is more likely to be used correctly.

A typical woman in the United States spends about 39 years—almost half of her lifespan of 80 years—at potential biological risk of pregnancy, during the time from menarche (at age 12.6) to natural menopause (at age 51.3).[51,52] What matters most to a woman when she considers a contraceptive method will ordinarily change over the course of her reproductive lifespan. Different reproductive stages are associated with distinct fertility goals and sexual behaviors (Table 3–5).[53] From menarche to first birth, the primary fertility goal is to postpone pregnancy and birth. Between the first birth and the time when a woman intends to have no more children, the primary goal is to space pregnancies leading to births. Between the time when a woman intends to have no more children and menopause, the goal is to cease childbearing altogether. The biggest demands on a contraceptive method are generated during the period between first intercourse and first birth, when the typical woman may have several sexual partners with periods of high coital frequency; the typical woman at this stage may attach great importance to preventing preg-

Table 3–5 The stages of reproductive life

	Adolescents/Young Adults		Later Reproductive Years	
	Menarche to First Intercourse	First Intercourse to First Birth	First Birth to Intend No More Children	Intend No More Children to Menopause
Fertility goals				
Births	postpone	postpone	space	stop
Ability to have children	preserve	preserve	preserve	irrelevant
Sexual behavior				
Number of partners	none	multiple?	one?	one?
Coital frequency	zero	moderate to high	moderate	moderate to low
Coital predictability	low	moderate to high	high	high
Importance of method characteristics				
Pregnancy prevention		high	moderate	high
PID prevention		high	moderate	low
Not coitus-linked		high	low	moderate
Reversibility		high	high	low
Most common methods				
Most common		pill	pill	sterilization
Next most common		condom	condom	pill, condom

Source: Forrest (1993).

nancy and STIs and to a method's reversibility and ease of use. In the last stage of her reproductive lifespan, from the time when a woman intends to have no more children to menopause, the most important factor is a method's efficacy at preventing pregnancy.

More than half the entire reproductive lifespan—20.4 years or 53% of the reproductive span of 38.7 years—is spent trying to avoid further childbearing, in the stage from the time when a woman intends to have no more children to menopause.[51,52] The typical woman accomplishes this goal via female or male sterilization. An additional 13.4 years or 35% of the reproductive span, from menarche to the first birth, is characterized by no desire to become pregnant. Thus, of a total reproductive span of 38.7 years during which a woman is potentially biologically at risk of conception, only 4.9 years (13% of the total), from the first birth to the time when a woman intends to have no more children, is characterized by any desire to become pregnant. Even this figure is exaggerated since a great fraction of this stage is spent in the pregnant or lactating state or trying to postpone the next pregnancy.

Pattern of sexual activity. In choosing their contraceptive method, women and men should consider their number of partners and their frequency of intercourse.

The number of partners affects an individual's risk of exposure to STIs. In more obvious cases, the individual will have more than one partner at any given time. Less obvious are the individuals who practice serial monogamy. That is, they have only one partner at a time; however, the relationships are not permanent, so at the end of one relationship, the individual will move on to a new partner. Indeed, having more than one partner in a lifetime is the norm, and it is not uncommon for unmarried men and women to have more than 1 partner per year. The practitioner recommending the use of male or female condoms must be prepared to take the time required to discuss risks of STIs, encourage behavioral change, and teach skills.

The frequency of intercourse also has bearing on a person's contraceptive method choice. For example, the woman who has infrequent intercourse may not wish to use a method that requires daily medication or continuous exposure to possible side effects posed by hormonal methods or IUDs. On the other hand, infrequent intercourse may also indicate that a client is at risk of intercourse at unpredictable times. These clients may need skills in "expecting the unexpected."

Pattern of childbearing. Couples should choose their contraceptive method based on the number of children they desire and the preferred timing of those births. For example, couples who plan on having a few children or having children early in their reproductive life cycle may have more flexible requirements about the spacing before and between pregnancies and may be more willing to risk a mistimed, but not unwanted, pregnancy. Such flexibility may mean that contraceptive method choices would not be limited to those with highest efficacy.

On the other hand, the couples who want only one child or want to delay childbearing until the woman is in her late 30s or early 40s may be less willing to choose any but the most highly effective methods. Among these couples, the reversible long-term methods may be more appealing than they would be for couples for whom a several-year span of protection is not an absolute necessity.

Access to medical care. Some people in our society have difficulty gaining access to the health care system: they do not understand the system, cannot afford care or find that the system shuns them. Others may find their access hampered by too long a wait at the clinic. Studies in other nations have shown that access has great bearing on contraceptive method compliance and choice.[54] Presumably, the degree of access can also influence women in the United States. Access can be eased for all clients by providing a full year's supply of contraceptives. While many clinicians do provide 13 cycles of pills, for example, most do not offer sufficient quantities of condoms.

Intimate partner violence. Women at risk of intimate partner violence probably cannot rely on their partners to use withdrawal or a male condom. A non-coitally dependent or a female-controlled coital method would probably be a better choice.

GOALS FOR COMMUNICATING ABOUT PERSONAL CONSIDERATIONS

Key concepts for discussing and teaching about contraceptive method choice and personal considerations include these:

1. **The patient decides which personal considerations matter.** Only the potential user can weigh all the elements for personal choice, and the clinician will not be able to predict what matters. Privacy? Lubrication? Light periods? What big sister uses? Do not guess; ask.

2. **It is a long way from the exam room to the bedroom.** We offer methods as medicines in a clinical setting, and then our patients go home and use them in a sexual setting, be it a bedroom, motel room, car seat, or tent. Remember to help your patient think through the sexual aspects of contraception.

3. **Give patients permission to make a second (or third) contraceptive method choice.** They may not like the first method at all and will need to know it is acceptable to come back and try something else. Besides, it is always good to know how to use several methods.

4. **Encourage your patients to talk about contraceptive issues with their partners.** How can one person decide if a method of contraception will be compatible with a couple's personal and sexual styles? Help your clients practice discussing contraception with their partners if this is new territory for them.

5. **Personal considerations change over time.** Teenagers and 35-year-olds will use different criteria as they evaluate their contraceptive method choices. Encourage patients to rethink their contraceptive method needs as life and sex and bodies change over time.

SUGGESTED READING

Brown SS, Eisenberg L. The best intentions: unintended pregnancy and the well-being of children and families. Washington DC: National Academy Press, 1995.

Harrison PF, Rosenfield A. Contraceptive research and development: looking to the future. Washington DC: National Academy Press, 1996.

REFERENCES

1. Gallen M, Lettenmaier C. Counseling makes a difference. Popul Rep 1987;15, Series J(35).
2. Mosher WD, Martinez GM, Chandra A, Abma JC, Wilson SJ. Use of contraception and use of family planning services in the United States: 1982–2002. Advance data from vital and health statistics, no 350. Hyattsville MD: National Center for Health Statistics, 2004.
3. Finer LB, Henshaw SK. Disparities in rates of unintended pregnancy in the United States, 1994 and 2001, Perspect Sex Reprod Health 2006;38:90–96.
4. Smith TW. Personal communication to James Trussell, December 13, 1993.
5. Grady WR, Klepinger DH, Nelson-Wally A. Contraceptive characteristics: the perceptions and priorities of men and women. Fam Plann Perspect 1999;31:168–175.
6. Trussell J, Grummer-Strawn L. Contraceptive failure of the ovulation method of periodic abstinence. Fam Plann Perspect 1990;22:65–75.
7. Trussell J, Kost K. Contraceptive failure in the United States: a critical review of the literature. Stud Fam Plann 1987;18:237–283.
8. Trussell J, Hatcher RA, Cates W, Stewart FH, Kost K. Contraceptive failure in the United States: an update. Stud Fam Plann 1990b;21:51–54.
9. World Health Organization (WHO). Comparing typical effectiveness of contraceptive methods. [Job Aid]. Geneva: World Health Organization, 2006. Available at: www.fhi.org/nr/shared/enFHI/Resources/EffectivenessChart.pdf.
10. Fu H, Darroch JE, Haas T, Ranjit N. Contraceptive failure rates: new estimates from the 1995 National Survey of Family Growth. Fam Plann Perspect 1999; 31:56–63.
11. Trussell J, Strickler J, Vaughan B. Contraceptive efficacy of the diaphragm, the sponge and the cervical cap. Fam Plann Perspect 1993;25:100–105, 135.
12. Frezieres RG, Walsh TL, Nelson AL, Clark VA, Coulson AH. Evaluation of the efficacy of a polyurethane condom: results from a randomized controlled clinical trial. Fam Plann Perspect 1999;31:81–87.
13. Walsh TL, Frezieres RG, Peacock K, Nelson AL, Clark VA, Bernstein L. Evaluation of the efficacy of a nonlatex condom: results from a randomized, controlled clinical trial. Perspect Sex Reprod Health 2003;35:79–86.
14. Steiner MJ, Dominik R, Rountree RW, Nanda K, Dorflinger LJ. Contraceptive effectiveness of a polyurethane condom and a latex condom: a randomized controlled trial. Obstet Gynecol 2003;101:539–547.
15. Farr G, Gabelnick H, Sturgen K, Dorflinger L. Contraceptive efficacy and acceptability of the female condom. Am J Public Health 1994;84:1960–1964.
16. Raymond:2004 Raymond EG, Chen PL, Luoto J. Contraceptive effectiveness and safety of five nonoxynol-9 spermicides: a randomized trial. Obstet Gynecol 2004; 103:430–439.
17. Mitchell AA, Van Bennekom CM, Louik C. A pregnancy-prevention program in women of childbearing age receiving isotretinoin. N Engl J Med 1995;333:101–106.
18. Speroff L, Glass RH, Kase NG. Clinical gynecologic endocrinology and infertility (Sixth Edition). Baltimore MD: Williams and Wilkins, 1999.
19. Kestelman P, Trussell J. Efficacy of the simultaneous use of condoms and spermicides. Fam Plann Perspect 1991;23:226–227, 232.
20. Trussell J, Vaughan B. Contraceptive failure, method-related discontinuation and resumption of use: results from the 1995 National Survey of Family Growth. Fam Plann Perspect 1999;31:64–72, 93.

21. Richwald GA, Greenland S, Gerber MM, Potik R, Kersey L, Comas MA. Effectiveness of the cavity-rim cervical cap: results of a large clinical study. Obstet Gynecol 1989; 74:143–148.
22. McIntyre SL, Higgins JE. Parity and use-effectiveness with the contraceptive sponge. Am J Obstet Gynecol 1986;155:796–801.
23. Menken J, Trussell J, Larsen U. Age and infertility. Science 1986;233:1389–1394.
24. Grady WR, Hayward MD, Yagi J. Contraceptive failure in the United States: estimates from the 1982 National Survey of Family Growth. Fam Plann Perspect 1986; 18:200–209.
25. Schirm AL, Trussell J, Menken J, Grady WR. Contraceptive failure in the United States: the impact of social, economic, and demographic factors. Fam Plann Perspect 1982;14:68–75.
26. Sivin I, Schmidt F. Effectiveness of IUDs: a review. Contraception 1987;36:55–84.
27. Vessey M, Lawless M, Yeates D. Efficacy of different contraceptive methods. Lancet 1982;1:841–842.
28. Trussell J, Westoff CF. Contraceptive practice and trends in coital frequency. Fam Plann Perspect 1980;12:246–249.
29. Steiner MJ, Hertz-Picciotto I, Raymond E, Trussell J, Wheeless A, Schoenbach V. Influence of cycle variability and coital frequency on the risk of pregnancy. Contraception 1999;60:137–143.
30. Davis HJ. The shield intrauterine device. A superior modern contraceptive. Am J Obstet Gynecol 1970;106:455–456.
31. Mintz M. At any cost: corporate greed, women, and the Dalkon shield. New York NY: Pantheon Books, 1985.
32. Trussell J. Methodological pitfalls in the analysis of contraceptive failure. Stat Med 1991;10:201–220.
33. Trussell J, Hatcher RA, Cates W, Stewart FH, Kost K. A guide to interpreting contraceptive efficacy studies. Obstet Gynecol 1990a;76:558–567.
34. Trussell J, Menken J. Life table analysis of contraceptive failure. In: Hermalin AI, Entwisle B (eds). The role of surveys in the analysis of family planning programs. Liege, Belgium: Ordina Editions, 1982:537–571.
35. Tietze C, Poliakoff SR, Rock J. The clinical effectiveness of the rhythm method of contraception. Fertil Steril 1951;2:444–450.
36. Trussell TJ, Faden R, Hatcher RA. Efficacy information in contraceptive counseling: those little white lies. Am J Public Health 1976;66:761–767.
37. Laudan L. The book of risks. New York: John Wiley and Sons, 1994.
38. Schwingl PJ, Ory HW, Visness CM. Estimates of the risk of cardiovascular death attributable to low-dose oral contraceptives in the United States. Am J Obstet Gynecol 1999;180:241–249.
39. Escobedo LG, Peterson HB, Grubb GS, Franks AL. Case-fatality rates for tubal sterilization in U.S. hospitals, 1979–1980. Am J Obstet Gynecol 1989;160:147–150.
40. Hajjeh RA, Reingold A, Weil A, Shutt K, Schuhat A, Perkins BA. Toxic sock syndrome in the United States, 1979–1996. Emerg Infect Dis 1999;5:807–810.
41. US Bureau of the Census. Statistical abstract of the United States: 2003. Washington DC:Government Printing Office, 2003. Table 11.
42. Berg CJ, Chang J, Callaghan WM, Whitehead SJ. Pregnancy-related mortality in the United States, 1991–1997. Obstet Gynecol 2003;101:289–296.
43. Saraiya M, Green CA, Berg CJ, Hopkins FW, Koonin LM, Atrash HK. Spontaneous abortion-related deaths among women in the United States–1981–1991. Obstet Gynecol 1999;94:172–176.
44. Summers C. Personal communication from Danco Laboratories, 6 November, 2006.
45. Bartlett LA, Berg CJ, Shulman HB, Zane SB, Green CA, Whitehead S, Atrash HK. Risk factors for legal induced abortion-related mortality in the United States. Obstet Gynecol 2004;103:729–737.

46. Burkman R, Schlesselman JJ, Zieman M. Safety concerns and health benefits associated with oral contraception. Am J Obstet Gynecol. 2004;190(4 Suppl):S5-S22.
47. Marchbanks PA, McDonald JA, Wilson HG, Folger SG, Mandel MG, Daling JR, Bernstein L, Malone KE, Ursin G, Strom BL, Norman SA, Wingo PA, Burkman RT, Berlin JA, Simon MS, Spirtas R, Weiss LK. Oral contraceptives and the risk of breast cancer. N Engl J Med. 2002;346:2025–2032.
48. Smith JS, Green J, Berrington de Gonzalez A, Appleby P, Peto J, Plummer M, Franceschi S, Beral V. Cervical cancer and use of hormonal contraceptives: a systematic review. Lancet. 2003;361:1159–1167.
49. Collaborative Group on Hormonal Factors in Breast Cancer. Breast cancer and hormonal contraceptives: collaborative reanalysis of individual data on 53,297 women with breast cancer and 100,239 women without breast cancer from 54 epidemiological studies. Lancet 1996;347:1713–1727.
50. Faculty of Family Planning and Reproductive Health Care Clinical Effectiveness Unit. FFPRHC Guidance (April 2002). The levonorgestrel-releasing intrauterine system (LNG-IUS) in contraception and reproductive health. J Fam Plann Reprod Health Care 2004;30:99–108.
51. The Alan Guttmacher Institute. Fulfilling the promise: public policy and U.S. family planning clinics. New York, NY: the Alan Guttmacher Institute, 2000.
52. Finer LB, Darroch JE. Special tabulations of the 1995 National Survey of Family Growth. New York, NY: the Alan Guttmacher Institute, 2001.
53. Forrest JD. Timing of reproductive life stages. Obstet Gynecol 1993;82:105–110.
54. Tsui AO, Ochoa LH. Service proximity as a determinant of contraceptive behaviour: evidence from cross-national studies of survey data. In: Philips JF, Ross JA (eds). Family planning programmes and fertility. Oxford, England: Clarendon Press, 1992:222–256.

Medical Eligibility Criteria

Kathryn M. Curtis, PhD*
Herbert B. Peterson, MD

- Evidence-based medical eligibility criteria for contraceptive use are necessary to improve safe access to and quality of family planning services.

- WHO's medical eligibility criteria are developed through a consensus process by an expert working group of international family planning experts, following a review of the best available evidence.

While most women can safely use any method of contraception, some women have health conditions that preclude the safe use of certain methods. Evidence-based guidelines regarding which women are medically eligible for contraceptive methods will help to assure that women are not exposed to inappropriate risks, while at the same time not denied access to methods that are medically appropriate. This, in turn, will improve access to and quality of family planning services. Past experience suggests that in the absence of such guidelines, unnecessary restrictions to contraceptive access may be imposed.

In 1994, the World Health Organization (WHO) initiated a process to develop appropriate medical eligibility criteria for widely used contraceptive methods. This process involved comparing existing eligibility criteria for contraceptive use from different agencies, preparing summaries of published medical and epidemiological literature relevant to medical eligibility criteria, and developing a draft classification framework. Two Expert Working Group meetings were convened by WHO in 1994 and 1995 to review the scientific evidence and to formulate recommendations. Publication of the first edition of *Improving Access to Quality Care in Family Planning: Medical Eligibility Criteria for Contraceptive Use* followed in 1996.

---

*The findings and conclusions in this chapter are those of the authors and do not necessarily represent the views of the Centers for Disease Control and Prevention.

The second and third editions of the *Medical Eligibility Criteria for Contraceptive Use* were published in 2000 and 2004, respectively. In the 2004 edition, three new contraceptive methods (combined hormonal contraceptive patch, combined hormonal vaginal ring, and etonogestrel implants) and three new conditions (depressive disorders, known thrombogenic mutations, and use of antiretroviral therapies) were added, increasing the current edition's recommendations to address 20 contraceptive methods and more than 75 medical conditions or characteristics.[1]

Since the publication of the first edition of the *Medical Eligibility Criteria for Contraceptive Use*, WHO has worked toward developing a series of "four cornerstones" of evidence-based family planning guidance (Figure 4–1). In 2001, WHO published the first edition of the *Selected Practice Recommendations for Contraceptive Use*; this document was revised in 2005.[2] Whereas the *Medical Eligibility Criteria for Contraceptive Use* provides guidelines regarding *who* can safely use contraceptive methods, the *Selected Practice Recommendations for Contraceptive Use* provides guidelines on *how* to safely and effectively use contraceptive methods, once they are deemed to be medically appropriate. Recommendations include instructions on when and how to start and use contraceptives and what to do in problem situations. These first two guidance documents are intended primarily for policy makers, program managers, and the scientific community for use in preparing service delivery guidelines, thus providing "guidance for guides." In 2005, WHO published the third cornerstone document, *Decision-Making Tool for Family Planning Clients and Providers*,[3] an interactive tool for facilitating communication between family planning clients and providers in choosing a contraceptive method. The fourth cornerstone, scheduled to be completed in 2007, will be a handbook for family planning providers and will include reference material on contraception. The decision-making tool and handbook are intended for use during family planning encounters to improve quality of care, thus providing "guidance for providers and clients." Both tools are derived primarily from the *Medical Eligibility Criteria for Contraceptive Use* and the *Selected Practice Recommendations for Contraceptive Use*, although they also include the best evidence from social science research on how to meet the needs of family planning clients. All four cornerstones are best interpreted and used in the broader context of reproductive and sexual health care. The complete text of the first three cornerstones can be found on WHO's family planning Web site at www.who.int/reproductive-health/family_planning.

METHODOLOGY

Recommendations for the *Medical Eligibility Criteria for Contraceptive Use* are periodically developed and revised using a systematic review process. Every 3 to 4 years, WHO convenes an Expert Working

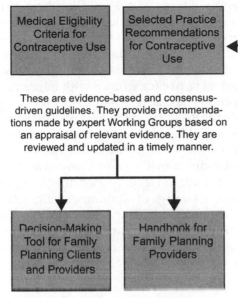

These are evidence-based and consensus-driven guidelines. They provide recommendations made by expert Working Groups based on an appraisal of relevant evidence. They are reviewed and updated in a timely manner.

These are tools that are derived primarily from the *Medical eligibility criteria*, the *Selected practice recommendations* and evidence from social science research on how to meet the needs of the family planning client. They will be updated as the guidelines are updated or as other evidence warrants.

Process for assuring that the guidelines remain current:

(1) Identify new, relevant evidence as soon as it becomes available through an ongoing comprehensive bibliographic search. (CIRE=Continuous identification of research evidence)

(2) Critically appraise the new evidence.

(3) Evaluate the new evidence in light of prior evidence.

(4) Determine whether the newly synthesized evidence is sufficient to warrant an update of existing recommendations.

(5) Provide electronic updates on the Department's web site as appropriate and determine the need to convene an expert Working Group to reassess guidelines formally.

Source: World Health Organization. Selected Practice Recommendations for Contraceptive Use. Geneva: WHO. 2005.

Figure 4–1 The four cornerstones of family planning guidance

Group of international family planning experts, including clinicians, epidemiologists, policy makers and program managers to review new scientific evidence. The Expert Working Group discusses the evidence and its implications for practice, and then reaches consensus on new recommendations and modifications to existing recommendations.

The most recent edition of the *Medical Eligibility Criteria for Contraceptive Use* is based on recommendations of an Expert Working Group meeting held at WHO on October 21–24, 2003, which brought together 36 participants from 18 countries, including representatives of many agencies and organizations. The group consisted of international family planning experts, professionals experienced in evidence identification and synthesis, and users of the medical eligibility criteria guidance. Using a system to identify new evidence on an on-going basis,[4] WHO identified 151 current recommendations for which new evidence was available since the publication of the second edition in 2000. Systematic reviews were conducted to appraise the body of evidence for these 151 recommendations as well as for 3 new conditions and 3 new contraceptive methods. A systematic, comprehensive search of bibliographic databases, such as MEDLINE, yielded all primary studies through August 2003 that described the use of contraceptive methods among women with certain conditions (e.g., the risk of stroke for women with migraines who use combined oral contraceptives). These systematic reviews were intended to identify direct evidence for the appropriateness of contraceptive method use by women with selected health conditions. When direct evidence for these recommendations was sought but not available, the Expert Working Group considered indirect evidence or theoretical considerations. The authors of the systematic reviews graded the strength and quality of the evidence using the Grades of Recommendation Assessment, Development, and Evaluation (GRADE) system.[5] Cost issues were considered primarily in terms of availability and access to contraceptive services. Potential resource constraints and programmatic implications of the recommendations were also considered by the Expert Working Group.

HOW TO USE THE RECOMMENDATIONS

The Expert Working Group used four categories to classify conditions affecting eligibility for the use of each contraceptive method (Table 4–1):

1. A condition for which there is no restriction for the use of the contraceptive method.

2. A condition where the advantages of using the method generally outweigh the theoretical or proven risks.

3. A condition where the theoretical or proven risks usually outweigh the advantages of using the method.

4. A condition which represents an unacceptable health risk if the contraceptive method is used.

USING THE CATEGORIES IN PRACTICE

For a method/condition combination classified as category 1, the contraceptive method can be used by women with the health condition. Classification of a method/condition as category 2 indicates that the method can generally be used, but careful follow-up may be required. For a method/condition classified as category 3, use of that method is not usually recommended unless other more appropriate methods are not available or acceptable. Providing contraception to a woman with a health condition classified as category 3 requires careful clinical judgement and access to clinical services; for such a woman, the severity of her condition and the availability, practicality, and acceptability of alternative methods should be taken into account. Careful follow-up will be required. For a method/condition classified as category 4, the method should not be used.

In settings where resources for clinical judgement are limited, such as in some community-based services, the four-category classification framework can be simplified into two categories (Table 4–1). In the simplified framework, a classification of Category 3 indicates that a woman is not medically eligible to use the contraceptive method. For example (Table 4–2), a smoker who is less than age 35 can generally use combined oral contraceptives (COCs) (Category 2). However, for a woman who is 35 years or older and who smokes less than 15 cigarettes per day, the use of COCs usually is not recommended unless other methods are not available or acceptable to her (Category 3). In a setting with limited access to clinical judgement, this woman should not use COCs. A woman who is 35 years or older and smokes 15 or more cigarettes per day should not use COCs in any setting (Category 4).

The tables at the end of this chapter present a summary of WHO's medical eligibility criteria for hormonal contraception, intrauterine devices, and barrier methods (Table 4–3); male and female sterilization (Table 4–4); and fertility awareness-based methods (Table 4–5).

Classification of Conditions For Sterilization Procedures

The Expert Working Group determined that while there are no medical conditions that would absolutely restrict a person's eligibility for surgical sterilization, some conditions or circumstances may require certain precautions (Table 4-4). For some of these conditions or circumstances, the theoretical or proven risks must be weighed against the benefits of a sterilization procedure, as well as the availability and acceptability of other long-term, highly effective, reversible contraceptive methods.

WHO has not addressed transcervical methods of sterilization in these recommendations.

WHO also notes that particular care must be taken to assure voluntary informed choice among clients undergoing sterilization, especially among young people, nulliparous women, men who have not yet been fathers, and clients with mental health problems. Careful counselling of all clients prior to sterilization should address the intended permanence of sterilization methods, as well as information on the availability of long-term, highly effective, reversible methods of contraception.

The following classification framework is used for conditions with regard to surgical sterilization procedures:

A = Accept:	There is no medical reason to deny sterilization to a person with this condition.
C = Caution:	The procedure is normally conducted in a routine setting, but with extra preparation and precautions.
D = Delay:	The procedure is delayed until the condition is evaluated and/or corrected. Alternative temporary methods of contraception should be provided.
S = Special:	The procedure should be undertaken in a setting with an experienced surgeon and staff, equipment needed to provide general anaesthesia, and other back-up medical support. For these conditions, the capacity to decide on the most appropriate procedure and anaesthesia regimen is also needed. Alternative temporary methods of contraception should be provided, if referral is required or there is otherwise any delay.

Classification of Conditions for Fertility Awareness-based Methods

While there are no medical conditions that are worsened with use of fertility awareness-based methods, some conditions or characteristics may make the use of these methods more difficult. In such cases, it may be recommended that the use of these methods be delayed until the condition is resolved or that special training is needed for correct use of the method. The following classification framework is used for conditions with regard to fertility awareness-based methods:

A = Accept:	There is no medical reason to deny the particular fertility awareness-based method to a woman in this circumstance.
C = Caution:	The method is normally provided in a routine setting, but with extra preparation and precautions. This usually means that special counselling may be needed to ensure correct use of the method by a woman in this circumstance.
D = Delay:	Use of this method should be delayed until the condition is evaluated or corrected. Alternative temporary methods of contraception should be offered.

NA = Not applicable

Contraceptive Method Initiation and Continuation

The Expert Working Group addressed medical eligibility criteria for initiating and continuing use of all contraceptive methods evaluated. Continuation criteria are clinically relevant whenever a woman develops a health condition while she is using a contraceptive method. If the Expert Working Group determined that categories for initiation and continuation differ, these difference are noted in the columns 'I = Initiation' and 'C = Continuation'; where I and C are not denoted, the category is the same for initiation and continuation of use.

Screening for Presence of Conditions

Conditions listed in the *Medical Eligibility Criteria for Contraceptive Use* represent either a person's characteristics (e.g., age, history of pregnancy) or a known pre-existing medical/pathological condition (e.g., diabetes, hypertension). Whether screening for conditions is needed and how such screening should be conducted will be determined by national and institutional health and service delivery environments. In many cases, client history will be an appropriate approach.

Clarification of the recommendations, comments, and citation of scientific evidence

In some cases, the Expert Working Group determined that a numeric classification did not capture the complete recommendation and that additional narrative clarification was needed. Recommendations for which the Expert Working Group added a clarification are noted by an asterisk in the summary tables included in this chapter. The clarifications themselves can be found on the WHO Web site. The complete text of the WHO document also contains comments on several of the recommendations, as well as a brief summary and complete citation of all the evidence reviewed by the Expert Working Group for each recommendation. The complete WHO document can be found on the WHO Web site: www.who.int/reproductive-health/publications/mec.

KEEPING CRITERIA UP TO DATE

WHO has initiated a process to keep up with new scientific evidence on medical eligibility criteria as it becomes available and, when necessary, provides guidance updates electronically based on this new evidence.[4] Electronic databases, such as POPLINE and MEDLINE, as well as relevant other sources, such as tables of contents of reproductive health-related journals, are searched on an on-going basis to identify newly published evidence related to the guidelines. When new, relevant evidence is found, a critical appraisal of the evidence is incorporated into an existing systematic review on the topic or a new systematic review is conducted. If the new evidence is sufficient to consider changing existing guidance, WHO's Team for Promoting Family Planning may choose to convene its Guidelines Steering Group. This group may, in turn, recommend an interim update in guidance pending the next Expert Working Group meeting. Family planning guidance updates are available on the WHO family planning Web site at www.who.int/reproductive-health/family_planning/updates.html.

REFERENCES

1. World Health Organization. Medical eligibility criteria for contraceptive use. Geneva: WHO, 2004.
2. World Health Organization. Selected practice recommendations for contraceptive use. Geneva: WHO, 2005.
3. World Health Organization and Info Project at Johns Hopkins Bloomberg School of Public Health. Decision-making tool for family planning clients and providers. Baltimore: Johns Hopkins University, 2005.
4. Mohllajee AP, Curtis KM, Flanagan RG, Rinehart W, Gaffield ML, Peterson HB. Keeping up with evidence a new system for WHO's evidence-based family planning guidance. Am J Prev Med 2005;28:483–490.
5. Grades of Recommendation, Assessment, Development, and Evaluation Working Group. Grading quality of evidence and strength of recommendations. BMJ 2004; 328:1490–1494.

Table 4–1 Four category classification framework for medical eligibility criteria for contraceptive use

Category	With Clinical Judgement	With Limited Clinical Judgement
1	Use method in any circumstances	Yes (Use the method)
2	Generally use the method	
3	Use of method not usually recommended unless other more appropriate methods are not available or not acceptable	No (Do not use the method)
4	Method not to be used	

Table 4–2 Example of medical eligibility criteria for smoking and combined oral contraceptive (COC) use

Smoking	COC	
	Clinical judgement	Limited clinical judgement
a) Age < 35	2	Yes
b) Age ≥ 35		
(i) < 15 cigarettes/day	3	No
(ii) ≥ 15 cigarettes/day	4	No

Table 4–3 Summary tables: hormonal contraception, intrauterine devices, and barrier methods

KEY:
COC Combined Oral Contraceptives
P/R Patch or Ring
POP Progestin–Only Pill
DMPA Depot Medroxyprogesterone Acetate
NET EN Norethisterone Enantate
LNG/ETG Levonorgestrel and Etonogestrel Implants
Cu IUD Copper IUD
LNG IUD Levonorgestrel IUD

C Male latex condoms, male polyurethane condoms, female condoms
S Spermicide (film, tablets, foam, gel)
D Diaphragm (with spermicide), cervical cap

I = Initiation, C = Continuation

PERSONAL CHARACTERISTICS AND REPRODUCTIVE HISTORY

CONDITION	COC	P/R	POP	DMPA NET-EN	LNG/ ETG Implants	Cu-IUD	LNG-IUD	C	S	D
PREGNANCY	NA*	NA*	NA*	NA*	NA*	4*	4*	NA*	NA*	NA*
AGE	Menarche to <40=1 ≥40=2	Menarche to <40=1 ≥40=2	Menarche to <18=1 18-45=1 >45=1	Menarche to <18=2 18-45=1 >45=2	Menarche to <18=1 18-45=1 >45=1	Menarche to <20=2 ≥20=1	Menarche to <20=2 ≥20=1	Menarche to <40=1 ≥40=1	Menarche to <40=1 ≥40=1	Menarche to <40=1 ≥40=1
PARITY										
a) Nulliparous	1	1	1	1	1	2	2	1	1	1
b) Parous	1	1	1	1	1	1	1	1	1	2*
BREASTFEEDING										
a) < 6 weeks postpartum	4	4	3*	3*	3*					
b) 6 weeks to < 6 months (primarily breastfeeding)	3	3	1	1	1					

* Please consult the full text of the WHO Medical Eligibility Criteria for a clarification to this classification.

(continued)

Table 4–3 Summary tables: hormonal contraception, intrauterine devices, and barrier methods—*(cont'd)*

CONDITION	COC	P/R	POP	DMPA NET-EN	LNG/ETG Implants	Cu-IUD	LNG-IUD	C	S	D
c) ≥ 6 months postpartum	2	2	1	1	1					
POSTPARTUM (non-breastfeeding women)										
a) < 21 days	3	3	1	1	1					
b) ≥ 21 days	1	1	1	1	1					
POSTPARTUM (breastfeeding or non-breastfeeding women, including post-caesarean section)										
a) < 48 hours						2	3			
b) ≥ 48 hours to < 4 weeks						3	3			
c) ≥ 4 weeks						1	1			
d) Puerperal sepsis						4	4			
POSTPARTUM										
a) < 6 weeks								1	1	N/A*
b) ≥ 6 weeks								1	1	1
POST-ABORTION										
a) First trimester	1*	1*	1*	1*	1*	1*	1*	1	1	1
b) Second trimester	1	1	1	1	1	2	2	1	1	1*
c) Immediate post-septic abortion	1	1	1	1	1	4	4	1	1	1

(continued)

* Please consult the full text of the WHO Medical Eligibility Criteria for a clarification to this classification.

Table 4–3 Summary tables: hormonal contraception, intrauterine devices, and barrier methods—*(cont'd)*

CONDITION	COC	P/R	POP	DMPA NET-EN	LNG/ ETG Implants	Cu-IUD	LNG-IUD	C	S	D
PAST ECTOPIC PREGNANCY	1	1	2	1	1	1	1	1	1	1
HISTORY OF PELVIC SURGERY (including caesarean section) (see also postpartum section)	1	1	1	1	1	1	1	1	1	1
SMOKING										
a) Age < 35	2	2	1	1	1	1	1	1	1	1
b) Age ≥ 35										
(i) <15 cigarettes/day	3	3	1	1	1	1	1	1	1	1
(ii) ≥15 cigarettes/day	4	4	1	1	1	1	1	1	1	1
OBESITY ≥30 kg/m² body mass index (BMI)	2	2	1	1	1	1	1	1	1	1
BLOOD PRESSURE MEASUREMENT UNAVAILABLE	NA*	NA*	NA*	NA*	NA*	NA*	NA*	NA*	NA*	NA*
CARDIOVASCULAR DISEASE										
MULTIPLE RISK FACTORS FOR ARTERIAL CARDIOVASCULAR DISEASE (such as older age, smoking, diabetes and hypertension)	3/4*	3/4*	2*	3*	2*	1	2	1	1	1

* Please consult the full text of the WHO Medical Eligibility Criteria for a clarification to this classification.

(continued)

Table 4–3 Summary tables: hormonal contraception, intrauterine devices, and barrier methods—(cont'd)

CONDITION	COC	P/R	POP	DMPA NET-EN	LNG/ETG Implants	Cu-IUD	LNG-IUD	C	S	D
HYPERTENSION										
a) History of hypertension where blood pressure CANNOT be evaluated (including hypertension during pregnancy)	3*	3*	2*	2*	2*	1	2	1	1	1
b) Adequately controlled hypertension, where blood pressure CAN be evaluated	3*	3*	1*	2*	1*	1	1	1	1	1
c) Elevated blood pressure levels (properly taken measurements)										
(i) systolic 140-159 or diastolic 90-99	3	3	1	2	1	1	1	1	1	1
(ii) systolic >160 or diastolic >100	4	4	2	3	2	1	2	1	1	1
d) Vascular disease	4	4	2	3	2	1	2	1	1	1
HISTORY OF HIGH BLOOD PRESSURE DURING PREGNANCY (where current blood pressure is measurable and normal)	2	2	1	1	1	1	1	1	1	1

* Please consult the full text of the WHO Medical Eligibility Criteria for a clarification to this classification.

(continued)

Table 4–3 Summary tables: hormonal contraception, intrauterine devices, and barrier methods—*(cont'd)*

CONDITION	COC	P/R	POP	DMPA NET-EN	LNG/ ETG Implants	Cu-IUD	LNG-IUD	C	S	D
DEEP VENOUS THROMBOSIS (DVT)/ PULMONARY EMBOLISM (PE)										
a) History of DVT/PE	4	4	2	2	2	1	2	1	1	1
b) Current DVT/PE	4	4	3	3	3	1	3	1	1	1
c) Family history (first-degree relatives)	2	2	1	1	1	1	1	1	1	1
d) Major surgery										
(i) with prolonged immobilization	4	4	2	2	2	1	2	1	1	1
(ii) without prolonged immobilization	2	2	1	1	1	1	1	1	1	1
e) Minor surgery without immobilization	1	1	1	1	1	1	1	1	1	1
KNOWN THROMBOGENIC MUTATIONS (e.g. Factor V Leiden; Prothrombin mutation; Protein S, Protein C and Antithrombin deficiencies)	4*	4*	2*	2*	2*	1*	2*	1*	1*	1*

* Please consult the full text of the WHO Medical Eligibility Criteria for a clarification to this classification.

(continued)

Table 4-3 Summary tables: hormonal contraception, intrauterine devices, and barrier methods—*(cont'd)*

CONDITION	COC	P/R	POP	DMPA NET-EN	LNG/ETG Implants	Cu-IUD	LNG-IUD	C	S	D
SUPERFICIAL VENOUS THROMBOSIS										
a) Varicose veins	1	1	1	1	1	1	1	1	1	1
b) Superficial thrombophlebitis	2	2	1	1	1	1	1	1	1	1
CURRENT AND HISTORY OF ISCHAEMIC HEART DISEASE	4	4	I 2 / C 3	3	I 2 / C 3	1	2	1	1	1
STROKE (history of cerebrovascular accident)	4	4	I 2 / C 3	3	I 2 / C 3	1	I 2 / C 3	1	1	1
KNOWN HYPERLIPIDAEMIAS (screening is NOT necessary for safe use of contraceptive methods)	2/3*	2/3*	2*	2*	2*	1*	2*	1*	1*	1*
VALVULAR HEART DISEASE										
a) Uncomplicated	2	2	1	1	1	1	1	1	1	1
b) Complicated (pulmonary hypertension, atrial fibrillation, history of subacute bacterial endocarditis)	4	4	1	1	1	2*	2*	1	1	2

* Please consult the full text of the WHO Medical Eligibility Criteria for a clarification to this classification.

(continued)

Table 4-3 Summary tables: hormonal contraception, intrauterine devices, and barrier methods—*(cont'd)*

CONDITION	COC	P/R	POP	DMPA NET-EN	LNG/ETG Implants	Cu-IUD	LNG-IUD	C	S	D
	I C	I C	I C	I C	I C	I C	I C			
NEUROLOGIC CONDITIONS										
HEADACHES										
a) Non-migrainous (mild or severe)	1* 2*	1* 2*	1*	1*	1* 1*	1*	1* 1*	1	1	1
b) Migraine										
(i) without aura										
Age <35	2* 3*	2* 3*	1* 2*	2*	2* 2*	1*	2* 2*	1	1	1
Age ≥35	3* 4*	3* 4*	1* 2*	2*	2* 2*	1*	2* 2*	1	1	1
(ii) with aura (at any age)	4* 4*	4* 4*	2* 3*	3*	2* 3*	1*	2* 3*	1	1	1
EPILEPSY	1*	1*	1*	1*	1*	1	1	1	1	1
DEPRESSIVE DISORDERS										
DEPRESSIVE DISORDERS	1*	1*	1*	1*	1*	1*	1*	1	1	1
REPRODUCTIVE TRACT INFECTIONS AND DISORDERS										
VAGINAL BLEEDING PATTERNS										
a) Irregular pattern *without* heavy bleeding	1	1	2	2	2	1	I C 1 1			
b) Heavy or prolonged bleeding (includes regular and irregular patterns)	1*	1*	2*	2*	2*	2*	1* 2*			

* Please consult the full text of the WHO Medical Eligibility Criteria for a clarification to this classification.

(continued)

Table 4–3 Summary tables: hormonal contraception, intrauterine devices, and barrier methods—(cont'd)

CONDITION	COC	P/R	POP	DMPA NET-EN	LNG/ETG Implants	Cu-IUD (I / C)	LNG-IUD (I / C)	C	S	D
UNEXPLAINED VAGINAL BLEEDING (suspicious for serious condition) Before evaluation	2*	2*	2*	3*	3*	4* / 2*	4* / 2*	1*	1*	1*
ENDOMETRIOSIS	1	1	1	1	1	2	1	1	1	1
BENIGN OVARIAN TUMOURS (including cysts)	1	1	1	1	1	1	1	1	1	1
SEVERE DYSMENORRHOEA	1	1	1	1	1	2	1	1	1	1
TROPHOBLAST DISEASE										
a) Benign gestational trophoblastic disease	1	1	1	1	1	3	3	1	1	1
b) Malignant gestational trophoblastic disease	1	1	1	1	1	4	4	1	1	1
CERVICAL ECTROPION	1	1	1	1	1	1	1	1	1	1
CERVICAL INTRAEPITHELIAL NEOPLASIA (CIN)	2	2	1	2	2	1	2	1	1	1*
CERVICAL CANCER (awaiting treatment)	2	2	1	2	2	4 / 2	4 / 2	1	2	1*

* Please consult the full text of the WHO Medical Eligibility Criteria for a clarification to this classification.

(continued)

CONDITION	COC	P/R	POP	DMPA NET-EN	LNG/ETG Implants	Cu-IUD	LNG-IUD	C	S	D
BREAST DISEASE										
a) Undiagnosed mass	2*	2*	2*	2*	2*	1	2	1	1	1
b) Benign breast disease	1	1	1	1	1	1	1	1	1	1
c) Family history of cancer	1	1	1	1	1	1	1	1	1	1
d) Cancer										
(i) current	4	4	4	4	4	1	4	1	1	1
(ii) past and no evidence of current disease for 5 years	3	3	3	3	3	1	3	1	1	1
ENDOMETRIAL CANCER	1	1	1	1	1	I 4 / C 2	I 4 / C 2	1	1	1
OVARIAN CANCER	1	1	1	1	1	I 1 / C 1	I 1 / C 1	1	1	1
UTERINE FIBROIDS										
a) Without distortion of the uterine cavity	1	1	1	1	1	1	1	1	1	1
b) With distortion of the uterine cavity	1	1	1	1	1	4	4	1	1	1

* Please consult the full text of the WHO Medical Eligibility Criteria for a clarification to this classification.

(continued)

Table 4–3 Summary tables: hormonal contraception, intrauterine devices, and barrier methods—*(cont'd.)*

CONDITION	COC	P/R	POP	DMPA NET-EN	LNG/ ETG Implants	Cu-IUD	LNG-IUD	C	S	D
ANATOMICAL ABNORMALITIES										
a) That distort the uterine cavity						4	4			NA*
b) That do not distort the uterine cavity						2	2			
PELVIC INFLAMMATORY DISEASE (PID)										
a) Past PID (assuming no current risk factors of STIs)										
(i) with subsequent pregnancy	1	1	1	1	1	1	1	1	1	1
(ii) without subsequent pregnancy	1	1	1	1	1	2	2	1	1	1
b) PID - current	1		1	1	1	4	2*	1	1	1
STIs										
a) Current purulent cervicitis or chlamydial infection or gonorrhoea	1		1	1	1	4	2*	1	1	1
b) Other STIs (excluding HIV and hepatitis)	1		1	1	1	2	2	1	1	1
c) Vaginitis (including trichomonas vaginalis and bacterial vaginosis)	1		1	1	1	2	2	1	1	1
d) Increased risk of STIs	1		1	1	1	2/3*	2/3*	1	1	1

*Please consult the full text of the WHO Medical Eligibility Criteria for a clarification to this classification.

(continued)

Table 4–3 Summary tables: hormonal contraception, intrauterine devices, and barrier methods—(cont'd)

CONDITION	COC	P/R	POP	DMPA NET-EN	LNG/ETG Implants	Cu-IUD		LNG-IUD		C	S	D
						I	C	I	C			
HIV/AIDS												
HIGH RISK OF HIV	1	1	1	1	1	2	2	2	2	1	4	3
HIV-INFECTED	1	1	1	1	1	2	2	2	2	1	4	3
AIDS	1*	1*	1*	1*	1*	3	2*	3	2*	1	4	3
Clinically well on ARV therapy	See ANTIRETROVIRAL THERAPY below					2	2	2	2			
OTHER INFECTIONS												
SCHISTOSOMIASIS												
a) Uncomplicated	1	1	1	1	1	1		1		1	1	1
b) Fibrosis of the liver	1	1	1	1	1	1		1		1	1	1
TUBERCULOSIS												
a) Non-pelvic	1*	1*	1*	1*	1*	1	1	1	1	1	1	1
b) Known pelvic	1*	1*	1	1	1	4	3	4	3	1	1	1
MALARIA	1	1	1	1	1	1		1		1	1	1
HISTORY OF TOXIC SHOCK										1	1	3
URINARY TRACT INFECTION										1	1	2

* Please consult the full text of the WHO Medical Eligibility Criteria for a clarification to this classification.

(continued)

Table 4-3 Summary tables: hormonal contraception, intrauterine devices, and barrier methods—*(cont'd)*

CONDITION	COC	P/R	POP	DMPA NET-EN	LNG/ ETG Implants	Cu-IUD	LNG-IUD	C	S	D
ENDOCRINE CONDITIONS										
DIABETES										
a) History of gestational disease	1	1	1	1	1	1	1	1	1	1
b) Non-vascular disease										
(i) non-insulin dependent	2	2	2	2	2	1	2	1	1	1
(ii) insulin dependent	2	2	2	2	2	1	2	1	1	1
c) Nephropathy/ retinopathy/ neuropathy	3/4*	3/4*	2	3	2	1	2	1	1	1
d) Other vascular disease or diabetes of >20 years' duration	3/4*	3/4*	2	3	2	1	2	1	1	1
THYROID DISORDERS										
a) Simple goitre	1	1	1	1	1	1	1	1	1	1
b) Hyperthyroid	1	1	1	1	1	1	1	1	1	1
c) Hypothyroid	1	1	1	1	1	1	1	1	1	1

* Please consult the full text of the WHO Medical Eligibility Criteria for a clarification to this classification.

(continued)

Table 4–3 Summary tables: hormonal contraception, intrauterine devices, and barrier methods—(cont'd)

CONDITION	COC	P/R	POP	DMPA NET-EN	LNG/ETG Implants	Cu-IUD	LNG-IUD	C	S	D
GASTROINTESTINAL CONDITIONS										
GALL-BLADDER DISEASE										
a) Symptomatic										
(i) treated by cholecystectomy	2	2	2	2	2	1	2	1	1	1
(ii) medically treated	3	3	2	2	2	1	2	1	1	1
(iii) current	3	3	2	2	2	1	2	1	1	1
b) Asymptomatic	2	2	2	2	2	1	2	1	1	1
HISTORY OF CHOLESTASIS										
a) Pregnancy-related	2	2	1	1	1	1	1	1	1	1
b) Past COC-related	3	3	2	2	2	1	2	1	1	1
VIRAL HEPATITIS										
a) Active	4	4*	3	3	3	1	3	1	1	1
b) Carrier	1	1*	1	1	1	1	1	1	1	1
CIRRHOSIS										
a) Mild (compensated)	3	3	2	2	2	1	2	1	1	1
b) Severe (decompensated)	4	4	3	3	3	1	3	1	1	1
LIVER TUMOURS										
a) Benign (adenoma)	4	4	3	3	3	1	3	1	1	1
b) Malignant (hepatoma)	4	4	3	3	3	1	3	1	1	1

* Please consult the full text of the WHO Medical Eligibility Criteria for a clarification to this classification.

(continued)

Table 4-3 Summary tables: hormonal contraception, intrauterine devices, and barrier methods—(cont'd)

CONDITION	COC	P/R	POP	DMPA NET-EN	LNG/ ETG Implants	Cu-IUD	LNG-IUD	Category C	S	D
ANAEMIAS										
THALASSAEMIA	1	1	1	1	1	2	1	1	1	1
SICKLE CELL DISEASE	2	2	1	1	1	2	1	1	1	1
IRON-DEFICIENCY ANAEMIA	1	1	1	1	1	2	1	1	1	1
DRUG INTERACTIONS										
DRUGS WHICH AFFECT LIVER ENZYMES										
a) Rifampicin	3*	3*	3*	2*	3*	1	1	1	1	1
b) Certain anticonvulsants (phenytoin, carbamazepine, barbiturates, primidone, topiramate, oxcarbazepine)	3*	3*	3*	2	3	1	1	1	1	1
ANTIBIOTICS (excluding rifampicin)										
a) Griseofulvin	2	2	2	1	2	1	1	1	1	1
b) Other antibiotics	1	1	1	1	1	1	1	1	1	1
ANTIRETROVIRAL THERAPY	2*	2*	2*	2*	2*	I 2/3* C 2	I 2/3* C 2	1	1	1
ALLERGIES										
ALLERGY TO LATEX								3*	1	3*

* Please consult the full text of the WHO Medical Eligibility Criteria for a clarification to this classification.

Table 4–4 **Surgical sterilization procedures**

KEY:	
A Accept	**D** Delay
C Caution	**S** Special

A. Female surgical sterilization

CONDITION	CATEGORY

PERSONAL CHARACTERISTICS AND REPRODUCTIVE HISTORY

PREGNANCY	D
YOUNG AGE	C*
PARITY	
a) Nulliparous	A
b) Parous	A
BREASTFEEDING	A
POSTPARTUM	
a) < 7 days	A
7 to < 42 days	D
≥ 42 days	A
b) Pre-eclampsia/ eclampsia	
(i) mild pre-eclampsia	A
(ii) severe pre-eclampsia/ eclampsia	D
c) Prolonged rupture of membranes: 24 hours or more	D
d) Puerperal sepsis, intrapartum or puerperal fever	D
e) Severe antepartum or postpartum haemorrhage	D
f) Severe trauma to the genital tract: cervical or vaginal tear at time of delivery	D
g) Uterine rupture or perforation	S*
POST-ABORTION	
a) Uncomplicated	A
b) Post-abortal sepsis or fever	D
c) Severe post-abortal haemorrhage	D
d) Severe trauma to the genital tract: cervical or vaginal tear at time of abortion	D
e) Uterine perforation	S*
f) Acute haematometra	D
PAST ECTOPIC PREGNANCY	A
SMOKING	
a) Age < 35 years	A
b) Age ≥ 35 years	
(i) < 15 cigarettes/day	A
(ii) ≥ 15 cigarettes/day	A

* Please consult the full text of the WHO Medical Eligibility Criteria for a clarification to this classification.

(continued)

Table 4–4 Surgical sterilization procedures—*(cont'd)*

CONDITION	CATEGORY
OBESITY	
≥ 30 kg/m² body mass index (BMI)	C*

CARDIOVASCULAR DISEASE

MULTIPLE RISK FACTORS FOR ARTERIAL CARDIOVASCULAR DISEASE (such as older age, smoking, diabetes and hypertension)	S

HYPERTENSION

For all categories of hypertension, classifications are based on the assumption that no other risk factors for cardiovascular disease exist. When multiple risk factors do exist, risk of cardiovascular disease may increase substantially. A single reading of blood pressure level is not sufficient to classify a woman as hypertensive.

a) Hypertension, adequately controlled	C
b) Elevated blood pressure levels (properly taken measurements)	
(i) systolic 140-159 or diastolic 90-99	C*
(ii) systolic ≥ 160 or diastolic ≥ 100	S*
c) Vascular disease	S
HISTORY OF HIGH BLOOD PRESSURE DURING PREGNANCY (where current blood pressure is measurable and normal)	A

DEEP VENOUS THROMBOSIS (DVT)/ PULMONARY EMBOLISM (PE)

a) History of DVT/PE	A*
b) Current DVT/PE	D
c) Family history of DVT/PE (first-degree relatives)	A
d) Major surgery	
(i) with prolonged immobilization	D
(ii) without prolonged immobilization	A
e) Minor surgery without immobilization	A
KNOWN THROMBOGENIC MUTATIONS (e.g., Factor V Leiden; Prothrombin mutation, Protein S, Protein C, and Antithrombin deficiencies)	A*

SUPERFICIAL VENOUS THROMBOSIS

a) Varicose veins	A
b) Superficial thrombophlebitis	A

CURRENT AND HISTORY OF ISCHAEMIC HEART DISEASE

a) Current ischaemic heart disease	D
b) History of ischaemic heart disease	C
STROKE (history of cerebrovascular accident)	C

* Please consult the full text of the WHO Medical Eligibility Criteria for a clarification to this classification.

(continued)

Table 4–4 Surgical sterilization procedures—*(cont'd)*

CONDITION	CATEGORY
KNOWN HYPERLIPIDAEMIAS	A*
VALVULAR HEART DISEASE	
a) Uncomplicated	C*
b) Complicated (pulmonary hypertension, atrial fibrillation, history of subacute bacterial endocarditis)	S*

NEUROLOGIC CONDITIONS

HEADACHES	
a) Non-migrainous (mild or severe)	A
b) Migraine	
(i) without aura	
Age < 35	A
Age ≥ 35	A
(ii) with aura (at any age)	A
EPILEPSY	C

DEPRESSIVE DISORDERS

DEPRESSIVE DISORDERS	C

REPRODUCTIVE TRACT INFECTIONS AND DISORDERS

VAGINAL BLEEDING PATTERNS	
a) Irregular pattern *without* heavy bleeding	A
b) Heavy or prolonged bleeding (includes regular and irregular patterns)	A
UNEXPLAINED VAGINAL BLEEDING (suspicious for serious condition)	
Before evaluation	D*
ENDOMETRIOSIS	S
BENIGN OVARIAN TUMOURS (including cysts)	A
SEVERE DYSMENORRHOEA	A
TROPHOBLAST DISEASE	
a) Benign gestational trophoblastic disease	A
b) Malignant gestational trophoblastic disease	D
CERVICAL ECTROPION	A
CERVICAL INTRAEPITHELIAL NEOPLASIA (CIN)	A
CERVICAL CANCER (awaiting treatment)	D

* Please consult the full text of the WHO Medical Eligibility Criteria for a clarification to this classification.

(continued)

Table 4–4 Surgical sterilization procedures—*(cont'd)*

CONDITION	CATEGORY
BREAST DISEASE	
a) Undiagnosed mass	A
b) Benign breast disease	A
c) Family history of cancer	A
d) Breast cancer	
(i) current	C
(ii) past and no evidence of current disease for 5 years	A
ENDOMETRIAL CANCER	D
OVARIAN CANCER	D
UTERINE FIBROIDS	
a) Without distortion of the uterine cavity	C
b) With distortion of the uterine cavity	C
PELVIC INFLAMMATORY DISEASE (PID)	
a) Past PID (assuming no current risk factors for STIs)	
(i) with subsequent pregnancy	A*
(ii) without subsequent pregnancy	C*
b) PID - current	D
STIs	
a) Current purulent cervicitis or chlamydial infection or gonorrhoea	D*
b) Other STIs (excluding HIV and hepatitis)	A
c) Vaginitis (including trichomonas vaginalis and bacterial vaginosis)	A
d) Increased risk of STIs	A

HIV/AIDS	
HIGH RISK OF HIV	A*
HIV-INFECTED	A*
AIDS	S*

OTHER INFECTIONS	
SCHISTOSOMIASIS	
a) Uncomplicated	A
b) Fibrosis of liver	C*
TUBERCULOSIS	
a) Non-pelvic	A
b) Known pelvic	S

* Please consult the full text of the WHO Medical Eligibility Criteria for a clarification to this classification.

(continued)

Table 4-4 Surgical sterilization procedures—*(cont'd)*

CONDITION	CATEGORY
MALARIA	A

ENDOCRINE CONDITIONS

DIABETES

a) History of gestational disease	A*
b) Non-vascular disease:	
(i) non-insulin dependent	C*
(ii) insulin dependent	C*
c) Nephropathy/retinopathy/neuropathy	S
d) Other vascular disease or diabetes of > 20 years' duration	S

THYROID DISORDERS

a) Simple goitre	A
b) Hyperthyroid	S
c) Hypothyroid	C

GASTROINTESTINAL CONDITIONS

GALL-BLADDER DISEASE

a) Symptomatic	
(i) treated by cholecystectomy	A
(ii) medically treated	A
(iii) current	D
b) symptomatic	A

HISTORY OF CHOLESTASIS

a) Pregnancy-related	A
b) Past COC-related	A

VIRAL HEPATITIS

a) Active	D*
b) Carrier	A*

CIRRHOSIS

a) Mild (compensated)	C*
b) Severe (decompensated)	S*

LIVER TUMOURS

a) Benign (adenoma)	C*
b) Malignant (hepatoma)	C*

* Please consult the full text of the WHO Medical Eligibility Criteria for a clarification to this classification.

(continued)

Table 4–4 Surgical sterilization procedures—*(cont'd)*

CONDITION	CATEGORY
ANAEMIAS	
THALASSAEMIA	C
SICKLE-CELL DISEASE	C
IRON-DEFICIENCY ANAEMIA	
a) Hb < 7g/dl	D*
b) Hb ≥ 7 to < 10g/dl	C*

OTHER CONDITIONS RELEVANT ONLY FOR FEMALE SURGICAL STERILIZATION

CONDITION	CATEGORY
LOCAL INFECTION	
Abdominal skin infection	D*
COAGULATION DISORDERS	S
RESPIRATORY DISEASES	
a) Acute (bronchitis, pneumonia)	D*
b) Chronic	
(i) asthma	S
(ii) bronchitis	S
(iii) emphysema	S
(iv) lung infection	S
SYSTEMIC INFECTION OR GASTROENTERITIS	D
FIXED UTERUS DUE TO PREVIOUS SURGERY OR INFECTION	S
ABDOMINAL WALL OR UMBILICAL HERNIA	S*
DIAPHRAGMATIC HERNIA	C
KIDNEY DISEASE	C
SEVERE NUTRITIONAL DEFICIENCIES	C
PREVIOUS ABDOMINAL OR PELVIC SURGERY	C
STERILIZATION CONCURRENT WITH ABDOMINAL SURGERY	
a) Elective	C
b) Emergency (without previous counselling)	D
c) Infectious condition	D
STERILIZATION CONCURRENT WITH CAESAREAN SECTION	A

* Please consult the full text of the WHO Medical Eligibility Criteria for a clarification to this classification.

(continued)

Table 4–4 Surgical sterilization procedures—*(cont'd)*

B. Male surgical sterilization

CONDITION	CATEGORY
PERSONAL CHARACTERISTICS AND REPRODUCTIVE HISTORY	
YOUNG AGE	C*
DEPRESSIVE DISORDERS	C
HIV/AIDS	
HIGH RISK OF HIV	A*
HIV-INFECTED	A*
AIDS	S*
ENDOCRINE CONDITIONS	
DIABETES	C
ANAEMIAS	
SICKLE-CELL DISEASE	A
OTHER CONDITIONS RELEVANT ONLY FOR MALE SURGICAL STERILIZATION	
LOCAL INFECTIONS	
a) scrotal skin infection	D
b) active STI	D
c) balanitis	D
d) epididymitis or orchitis	D
COAGULATION DISORDERS	S
PREVIOUS SCROTAL INJURY	C
SYSTEMIC INFECTION OR GASTROENTERITIS	D
LARGE VARICOCELE	C
LARGE HYDROCELE	C
FILARIASIS; ELEPHANTIASIS	D
INTRASCROTAL MASS	D
CRYPTORCHIDISM	C*
INGUINAL HERNIA	S

* Please consult the full text of the WHO Medical Eligibility Criteria for a clarification to this classification.

Table 4–5 Fertility awareness-based methods

KEY:

SYM Symptoms-based methods   **A** Accept

CAL Calendar-based methods   **C** Caution

                                       D Delay

                                       NA Not applicable

Women with conditions which make pregnancy an unacceptable risk should be advised that fertility awareness-based methods may not be appropriate for them because of their relatively-higher typical-use failure rates.

	CATEGORY	
CONDITION	SYM	CAL

PERSONAL CHARACTERISTICS AND REPRODUCTIVE HISTORY

PREGNANCY	NA	
LIFE STAGE		
a) Post-menarche	C*	C*
b) Peri-menopause	C*	C*
BREASTFEEDING		
a) < 6 weeks postpartum	D	D
b) ≥ 6 weeks	C	D
c) After menses begin	C	C
POSTPARTUM (in non-breastfeeding women)		
a) < 4 weeks	D	D
b) ≥ 4 weeks	A	D
POST-ABORTION	C	D

REPRODUCTIVE TRACT INFECTIONS AND DISORDERS

IRREGULAR VAGINAL BLEEDING	D	D
VAGINAL DISCHARGE	D	A

OTHER

USE OF DRUGS WHICH AFFECT CYCLE REGULARITY, HORMONES AND/OR FERTILITY SIGNS	C/D	C/D
DISEASES WHICH ELEVATE BODY TEMPERATURE		
a) Chronic diseases	C	A
b) Acute diseases	D	A

* Please consult the full text of the WHO Medical Eligibility Criteria for a clarification to this classification.

Abstinence and the Range of Sexual Expression

Deborah Kowal, MA, PA

- Abstinence can be primary or secondary. Primary abstainers have not had a sexual experience with another person. Secondary abstainers are sexually experienced persons who become sexually inactive.

- Abstinence, or celibacy, may be voluntary or involuntary. Many abstainers engage in other forms of sexual intimacy.

- The care provider's role is one of support: encouraging the use of abstinence when it is chosen or, when it is involuntary, counseling about relationships or other forms of sexual expression.

Historically, sexual abstinence has probably been the single most important factor in curtailing human fertility.[1] In the United States of the 21st century, however, there is a lack of consensus about what abstinence does, and does not, entail.[2] Some people define abstinence as refraining from all sexual behavior, including masturbation. Some people define abstinence as refraining from sexual behavior involving genital contact. Others define it as refraining from penetrative sexual practices. Still others would offer different definitions.

Asking clients what they define as abstinence is an important question with clinical implications. In a study of high-school students who consider themselves virgins, 30% had engaged in heterosexual masturbation of or by a partner, 9% had engaged in fellatio with ejaculation, and 10% had engaged in cunnilingus.[3] More than half (59%) of college undergraduates in another study responded that oral-genital contact did not constitute having "had sex" with a partner, and 19% said the same about penile-anal intercourse.[4]

While allowing that individuals have personal definitions regarding what is meant by abstinence, the authors of *Contraceptive Technology* use situational definitions. For purposes of contraception, abstinence is defined as refraining from penile-vaginal intercourse. For purposes of protection from sexually transmitted infections (STIs), abstinence is defined as refraining from those acts that permit exposure to infectious lesions or secretions.

Abstinence can be primary or secondary. Primary abstainers have never had sexual intercourse with another person. Primary abstinence is not uncommon among young persons. One in three (36%) of males and females ages 15 to 19 years report never having had sexual contact with someone of the opposite or same sex, according to the 2002 National Survey of Family Growth (NSFG).[5] Sexual contact was defined as vaginal, oral, or anal sex. As regards the risk of pregnancy, 47% of teen females and 51% of teen males reported never having had penile-vaginal intercourse. Among adults, primary abstinence is rare. Only 3% of persons age 25 to 44 years report having had no sexual contact with someone of the opposite sex, although some will have had same-sex experience. The percentage of persons who have not had penile-vaginal intercourse ranges from 12% among 20 to 24 year olds and from 2% to 5% for those 25 to 44 years.

Secondary abstainers are sexually experienced but for various reasons no longer engage in behaviors they consider as "having sex." Among sexually experienced women age 15 to 44 years, 4% to 9%, depending on age group, report that they had not had sexual contact with a man in the 12 months prior to the interview. Among men, those percentages are 5% to 7%. (See Table 5–1.) Whether these individuals deliberately chose to abstain, merely had a brief lapse in a relationship, or had other reasons for not having had sexual intercourse is not known.

At a number of times throughout their lives, people of all ages may become abstinent. It may be useful to think about abstinence in terms of duration. *Primary abstinence* may be practiced for a long time, until engagement or marriage, for example. For those who have been sexually

Table 5–1 Percentage of women age 15–44 who report having had no sexual contact in the 12 months prior to NSFG interview, 2005

AGE	15–44	15–19	20–24	25–29	30–34	35–39	40–44
Never had sexual contact	8.4	36.7	8.7	2.5	1.8	1.0	1.3
Has had sexual contact but not in 12 months before interview	6.9	8.1	4.7	4.4	6.1	8.2	9.2
Total with no sexual contact in 12 months before interview	15.3	44.8	13.4	6.9	7.9	9.2	10.5

Source: Mosher, et al. (2005).[5]

experienced, some may also practice *secondary abstinence* a long time, in what some refer to as secondary virginity. The idea of *abstinence "for a while"* is useful until effective contraception is achieved, while waiting for tests for sexually transmitted infections and agreement about protection, or during the 2 to 6 weeks postpartum. For many individuals, *abstinence "right now, tonight or today"* is the ever-available backup method of contraception and protection. Hatcher estimates that "each night there are some 10 million acts of intercourse by couples not wanting to become pregnant, and 700,000 of those acts of intercourse are completely unprotected." Persons engaging in those latter 700,000 acts of intercourse would have been better served by abstinence.[6]

For those who deliberately choose to abstain, your role as care provider is to support the choice of abstinence and to teach negotiation and planning skills for using abstinence effectively and safely. For those who reluctantly choose to abstain, it is important that they see abstinence as normal, common, and acceptable—and reversible. In some cases, abstinence is involuntary.[7] These individuals may require help if they feel abstinence stems from a dysfunction. They may abstain for a range of reasons:

- Unhappiness with a relationship, or an estranged relationship
- Fear of sexually transmitted infection
- Increased age
- Presence of preschoolers
- Poor health, illness, or injury
- Pregnancy or recent childbirth

Counsel patients who abstain, whether voluntarily or involuntarily, that they are still sexual human beings, and explore with them the range of sexual expression (see next section). Because opportunities may arise for having sex and because resolve may weaken, educate all abstemious persons about the other methods of contraception and safer sex available to them, including the following:

- Effective over-the-counter products
- Prescription methods
- Emergency contraception options
- Safer-sex practices

THE RANGE OF SEXUAL EXPRESSION

Although abstinence has become associated with saying "no," viewed from another perspective, abstinence can mean saying "yes" to a number of other sexual activities. For some people, only penile penetration of the vagina equals intercourse. Most people, however, have a more expansive view of sexual expression, and other activities give them pleasure and meaning. Holding hands, kissing, massage, solo masturbation, mutual masturbation, dancing, oral-genital sex, fantasy, and erotic books and movies all fit along the sexual continuum, as do many other activities. Taste, smell, vision, and hearing may matter as much as touch for erotic pleasure. All human beings need touching—for nurture, for solace, for communication, for simple affection. Most human beings enjoy erotic touching as well, a specialized language of sexual gratification and more intimate forms of affection.

INDICATIONS FOR ABSTINENCE OR OTHER FORMS OF SEXUAL EXPRESSION

Consider discussing abstinence even with patients who currently engage in intercourse and other sexual behaviors. At some point in their lives, they may choose to become abstinent, removing themselves at least for a while from the health risks of intercourse. You can help people learn that the door between abstinence and sexual activity opens in both directions.

Contraception. When the only goal of abstinence is to avoid unwanted pregnancy, then all forms of sexual expression are available to a couple except for penis-in-vagina intercourse.

STI protection. When a goal of abstinence is to avoid STIs, then not only penile-vaginal, but also oral-genital sex, anal intercourse, and other practices that expose the partner to pre-ejaculatory fluid, semen, cervical-vaginal secretions, or blood must be reconsidered. Some couples avoid these practices altogether, and others use condoms, latex dams, or other barriers to inhibit body fluid transmission during these practices. The care provider's role is to offer factual, explicit guidance on safer-sex options. (See Chapter 21 on Reproductive Tract Infections.)

Lack of partner. Patients may be abstinent if they lack a partner or their partner becomes celibate, for any number of reasons. The care provider can give these individuals permission to engage in auto-gratification or, if needed, refer them for counseling if they are dissatisfied with their celibacy.

Medical reasons. Some situations in which insertive sex may be ill-advised and alternatives recommended include the following:

- Known or suspected STI (also avoid other sexual practices that transmit pre-ejaculatory fluid, semen, cervical-vaginal secretions, and blood)

- Post-operative pain or tenderness, such as from episiotomy, hemorrhoidectomy, vasectomy, and other procedures
- Pelvic, vaginal, or urinary tract infection
- Gastrointestinal illness or infection
- Dyspareunia or other pelvic pain
- Undiagnosed postcoital bleeding
- Late third trimester of pregnancy, postpartum, or postabortion
- Postmyocardial infarction
- Certain disabling physical conditions
- Known or suspected allergic sensitization to a partner's semen

Sex therapy. Therapy for a variety of sexual problems may include exploration of avenues of sexual gratification other than intercourse. Temporarily forbidding intercourse takes performance pressure off couples struggling with erection difficulty, orgasm difficulty, or rapid ejaculation.

INSTRUCTIONS FOR USING ABSTINENCE FOR CONTRACEPTION OR STI PROTECTION

1. Decide what you want to do about sex at a time when you feel clearheaded, sober, and good about yourself. If you have a partner, decide together at a time when you feel close to each other but not sexual. For example, try talking while you take a walk and hold hands.

2. Decide in advance what sexual activities you will say "yes" to and discuss these with your partner.

3. Tell your partner, very clearly and in advance—not at the last minute—what activities you will not do.

4. Avoid high-pressure sexual situations; do not get drunk or high.

5. If you say "no," say it so it is clear that you mean it.

6. Learn more about your body and how to keep it healthy.

7. Learn about contraception and safer sex, so you will be ready if you change your mind. Always keep condoms on hand.

8. Refrain from intercourse if you do not have a contraceptive method available. Learn about emergency contraception in case you have intercourse when you did not expect it. If you

need information about emergency contraception, call 1–888-NOT-2-LATE.

> **Emergency Contraceptive Pills:** Treatment initiated within 72 hours after unprotected intercourse reduces the risk of pregnancy by at least 75%.

REFERENCES

1. Hajnal J. European marriage patterns in perspective. In: Glass DV, Eversley DEC (eds). Population in history: essays in historical demography. London: Aldine, 1986:101.
2. Remez L. Oral sex among adolescents: is it sex or is it abstinence? Fam Plann Perspect 2000;32:298–304.
3. Schuster MA, Bell RM, Kanouse DE. The sexual practices of adolescent virgins: genital sexual activities of high school students who have never had vaginal intercourse. Am J Publ Health 1996:86:1570–1576.
4. Sanders SA, Reinisch JM. Would you say you "had sex" if ...? JAMA 1999; 281:275–277.
5. Mosher WD, Chandra A, Jones J. Sexual behavior and selected health measures: men and women 15–44 years of age, United States, 2002. Advance data from vital and health statistics: no. 362. Hyattsville MD: National Center for Health Statistics, 2005.
6. Hatcher RA. Personal communication, April 19, 2006.
7. Donnelly D, Burgess E, Anderson S, Davis R, Dillard J. Involuntary celibacy: a life course analysis. J Sex Research 2001;38:159–169.

Emergency Contraception

Felicia Stewart, MD
James Trussell, PhD
Paul F.A. Van Look, MD, PhD, FRCOG

- Emergency contraceptive pills containing levonorgestrel alone reduce the risk of pregnancy after unprotected intercourse by 89%. If a levonorgestrel-only product is not available, pills containing a combination of ethinyl estradiol and either norgestrel or levonorgestrel can be provided to reduce the risk by 74%. Emergency insertion of a copper-releasing IUD reduces the risk of pregnancy by more than 99%.

- There are no medical contraindications to treatment with emergency contraceptive pills (ECPs), except pregnancy. If a woman is already pregnant, treatment is ineffective but will not be harmful to a pregnancy.

- Providing information about emergency contraception, treatment when needed, and advance prescription/provision for women who want to have ECPs on hand have become accepted "standards of care" in the United States.

Given the chance, most women would prefer to prevent an unplanned pregnancy rather than decide what to do once one occurs. In some instances, unintended pregnancy is entirely unexpected, such as when a woman conceives while wearing an IUD or following sterilization. Often, however, unintended pregnancies occur after contraceptive mishap or failure that was recognized at the time it occurred. Typical examples of such situations include breakage or slippage of a barrier method, missing hormonal contraceptive pills during risky days of the cycle, being too late for a contraceptive injection, or erring in practicing coitus interruptus or abstinence. In these instances, as well as in all situations in which sexual intercourse was unprotected, including rape, emergency contraception offers a second chance to avoid unintended pregnancy.

Emergency contraceptives are methods women can use after intercourse to prevent pregnancy.[1] Two dedicated emergency contraceptive products have been approved by the U.S. Food and Drug Administration (FDA) for use in the U.S.:

- Plan B, containing two tablets of levonorgestrel (750 mcg) was approved in 1999; in 2006, it was switched from prescription to over-the-counter for those age 18 and over but remains prescription only for females age 17 and younger.

- Preven, containing two doses of ethinyl estradiol (100 mcg) combined with levonorgestrel (500 mcg), was approved in 1998 but withdrawn from the market in 2004.

Other options include use of the following:

- Ordinary combined oral contraceptive pills containing ethinyl estradiol and either norgestrel or levonorgestrel (See Table 6–1)

- Progestin-only pills providing a hormone dose comparable to the regimen in a dedicated product (see Table 6–1)

- Insertion of a copper-releasing intrauterine device (IUD)

Oral regimens (called ECPs, for emergency contraceptive pills) involve one or two doses. Initiate treatment as soon as possible after unprotected intercourse, and definitely within 120 hours. When using a two-dose regimen, the woman must take the second dose 12 hours after the first. In describing these methods, terms such as "postcoital" contraception and "morning-after" pills are not recommended, because they may be misleading: treatment can be initiated sooner than the morning after or later—as long as 120 hours (5 days) after intercourse.

HISTORY

Use of high-dose postcoital estrogen began in the 1960s as a treatment for rape victims.[2,3] The combined estrogen-progestin regimen (Yuzpe regimen) was introduced in the 1970s[4,5] and soon replaced the high-dose estrogen approach. Postcoital insertion of a copper-releasing IUD for emergency contraception was first reported in 1976.[6]

Pills containing progestin alone have been used for intermittent contraception in China,[7] and tablets containing 750 mcg levonorgestrel were marketed for this purpose in several countries under the trade name Postinor. Although its low efficacy has made this approach unsuitable for ongoing postcoital use,[8] single or infrequent use for emergency contraception is effective. Before 1999, when the levonorgestrel emergency contraceptive product was approved by the FDA, no single levonorgestrel tablet of similar hormone content was available in the United States. Providing an equivalent dose using available progestin-only birth control pills required 20 Ovrette tablets for each ECP dose of 750 mcg levo-

Table 6–1 Twenty-three OCs that can be used for emergency contraception in the United States[a]

Brand	Company	Pills per Dose[b]	Ethinyl Estradiol per Dose (μg)	Levonorgestrel per Dose (mg)[c]
		Progestin-only pills: take one dose[b]		
Plan B	Barr/Duramed	2 white pills	0	1.5
		Combined progestin and estrogen pills: take two doses 12 hours apart		
Alesse	Wyeth-Ayerst	5 pink pills	100	0.50
Aviane	Barr/Duramed	5 orange pills	100	0.50
Cryselle	Barr/Duramed	4 white pills	120	0.60
Enpresse	Barr/Duramed	4 orange pills	120	0.50
Jolessa	Barr/Duramed	4 pink pills	120	0.60
Lessina	Barr/Duramed	5 pink pills	100	0.50
Levlen	Berlex	4 light-orange pills	120	0.60
Levlite	Berlex	5 pink pills	100	0.50
Levora	Watson	4 white pills	120	0.60
Lo/Ovral	Wyeth-Ayerst	4 white pills	120	0.60
Low-Ogestrel	Watson	4 white pills	120	0.60
Lutera	Watson	5 white pills	100	0.50
Nordette	Wyeth-Ayerst	4 light-orange pills	120	0.60
Ogestrel	Watson	2 white pills	100	0.50
Ovral	Wyeth-Ayerst	2 white pills	100	0.50
Portia	Barr/Duramed	4 pink pills	120	0.60
Quasense	Watson	4 white pills	120	0.60
Seasonale	Barr/Duramed	4 pink pills	120	0.60
Seasonique	Barr/Duramed	4 light-blue-green pills	120	0.60
Tri-Levlen	Berlex	4 yellow pills	120	0.50
Triphasil	Wyeth-Ayerst	4 yellow pills	120	0.50
Trivora	Watson	4 pink pills	120	0.50

Notes:

[a] Plan B is the only dedicated product specifically marketed for emergency contraception. Alesse, Aviane, Cryselle, Enpresse, Jolessa, Lessina, Levlen, Levlite, Levora, Lo/Ovral, Low-Ogestrel, Lutera, Nordette, Ogestrel, Ovral, Portia, Quasense, Seasonale, Seasonique, Tri-Levlen, Triphasil, and Trivora have been declared safe and effective for use as ECPs by the U.S. FDA.[17] Worldwide, about 50 emergency contraceptive products are specifically packaged, labeled, and marketed. For example, Gedeon Richter and HRAPharma are marketing in many countries the levonorgestrel-only products Postinor-2 and Norlevo, respectively, each consisting of a two-pill strip with each pill containing 0.75 mg levonorgestrel. Levonorgestrel-only ECPs are available either over-the-counter or from a pharmacist without having to see a clinician in 43 countries.

[b] The label for Plan B says to take one pill within 72 hours after unprotected intercourse, and another pill 12 hours later. However, recent research has found that both Plan B pills can be taken at the same time. Research has also shown that that all of the brands listed here are effective when used within 120 hours after unprotected sex.

[c] The progestin in Cryselle, Lo/Ovral, Low-Ogestrel, Ogestrel, and Ovral is norgestrel, which contains two isomers, only one of which (levonorgestrel) is bioactive; the amount of norgestrel in each tablet is twice the amount of levonorgestrel.

norgestrel (each Ovrette tablet contains 75 mcg norgestrel, equivalent to 37.5 mcg levonorgestrel; Ovrette is no longer marketed in the United States). Safety of emergency use of pills containing norethindrone has been documented in one study, which found an efficacy slightly lower than that for levonorgestrel pills,[9] but no published studies are available for pills containing other progestins such as gestodene or etonorgestrel; such pills should not be used in routine practice.

In the future, antiprogestins may be another option for emergency contraception. This family of compounds, which includes mifepristone (Mifeprex, also known as RU-486), blocks the effects of progesterone by binding to its receptors. Antiprogestin effects prevent or stop ovulation and disrupt luteal-phase events and endometrial development, depending on whether the drug is administered before or after ovulation.[10] A single 10 milligram (mg) dose of mifepristone, initiated within 120 hours after unprotected intercourse,[11-14] is highly effective in preventing pregnancy. Mifepristone is more effective and causes less nausea and vomiting and fewer side effects than the Yuzpe regimen.[11,15-17] In contrast, mifepristone and the levonorgestrel regimen have equivalent efficacy and side effects, except that the next period is more often delayed after taking mifepristone.[13,14,18]

Older methods for emergency contraception, no longer recommended, include high-dose estrogen or danazol. Treatment with diethylstilbestrol (DES), 25 mg to 50 mg, or ethinyl estradiol, 5 mg to 10 mg given daily for 5 days, provides efficacy similar to the Yuzpe method[19,20] but with a high incidence of nausea and vomiting. Studies of danazol, an androgenic and progestogenic steroid, were initially promising,[21] but this approach was abandoned when a subsequent study found an unacceptably low efficacy.[16]

FUTURE POTENTIAL FOR EMERGENCY CONTRACEPTIVE USE

Wider use of emergency contraception could prevent a substantial proportion of the millions of unplanned pregnancies that occur every year. Educate women about this option during routine visits, provide information materials, provide to those age 17 and younger a prescription or pills in advance for later use if needed, and make certain that office procedures call for prompt response to any request for emergency contraceptive help when someone calls for advice or to make an appointment.

Emergency contraception is nearly always cost-effective. Use of combined or progestin-only ECPs reduces expenditures on medical care by preventing unintended pregnancies, which are very costly. In the United States, insertion of a copper T IUD is not cost-saving when used solely as an emergency contraceptive. However, it becomes cost-effective if it is used as an ongoing method of contraception for as little as four months after emergency insertion; the copper IUD can provide continuous contraceptive protection for up to 10 years thereafter, producing considerable savings.[22] ECPs are cost-effective regardless of whether they are provided when the emergency arises or provided beforehand as a routine preventive measure.[23-27]

That many hospital emergency departments do not provide emergency contraceptive services to women who have been raped is a tragic example of neglected preventive health care.[28] Legal precedent also indicates that this failure constitutes inadequate care and confers to a woman in this situation the standing to sue the hospital.[29] Of the 683,000 rapes identified by the 1992 National Women's Study, only 17% of the women involved received medical care within the first week, and only half of these women recalled being counseled about the possibility of pregnancy. As many as 22,000 pregnancies resulting annually from rape could be prevented by appropriate care. In addition, such care could provide testing and prophylaxis for sexually transmitted infection (STI).[30]

One concern often voiced about making ECPs more widely available is that women who know they can use ECPs might become less diligent with their ongoing contraceptive method. If used as a sole method, repeated ECP therapy would be far less effective than most other contraceptive methods. For a typical woman who used combined ECPs repeatedly as her sole method for a year, the risk of pregnancy would exceed 35%; if she used progestin-only ECPs, she would still have a 20% chance of pregnancy.[31] Therefore, repeated ECP use would not be a rational contraceptive strategy. Also, side effects such as nausea and vomiting that are quite common with combined ECP use are likely to dissuade women from adopting ECP as a principal strategy. Even if ECP availability did adversely affect regular contraceptive use, women are nevertheless entitled to know about all contraceptive options and make decisions themselves about method use.[32]

Reported evidence demonstrates that making ECPs more widely available does not increase risk-taking[33-43] and that women who are the most diligent about ongoing contraceptive use are those most likely to seek emergency treatment.[44] For example, in a recent study considering the effect of advance ECP provision on regular methods of birth control, teens receiving emergency contraception supplies in advance were more likely to use ECPs when needed but did not report higher frequencies of unprotected sex and did not use condoms or hormonal contraception less often.[36] Another study demonstrated that educating teens about ECPs does not increase their sexual activity levels or use of EC but increased their knowledge about proper administration of the drugs.[45]

On the other hand, no published study has yet demonstrated that increasing access to ECPs can reduce pregnancy or abortion rates in a population, although one demonstration project[46] and three clinical trials[38,39,43] were specifically designed to address this issue. The explanation for this result is that even when provided with ECPs in advance, women do not use the treatment often enough after the most risky incidents to result in a substantial population impact.

Many policy initiatives have been undertaken to encourage greater awareness and use of emergency contraception. In 1997, when providing emergency contraception involved evidence-based use of tablets from oral contraceptive pill packets for a non-approved indication, the FDA reviewed relevant research and published the following statement in the Federal Register:[47]

> "Summary: The Food and Drug Administration (FDA) is announcing that the Commissioner of Food and Drugs (the Commissioner) has concluded that certain combined oral contraceptives containing ethinyl estradiol and norgestrel or levonorgestrel are safe and effective for use as postcoital emergency contraception.... The Commissioner bases this conclusion on FDA's review of the published literature concerning this use, FDA's knowledge of the safety of combined oral contraceptives as currently labeled, and on the unanimous conclusion that these regimens are safe and effective made by the agency's Advisory Committee for Reproductive Health Drugs at its June 28, 1996 meeting."

This action provided reassurance for providers about using ordinary oral contraceptive products containing ethinyl estradiol and either norgestrel or levonorgestrel for this unlabeled indication. In 1996, an American College of Obstetricians and Gynecologists (ACOG) Practice Pattern detailed the use of emergency oral contraception,[48] and in 2001 and 2005, ACOG Practice Bulletins updated information about emergency contraception and recommended that clinicians consider giving an advance prescription for emergency contraception at the time of a routine gynecologic visit.[49,50]

Clinical guidelines that include emergency contraception options have been released by the American College of Obstetricians and Gynecologists,[51] the International Planned Parenthood Federation[51] and the Royal College of Obstetricians and Gynaecologists,[52] and levonorgestrel-only ECPs were added by the World Health Organization (WHO) to its WHO Model List of Essential Medicines.[53] In its clinical standards and guidelines, the Planned Parenthood Federation of America now includes advance provision of ECPs for later use (adopted in 1996) or a prescription given over the telephone (adopted in 1998). Family planning clinics in the federally funded Title X program received explicit authorization to provide emergency contraceptive treatment in April 1997.[54] The feasibility of providing emergency contraceptives as a service to members of a large health maintenance organization (HMO) was documented in a demonstration project involving more than 100 providers at Kaiser Permanente medical offices in San Diego.[55] An innovative program in the state of Washington has shown that pharmacists can effectively provide emergency contraceptives directly to patients.[56,57] A similar pharmacist program began in California in 2002 and was adopted in the United Kingdom in January, 2001.[58] Practical steps such as these to increase timely access may be of special importance for teen women. Young women have high rates of unintended pregnancy and are likely to face significant financial and confidentiality obstacles in obtaining services.[59]

The importance of timely access underlay the decision in France in 1999 to make ECPs available from pharmacists and in 2000 to provide ECPs free to young women who need treatment. Norway (2000), Sweden (2001), the Netherlands (2004), India (2005), and the United States (2006, for those aged 18 and over) have changed ECP status from prescription to over-the-counter (OTC). Levonorgestrel-only ECPs are also available from pharmacists in ten U.S. states (Alaska, California, Hawaii, Maine, Massachusetts, Montana, New Hampshire, New Mexico, Vermont, and Washington State), Aruba, Australia, Belgium, Benin, Burkina Faso, Cameroon, Canada, China, Congo, Denmark, Estonia, Finland, France, French Polynesia, Gabon, Ghana, Greece, Guinea-Conakry, Iceland, Israel, Jamaica, Latvia, Libya, Luxembourg, Mali, Mauritania, Mauritius, New Zealand, Niger, Portugal, Senegal, Slovakia, South Africa, Sri Lanka, Switzerland, Togo, Tunisia, and the United Kingdom.

Changing ECPs from prescription to OTC in the United States has been recommended by respected reproductive health leaders[60,61] and endorsed by many professional organizations including ACOG and the American Medical Association (AMA).[61] In December 2003, an FDA advisory committee voted 23 to 4 to approve a switch for Plan B from prescription to OTC, but the FDA rejected an OTC switch in May 2004 in an unprecedented repudiation of such an overwhelmingly positive advisory committee recommendation. The independent Government Accountability Office concluded that the decision process was highly unusual and that the decision was made with atypical involvement from top agency officials and may well have been made months before it was formally announced.[62] Barr Laboratories submitted an amended application in July 2004 to make Plan B a prescription drug for females younger than 16 years and OTC for women and men 16 and older. The FDA had until January 21, 2005 to respond. On August 26, 2005, the FDA announced that Plan B was safe for OTC use by women age 17 and older, but the FDA announced an indefinite delay in reaching a decision, citing three concerns: (1) Can Plan B be both prescription-based and OTC depending on age? (2) Can prescription and OTC versions of the same drug be marketed in the same package, and (3) Can an age restriction be enforced? The FDA failed to articulate clear criteria or an explicit timetable for a final decision. This indefinite delay was heavily criticized.[63] Finally, on August 24, 2006, the FDA approved the nonprescription sale of Plan B for women and men age 18 and older. Younger women will still need a prescription to buy the drug, and it will be kept behind the pharmacy counter, not on the shelf. The FDA decision is a qualified victory for women. Access is limited by whether a pharmacist is on duty and willing to dispense Plan B, and the lack of privacy may be a barrier to access for women who are embarrassed to ask a pharmacist for the drug. Further, the prescription requirement for young women obstructs timely access for many of the women most at risk for unintended pregnancy. Even so, nonprescription availability will facilitate access even for women aged 17 and younger, many of whom will likely circumvent the prescription requirement by getting parents, siblings, or older friends to buy it for them. The age cutoff was chosen not based on any medical evidence that young women could not use emergency contraceptive pills safely or correctly, but rather, according to the FDA's Steven Galson, because it was easy for pharmacists to remember and enforce, since it is the same age limit placed on tobacco and nicotine-replacement products.

MECHANISM OF ACTION
EMERGENCY CONTRACEPTIVE PILLS

Several clinical studies have shown that combined ECPs containing the estrogen ethinyl estradiol and the progestin levonorgestrel can inhibit or delay ovulation.[64-67] This is an important mechanism of action and may explain combined ECP effectiveness when used during the first half of the menstrual cycle, before ovulation has occurred. Some studies have shown histologic or biochemical alterations in the endometrium after treatment with the regimen, leading to the conclusion that combined ECPs may act by impairing endometrial receptivity to implantation of a fertilized egg.[65,68-70] However, other more recent studies have found no such effects on the endometrium.[64,71,72] Additional possible mechanisms include interference with corpus luteum function; thickening of the cervical mucus resulting in trapping of sperm; alterations in the tubal transport of sperm, egg, or embryo; and direct inhibition of fertilization.[73-76] No clinical data exist regarding the last three of these possibilities. Nevertheless, statistical evidence on the effectiveness of combined ECPs suggests that there must be a mechanism of action other than delaying or preventing ovulation.[77] However, the effectiveness of combined ECPs was probably overestimated in that study, in which case the results would be less persuasive.[78]

Early treatment with ECPs containing only the progestin levonorgestrel has been shown to impair the ovulatory process and luteal function;[79-83] no effect on the endometrium was found in two studies,[80,81] but in another study levonorgestrel taken before the LH surge altered the luteal phase secretory pattern of glycodelin in serum and the endometrium.[84] Levonorgestrel also interferes with sperm migration and function at all levels of the genital tract.[85] Studies in the rat and the Cebus monkey demonstrate that levonorgestrel administered in doses that inhibit ovulation has no postfertilization effect that impairs fertility.[76,86,87] Whether these results can be extrapolated to women is unknown.

Based on those animal studies and on their own studies in women (including one in which no pregnancies were observed when levonorgestrel-only ECPs were taken before the day of ovulation whereas 4–5 would have been expected and three pregnancies were observed when ECPs were taken after ovulation when 3–4 would have been expected[88]), Croxatto and colleagues have argued that most if not all of the contraceptive effect of both combined and levonorgestrel only ECPs can be explained by inhibited or dysfunctional ovulation. Based on their studies on human and animals, some are tempted to conclude that there is no post-fertilization effect.[89] It is unlikely that this question can ever be unequivocally answered, and we therefore cannot conclude that ECPs never prevent pregnancy after fertilization. Even if there were an accurate test for fertilization, a finding that some fertilized eggs do not implant after ECPs are taken would not mean that ECPs can work after fertilization, since many, if not most, fertilized eggs naturally do not implant. Nevertheless, even if in some cases ECPs work by inhibiting implantation of a fertilized egg, these probably would be outnumbered by other cases where fertilization of an egg that would not have implanted naturally is prevented because ECPs inhibited ovulation. ECPs do not interrupt an established pregnancy, defined by medical authorities such as the FDA, the National Institutes of Health[90] and ACOG[91] as beginning with implantation. Therefore, ECPs are not abortifacient.[92] To make an informed choice, women must know that ECPs—like all regular hormonal contraceptives such as the birth control pill, Implanon, Evra, NuvaRing, and Depo-Provera,[93] and even like the lactational amenorrhea method[94]— may prevent pregnancy by delaying or inhibiting ovulation, inhibiting fertilization, or inhibiting implantation of a fertilized egg in the endometrium. At the same time, however, all women should be informed that the best available evidence is consistent with the hypothesis that Plan B's ability to prevent pregnancy can be fully accounted for by mechanisms that do not involve interference with post-fertilization events.[120]

COPPER-RELEASING IUDS

When used as a regular method of contraception, copper-releasing IUDs act primarily to prevent fertilization. Copper IUD use for emergency contraception may involve the same mechanism in some cases. Emergency insertion of a copper IUD is significantly more effective than use of ECPs, reducing the risk of pregnancy following unprotected intercourse by as much as 99%.[95,96] This very high level of effectiveness implies that emergency insertion of a copper IUD must also be able to prevent pregnancy after fertilization. (See Chapter 7 on Intrauterine Contraception.)

EFFECTIVENESS

The effectiveness of a preventive therapy is best measured by comparing the probability that the condition will occur if the therapy is used to the probability that it will occur without treatment. For many preventive therapies, such as vaccines, these probabilities are often determined in a randomized clinical trial comparing treatment to a placebo. In the case of emergency contraception, however, efficacy was demonstrated initially in noncomparative observational studies, and, thereafter, use of a placebo was felt to be unethical. Therefore, the chance that pregnancy would occur in the absence of emergency contraception is estimated indirectly using published data on the probability of pregnancy on each day of the menstrual cycle.[97,98] This estimate is compared to the actual number of pregnancies observed after treatment in observational treatment trials. Effectiveness is calculated as 1-[O/E], where O and E are the observed and expected number of pregnancies, respectively.

Calculation of effectiveness, and particularly the denominator of the fraction, involves many assumptions that are difficult to validate. Therefore, reported figures on the efficacy of emergency contraception may be underestimates or, of more concern, overestimates. Yet, precise estimates of efficacy may not be highly relevant to many women who have had unprotected intercourse, since ECPs are often the only available treatment. A more important consideration for most ECP clients may be the fact that data from both clinical trials and studies on the mechanism of action clearly show that at least the levonorgestrel regimen of ECPs is more effective than doing nothing.[99]

Eight studies of the levonorgestrel regimen that included a total of more than 9,500 women reported estimates of effectiveness (reduction in a woman's chance of pregnancy) between 59% and 94%.[13,14,18,100–103,121] A meta-analysis of eight studies of the combined regimen including more than 3,800 women concluded that the regimen prevents about 74% of expected pregnancies; the proportion ranged from 56% to 89% in the different studies.[104] A more recent analysis using possibly improved methodology estimated effectiveness at 53% and 47% in two of the largest trials of the combined regimen.[78] Combined data from two randomized trials that directly compared the two regimens showed a relative risk of pregnancy of 0.51 (95% confidence limits 0.31, 0.83), indicating that the chance of pregnancy among women who received the levonorgestrel regimen was about half that among those who received the combined regimen.[99,102,103]

Several studies have indicated that both regimens are more effective the sooner after sex the pills are taken.[13,17,100,103,105,106] Other studies of both regimens have not found this time effect,[9,14,18,101,102,107–109,121] although sample sizes were often small. The initial studies showed that these regimens are effective when used up to 72 hours after intercourse.[4,103] Consequently, some product package instructions, including that for Plan B, and older guidelines advise use only within that time frame. However, more recent studies indicate that the regimens continue to be moderately effective if started between 72 and 120 hours.[13,101,108,109] No data are available establishing efficacy if ECPs are taken more than 120 hours after intercourse.

Over 9,400 postcoital insertions of copper-bearing IUDs are known to have been carried out since the practice was introduced in 1976. With only 10 failures, this approach probably has a pregnancy rate no higher than 0.2%.[95,96] The effectiveness of using a levonorgestrel-releasing IUD (LNg-20) for emergency contraception has not been studied and is not recommended.

In the case of progestin-only ECPs, new evidence suggests that providing both doses (a total of 1,500 mcg levonorgestrel) at the same time is as effective as and causes no more side effects than taking two doses 12 hours apart.[13,100] (Another study found that two 750 mcg doses 24 hours apart were just as effective as two 750 mcg doses 12 hours apart.[101]

A DVANTAGES AND INDICATIONS

Emergency contraceptives are the only methods a couple can use to prevent pregnancy after unprotected sexual intercourse or after a contraceptive "accident." Emergency contraception also is an essential part of treatment, and standard of care, following sexual assault for women who were not protected by an effective contraceptive method when the assault occurred.[110] Emergency contraception may be an appropriate option in the following circumstances:[92,111]

- No contraceptive was used when intercourse took place.

- A male condom slipped, broke, or leaked.

- A woman's female condom, diaphragm, or cervical cap was inserted incorrectly, dislodged during intercourse, removed too early, or found to be torn.

- A woman missed too many combined oral contraceptive pills (COCs) at the wrong time. Because combined pills act by suppressing ovulation, the risk of conception occurs some days after the missed pills when follicular development, freed from the inhibition by the oral contraceptive, is sufficient to allow ovulation. Ovulation is unlikely if only a few pills have been missed during a pill cycle. Advise a woman who misses 3 or more consecutive pills containing 30 to 35 mcg ethinyl estradiol or who misses 2 or more consecutive pills containing 20 mcg or less ethinyl estradiol during the last week of a pill pack simply to finish the active pills in her current pack and start a new pack the next day with no break for the placebo pills. (Note: no matter how many pills have been missed, treatment is reasonable if the woman is worried or wishes to avoid even a small risk of pregnancy.) Missing pills during the first week, however, is riskier. Recommend emergency contraception to COC users in the following circumstances:

  — 3 or more consecutive COCs containing 30 to 35 mcg ethinyl estradiol missed during the first week of a pill pack, including when a new pack is started 3 or more days late

  — 2 or more consecutive COCs containing 20 mcg or less ethinyl estradiol missed during the first week of a pill pack, including when a new pack is started 2 or more days late

- A woman who is having menstrual periods or who is breastfeeding and amenorrheic but more than six months postpartum is 3 or more hours late taking a progestin-only pill. In contrast to combined pills, progestin-only pills do not consistently suppress ovulation, and the risk of pregnancy after missing progestin-only pills is greater and more immediate than is the case with missed combined pills.

- A woman is more than 7 days late in getting a monthly combined contraceptive injection.

- A woman is more than 14 days late in getting a 3-month progestin-only contraceptive injection, or the date or type of the previous injection is unknown.

- A woman was 2 or more days late starting a new vaginal ring cycle.

- A woman was 2 or more days late starting a new patch cycle.

- A female condom was inserted or removed incorrectly leading to spillage of semen, or the penis was inserted mistakenly between the female condom and the vaginal wall resulting in intravaginal ejaculation.

- The couple erred in practicing coitus interruptus (ejaculation in vagina or on external genitalia).

- The couple erred in practicing periodic abstinence (sexual intercourse on a fertile day of the cycle).

- An IUD was partially or totally expelled or has been removed 7 days or less after the last act of intercourse.

- A woman was exposed to a possible teratogen such as retinoic acid or a cytotoxic drug when she was not protected by effective contraception.

Because it provides extremely high emergency contraceptive efficacy for at least 5 days after intercourse, the IUD may be an especially useful option for women who present 4 or 5 days after unprotected intercourse. It may also be a good choice for the woman who wishes to continue using an IUD as her long-term method of contraception.

SIDE EFFECTS
HORMONAL METHODS

Nausea and vomiting. Following treatment with combined estrogen-progestin ECPs, nausea occurs in about 50% of women, and vomiting in about 20%. These side effects are about half as common following treatment with progestin-only ECPs.[103] Other reported complaints include fatigue, breast tenderness, headache, abdominal pain, and dizziness. Side effects subside within a day or two after treatment is completed. Routine use of the anti-nausea medication meclizine 1 hour before the first ECP dose may help reduce nausea and vomiting.[112]

There is no research to indicate whether it is necessary to repeat the ECP dose if the woman vomits within 2 hours after taking ECPs. Some practitioners take the view that a replacement dose should be given orally, or in the opinion of some, vaginally to prevent the tablets from being vomited a second time. Other providers, believing that nausea and vomiting are evidence of an estrogen-mediated effect on the central nervous system and thus of absorption of the drugs, conclude that a replacement dose is not necessary unless an ECP tablet is visible in the vomitus.

Ectopic pregnancy. Available evidence suggests that ECPs do not increase the chance that a pregnancy following ECP use will be ectopic; moreover, like all contraceptive methods, ECPs reduce the absolute risk of ectopic pregnancy by preventing pregnancy in general.[113] However, ectopic pregnancy can occur following ECP treatment. Keep this possibility in mind whenever a treatment failure occurs.

Menstrual changes. Two studies have been specifically designed to assess the effects of ECPs consisting of 1.5 mg levonorgestrel in a single dose on bleeding patterns. The first study found that when taken in the first three weeks of the menstrual cycle, ECPs significantly shortened that cycle as compared both to the usual cycle length and to the cycle duration in a comparison group of similar women who had not taken ECPs. The magnitude of this effect was greater the earlier the pills were taken. This regimen taken later in the cycle had no effect on cycle length, but it did cause prolongation of the next menstrual period. The ECPs had no effect on the duration of the post-treatment menstrual cycle, but the second period was prolonged. Intermenstrual bleeding was uncommon after ECP use, although more common than among women who had not taken ECPs.[114] The second study compared the baseline cycle with the treatment and post-treatment cycles. Cycle length was significantly shortened by one day when ECPs were taken in the preovulatory phase of the cycle and was significantly lengthened by two days when ECPs were taken in the postovulatory phase. No difference in cycle length was observed for women who took ECPs during the periovulatory phase of the cycle (from two days before to two days after the expected day of ovulation). Menstrual period duration increased significantly when ECPs were taken in the periovulatory or postovulatory phase in both the treatment and post-treatment cycles. The duration of the post-treatment menstrual cycle remained significantly longer when ECPs were taken in the postovulatory phase. During the treatment cycle, 15% of women experienced intermenstrual bleeding; this was significantly more common when ECPs were taken in the preovulatory phase.[115]

COPPER-RELEASING IUD

Side effects after emergency insertion of an IUD are similar to those seen after routine insertion at other times and include abdominal discomfort and vaginal bleeding or spotting. (See Chapter 7 on Intrauterine Contraception.)

CAUTIONS

There are no evidence-based medical contraindications to the use of ECPs, with the exception of pregnancy.[48,49,116] The reason ECPs should not be used in pregnancy is not because they are thought to be harmful, but because they are ineffective. The advantages of ECP use generally outweigh the theoretical risks even for women who have one or more contraindications to the ongoing use of combined oral contraceptives, such as a history of heart disease, acute focal migraine, or severe liver disease. Use of progestin-only emergency treatment, however, may be preferable to use of combined estrogen-progestin ECPs for a woman who has a history of thromboembolic disease and wishes to be treated.

Few adverse events have been reported for women using emergency contraception. The Committee on Safety of Medicines in the United Kingdom reviewed all problems reported during the first 13 years of use of the combination estrogen-progestin ECP product available there (PC4) and among 4 million uses found 61 pregnancies, 3 cases of venous thrombosis (including one death), and 3 cases of cerebrovascular disorder. The Committee further concluded that none of the 6 vascular cases could be definitely linked to ECP use because of the significant time delay in their onset.[73]

In the United States, the labeling for Plan B includes three contraindications:

- pregnancy
- hypersensitivity to any component of the product
- undiagnosed abnormal genital bleeding

Breastfeeding women. During the first 6 weeks postpartum, women who are fully breastfeeding and amenorrheic have little risk of pregnancy. After the first 6 weeks postpartum, initiation of progestin-only oral contraceptives is recommended without caution for breastfeeding women,[116] and use of progestin-only ECPs is not contraindicated.[116] Progestin from pills taken by the mother does appear at low levels in breast milk (1–6% of the maternal serum level), but no adverse effects on the quality or quantity of milk, or on the infant, have been identified (see Chapter 18). Ongoing use of contraceptive pills containing estrogen is recommended only with caution for breastfeeding women from 6 weeks through 6 months postpartum. During this interval, if emergency contraception is needed, use of a progestin-only option may be preferable to a combined estrogen and progestin product.

Drug interactions. Although medications such as phenytoin for treatment of epilepsy or rifampin for treatment of tuberculosis could theoretically reduce the effectiveness of ECPs, whether they actually reduce treatment effectiveness of combined or progestin-only ECPs is not known. Consider increasing the amount of hormone administered in the ECPs, either by increasing the amount of hormone in one or both doses, or by giving an extra dose. No significant interactions have been found with concurrent use of other antibiotics (see Chapter 11 on Combined Oral Contraceptives).

Eligibility criteria and contraindications for emergency insertion of an IUD are the same as for insertion at other times. (See Chapter 7 on Intrauterine Contraception.) A particular concern is the risk of pelvic inflammatory disease, particularly in women requesting emergency contraception after unprotected intercourse with a new sexual partner and in victims of sexual assault, when the risk of STI may be high.

PROVIDING EMERGENCY CONTRACEPTION

If progestin-only ECPs are immediately available, providing this option is preferable to providing combined estrogen-progestin ECP treatment. There is evidence that the progestin-only option is more effective and that the incidence of nausea and vomiting is significantly lower.[103] Availability, however, is an important consideration, because treatment may be most effective when initiated promptly.[117]

Although pregnancy can result from intercourse only during the fertile phase of the cycle, any woman requesting emergency contraception after unprotected intercourse should be offered treatment unless there are sound medical grounds for not doing so. For example, a woman may present more than 72 hours (the currently labeled time window for ECPs) after unprotected intercourse. In this case, offering ECPs should be considered: treatment effectiveness through 120 hours has been documented.[13,101,108,109] Unless the woman is already pregnant and has a positive pregnancy test, it is also illogical to withhold treatment in situations involving more than one unprotected coital exposure or exposure on a low-risk day. In reviewing the cycle day when exposure occurred, you may determine whether the risk of pregnancy is likely to be high or low, but what matters most is how the woman feels about her risk, no matter whether it is likely to be high or low. Also, it is important to remember that determining pregnancy risk is not always straightforward. The risk is low except for the 5 days just before ovulation and on the day of ovulation (see Figure 6–1, graph 1).[118] The problem is that neither the woman nor her clinician is likely to know for sure which day ovulation occurs. What will be known is menstrual period dates. Plotting pregnancy probability versus menstrual period dates (see Figure 6–1, graph 2) shows that late (or early) ovulation is common enough that pregnancy risk is above 1% beginning as early as cycle day 7 and continuing until at least day 39.[118]

COUNSELING

In counseling women who seek emergency contraceptive treatment, remember this is often a difficult and stressful situation. Be respectful of the woman and responsive to her needs. Explain reporting requirements for statutory rape if applicable, and otherwise reassure the woman that all information will be kept confidential. Be as supportive as possible of the woman's choices and refrain from making judgmental comments or

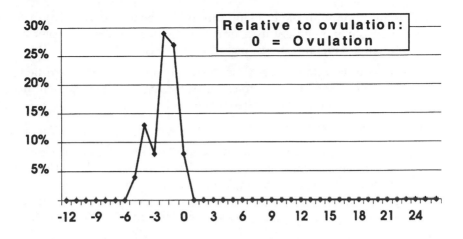

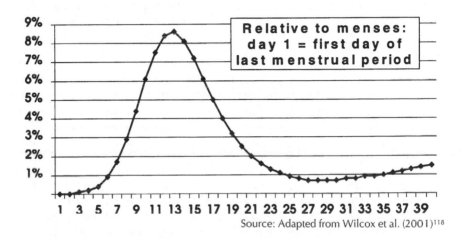

Source: Adapted from Wilcox et al. (2001)[118]

Figure 6–1 Pregnancy probability by cycle day

indicating disapproval through body language or facial expressions. Supportive attitudes will help improve compliance and set the stage for effective follow-up counseling about regular contraceptive use and prevention of STI.

After unprotected intercourse, some women may feel particularly anxious about becoming pregnant and missing the 120-hour window of opportunity for ECPs. They may feel embarrassed about failing to use regular contraception effectively. Rape survivors will feel traumatized. Women may be very concerned about possible infection, especially in cases of rape. Counsel women and provide STI diagnostic services (or referrals) and information about preventive measures. Women must understand that emergency contraception offers no protection against STIs, including infection with the human immunodeficiency virus (HIV). Additional emergency treatment measures may be needed. (See Chapter 21 on Reproductive Tract Infections, including HIV/AIDS.)

Women who would not plan to have an abortion in case of treatment failure can be reassured that pregnancies occurring despite treatment do not have an increased risk of adverse outcome.

Other issues may also arise:

Frequent use. Emphasize that ECPs are for emergency use only. They are not recommended for routine use because they are less effective than regular contraceptives. (Note: Although not recommended, repeated ECP use is not known to pose health risks to users, and concern about this risk is not a logical reason for denying women access to treatment.)

Use after 72 hours. Although most studies of ECP treatment have specified treatment within 72 hours, more recent studies have demonstrated efficacy of giving ECPs up to 120 hours after unprotected intercourse.[13,101,108,109]

Use after multiple acts of unprotected intercourse. If more than 120 hours have elapsed since the time of the first unprotected exposure, ECPs may be less effective in preventing pregnancy that resulted from the first exposure. Providing ECPs, however, would not be expected to disrupt or harm subsequent pregnancy development and would reduce the risk that pregnancy would result from later exposures that did occur within the preceding 120 hours.

Ongoing contraception refused. Women requesting emergency contraception should be offered information and services for regular contraception. Not all of them, however, will want contraceptive counseling. Thus, while counseling about regular contraceptives is recommended, it should not be a prerequisite for providing emergency treatment. If the reason for requesting emergency contraception is that the regular contraceptive method failed, discuss the reasons for failure and how it can be prevented in the future.

BEFORE PROVIDING EMERGENCY CONTRACEPTIVE TREATMENT

Exclude the possibility that a woman may already be pregnant: assess the date of the last menstrual period and whether it was normal. Establish the time of the first episode of unprotected intercourse to determine whether a pregnancy test before treatment may be indicated, and assess the time of the most recent episode of unprotected intercourse to ensure she is within the treatment time frame (120 hours for ECPs or insertion of a copper-releasing IUD). Ask if the woman is currently using a regular

Table 6–2 Anti-nausea treatment options

Drug	Dose	Timing of Administration
Non-prescription Drugs		
Meclizine hydrochloride (Dramamine II, Bonine)	One or two 25 mg tablets	1 hour before first ECP dose; repeat if needed in 24 hours
Diphenhydramine Hydrochloride (Benadryl)	One or two 25 mg tablets	1 hour before first ECP dose; repeat as needed every 4–6 hours
Dimenhydrinate (Dramamine)	One or two 50 mg tablets or 4–8 teaspoons liquid	30 minutes to 1 hour before first ECP dose; repeat as needed every 4–6 hours
Cyclizine hydrochloride (Marezine)	One 50 mg tablet	30 minutes before first ECP dose; repeat as needed every 4–6 hours
Prescription Drugs		
Meclizine hydrochloride (Antivert)	One or two 25 mg tablets	1 hour before first ECP dose; repeat if needed in 24 hours
Trimethobenzamide hydrochloride (Tigan)	One 250 mg tablet or 200 mg suppository	1 hour before first ECP dose; repeat as needed every 6–8 hours
Promethazine hydrochloride (Phenergan)	One 25 mg tablet or suppository	30 minutes to 1 hour before first ECP dose; repeat as needed every 8–12 hours

Source: Trussell et al. (2004)[31]

method of contraception. This question can be a good starting point for a discussion of regular contraceptive use and how to use methods correctly.

Make certain the woman does not want to become pregnant and understands there is still a chance of pregnancy even after treatment. Describe common side effects. Advance counseling about possible side effects helps women know what to expect and may lead to greater tolerance. If the patient will be using a combined estrogen-progestin ECP option, provide meclizine or another anti-nausea medication or recommend an OTC product to be taken 1 hour before starting ECP treatment (see Table 6–2).[31]

A pregnancy test may be helpful if there is some doubt about whether she is already pregnant from intercourse in the past (more than 1 week earlier). If the test is positive, ECP treatment will not be effective. A negative test, however, does not mean that ECPs are unnecessary. Rather, this is the situation when ECPs can work to reduce the risk of pregnancy. Unless there is a doubt about pregnancy from intercourse more than 1 week ago, it makes more sense to provide ECPs; use a pregnancy test only after the next period fails to come on time.[119]

Make sure the woman understands that ECPs will not protect her from pregnancy if she engages in unprotected intercourse in the days or weeks following treatment. This is a common misperception. If the woman wishes to use COCs as an ongoing method, she can take one oral contraceptive tablet the day after emergency treatment is completed and then continue with daily pills, as if the ECP treatment days had been the beginning of a new pill cycle. If the woman does not want to continue using oral contraceptives, but needs contraceptive protection, she can begin the injectable, the vaginal contraceptive ring, or the patch immediately after ECP treatment, or she can use a barrier method, such as condoms, for the remainder of her cycle. A different contraceptive method, such as intrauterine contraception, can be initiated at the beginning of her next cycle (see Table 6–3).

Because ECPs can delay ovulation, a woman could be at risk of pregnancy in the first few days after treatment. Women should abstain from having intercourse or use an effective method of contraception for the remainder of the treatment cycle and thereafter.

EMERGENCY CONTRACEPTION TREATMENT REGIMENS

Emergency contraceptive pills. For maximum effectiveness, ECP treatment should be started as soon as possible after unprotected intercourse, and within 120 hours. Progestin-only ECP treatment (two tablets of 750 mcg levonorgestrel taken together as one 1,500 mcg dose) is more effective and causes significantly less nausea and vomiting than does treatment with combined estrogen-progestin ECP options (100 to 120 mcg ethinyl estradiol and 500 to 600 mcg levonorgestrel in each dose).

Combined estrogen-progestin treatment involves two doses taken 12 hours apart. If necessary, adjust the timing for the second dose by a few hours to avoid a middle-of-the-night dose. Drugs and doses are shown in Table 6–1.

Intrauterine devices. The copper-bearing IUD as an emergency contraceptive method can be inserted up to 5 days after ovulation. Thus, if a woman had unprotected intercourse 3 days before the day ovulation is estimated to have occurred in that cycle, the IUD could, in principle, be inserted up to 8 days after the intercourse. Most family planning providers, however, limit insertion to the first 5 days after intercourse because it is difficult to estimate reliably the day of ovulation. If emergency IUD insertion is planned, but cannot be carried out immediately, provide ECP treatment when the woman is initially evaluated. Even if the ECP effectiveness is not optimal because of an interval longer than 72 hours since unprotected intercourse, it may help reduce the risk of pregnancy. If IUD

Table 6–3 Initiating ongoing contraception after ECP use

Because ECPs can delay ovulation, a woman could be at risk of pregnancy until the next menstrual period after treatment. Women should use an effective method of contraception for the remainder of the treatment cycle and thereafter.

Method	When to Initiate
Condom	Can be used immediately
Diaphragm	Can be used immediately
Spermicide	Can be used immediately
Sponge	Can be used immediately
Combined Oral Contraceptives (COCs)	Initiate a new pack, either according to manufacturer's instructions after beginning the next menstrual cycle, or begin taking one COC tablet daily the day after ECP treatment is completed. Women using Levlen, Levora, Lo/Ovral, Low-Ogestrel, Nordette, or Portia for emergency contraception can continue taking one pill per day from the same pack; women using other brands can begin a new pack the day after ECP treatment is completed; abstain from intercourse or use backup protection for the first seven days
Progestin-only Pills (POPs)	Initiate a new pack, either according to manufacturer's instructions after beginning the next menstrual cycle, or begin taking one POP tablet daily the day after ECP treatment is completed. If starting immediately after ECP use, abstain from intercourse or use backup protection in addition to POPs for the first 2 days of the POP pack.
Vaginal Ring	Initiate the day after ECP treatment is completed or within 5 days of beginning the next menstrual period. If starting immediately after ECP use, abstain from intercourse or use backup protection in addition to the ring for the first 7 days.
Contraceptive Patch	Initiate the day after ECP treatment is completed or within 5 days of beginning the next menstrual period. If starting immediately after ECP use, abstain from intercourse or use backup protection in addition to the patch for the first 7 days.
Three-Month Injectable	Initiate the day ECP treatment is initiated or the day after ECP treatment is completed or within 7 days of beginning the next menstrual period. If starting immediately after ECP use, abstain from intercourse or use backup protection for the first 7 days.
Implants	Initiate within 7 days of beginning the next menstrual period
Intrauterine Contraception	Initiate during the next menstrual period (If the patient intends to use an IUD for ongoing contraception, consider inserting a copper-releasing IUD for emergency contraception treatment.)
Fertility Awareness Methods	Initiate after onset of the next normal menstrual period and after the patient has been trained in using the method
Sterilization	Perform the operation any time after beginning the next menstrual period

insertion is subsequently not feasible, or does not occur, the patient will at least have had the possible benefit of ECP treatment.

AFTER PROVIDING EMERGENCY CONTRACEPTIVE TREATMENT

If the woman has already adopted a method of contraception for regular use and wishes to continue using this method, no follow-up is needed unless she does not have a normal menstrual period within 3 weeks, suspects she may be pregnant, or has other reasons for concern. If a follow-up appointment is indicated, be sure to record information about the woman's menstrual periods and any other bleeding she has experienced to verify that she is not pregnant. If there is any doubt, perform a pregnancy test. Also, review her contraceptive options as appropriate and provide a method if she has not already initiated one.

If emergency contraception has failed and the woman is pregnant, advise her of the possible options and provide appropriate referral information. If she decides to continue the pregnancy, reassure her that there is no evidence of any teratogenic effect following the use of ECPs. Pregnancy following emergency insertion of a copper IUD should be managed the same way as IUD-associated pregnancy following routine insertion (see Chapter 7 on Intrauterine Contraception).

ESTABLISHING EMERGENCY CONTRACEPTIVE SERVICES

Additional information and materials that may be of help in establishing emergency contraception services are available from the following sources:

- Information about emergency contraception method options and access to the U.S. directory of providers via internet: www.NOT-2-LATE.com or ec.princeton.edu.

- Toll-free telephone information about method options and referral to providers listed in the directory nearest the caller's telephone area code: call 1–888-NOT-2-LATE.

- Information about enrolling as a provider in the U.S. directory: ec.princeton.edu/questions/ecsignup.html.

- *Emergency Contraception.* ACOG Practice Bulletin, Number 69. Washington DC: The American College of Obstetricians and Gynecologists, December 2005. To order, call 508–750–8400. Also available in *Obstet Gynecol* 2005;106:1443–1451.

- *Emergency Contraception: Common Legal Questions about Prescribing, Dispensing, Repackaging, and Advertising.* New York NY:

Center for Reproductive Rights, 2002. www.crlp.org/pdf/pub_bp_ec_commonlegal.pdf.

- Information for pharmacists interested in provision of emergency contraception through collaborative practice agreements, and CME accredited, on-line self-instruction: American Pharmaceutical Association, 2215 Constitution Avenue NW, Washington, D.C. 20037. www.aphanet.org.

INSTRUCTIONS FOR USING EMERGENCY CONTRACEPTION

Instructions for women who have emergency insertion of an IUD are the same as for IUD insertion at other times (see Chapter 7 on Intrauterine Contraception).

Women provided with ECPs should receive medication labeling that identifies the specific product prescribed and the number of tablets needed for each dose (see Table 6–1). Give the following instructions to women to ensure correct use.

1. **If you are taking progestin-only ECPs,** swallow the two Plan B tablets as one dose as soon as possible within 120 hours after unprotected sex. Do not take any extra pills. More pills will not decrease the risk of pregnancy any further.

2. **If you are taking combined estrogen-progestin ECPs,** swallow the first dose as soon as possible within 120 hours after unprotected sex. Do not take any extra pills. More pills will not decrease the risk of pregnancy any further but may increase the risk of nausea, possibly causing you to vomit.

    Swallow the second dose 12 hours after taking the first dose. If necessary, you can delay the second dose by a few hours to avoid having to take your second dose in the middle of the night.

    Take anti-nausea medication 1 hour before the first dose. About one-half of women who use combined ECPs have temporary nausea. It is usually mild and should stop in a day or so. If you vomit within 2 hours after taking a dose, call your clinician. You may need to repeat a dose.

3. **If your period does not start within 3 weeks, see your clinician for an exam and pregnancy test.** Your next period may start a few days earlier or later than usual. If you think you may be pregnant, see your clinician at once, whether or not you plan to continue the pregnancy.

4. **Do not have unprotected intercourse in the days or weeks following treatment.**   ECPs will not protect you from pregnancy if you do so. Continue or start taking normal birth control pills, one tablet daily, or use a vaginal ring, contraceptive patches, injectable contraceptive, or a barrier method such as a condom for the remainder of your cycle. After your menstrual period, continue using pills, patches, rings, or condoms, or begin another method of contraception.

5. As soon as you possibly can, **begin using a method of birth control** you will be able to use on an ongoing basis. Emergency contraceptive pills **are not as effective** as other forms of contraception. They are meant for one-time, emergency protection. Discuss with your clinician which method may suit you best and when you can start it.

REFERENCES

1. Anonymous. Consensus statement on emergency contraception. Contraception 1995;52:211–213.
2. Morris JM, Van Wagenen G. Compounds interfering with ovum implantation and development. 3. The role of estrogens. Am J Obstet Gynecol 1966;96:804–815.
3. Van Look PF, von Hertzen H. Emergency contraception. Br Med Bull 1993;49:158–170.
4. Yuzpe AA, Lancee WJ. Ethinylestradiol and dl-norgestrel as a postcoital contraceptive. Fertil Steril 1977;28:932–936.
5. Yuzpe AA, Smith RP, Rademaker AW. A multicenter clinical investigation employing ethinyl estradiol combined with dl-norgestrel as postcoital contraceptive agent. Fertil Steril 1982;37:508–513.
6. Lippes J, Malik T, Tatum HJ. The postcoital copper-T. Adv Plan Parent 1976;11:24–29.
7. Lei H, Hu Z-Y. The mechanisms of action of vacation pills. In: Chang C, Griffin D, Woolman A (eds). Recent advances in fertility regulation: proceedings of a Symposium organized by the Ministry of Public Health of the People's Republic of China, and the World Health Organization's Special Programme of Research, Development and Research Training in Human Reproduction: Beijing, 2–5 September, 1980. Geneva: Atar, 1981.
8. Task Force on Post-Ovulatory Methods for Fertility Regulation. Efficacy and side effects of immediate postcoital levonorgestrel used repeatedly for contraception. Contraception 2000;61:303–308.
9. Ellertson C, Webb A, Blanchard K, et al. Modifying the Yuzpe regimen of emergency contraception: A multi-center randomized, controlled trial. Obstet Gynecol 2003;101:1160–1167.
10. Van Look PF, von Hertzen H. Clinical uses of antiprogestogens. Hum Reprod Update 1995;1:19–34.
11. Van Look PFA. Emergency contraception: the Cinderella of family planning. In: Rodríguez-Armas O, Hédon B, Daya S (eds). Infertility and contraception: a textbook for clinical practice. New York: Parthenon, 1998:209–216.
12. Task Force on Postovulatory Methods of Fertility Regulation. Comparison of three single doses of mifepristone as emergency contraception: a randomised trial. Lancet 1999;353:697–702.

13. von Hertzen H, Piaggio G, Ding J, Chen J, Song S, Bártfai G, Ng E, Gemzell-Danielsson K, Oyunbileg A, Wu S, Cheng W, Lüdicke F, Pretnar-Darovec A, Kirkman R, Mittal S, Khomassuridze A, Apter D, Peregoudov A. Low dose mifepristone and two regimens of levonorgestrel for emergency contraception: a WHO multicentre randomised trial. Lancet 2002;360:1803–1810.

14. Hamoda H, Ashok PW, Stalder C, Flett GM, Kennedy E, Templeton A. A randomized trial of mifepristone (10 mg) and levonorgestrel for emergency contraception. Obstet Gynecol 2004;104:1307–1313.

15. Glasier A, Thong KJ, Dewar M, Mackie M, Baird DT. Mifepristone (RU 486) compared with high-dose estrogen and progestogen for emergency postcoital contraception. N Engl J Med 1992;327:1041–1044.

16. Webb AM, Russell J, Elstein M. Comparison of Yuzpe regimen, danazol, and mifepristone (RU486) in oral postcoital contraception. BMJ (Clinical Research Ed.) 1992;305:927–931.

17. Ashok PW, Stalder C, Wagaarachchi PT, Flett GM, Melvin L, Templeton A. A randomised study comparing a low dose of mifepristone and the Yuzpe regimen for emergency contraception. BJOG 2002;109:553–560.

18. Wu S, Wang C, Wang Y, Cheng W, Zuo S, Li H Xu X, Wang R, Dong J. A randomized, double-blind, multicenter study on comparing levonorgestrel and mifepristone for emergency contraception. J Reprod Med 1999;8(suppl 1):43–46.

19. Morris JM, Van Wagenen G. Postcoital oral contraception. In: Hankinson R, Kleinman R, Esckstein P, Romero H (eds). Proceedings of the Eighth International Conference of the International Planned Parenthood Federation, April 9–15, 1967. Santiago, Chile and London: International Planned Parenthood Federation, 1967.

20. Van Look F. Postcoital contraception: a cover-up story. In: Diczfalusy E, Bygdeman M (eds). Fertility regulation today and tomorrow. Vol 36. New York: Raven Press, 1987.

21. Zuliani G, Colombo UF, Molla R. Hormonal postcoital contraception with an ethinylestradiol-norgestrel combination and two danazol regimens. Europ J Obstet Gynecol Reprod Biology 1990;37:253–260.

22. Trussell J, Leveque JA, Koenig JD, London R, Borden S, Henneberry J, LaGuardia KD, Stewart F, Wilson TG, Wysocki S, Strauss M. The economic value of contraception: a comparison of 15 methods. Am J Public Health 1995;85:494–503.

23. Trussell J, Koenig J, Ellertson C, Stewart F. Preventing unintended pregnancy: the cost-effectiveness of three methods of emergency contraception. Am J Public Health 1997;87:932–937.

24. Trussell J, Koenig J, Stewart F, Darroch JE. Medical care cost savings from adolescent contraceptive use. Fam Plann Perspect 1997;29:248–255, 295.

25. Trussell J, Wiebe E, Shochet T, Guilbert É. Cost savings from emergency contraceptive pills in Canada. Obstet Gynecol 2001;97:789–793.

26. Trussell J, Shochet T. Cost-effectiveness of emergency contraceptive pills in the public sector in the USA. Expert Rev Pharmacoeconomics Outcomes Res 2003;3:433–440.

27. Trussell J, Calabretto H. Cost savings from use of emergency contraceptive pills in Australia. Aust N Z J Obstet Gynaecol 2005;45:308–311.

28. Harrison T. Availability of emergency contraception: a survey of hospital emergency department staff. Ann Emerg Med 2005;46:105–110.

29. Goldenring JM, Allred G. Post-rape care in hospital emergency rooms. Am J Public Health 2001;91:1169–1170.

30. Stewart FH, Trussell J. Prevention of pregnancy resulting from rape: a neglected preventive health measure. Am J Prevent Med 2000;19:228–229.

31. Trussell J, Ellertson C, Stewart F, Raymond EG, Shochet T. The role of emergency contraception. Am J Obstet Gynecol 2004;190:S30-S38.

32. Shelton JD. Repeat emergency contraception: facing our fears. Contraception 2002;66:15–17.

33. Glasier A, Baird D. The effects of self-administering emergency contraception. N Engl J Med 1998;339:1–4.
34. Raine T, Harper C, Leon K, Darney P. Emergency contraception: advance provision in a young, high-risk clinic population. Obstet Gynecol 2000;96:1–7.
35. Jackson RA, Schwarz EB, Freedman L, Darney P. Advance supply of emergency contraception: effect on use and usual contraception?a randomized trial. Obstet Gynecol 2003;102:8–16.
36. Gold MA, Wolford JE, Smith KA, Parker AM. The effects of advance provision of emergency contraception on Adolescent women's sexual and contraceptive behaviors. J Pediatr Adolesc Gynecol 2004;17:87–96.
37. Lo SS, Fan SYS, Ho PC, Glasier AF. Effect of advanced provision of emergency contraception on women's contraceptive behavior: a randomized controlled trial. Hum Reprod 2004;19:2404–410.
38. Raine TR, Harper CC, Rocca CH, Fischer R, Padian N, Klausner JD, Darney PD. Direct access to emergency contraception through pharmacies and effect on unintended pregnancy and STIs: a randomized controlled trial. JAMA 2005;293:54–62.
39. Hu X, Cheng L, Hua X, Glasier A. Advanced provision of emergency contraception to postnatal women in China makes no difference in abortion rates: a randomized controlled trial. Contraception 2005;72:111–116.
40. Belzer M, Sanchez K, Olson J, Jacobs AM, Tucker D. Advance supply of emergency contraception: a randomized trial in adolescent mothers. J Pediatr Adolesc Gynecol. 2005;18:347–354.
41. Trussell J, Raymond E, Stewart FH. Advance supply of emergency contraception: a randomized trial in adolescent mothers [Letter to the editor]. J Pediatr Adolesc Gynecol. 2006;19:251.
42. Walsh TL, Frezieres RG. Patterns of emergency contraception use by age and ethnicity from a randomized trial comparing advance provision and information only. Contraception 2006;74:110–117.
43. Raymond EG, Stewart F, Weaver M, Monteith C, Van Der Pol B. Impact of increased access to emergency contraceptive pills: a randomized controlled trial. Obstet Gynecol 2006;108:1098–1106.
44. Kosunen E, Sihvo S, Hemminki E. Knowledge and use of hormonal emergency contraception in Finland. Contraception 1997;55:153–157.
45. Graham A, Moore L, Sharp D, Diamond I. Improving teenagers' knowledge of emergency contraception: cluster randomized controlled trial of a teacher led intervention. Br Med J 2002;234(7347):1179–1184.
46. Glasier A, Fairhurst K, Wyke S, Ziebland S, Seaman P, Walker J, Lakha F. Advanced provision of emergency contraception does not reduce abortion rates. Contraception 2004;69:361–366.
47. Food and Drug Administration. Prescription drug products; certain combined oral contraceptives for use as postcoital emergency contraception. Federal Regist 1997;62:8610–8612.
48. Emergency oral contraception. ACOG Practice Patterns #3. Washington DC: American College of Obstetricians and Gynecologists, 1996.
49. Emergency oral contraception. ACOG Practice Bulletin, Number 25. Washington DC: American College of Obstetricians and Gynecologists, 2001.
50. Emergency contraception. ACOG Practice Bulletin, Number 69. Washington DC: The American College of Obstetricians and Gynecologists, December 2005. Also available in Obstet Gynecol 2005;106:1443–1451.
51. International Planned Parenthood Federation (IPPF). IMAP statement on emergency contraception. IPPF Medical Bulletin 2004;38:1–3.
52. Faculty of Family Planning and Reproductive Health Care Clinical Effectiveness Unit. FFPRHC Guidance April 2006. Emergency contraception. J Fam Plann Reprod Health Care 2006;32:121–128.

53. World Health Organization. The selection and use of essential medicines. Report of the WHO Expert Committee 2002 (including the 12th model list of essential medicines. Geneva: World Health Organization, 2003. (WHO Technical Report Series No. 914.)

54. Kring T. Emergency contraception. Washington DC: Department of Health and Human Services, Office of Population Affairs, 1997. Report Number 97–2.

55. Beckman LJ, Harvey SM, Sherman CA, Petitti DB. Changes in providers' views and practices about emergency contraception with education. Obstet Gynecol 2001;97:942–946.

56. Wells ES, Hutchings J, Gardiner JS, Winkler JL, Fuller DS, Downing D, Shafer R. Using pharmacies in Washington State to expand access to emergency contraception. Fam Plann Perspect 1998;30:288–290.

57. Gardner JS, Hutchings J, Fuller TS, Downing D. Increasing access to emergency contraception through community pharmacies: lessons from Washington State. Fam Plann Perspect 2001;33:172–175.

58. Harrison-Woolrych M, Howe J, Smith C. Improving access to emergency contraception. BMJ (Clinical Research Ed.) 2001;322(7280):186–187.

59. Gold MA. Prescribing and managing oral contraceptive pills and emergency contraception for adolescents. Pediatr Clin N Am 1999;46:695–718.

60. Grimes DA. Emergency contraception and fire extinguishers: a prevention paradox. Am J Obstet Gynecol 2002;187:1536–1538.

61. Grimes DA, Raymond EG, Scott Jones B. Emergency contraception over-the-counter: the medical and legal imperatives. Obstet Gynecol 2001;98:151–155.

62. Decision process to deny initial application for over-the-counter marketing of the emergency contraceptive drug Plan B was unusual. Washington DC: Government Accountability Office, 2004.

63. Wood AJJ, Drazen JM, Greene MF. A sad day for science at the FDA. N Engl J Med 2005;353:1197–1198.

64. Swahn ML, Westlund P, Johannisson E, Bygdeman M. Effect of post-coital contraceptive methods on the endometrium and the menstrual cycle. Acta Obstet Gynecol Scand 1996;75:738–744.

65. Ling WY, Robichaud A, Zayid I, Wrixon W, MacLeod SC. Mode of action of dl-norgestrel and ethinylestradiol combination in postcoital contraception. Fertil Steril 1979;32:297–302.

66. Rowlands S, Kubba AA, Guillebaud J, Bounds W. A possible mechanism of action of danazol and an ethinylestradiol/norgestrel combination used as postcoital contraceptive agents. Contraception 1986;33:539–545.

67. Croxatto HB, Fuentalba B, Brache V, Salvatierra AM, Alvarez F, Massai R, Cochon L, Faundes A. Effects of the Yuzpe regimen, given during the follicular phase, on ovarian function. Contraception 2002;65:121–128.

68. Kubba AA, White JO, Guillebaud J, Elder MG. The biochemistry of human endometrium after two regimens of postcoital contraception: a dl-norgestrel/ethinylestradiol combination or danazol. Fertil Steril 1986;45:512–516.

69. Ling WY, Wrixon W, Zayid I, Acorn T, Popat R, Wilson E. Mode of action of dl-norgestrel and ethinylestradiol combination in postcoital contraception. II. Effect of postovulatory administration on ovarian function and endometrium. Fertil Steril 1983;39:292–297.

70. Yuzpe AA, Thurlow HJ, Ramzy I, Leyshon JI. Post coital contraception—a pilot study. J Reprod Med 1974;13:53–58.

71. Taskin O, Brown RW, Young DC, Poindexter AN, Wiehle RD. High doses of oral contraceptives do not alter endometrial $\alpha 1$ and $\alpha \nu \beta 3$ integrins in the late implantation window. Fertil Steril 1994;61:850–855.

72. Raymond EG, Lovely LP, Chen-Mok M, Seppälä M, Kurman RJ, Lessey BA. Effect of the Yuzpe regimen of emergency contraception on markers of endometrial receptivity. Hum Reprod 2000;15:2351–2355.

73. Glasier A. Emergency postcoital contraception. N Engl J Med 1997;337:1058–1064.
74. Ling WY, Wrixon W, Acorn T, Wilson E, Collins J. Mode of action of dl-norgestrel and ethinylestradiol combination in postcoital contraception. III. Effect of preovulatory administration following the luteinizing hormone surge on ovarian steroidogenesis. Fertil Steril 1983;40:631–636.
75. Croxatto HB, Devoto L, Durand M, Ezcurra E, Larrea F, Nagle C, Ortiz ME, Vantman D, Vega M, von Hertzen H. Mechanism of action of hormonal preparations used for emergency contraception: a review of the literature. Contraception 2001;63:111–121.
76. Croxatto HB, Ortiz ME, Müller AL. Mechanisms of action of emergency contraception. Steroids 2003;68:1095–1098.
77. Trussell J, Raymond EG. Statistical evidence concerning the mechanism of action of the Yuzpe regimen of emergency contraception. Obstet Gynecol 1999;93:872–876.
78. Trussell J, Ellertson C, von Hertzen H, Bigrigg A, Webb A, Evans M, Ferden S. Leadbetter C. Estimating the effectiveness of emergency contraceptive pills. Contraception 2003;67:259–265.
79. Hapangama D, Glasier AF, Baird DT. The effects of peri-ovulatory administration of levonorgestrel on the menstrual cycle. Contraception 2001;63:123–129.
80. Durand M, del Carmen Cravioto M, Raymond EG, Durán-Sánchez O, De la Luz Cruz-Hinojosa L, Castell-Rodríguez A, Schiavon R, Larrea F. On the mechanisms of action of short-term levonorgestrel administration in emergency contraception. Contraception 2001;64:227–234.
81. Marions L, Hultenby K, Lindell I, Sun X, Ståbi B, Gemzell Danielsson K. Emergency contraception with mifepristone and levonorgestrel: mechanism of action. Obstet Gynecol 2002;100:65–71.
82. Marions L, Cekan SZ, Bygdeman M, Gemzell-Danielsson K. Effect of emergency contraception with levonorgestrel or mifepristone on ovarian function. Contraception 2004;69:373–377.
83. Croxatto HB, Brache V, Pavez M, Cochon L, Forcelledo ML, Alvarez F, Massai R, Faundes A, Salvatierra AM. Pituitary-ovarian function following the standard levonorgestrel emergency contraceptive dose or a single 0.75-mg dose given on the days preceding ovulation. Contraception 2004;70:442–450.
84. Durand M, Sépala M, del Carmen Cravioto M, Koistinen H, Koistinen R, González-Macedo J, Larrea F. Late follicular phase administration of levonorgestrel as an emergency contraceptive changes the secretory pattern of glycodelin in serum and endometrium during the luteal phase of the menstrual cycle. Contraception 2005;71:451–457.
85. Kesserü E, Garmendia F, Westphal N, Parada J. The hormonal and peripheral effects of d-norgestrel in postcoital contraception. Contraception 1974;10:411–424.
86. Müller AL, Llados CM, Croxatto HB. Postcoital treatment with levonorgestrel does not disrupt postfertilization events in the rat. Contraception 2003;67:415–419.
87. Ortiz ME, Ortiz RE, Fuentes MA, Parraguez VH, Croxatto HB. Postcoital administration of levonorgestrel does not interfere with post-fertilization events in the new-world monkey Cebus apella. Hum Reprod 2004;19:1352–1356.
88. Novikova N, Weisberg E, Stanczyk FZ, Croxatto HB, Fraser, IS. Effectiveness of levonorgestrel emergency contraception given before or after ovulation—a pilot study. Contraception 2007;75, in press.
89. Anonymous. Emergency contraception's mode of action clarified. Popul Briefs 2005;11:3 Available at www.popcouncil.org/pdfs/popbriefs/pbmay05.pdf (accessed March 23, 2006).
90. OPRR Reports: Protection of Human Subjects. Code of Federal Regulations 45CFR 46, March 8, 1983.
91. Hughes EC (ed), Committee on Terminology, The American College of Obstetricians and Gynecologists, Obstetric-Gynecologic Terminology. Philadelphia PA: F.A. Davis Company, 1972.

92. Levonorgestrel for emergency contraception. Fact sheet. Geneva, World Health Organization, March 2005.

93. Statement on Contraceptive Methods. Washington DC: American College of Obstetricians and Gynecologists, July 1998.

94. Díaz S, Cárdenas H, Brandeis A, Miranda P, Salvatierra AM, Croxatto HB. Relative contributions of anovulation and luteal phase defect to the reduced pregnancy rate of breastfeeding women. Fertil Steril 1992;58:498–503.

95. Trussell J, Ellertson C. Efficacy of emergency contraception. Fertility Control Reviews 1995;4:8–11.

96. Zhou L, Xiao B. Emergency contraception with Multiload Cu-375 SL IUD: a multicenter clinical trial. Contraception 2001;64:107–112.

97. Dixon GW, Schlesselman JJ, Ory HW, Blye RP. Ethinyl estradiol and conjugated estrogens as postcoital contraceptives. JAMA 1980;244:1336–1339.

98. Wilcox AJ, Weinberg CR, Baird DD. Timing of sexual intercourse in relation to ovulation. Effects on the probability of conception, survival of the pregnancy, and sex of the baby. N Engl J Med 1995;333:1517–1521.

99. Raymond E, Taylor D, Trussell J, Steiner MJ. Minimum effectiveness of the levonorgestrel regimen of emergency contraception. Contraception 2004;69:79–81.

100. Arowojolu AO, Okewole IA, Adekunle AO. Comparative evaluation of the effectiveness and safety of two regimens of levonorgestrel for emergency contraception in Nigerians. Contraception 2002;66:269–273.

101. Ngai SW, Fan S, Li S, Cheng L, Ding J, Jing X, Ng EHY, Ho PC. A randomized trial to compare 24h versus 12h double dose regimen of levonorgestrel for emergency contraception. Hum Reprod 2004;20:307–311.

102. Ho PC, Kwan MS. A prospective randomized comparison of levonorgestrel with the Yuzpe regimen in post-coital contraception. Hum Reprod 1993;8:389–392.

103. Task Force on Postovulatory Methods of Fertility Regulation. Randomised controlled trial of levonorgestrel versus the Yuzpe regimen of combined oral contraceptives for emergency contraception. Lancet 1998;352:428–433.

104. Trussell J, Rodríguez G, Ellertson C. Updated estimates of the effectiveness of the Yuzpe regimen of emergency contraception. Contraception 1999;59:147–151.

105. Kane LA, Sparrow MJ. Postcoital contraception: a family planning study. N Z Med J 1989;102:151–153.

106. Piaggio G, von Hertzen H, Grimes DA, Van Look PFA. Timing of emergency contraception with levonorgestrel or the Yuzpe regimen. Lancet 1999;353:721.

107. Trussell J, Ellertson C, Rodríguez G. The Yuzpe regimen of emergency contraception: how long after the morning after? Obstet Gynecol 1996;88:150–154.

108. Rodrigues I, Grou F, Joly J. Effectiveness of emergency contraception pills between 72 and 120 hours after unprotected sexual intercourse. Am J Obstet Gynecol 2001;184:531–537.

109. Ellertson C, Evans M, Ferden S, Leadbetter C, Spears A, Johnstone K, Trussell J. Extending the time limit for starting the Yuzpe regimen of emergency contraception to 120 hours. Obstet Gynecol 2003;101:1168–1171.

110. Feldhaus KM. A 21st-century challenge: improving the care of the sexual assault victim. Ann Emerg Med 2002;39:653–655.

111. Selected practice recommendations for contraceptive use. Second Edition. Geneva: World Health Organization, 2005.

112. Raymond EG, Creinin MD, Barnhart KT, Lovvorn AE, Rountree RW, Trussell J. Meclizine for prevention of nausea associated with use of emergency contraceptive pills: a randomized trial. Obstet Gynecol 2000;95:271–277.

113. Trussell J, Hedley A, Raymond E. Ectopic pregnancy following use of progestin-only ECPs [letter]. J Fam Plann Reprod Health Care 2003;29:249.

114. Raymond EG, Goldberg A, Trussell J, Hays M, Roach E, Taylor D. Bleeding patterns after use of levonorgestrel emergency contraceptive pills. Contraception 2006;73:376–381. Erratum. Contraception 2006;74:349–350.

115. Gainer E, Kenfack B, Mboudou E, Doh AS, Bouyer J. Menstrual bleeding patterns following levonorgestrel emergency contraception. Contraception 2006;74:118–124.
116. Medical eligibility criteria for contraceptive use: Third Edition. Geneva: World Health Organization, 2004.
117. Ellertson C, Blanchard K, Webb A, Bigrigg A, Haskell S. Emergency contraception. Lancet 1998;352(9138):1477.
118. Wilcox AJ, Dunson DB, Weinberg CR, Trussell J, Baird DD. Likelihood of conception with a single act of intercourse: providing benchmark rates for assessment of post-coital contraceptives. Contraception 2001;63:211–215.
119. Grimes DA, Raymond EG. Bundling a pregnancy test with the Yuzpe regimen of emergency contraception. Obstet Gynecol 1999;94:471–473.

LATE REFERENCES

120. Davidoff F, Trussell J. Plan B and the politics of doubt. J Am Med Assoc 2006;296:1775–1778.
121. Creinin MD, Schlaff W, Archer DF, Wan L, Frezieres R, Thomas M, Rosenberg M, Higgins J. Progesterone receptor modulator for emergency contraception: a randomized controlled trial. Obstet Gynecol 2006;108:1089–1097.

Intrauterine Devices (IUDs)

David A. Grimes, MD

- The Cu T 380A and levonorgestrel-releasing intrauterine system rival surgical sterilization in efficacy.

- Continuation rates are high compared with other reversible contraceptives.

- Intrauterine contraception provides long-term protection against pregnancy yet is promptly reversible.

- The risk of upper-genital-tract infection is negligible; prophylactic antibiotics are not indicated.

- The levonorgestrel IUD can be used to treat heavy bleeding and to protect the endometrium during estrogen therapy in the menopause.

Intrauterine contraception is enjoying a renaissance in the United States and elsewhere, due in part to the growing good news about safety, efficacy, and non-contraceptive therapeutic benefits. For example, in 2005, the U.S. Food and Drug Administration approved liberalized package labeling for the copper T 380A. The revised labeling does not proscribe insertion in nulliparous women or in those with more than one sexual partner; insertion immediately after an abortion or delivery is also deemed appropriate. Much of this scientific evidence is summarized in two important reviews.[1,2]

Nevertheless, opinions about IUDs in the United States remain paradoxical. Surveys among women reveal that a minority have a favorable view of IUDs... except those using them. Among women using an IUD for contraception, 99% reported being "very" or "somewhat satisfied" with the method. In contrast, 92% of implant users and 91% of oral contraceptive users held these views.[3] An important responsibility for health care providers—and the media—is to provide correct information to consumers and professionals. This, in turn, will increase the availability and use of this excellent method. In Turkey, the media made a large impact,

Copper T 380A IUD

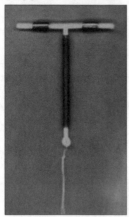

Levonogestrel IUS

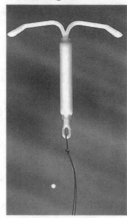

Figure 7–1 Two IUDs available in the United States

with an information campaign leading to a 30% increase in IUD use.[4] Direct-to-consumer advertising in the United States has been temporally associated with substantial growth in IUD use.

OPTIONS IN THE UNITED STATES

Two highly effective intrauterine contraceptives are available in the United States: the Copper T 380A (ParaGard®, Duramed Pharmaceuticals, Inc., Cincinnati, Ohio), and the levonorgestrel intrauterine system (Mirena®, Berlex Inc., Montville, New Jersey) (Figure 7–1).

Introduced in the United States in 1988, the TCu 380A is made of polyethylene with barium sulfate added to create x-ray visibility. Fine copper wire is wound around the vertical stem of the T. Each of the two horizontal arms has a sleeve of copper as well. The combined copper surface area of the wire and sleeves is 380 +/- 23 mm^2. The device measures 36 mm tall and 32 mm wide. The bottom of the vertical stem has a 3 mm bulb into which a monofilament polyethylene string is tied; these two strands enable easy removal of the device. Throughout the world, tens of millions of Copper T 380A IUDs have been distributed in 70 countries. The approved duration of use of the device is ten years, although data indicate high effectiveness as long as 12 years.[5]

The levonorgestrel intrauterine system was approved for use in the United States in 2000 and first sold in 2001. This system has been available in Europe for a decade, and several million women have used it to date. The system releases levonorgestrel directly into the endometrial cavity at an initial rate of 20 mcg per day. This release rate was selected to provide high contraceptive effectiveness while minimizing side effects. The rate declines to about 14 mcg per day after 5 years, which is still in the therapeutic range.

The approved life span of the levonorgestrel system is 5 years, although the protection with the system in place may last at least 7 years.[6] The product is based on a NOVA T model polyethylene frame, with a cylinder of a polydimethylsiloxane-levonorgestrel mixture molded around its vertical arm. The cylinder is coated with a membrane that regulates the release of the hormone. Measuring 32 mm in both height and width, the T-shaped frame contains barium sulfate for visibility on X-ray. The base of the vertical stem has dark monofilament polyethylene threads to assist with removal.

Small amounts of levonorgestrel are systemically absorbed, and, thus, some systemic side effects can occur. However, the daily dose of levonorgestrel is about 10% that with an oral contraceptive containing 150 mcg levonorgestrel, and the mean plasma concentration only 5%. Moreover, the plasma concentrations of levonorgestrel are lower than those achieved with either the subdermal levonorgestrel implants or the progestin-only pill.

EFFECTIVENESS

While contraceptive effectiveness is discussed in more detail in Chapter 27, a simple formula explains why today's IUDs provide superior contraception (Figure 7–2). The effectiveness in the community of any contraceptive is related to a number of factors. These include the inherent ability of the method to prevent pregnancy (efficacy) and the user's compliance (adherence to the regimen, such as pill taking) and continuation (ongoing use over time). Factors influencing effectiveness include a woman's fecundability (reflecting age, body mass index, prior salpingitis, etc.) and frequency of coitus. Although combined oral contraceptives have excellent efficacy, compliance is only fair—as is continuation. Hence, the contraceptive effectiveness of combined oral contraceptives falls in the middle tier.[7] In contrast, IUDs have excellent efficacy and users exhibit high compliance and high continuation rates (about 85% to 90% at one year). This translates into superior protection against unintended pregnancy.

Both of the intrauterine contraceptives in the United States rank in the top tier of contraceptive effectiveness (along with surgical sterilization, implants, and injectable contraceptives).[7] In combined World Health Organization and Population Council trials, the first-year discontinuation rate of the TCu 380A for accidental pregnancy was only 0.7 per 100 women, and even lower rates occurred in years two through ten.[8] In World Health Organization trials, the cumulative 12-year failure rate with the TCu 380A was 2.2 pregnancies per 100 women.[5] In three trials

Determinants of
Contraceptive Effectiveness

$$\text{Contraceptive effectiveness} \approx \frac{\text{Efficacy} \times \text{compliance* } \times \text{continuation*}}{\text{Fecundability} \times \text{coital frequency*}}$$

* Factors amenable to control by the woman

Figure 7–2 A simple formula of contraceptive effectiveness

conducted by Leiras, the Finnish manufacturer of the levonorgestrel system, the first-year cumulative failure rate was 0.14 per 100 women, and the cumulative five-year failure rate was only 0.71 per 100 women. In the Population Council's randomized trial of the levonorgestrel intrauterine system vs. the TCu 380A, the seven-year cumulative failure rates were 1.1 and 1.4 per 100 women, respectively.[6] In contrast, the overall ten-year failure rate with all methods of tubal sterilization in the United States is 1.9 per 100 women.[9] Thus, contemporary intrauterine contraceptives rival the effectiveness of tubal sterilization.

MECHANISM OF ACTION

IUDs work primarily by preventing sperm from fertilizing ova.[10] Stated alternatively, IUDs are not abortifacients.[11] The TCu 380A causes an increase in copper ions, enzymes, prostaglandins, and white blood cells (macrophages) in uterine and tubal fluids; these impair sperm function and prevent fertilization. The levonorgestrel intrauterine system may have an array of contraceptive actions, including thickening the cervical mucus, inhibiting sperm capacitation and survival, and suppressing the endometrium. The system has a local effect in the endometrium causing release of foreign-body mediators. In addition, some women do not ovulate as a result of systemic absorption of levonorgestrel.[12]

Two lines of evidence indicate that IUDs work earlier in the reproductive process than previously thought.[11] First, sensitive assays for early pregnancy do not reveal "chemical pregnancies."[13,14] Second, and more compelling, are tubal flushing studies. Investigators have studied women undergoing Pomeroy tubal sterilization at mid-cycle. The fallopian tubes were then flushed and the fluid examined with a microscope to look for sperm and fertilized eggs. In women not using contraception, eggs were recovered in about half of the women. In women using IUDs, no fertilized, normally-dividing eggs were recovered.[15] As discussed below, IUD users have a marked decrease in the risk of ectopic pregnancies, which implies that IUDs inhibit fertilization.

A DVANTAGES OF INTRAUTERINE CONTRACEPTION

- Highly effective
- Protective against ectopic pregnancy
- Long-lasting
- Convenient
- Well-liked by users
- Safer than previously thought
- Cost-effective

Intrauterine contraception is "first-line" family planning. One office visit can provide a decade or more of superb contraception, at a low daily cost. Few methods are as convenient: the need for daily pill taking or use of barrier methods is obviated. Fertility rebounds promptly upon discontinuation. Modern intrauterine contraceptives have an enviable safety record.

Not only are contemporary intrauterine contraceptives effective against intrauterine pregnancies, they also prevent extrauterine pregnancies as well. The notion that intrauterine contraceptives increase the risk of ectopic pregnancy was debunked long ago.[16] Both the copper and levonorgestrel-releasing contraceptives dramatically reduce a woman's risk of an ectopic pregnancy, compared with use of no contraception.[6,27] For example, in the World Health Organization trials of the TCu 380A, the 12-year cumulative discontinuation rate for ectopic pregnancy was only 0.4 per 100 women.[5]

In addition, intrauterine contraception is often an excellent choice for women who cannot use oral contraceptives because of medical disorders.[18] Women who are poor surgical candidates for sterilization (e.g., because of obesity or severe asthma) are often ideal candidates for this method. Similarly, IUDs may be useful for women with HIV infection.

Cancer Protection

One of the most intriguing aspects of intrauterine contraception is the evolving story of cancer prophylaxis. Seven case-control studies around the world have examined the potential association between non-medicated or copper IUD use and development of endometrial cancer.[19] Six of the seven found protection against endometrial cancer from devices, and the effect was statistically significant in two (including the Cancer and Steroid Hormone Study of the Centers for Disease Control and Prevention). The only study not to find benefit related to a steel ring used in China, which is not relevant to Western practice. While the mechanism of action is unknown, it may relate to the altered endometrium associated with intrauterine contraception. Similarly, progestin-releasing intrauterine contraceptives should also protect against this cancer,[20] as is true of contraceptives that deliver a progestin systemically.[21] Indeed, the levonorgestrel device has been used to treat endometrial hyperplasia and adenocarcinoma.[22] Two studies have addressed cervical cancer,[23,24] and both found a 40% reduction in risk associated with IUDs, which was not statistically significant.

MEDICAL BENEFITS OF THE LEVONORGESTREL INTRAUTERINE SYSTEM

Topical delivery of progestin to the uterine cavity has exciting therapeutic uses aside from contraception. Some are well-established and approved indications overseas, while others are still being explored. Although average menstrual blood loss increases among users of the TCu 380A, the opposite occurs among users of the levonorgestrel system. Overall blood loss drops about 90%, and 20% or more women stop bleeding altogether. This translates into clinically important increases in hemoglobin and iron stores. Some evidence supports a benefit in treating heavy bleeding associated with adenomyosis[25] and leiomyomas.[26]

Indeed, the levonorgestrel system can be used to treat heavy menses, not just prevent them. Trials have compared this approach to medical treatments with an oral progestin, a nonsteroidal anti-inflammatory drug, or tranexamic acid (not available in the United States). The levonorgestrel system proved superior to the other alternatives. In addition, this system has been found an acceptable (and inexpensive) alternative to endometrial ablation or hysterectomy.[2]

Another logical use of the levonorgestrel intrauterine system is as part of hormone replacement therapy in menopause. Many women suffer from unpleasant side effects of oral progestins given along with estrogen. In addition, nuisance bleeding is the primary reason women abandon hormone replacement therapy. Use of the levonorgestrel system leads to profound suppression of the endometrium, which then ceases to bleed.[27] Lack of uterine bleeding during hormone replacement therapy is desirable for the woman and her clinician.

DISADVANTAGES OF INTRAUTERINE CONTRACEPTION

- Menstrual disturbances
- Cramping and pain
- Spontaneous expulsion

- Perforation
- String problems
- Pregnancy complications
- Upper-genital-tract infection
- Actinomyces-like organisms seen on Papanicolaou smear

Menstrual Problems

Bleeding problems constitute one of the more common IUD complications. Altered bleeding patterns may be a normal side-effect of intrauterine contraception or may signal pregnancy, infection, or partial expulsion. Irregular bleeding is common in the early months of intrauterine contraception with either device. Women using the TCu 380A usually have heavier menses, and irregular bleeding can occur during early use. Irregular but light bleeding or spotting is the norm in the early months of the levonorgestrel intrauterine system, since endometrial suppression takes several months to achieve. Thereafter, a marked decrease in bleeding occurs. Women should be thoroughly counseled about these effects, which tend to be self-limiting.

Excessive bleeding with the TCu 380A can be treated with non-steroidal anti-inflammatory drugs;[30] trials have not demonstrated the superiority of one product over another. Since local prostaglandin production is involved with excessive bleeding, any prostaglandin synthetase inhibitor should help; in contrast, aspirin and acetaminophen do not. Starting in advance of menses does not give better results than starting with the onset of flow. If hemoglobin levels drop, oral iron supplementation can be started.

Not all nuisance bleeding can be attributed to the contraceptive. For example, other gynecologic disorders, such as endometrial polyps, may be responsible. Alternatively, an accidental pregnancy (including an ectopic pregnancy) can present with bleeding. In addition, bleeding may accompany endometritis. Of note, with the use of small catheters, the endometrium can be biopsied with the device remaining in place. Persistent abnormal bleeding requires clinical evaluation. If no explanation is found and if the woman's threshold for tolerance is passed, the device can be removed.

Cramping and Pain

Discomfort may be felt at the time of IUD insertion and may be followed by cramping pain over the next 10 to 15 minutes. One approach is preventive therapy with oral non-steroidal anti-inflammatory drugs, local anesthesia, or both. Prophylactic administration of a non-steroidal anti-inflammatory drug around the time of insertion has not been found to be helpful. The most common analgesia approach used for insertion in the United Kingdom is intrauterine anesthesia with a solution of 2% lidocaine (Instillagel), which is not commercially available in the United States.[2,31] For paracervical anesthesia, use of a long-acting local anesthetic, such as bupivacaine, may be preferable to shorter-acting drugs, such as lidocaine. Should a woman have pain or vasovagal symptoms immediately after insertion, a paracervical block can be placed at that time. Rarely, the IUD needs to be removed at the insertion visit. Pain that develops later may reflect threatened or partial expulsion, dislodgment, infection, or a complicated pregnancy.

Expulsion

Between 2% to 10% of IUD users spontaneously expel their IUD within the first year. An IUD expulsion can occur without the woman detecting it. Nulliparity, an abnormal amount of menstrual flow, and severe dysmenorrhea are risk factors for Cu T 380A expulsion.[32] A woman who has expelled one IUD has a 30% chance of subsequent expulsions.[33]

The symptoms of an IUD expulsion include unusual vaginal discharge, cramping or pain, intermenstrual spotting, postcoital spotting, dyspareunia (for the man or the woman), absence or lengthening of the IUD string, and presence of the hard plastic of the IUD at the cervical os or in the vagina.[34] If the menstrual period is delayed, check for IUD strings. A missed period may be the first indication of a "silent" expulsion. If the woman is not pregnant, another IUD can be replaced immediately.

Perforation

Perforation of the uterus can occur at the time of IUD insertion; no evidence supports that notion that IUDs "migrate" outside the uterus thereafter. The most important determinant of the risk of perforation is the skill of the person doing the insertion ("the magic is in the magician, and not in the wand"). In experienced hands, this risk is 1 per 1,000 insertions or less.[11]

Copper-bearing IUDs found to be outside the endometrial cavity should be removed promptly. Copper in the peritoneal cavity induces adhesion formation, which may involve the adnexa, omentum, and bowel. Laparoscopy is the preferred approach for removal. In contrast, non-medicated and progestin-bearing devices do not evoke similar intraperitoneal adhesions. No clear medical indication exists for removal of T-shaped IUDs not containing copper,[35] although this is commonly done.

String Problems

Missing strings may signal an unsuspected perforation or spontaneous expulsion; alternatively, some strings ascend into the endometrial cavity and descend without known explanation. Ultrasound examination can quickly confirm the presence of an IUD within the endometrial cavity. Should the device be present but no strings visible and should the woman request its removal, a cotton swab or endometrial biopsy instrument can sometimes tease the strings from the endometrium to the endocervix.

Removal of a T-shaped device without visible strings has two prerequisites: the patient's comfort and cervical dilation. A paracervical block or intrauterine instillation of anesthetic administered before manipulation, supplemented by an oral analgesic, can decrease the pain associated with the procedure. Second, osmotic dilators left in the os overnight, or misoprostol 400 mcg (vaginally or orally), will dilate the cervix. Gentle exploration with an alligator forceps usually yields the device quickly; if not, ultrasound guidance may be helpful. Rarely are the expense and inconvenience of hysteroscopy required for IUD removal.

Several mechanical problems relate to string length. If the male partner complains of penile discomfort from the string being cut too short, one option is to cut the strings off even shorter within the endocervical canal. This may eliminate the barb-like sensation and obviate the need to replace the IUD. If the strings initially are too long, simply trim them. If the strings become longer at a later time, check for partial expulsion of the IUD.

Pregnancy

If a woman becomes pregnant with an IUD in place, confirm that the pregnancy is intrauterine and not ectopic. Remove the IUD promptly, regardless of her plans for the pregnancy. Early removal reduces the risk of spontaneous miscarriage or preterm delivery should the woman plan to continue the pregnancy.[11,36] If the woman plans to continue the pregnancy, she should be alerted to look for symptoms of an influenza-like syndrome, which might be manifestations of a septic spontaneous abortion. A copper or non-medicated IUD in place during pregnancy carries no known risk of teratogenesis. If the woman plans to have an induced abortion, remove the IUD promptly rather than wait for removal at the time of abortion.

Upper-genital-tract Infection

The risk of upper-genital-tract infection has been exaggerated due to flaws in early IUD research. Rigorous studies[37,38] and reviews of the literature[39] have established that the risk of infection and infertility among IUD users is very low.

Both epidemiological[40] and bacteriological evidence[41] indicates that the insertion process, and not the device or its string, poses the transient risk of infection. In the vagina, "strict asepsis " (widely recommended for the insertion process) is an oxymoron. No procedure that requires traversing the cervical canal can be devoid of all pathogenic organisms. Although sterile technique should be used, endocervical bacteria are routinely introduced to the endometrial cavity regardless of technique.[41]

Antibiotic prophylaxis should not be routinely used before insertion.[42] Strong evidence supports the benefit of prophylactic antibiotics around the time of induced abortion;[43] by analogy, the same might hold for endometrial contamination at IUD insertion.[44] A large randomized controlled trial in Los Angeles County evaluated the potential benefit of prophylactic azithromycin given before IUD insertion.[37] Overall, no benefit was evident. The more important finding, however, was that salpingitis was rare with or without prophylaxis: only one women out of about a thousand in each group developed salpingitis in the early months of IUD use.

International experience with IUDs has been similarly favorable. In large World Health Organization-sponsored trials of IUDs, the risk of upper-genital-tract infection was limited to the first 20 days after insertion.[38] Afterwards, the risk returned to a low level and remained there for years. Both a randomized controlled trial and cohort studies have revealed that the monofilament string does not increase the risk of upper-genital-tract infection.[39]

Early assessments of the risk of tubal infertility among IUD users appear exaggerated as well.[45,46] Recent follow-up studies of IUD users discontinuing their contraception have found no significant differences in return to fertility, whether the IUD was removed because of a desire for pregnancy or because of problems with the IUD. This was true in both New Zealand[47] and Norway.[48] Indeed, the common problem among women who had had their IUDs removed was *excess* fertility, leading to induced abortions and unplanned births. Moreover, in a Mexican case-control study,[49] prior copper IUD use was not significantly related to documented tubal pathology, whereas the presence of *Chlamydia* antibodies was. Again, this underscores the point that sexually transmitted diseases, not contraception, cause salpingitis.

Little is known about the potential effect of an IUD on acquiring a cervical or vaginal sexually transmitted infection. Fair evidence refutes an increased risk of chlamydial infection, but no evidence is available concerning gonorrhea.[39] Women who harbor sexually transmitted infections in their cervices have an increased risk of upper-genital tract infection, regardless of their IUD status. However, whether the IUD contributes in any way to that risk is unknown. No study to date has used the appropriate comparison group: women with an STI not having an IUD insertion. The comparison group has always been women with an IUD but without an STI, which addresses a different question.

Upper-genital-tract infection needs prompt treatment and follow-up. Accurate diagnosis is often difficult. Widely used diagnostic criteria for acute salpingitis[50] have been found invalid,[51] and atypical salpingitis may be more common. Hence, when in doubt, treat.

The Centers for Disease Control and Prevention has published recommendations for both inpatient and outpatient therapy of upper-genital-tract infection (Chapter 21 on Reproductive Tract Infections).[52] All involve two antibiotics in order to provide an adequate spectrum of coverage. Male partners of women thought to have salpingitis should be examined and treated presumptively according to guidelines. Some clinicians recommend IUD removal along with antibiotics. However, evidence for this recommendation is limited.[2] Indeed, one small randomized controlled trial showed no benefit of IUD removal as an adjunct to antibiotic therapy.[53]

Actinomyces-like Organisms Seen on Papanicolaou Smear

Several decades ago, a pseudo-epidemic of genital actinomycosis occurred among IUD users. Cytologists and cytopathologists[54] began reporting *Actinomyces*-like organisms on routine cytology smears, creating alarm and confusion. Current evidence supports the following points:[55]

- The Papanicolaou smear is an invalid test for *Actinomyces*

- The presence of *Actinomyces*-like organisms on Papanicolaou smear does not predict clinical illness

- *Actinomyces* species are normal inhabitants of the female genital tract

- Vaginal culture is not helpful in diagnosing actinomycosis

- Pelvic actinomycosis is a very rare, serious, and poorly understood infection

An asymptomatic IUD user who has "*Actinomyces*-like organisms" reported on Papanicolaou smear should be apprised of this, and the above information conveyed. If she is asymptomatic, nothing more need be done. If she is symptomatic, the device should be removed and a course of oral antibiotics given. The reason for removal is that, unlike usual gynecological pathogens, this genus of bacterium preferentially grows on foreign bodies. *Actinomyces* species are sensitive to a variety of antibiotics, including penicillin.

PROVIDING THE IUD
SPECIAL POPULATIONS

Women Who Have Not Been Pregnant

Although "nulliparity" is often cited as a relative contraindication to IUD use, the real issue appears to be "nulligravidity," i.e., never having been pregnant before. Uterine enlargement by pregnancy, even one ended through miscarriage or induced abortion, seems to promote successful IUD use. Concerning the risk of upper-genital-tract infection, number of recent sex partners appears to be more important than age or parity *per se*.[56] After its review of the evidence, the World Health Organization[57] listed nulliparity as category 2, meaning that, in general, the benefits of IUD use outweigh the potential or known risks. However, the WHO noted that nulliparity is related to an increased risk of expulsion.

Women who have not been pregnant may have a higher rate of mechanical problems with IUDs than other women, related to the small diameter of the cervical canal or size of the endometrial cavity. Several steps can facilitate the insertion and thus minimize the risk of a vasovagal reaction. Cervical priming with misoprostol 400 mcg either a few hours or the night before insertion can open the canal. Similarly, one or more osmotic dilators, such as laminaria, when left in overnight can gently dilate the canal to a small diameter. Prophylaxis with an oral nonsteroidal anti-inflammatory drug and paracervical[58] or intrauterine anesthesia[2] may help as well.

Women Infected with Human Immunodeficiency Virus

IUD use appears safe and effective for selected HIV-infected women who have access to medical care. Because of theoretical increases in the risk of pelvic inflammatory disease among users or female-to-male transmission of HIV to an uninfected partner, several major international medical organizations have discouraged IUD use among such women. In contrast, a cohort study in Nairobi has shown no significant increase in the risk of complications, including infection, in the early months of IUD use, as compared with uninfected IUD users.[59] The women continued using the IUD safely for two years.[60] Moreover, viral shedding of HIV did not increase in these IUD users.[61] In light of this new evidence, the World Health Organization revised its recommendation for HIV-infected women to make the copper and levonorgestrel IUDs category 2[62] (Chapter 4 on Medical Eligibility Criteria).

Women with Heart Valve Abnormalities or Shunts

The risk of infectious complications, such as bacterial endocarditis, following IUD insertion or removal is unknown but presumably negligible among women with heart valve abnormalities or shunts. No bacteremia has been found after manipulation of an IUD in the absence of obvious infection.[63] Hence, no evidence suggests that antibiotic prophylaxis is warranted. Bacteremia after removal of an "infected IUD" is controversial, and prophylaxis may be reasonable.[64] Should prophylaxis be desired, patients deemed at high risk (e.g., prosthetic heart valve) should receive parenteral ampicillin and gentamicin. For those at moderate risk (e.g., rheumatic heart disease), a single oral dose of amoxicillin 2 g can be given one hour before insertion or removal.[64]

Women with Diabetes

Good evidence supports the use of copper-bearing IUDs for women with Type 1 and 2 diabetes.[65–68] Earlier concerns about possible decreased contraceptive effectiveness and increased risk of infection have now been allayed. A recent rigorous trial of the levonorgestrel device used by women with Type 1 diabetes has confirmed no adverse effect on glucose metabolism or insulin requirements;[69] hence, the current World Health Organization category 2 rating for the levonorgestrel device needs to be revised.[62]

Women Who Have New Sexual Partners

Women who are at risk of acquiring sexually transmitted diseases from a new partner or partners should be advised to use condoms. This advice should be independent of the contraceptive she uses.

Women Who Acquire Chlamydial Infection or Gonorrhea

Standard treatment and counseling of the woman and her partner(s) is indicated.[70] No evidence suggests that an IUD should be removed in this setting.

COUNSELING ABOUT THE IUD

- Make all presentations, counseling, and educational materials (handouts, flipcharts, and posters) compatible with the language, culture, and education of the patient. Manufacturers provide Patient Package Inserts in Spanish and several other foreign languages.

- During the initial visit, help her select a method, then provide additional counseling after the IUD insertion to educate her about IUD use.

- Let women handle and examine sample IUDs. Many are surprised at how small IUDs are.

Myths and Misconceptions about the IUD

Myth	Fact
IUDs are abortifacients.	IUDs prevent fertilization and thus are true contraceptives.
IUDs increase the risk of ectopic pregnancy.	IUDs significantly reduce a woman's risk of an ectopic pregnancy, compared with her risk if not using contraception. Should a pregnancy occur with an IUD in place, the ratio of ectopic to intrauterine pregnancies may be increased.
IUDs expose the provider to medicolegal risk.	In past decades, product liability suits against manufacturers alleged inherently unsafe products and/or failure to warn of risks. Today, both IUDs have been judged safe by the Food and Drug Administration. Package inserts and patient brochures provide extensive information about risks and benefits. Hence, litigation related to IUDs has virtually disappeared.
IUDs increase the risk of PID.	The IUD itself appears to have no effect on the risk of upper-genital-tract infection. Rather, the insertion process carries a small, transient risk in some women. The risk of PID in appropriately selected IUD candidates is so small that prophylactic antibiotics are not warranted.

- Be aware of the local myths and misconceptions about IUDs (e.g., that the IUD can "float off" and lodge in distant parts of the body, such as heart and brain). Address these sensitively but directly (See Myths and Misconceptions About the IUD, above).

- Use a standard checklist to remember important information to tell the user.

- Ask the woman to repeat important information.

- Give each woman an identification card with the name and picture of her IUD, date of insertion, and date recommended for removal.

PROVIDER TRAINING

With appropriate training, a broad range of clinical personnel including nurses, nurse-midwives, physician assistants, and paramedical personnel can safely insert the IUD. Practice IUD insertions first on a model, then counsel women and insert an adequate number of IUDs under supervision to demonstrate your proficiency. Rather than an absolute number requirement, a level of proficiency in varying insertion situations (different uterine positions) should be the criterion for certification. Because the levonorgestrel system has a different insertion device and process than the TCu 380, clinicians should be trained before beginning to insert these.

INSERTION TIMING

No scientific reason supports the common practice of inserting the IUD only during menstrual bleeding.[11,71] The inconvenience and cost to the woman caused by such a policy can be substantial. Allowing insertion during the entire menstrual cycle gives the woman and her provider more flexible appointment times. An IUD can be inserted at any time during the menstrual cycle, provided reasonable assurance exists that the woman is not pregnant. Sensitive pregnancy tests can assist here.

Extensive experience overseas has shown the safety and feasibility of IUD insertion immediately after abortion or delivery. A recent systematic review[72] of randomized controlled trials of immediate post-abortal insertion showed low rates of perforation and pelvic inflammatory disease. Only one trial directly compared immediate vs. delayed insertion of the Copper 7 IUD. The performance of the Copper 7 inserted immediately was inferior to that of delayed insertion, unrelated to recent pregnancy, although the difference was not statistically significant. Of note, however, 42% of women scheduled to return for delayed insertion did not return. Insertion of IUDs after second-trimester abortions were associated with high expulsion rates. A trial in progress with insertion under ultrasound guidance after dilation and evacuation abortion (D&E) will provide a much needed update. Evidence is insufficient to compare post-abortal vs. delayed interval insertion of IUDs.

Insertion of IUDs immediately after delivery is popular in many countries, including China, Mexico, and Egypt. Another systematic review[73] of randomized controlled trials found no direct comparisons of immediate vs. delayed vs. interval insertion. Nevertheless, immediate insertions appeared both safe and practical. Advantages of this practice include convenience, high motivation, and assurance that the woman is not pregnant. On the other hand, expulsions appear to be higher than with interval insertions. Modifications to existing IUDs did not improve performance. Whether insertion was done by hand or by instrument made little difference in subsequent outcomes. Trials now underway in the United States may provide new guidance in the years ahead.

A case-control study from the United States suggested a dramatic increase in the risk of IUD perforation if the woman was breastfeeding.[74] However, other large cohort studies have not confirmed this conclusion.[75] Thus, breastfeeding is not a contraindication to IUD insertion.[76]

INSERTION TECHNIQUE

Review the IUD insertion procedure with the woman.

Perform a careful pelvic examination before IUD insertion. Confirm the direction of the uterus and its axial length. In general, a length of 6 to 9 cm leads to successful use; a shorter length may increase the risk of expulsion and other mechanical problems. Anatomic abnormalities that distort the uterine cavity, such as a bicornuate uterus or submucous leiomyomas, are considered contraindications. More detailed information is available in the World Health Organization's *Medical Eligibility Criteria for Contraception Use* (Chapter 4).

Always insert an IUD slowly and gently. Read and follow the manufacturer's instructions on insertion. Detailed handbooks and videos from manufacturers are available on insertion, withdrawal, and management techniques.

General preparation

1. Perform a careful bimanual examination to exclude pelvic infection and to identify the position of the uterus. An unrecognized retroflexed uterus increases the possibility of uterine perforation at the time of the IUD insertion.

2. Most clinicians wash the cervix and vagina with an antiseptic, such as povidone-iodine. However, no evidence supports this practice,[2] and its effect on bacterial colony counts in the endocervix is minimal.[77]

3. If appropriate, inject a paracervical block. If lidocaine is used, the upper limit should be 2 mg per pound or 4.5 mg per kg, not to exceed 300 mg of lidocaine plain. If bupivacaine is used, a common dose is 20cc of 0.25% bupivacaine. An alternative is to instill lidocaine in the uterine cavity.[2]

4. Anesthetize the cervix at the 12:00 position. Grasp the anterior lip of the cervix with a tenaculum about 1.5 to 2.0 cm from the os. Close the single-tooth tenaculum slowly. Before sounding the uterus, straighten the axis of the uterus by applying traction to the tenaculum.

PARAGARD INSERTION INSTRUCTIONS

How to load and place ParaGard:

Do not bend the arms of ParaGard earlier than 5 minutes before it is to be placed in the uterus. Use aseptic technique when handling ParaGard and the part of the insertion tube that will enter the uterus.

Step 1. Load ParaGard into the insertion tube by folding the two horizontal arms of ParaGard against the stem and push the tips of the arms securely into the inserter tube.

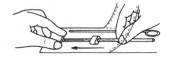

Figure 7–3 Step 1

If you do not have sterile gloves, you can do STEPS 1 and 2 while ParaGard is in the sterile package. First, place the package face up on a clean surface. Next, open at the bottom end (where arrow says OPEN). Pull the solid white rod partially from the package so it will not interfere with assembly. Place thumb and index finger on top of package on ends of the horizontal arms. Use other hand to push insertion tube against arms of ParaGard (shown by arrow in Figure 7–3). This will start bending the T arms.

Step 2. Bring the thumb and index finger closer together to continue bending the arms until they are alongside the stem. Use the other hand to withdraw the insertion tube just enough so that the inser-

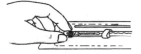

Figure 7–4 Step 2

tion tube can be pushed and rotated onto the tips of the arms. Your goal is to secure the tips of the arms inside the tube (Figure 7 4). Insert the arms no further than necessary to insure retention. Introduce the solid white rod into the insertion tube from the bottom, alongside the threads, *until it touches the bottom of the ParaGard.*

Step 3. Grasp the insertion tube at the open end of the package; adjust the blue flange so that the distance from the top of the ParaGard (where it protrudes from the inserter) to the blue flange is the same as the uterine depth that you mea-

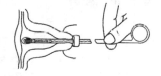

Figure 7–5 Step 3

sured with the sound. Rotate the insertion tube so that the horizontal arms of the T and the long axis of the blue flange lie in the same horizontal plane (Figure 7–5). Now pass the loaded insertion tube through the cervical canal until ParaGard just touches the fundus of the uterus. The blue flange should be at the cervix in the horizontal plane.

Step 4. To release the arms of ParaGard, hold the solid white rod steady and withdraw the insertion tube no more than one centimeter This releases the arms of ParaGard high in the uterine fundus (Figure 7–6).

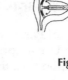

Figure 7–6 Step 4

Step 5. Gently and carefully move the insertion tube upward toward the top of the uterus, until slight resistance is felt. This will ensure placement of the T at the highest possible position within the uterus (Figure 7–7).

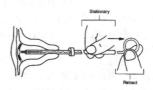

Figure 7–7 Step 5

Step 6. Hold the insertion tube steady and withdraw the solid white rod (Figure 7–8).

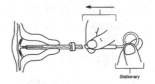

Figure 7–8 Step 6

Step 7. Gently and slowly withdraw the insertion tube from the cervical canal. Only the threads should be visible protruding from the cervix. (Figure 7–9). Trim the threads so that 3 to 4 cm protrude into the vagina. Note the length of the threads in the patient's records.

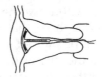

Figure 7–9 Step 7

If you suspect that ParaGard is not in the correct position, check placement (with ultrasound, if necessary). If ParaGard is not positioned completely within the uterus, remove it and replace it with a new ParaGard. Do not reinsert an expelled or partially expelled ParaGard.

CAUTION

Instrumentation of the cervical os may result in vasovagal reactions, including fainting. Have the patient remain supine until she feels well, and have her get up with caution.

MIRENA INSERTION INSTRUCTIONS

The following insertion instructions for the levonorgestrel intrauterine system are reproduced from the package insert with permission.

Insertion Procedure

- Open the sterile package.
- Place sterile gloves on your hands.
- Pick up the inserter containing Mirena.
- Carefully release the threads from behind the slider, so that they hang freely.
- Make sure that the slider is in the furthest position away from you (positioned at the top of the handle nearest the IUS).
- While looking at the insertion tube, check that the arms of the system are horizontal. If not, align them on a sterile surface (Figure 7–10) or with sterile gloved fingers.

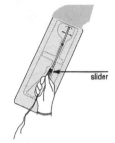

Figure 7–10 Checking that the arms of the system are horizontal

- Pull on both threads to draw the Mirena system into the insertion tube (Figure 7–11a).
- Note that the knobs at the ends of the arms now cover the open end of the inserter (Figure 7–11b).

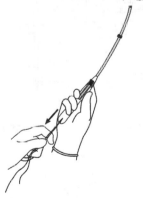

Figure 7–11a MIRENA system being drawn into the insertion tube

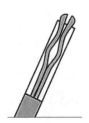

Figure 7–11b The knobs at the ends of the arms

- Fix the threads tightly in the cleft at the end of the handle (Figure 7–12).

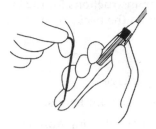

Figure 7–12 Threads are fixed tightly in the cleft

Set the flange to the depth measured by the sound, as indicated in Figure 7–13.

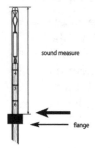

sound measure

flange

Figure 7–13 Flange adjusted to sound depth

Mirena is now ready to be inserted.

Hold the slider firmly in the furthermost position (at the top of the handle). Grasp the cervix with the tenaculum and apply gentle traction to align the cervical canal with the uterine cavity. Gently insert the inserter into the cervical canal and advance the insertion tube into the uterus until the flange is situated at a distance of about 1.5–2 cm from the external cervical os to give sufficient space for the arms to open (Figure 7–14).

NOTE! Do not force the inserter.

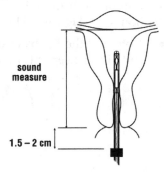

sound
measure

1.5 – 2 cm

Figure 7–14 Inserting MIRENA

While holding the inserter steady release the arms of Mirena (Figure 7–15a) by pulling the slider back until the top of the slider reaches the mark (raised horizontal line on the handle) (Figure 7–15b).

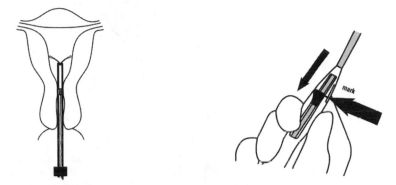

Figure 7–15a The arms of the MIRENA being released **Figure 7–15b** Pulling the slider back to reach the mark

Push the inserter gently into the uterine cavity until the flange touches the cervix. Mirena should now be in the fundal position (Figure 7–16).

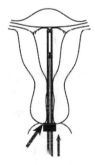

Figure 7–16 MIRENA in the fundal position

Holding the inserter firmly in position release Mirena by pulling the slider down all the way. The threads will be released automatically (Figure 7–17)

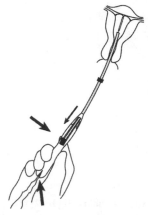

Figure 7–17 Releasing MIRENA and withdrawing the inserter

Remove the inserter from the uterus. Cut the threads to leave about 2–3 cm visible outside the cervix (Figure 7–18)

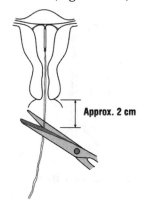

Approx. 2 cm

Figure 7–18 Cutting the threads

IUD REMOVAL

When removing an IUD, apply gentle, steady traction and remove the IUD slowly. If you cannot remove the IUD with gentle traction, a paracervical block may make the removal easier and less painful. After placing the block, use a tenaculum to steady the cervix and straighten the anteversion or retroversion of the uterus and try again. If this technique does not work, dilate the cervix to a small amount with misoprostol, osmotic dilators, or rigid dilators. (Dilators should always be available in a family planning clinic using IUDs).

Managing Problems and Follow-Up

MPlan for a follow-up visit after the woman's next menses. Check that the IUD is still in place and that no signs of infection are evident. Further routine visits are not required;[78,79] however, encourage women to return at any time that they have problems, questions, or concerns. In particular, encourage revisits if they cannot feel the IUD strings, the strings seem too long, or the plastic IUD is palpable in the cervix.

The one-month visit can be strategically important in identifying women at increased risk of quitting prematurely. Women with intermenstrual bleeding or spotting and those with excessive menstrual flow are significantly more likely to discontinue than are other women.[80] Hence, at the first follow-up visit, intervention with counseling and non-steroidal anti-inflammatory drugs may help.

In summary, IUDs are enjoying a comeback. Nevertheless, the United States remains an anomaly. Worldwide, the IUD is the most commonly used reversible method of contraception today, eclipsing oral contraceptives by a large margin.[81] Not so in the United States. Although an IUD renaissance is underway, much work remains to be done.

References

1. American College of Obstetricians and Gynecologists. ACOG practice bulletin. Clinical management guidelines for obstetrician-gynecologists. Number 59, January 2005. Intrauterine device. Obstet Gynecol 2005;105:223–232.
2. Penney G, Brechin S, de Souza A, Bankowska U, Belfield T, Gormley M, et al. FFPRHC Guidance (January 2004). The copper intrauterine device as long-term contraception. J Fam Plann Reprod Health Care 2004;30:29–41; quiz 42.
3. Forrest JD. U.S. women's perceptions of and attitudes about the IUD. Obstet Gynecol Surv 1996;51:S30–34.
4. Trieman K, Liskin L, Kols A, et al. IUDs—an update. Popul Rep 1995;Series B, No. 5.
5. World Health Organization. Long-term reversible contraception. Twelve years of experience with the TCu380A and TCu220C. Contraception 1997;56:341–352.
6. Sivin I, Stern J, Coutinho E, Mattos CE, el Mahgoub S, Diaz S, et al. Prolonged intrauterine contraception: a seven-year randomized study of the levonorgestrel 20 mcg/day (LNg 20) and the Copper T380 Ag IUDS. Contraception 1991;44:473–480.
7. Steiner MJ, Dalebout S, Condon S, Dominik R, Trussell J. Understanding risk: a randomized controlled trial of communicating contraceptive effectiveness. Obstet Gynecol 2003;102:709–717.
8. Sivin I, Schmidt F. Effectiveness of IUDs: a review. Contraception 1987;36:55–84.
9. Peterson HB, Xia Z, Hughes JM, Wilcox LS, Tylor LR, Trussell J. The risk of pregnancy after tubal sterilization: findings from the U.S. Collaborative Review of Sterilization. Am J Obstet Gynecol 1996;174:1161–1168; discussion 1168–1170.
10. Rivera R, Yacobson I, Grimes D. The mechanism of action of hormonal contraceptives and intrauterine contraceptive devices. Am J Obstet Gynecol 1999; 181:1263–1269.
11. World Health Organization. Mechanism of action, safety and efficacy of intrauterine devices: technical report series 753. Geneva: World Health Organization, 1987.
12. Barbosa I, Olsson SE, Odlind V, Goncalves T, Coutinho E. Ovarian function after seven year's use of a levonorgestrel IUD. Adv Contracept 1995;11:85–95.

13. Segal SJ, Alvarez-Sanchez F, Adejuwon CA, Brache de Mejia V, Leon P, Faundes A. Absence of chorionic gonadotropin in sera of women who use intrauterine devices. Fertil Steril 1985;44:214–218.
14. Wilcox AJ, Weinberg CR, Armstrong EG, Canfield RE. Urinary human chorionic gonadotropin among intrauterine device users: detection with a highly specific and sensitive assay. Fertil Steril 1987;47:265–269.
15. Alvarez F, Brache V, Fernandez E, Guerrero B, Guiloff E, Hess R, et al. New insights on the mode of action of intrauterine contraceptive devices in women. Fertil Steril 1988;49:768–773.
16. Ory HW. Ectopic pregnancy and intrauterine contraceptive devices: new perspectives. The Women's Health Study. Obstet Gynecol 1981;57:137–144.
17. Franks AL, Beral V, Cates W Jr, Hogue CJ. Contraception and ectopic pregnancy risk. Am J Obstet Gynecol 1990;163:1120–1123.
18. Nelson AL. Intrauterine device practice guidelines: medical conditions. Contraception 1998;58:59S-63S; quiz 72S.
19. Hubacher D, Grimes DA. Noncontraceptive health benefits of intrauterine devices: a systematic review. Obstet Gynecol Surv 2002;57:120–128.
20. Gardner FJ, Konje JC, Abrams KR, Brown LJ, Khanna S, Al-Azzawi F, et al. Endometrial protection from tamoxifen-stimulated changes by a levonorgestrel-releasing intrauterine system: a randomised controlled trial. Lancet 2000;356:1711–1717.
21. World Health Organization. Depot-medroxyprogesterone acetate (DMPA) and risk of endometrial cancer. The WHO Collaborative Study of Neoplasia and Steroid Contraceptives. Int J Cancer 1991;49:186–190.
22. Bahamondes L, Ribeiro-Huguet P, de Andrade KC, Leon-Martins O, Petta CA. Levonorgestrel-releasing intrauterine system (Mirena) as a therapy for endometrial hyperplasia and carcinoma. Acta Obstet Gynecol Scand 2003;82:580–582.
23. Lassise DL, Savitz DA, Hamman RF, Baron AE, Brinton LA, Levines RS. Invasive cervical cancer and intrauterine device use. Int J Epidemiol 1991;20:865–870.
24. Parazzini F, La Vecchia C, Negri E. Use of intrauterine device and risk of invasive cervical cancer. Int J Epidemiol 1992;21:1030–1031.
25. Fedele L, Bianchi S, Raffaelli R, Portuese A, Dorta M. Treatment of adenomyosis-associated menorrhagia with a levonorgestrel- releasing intrauterine device. Fertil Steril 1997;68:426–429.
26. Grigorieva V, Chen-Mok M, Tarasova M, Mikhailov A. Use of a levonorgestrel-releasing intrauterine system to treat bleeding related to uterine leiomyomas. Fertil Steril 2003;79:1194–1198.
27. Pakarinen P, Toivonen J, Luukkainen T. Therapeutic use of the LNG IUS, and counseling. Semin Reprod Med 2001;19:365–372.
28. Hurskainen R, Teperi J, Rissanen P, Aalto AM, Grenman S, Kivela A, et al. Quality of life and cost-effectiveness of levonorgestrel-releasing intrauterine system versus hysterectomy for treatment of menorrhagia: a randomised trial. Lancet 2001;357:273–277.
29. Marjoribanks J, Lethaby A, Farquhar C. Surgery versus medical therapy for heavy menstrual bleeding. Cochrane Database Syst Rev 2003;CD003855.
30. Ylikorkala O. Prostaglandin synthesis inhibitors in menorrhagia, intrauterine contraceptive device-induced side effects and endometriosis. Pharmacol Toxicol 1994;75 Suppl 2:86–88.
31. Tolcher R. Intrauterine techniques: contentious or consensus opinion? J Fam Plann Reprod Health Care 2003;29:21–24.
32. Zhang J, Feldblum PJ, Chi IC, Farr MG. Risk factors for copper T IUD expulsion: an epidemiologic analysis. Contraception 1992;46:427–433.
33. Bahamondes L, Diaz J, Marchi NM, Petta CA, Cristofoletti ML, Gomez G. Performance of copper intrauterine devices when inserted after an expulsion. Hum Reprod 1995;10:2917–2918.
34. Gruber A, Rabinerson D, Kaplan B, Pardo J, Neri A. The missing forgotten intrauterine contraceptive device. Contraception 1996;54:117–119.

35. Adoni A, Ben Chetrit A. The management of intrauterine devices following uterine perforation. Contraception 1991;43:77–81.
36. Foreman H, Stadel BV, Schlesselman S. Intrauterine device usage and fetal loss. Obstet Gynecol 1981;58:669–677.
37. Walsh T, Grimes D, Frezieres R, Nelson A, Bernstein L, Coulson A, et al. Randomised controlled trial of prophylactic antibiotics before insertion of intrauterine devices. IUD Study Group. Lancet 1998;351:1005–1008.
38. Farley TM, Rosenberg MJ, Rowe PJ, Chen JH, Meirik O. Intrauterine devices and pelvic inflammatory disease: an international perspective. Lancet 1992;339:785–788.
39. Grimes DA. Intrauterine device and upper-genital-tract infection. Lancet 2000; 356:1013–1019.
40. Lee NC, Rubin GL, Ory HW, Burkman RT. Type of intrauterine device and the risk of pelvic inflammatory disease. Obstet Gynecol 1983;62:1–6.
41. Mishell DR Jr, Bell JH, Good RG, Moyer DL. The intrauterine device: a bacteriologic study of the endometrial cavity. Am J Obstet Gynecol 1966;96:119–126.
42. Grimes DA, Schulz KF. Prophylactic antibiotics for intrauterine device insertion: a metaanalysis of the randomized controlled trials. Contraception 1999;60:57–63.
43. Sawaya GF, Grady D, Kerlikowske K, Grimes DA. Antibiotics at the time of induced abortion: the case for universal prophylaxis based on a meta-analysis. Obstet Gynecol 1996;87:884–890.
44. Sinei SK, Schulz KF, Lamptey PR, Grimes DA, Mati JK, Rosenthal SM, et al. Preventing IUCD-related pelvic infection: the efficacy of prophylactic doxycycline at insertion. Br J Obstet Gynaecol 1990;97:412–419.
45. Daling JR, Weiss NS, Metch BJ, Chow WH, Soderstrom RM, Moore DE, et al. Primary tubal infertility in relation to the use of an intrauterine device. N Engl J Med 1985; 312:937–941.
46. Cramer DW, Schiff I, Schoenbaum SC, Gibson M, Belisle S, Albrecht B, et al. Tubal infertility and the intrauterine device. N Engl J Med 1985;312:941–947.
47. Wilson JC. A prospective New Zealand study of fertility after removal of copper intrauterine contraceptive devices for conception and because of complications: a four-year study. Am J Obstet Gynecol 1989;160:391–396.
48. Skjeldestad F, Bratt H. Fertility after complicated and non-complicated use of IUDs. A controlled prospective study. Adv Contracept 1988;4:179–184.
49. Hubacher D, Lara-Ricalde R, Taylor DJ, Guerra-Infante F, Guzman-Rodriguez R. Use of copper intrauterine devices and the risk of tubal infertility among nulligravid women. N Engl J Med 2001;345:561–567.
50. Hager WD, Eschenbach DA, Spence MR, Sweet RL. Criteria for diagnosis and grading of salpingitis. Obstet Gynecol 1983;61:113–114.
51. Hadgu A, Westrom L, Brooks CA, Reynolds GH, Thompson SE. Predicting acute pelvic inflammatory disease: a multivariate analysis. Am J Obstet Gynecol 1986; 155:954–960.
52. Centers for Disease Control and Prevention. Sexually transmitted disease treatment guidelines, 2006. MMWR 2006;55 (RR-11).
53. Soderberg G, Lindgren S. Influence of an intrauterine device on the course of an acute salpingitis. Contraception 1981;24:137–143.
54. Gupta PK, Hollander DH, Frost JK. Actinomycetes in cervico-vaginal smears: an association with IUD usage. Acta Cytol 1976;20:295–297.
55. Lippes J. Pelvic actinomycosis: a review and preliminary look at prevalence. Am J Obstet Gynecol 1999;180:265–269.
56. Dardano KL, Burkman RT. The intrauterine contraceptive device: an often-forgotten and maligned method of contraception. Am J Obstet Gynecol 1999;181:1–5.
57. World Health Organization. Improving access to quality care in family planning. Medical eligibility criteria for contraceptive use. 2nd edition. Geneva, Switzerland: World Health Organization, 2000.

58. Thiery M. Pain relief at insertion and removal of an IUD: a simplified technique for paracervical block. Adv Contracept 1985;1:167–170.

59. Sinei SK, Morrison CS, Sekadde-Kigondu C, Allen M, Kokonya D. Complications of use of intrauterine devices among HIV-1-infected women. Lancet 1998;351:1238–41.

60. Morrison CS, Sekadde-Kigondu C, Sinei SK, Weiner DH, Kwok C, Kokonya D. Is the intrauterine device appropriate contraception for HIV-1-infected women? BJOG 2001;108:784–790.

61. Richardson BA, Morrison CS, Sekadde-Kigondu C, Sinei SK, Overbaugh J, Panteleeff DD, et al. Effect of intrauterine device use on cervical shedding of HIV-1 DNA. AIDS 1999;13:2091–2097.

62. World Health Organization. Medical eligibility criteria for contraceptive use, third edition. www.who.int/reproductive-health/publications/mec/srhcare.html, accessed February 11, 2005.

63. Durack DT. Prevention of infective endocarditis. N Engl J Med 1995;332:38–44.

64. Dajani AS, Taubert KA, Wilson W, Bolger AF, Bayer A, Ferrieri P, et al. Prevention of bacterial endocarditis. Recommendations by the American Heart Association. Circulation 1997;96:358–366.

65. Kjos SL, Ballagh SA, La Cour M, Xiang A, Mishell DR Jr. The copper T380A intrauterine device in women with type II diabetes mellitus. Obstet Gynecol 1994; 84:1006–1009.

66. Skouby SO, Molsted-Pedersen L, Petersen KR. Contraception for women with diabetes: an update. Baillieres Clin Obstet Gynaecol 1991;5:493–503.

67. Kimmerle R, Heinemann L, Berger M. Intrauterine devices are safe and effective contraceptives for type I diabetic women. Diabetes Care 1995;18:1506–1507.

68. Petersen KR, Skouby SO, Jespersen J. Contraception guidance in women with pre-existing disturbances in carbohydrate metabolism. Eur J Contracept Reprod Health Care 1996;1:53–59.

69. Rogovskaya S, Rivera R, Grimes DA, Chen PL, Pierre-Louis B, Prilepskaya V, et al. Effect of a levonorgestrel intrauterine system on women with type 1 diabetes: a randomized trial. Obstet Gynecol 2005;105:811–815.

70. Centers for Disease Control and Prevention. 1998 guidelines for the treatment of sexually transmitted diseases. MMWR 1998;47 (No. RR-1):1–116.

71. White MK, Ory HW, Rooks JB, Rochat RW. Intrauterine device termination rates and the menstrual cycle day of insertion. Obstet Gynecol 1980;55:220–224.

72. Grimes DA, Schulz KF, Stanwood N. Immediate post-abortal insertion of intrauterine devices. Cochrane Database Syst Rev 2000;2.

73. Grimes DA, Schulz K , van Vliet H, Stanwood N. Immediate post-partum insertion of intrauterine devices. Cochrane Database Syst Rev 2001;2.

74. Heartwell SF, Schlesselman S. Risk of uterine perforation among users of intrauterine devices. Obstet Gynecol 1983;61:31–66.

75. Chi IC, Potts M, Wilkens LR, Champion CB. Performance of the copper T-380A intrauterine device in breastfeeding women. Contraception 1989;39:603–618.

76. Chi IC, Wilkens LR, Champion CB, Machemer RE, Rivera R. Insertional pain and other IUD insertion-related rare events for breastfeeding and non-breastfeeding women–a decade's experience in developing countries. Adv Contracept 1989; 5:101–119.

77. Osborne NG, Wright RC. Effect of preoperative scrub on the bacterial flora of the endocervix and vagina. Obstet Gynecol 1977;50:148–151.

78. Hubacher D, Fortney J. Follow-up visits after IUD insertion. Are more better? J Reprod Med 1999;44:801–806.

79. Janowitz B, Hubacher D, Petrick T, Dighe N. Should the recommended number of IUD revisits be reduced? Stud Fam Plann 1994;25:362–367.

80. Stanback J, Grimes D. Can intrauterine device removals for bleeding or pain be predicted at a one-month follow-up visit? A multivariate analysis. Contraception 1998; 58:357–360.

81. Population Reference Bureau. Family planning worldwide. 2002 data sheet. www.prb.org/Template.cfm?Section=PRB&template=/Content/ContentGroups/ Datasheets/Family_Planning_Worldwide_2002_Data_Sheet.htm, accessed February 11, 2005.

Contraceptive Implants

Elizabeth G. Raymond, MD, MPH

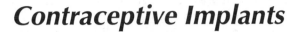

- Implants are thin rods or tubes containing a progestin hormone. They are inserted under the skin of a woman's arm.

- Marketed implants provide contraception for at least 3 years. Their efficacy is comparable to that of sterilization.

- Implants cause menstrual cycle irregularities in most users.

- Implants are particularly suitable for women who desire safe, extremely effective, long-term, maintenance-free, reversible contraception.

- Like other progestin-only contraceptives, implants may be of special interest to women who cannot use a contraceptive that contains estrogen.

- As of this writing, the only implant available in the United States is Implanon, a single rod that provides contraception for 3 years.

Contraceptive implants consist of one or more thin tubes or rods containing a progestin hormone. They are inserted just under the skin of a woman's arm and provide effective contraception for at least 3 years. Implants currently available are not biodegradable, and therefore removal is generally recommended when the period of efficacy expires. They may be removed earlier if the patient desires fertility or another contraceptive method. Contraceptive implants are now approved in more than 60 countries and have been used by at least 11 million women worldwide.[1]

As of this writing, the only implant available in the United States is a single rod implant called Implanon. Implanon has been used in Asia, Europe, and Australia since 1998. The Implanon rod is 4 cm long and 2 mm in diameter and contains 68 mg etonogestrel (also called 3-keto-desogestrel), which is the main active metabolite of desogestrel, a progestin used in many oral contraceptive pills. Implanon is intended to provide contraception for 3 years after insertion.

Two other implants have been approved by the U.S. Food and Drug Administration (FDA) but are not currently being distributed here:

- *Norplant.* The Norplant system consists of 6 flexible capsules containing a total of 216 mg levonorgestrel. Each capsule is 3.4 cm long and 2.4 mm in diameter. It provides highly effective contraception for at least 7 years after insertion. First approved in Finland in 1983,[2] Norplant was approved by the FDA in 1990 and marketed in the United States until 2002. In that year, the U.S. distributor stopped selling it, citing limitations in product component supplies. Some U.S. women may still have Norplant in situ. A Chinese implant system (Sinoplant I) designed to be identical to Norplant has been used in China.

- *Jadelle.* Formerly called Norplant II, Jadelle consists of two rods 4.3 cm long and 2.5 mm in diameter, each containing 75 mg levonorgestrel. Jadelle is effective for at least 5 years. It was approved by the FDA in 1996 but has never been sold in this country. It is available elsewhere in the world, however. A Chinese version of Jadelle (Sinoplant II) is currently used in several countries in Asia.

Several other progestin-releasing implants are in various phases of development, including a one-year implant containing nomegestrol acetate (Uniplant) invented in Brazil and a two-year implant containing nestorone being studied by the Population Council. (See Chapter 19 on Contraceptive Research and Development.) Developers currently have no concrete plans to commercialize these products.

Because Implanon is the implant now available in the United States, it is the focus of this chapter. Most of the published data on Implanon were derived from studies sponsored by Organon, the pharmaceutical company that manufactures and markets the product. Unfortunately, some of these studies were found after publication to have included possibly invalid data.[3] A list of publications that included data from these studies was obtained from the company. Data from these publications, as well as conclusions of review articles based on them, were not used in writing this chapter.

EFFECTIVENESS

Implants are among the most effective of the available contraceptive methods; from a clinical viewpoint, their efficacy is essentially indistinguishable from that of sterilization and intrauterine devices.[4] Because implants allow no possibility of user error, all pregnancies occurring in implant users are method failures. To date, no pregnancies have been observed in prospective follow-up studies of Implanon, which included a total of more than 2,467 women-years of exposure.[5-11] However, in

2005, a case-series of 134 pregnancies was reported after Implanon insertion in Australia. Of these pregnancies, 46 were apparently conceived before the women had Implanon inserted, 19 were attributed to insertion outside the recommended time of the menstrual cycle, 3 to expulsion of the implants, 8 to interactions with other drugs, and 13 to method failures for unknown reasons. Based on data on Implanon sales in Australia, the authors estimated an approximate failure rate of 1/1000 insertions.[12]

Whether user characteristics, such as body weight, might reduce the efficacy of Implanon is unknown.

Implanon is marketed with a duration of action of 3 years, although fewer than 500 women in valid published trials used the method for that long. Pharmacokinetic data from Implanon users show stable serum concentrations of etonorgestrel out to 36 months,[13] suggesting that the method may be effective for longer than that. (See Figure 8–1.) Two small studies found no pregnancies among women in the fourth year of Implanon use.[9,20]

MECHANISM OF ACTION

Small studies have shown that Implanon suppresses ovulation in almost all users throughout the first 3 years after insertion. One study of 244 scans in 188 women who had had Implanon inserted 0 to 20 months (median 3 months) earlier found one ovulation at 16 months[14]; a smaller study documented two ovulations in 1 of 16 women at 30 and 33 months

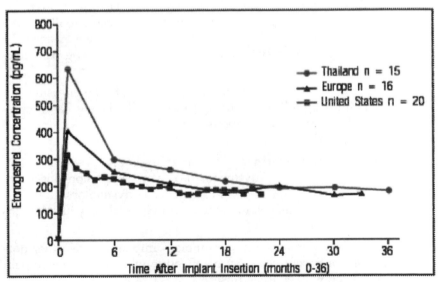

Source: Organon USA, Inc., with permission.

Figure 8–1 Serum etonogestrel concentrations in Implanon users

after insertion.[13] Implanon also alters endometrial structure, and it changes cervical mucus in a way that may impede sperm penetration.[14] These mechanisms may contribute to the method's protective effect if ovulation does occur.

On average, estradiol levels in Implanon users tend to decrease to the range of the early follicular phase immediately after insertion and then rise slowly, reflecting increasing follicular activity. Among individual women, however, one study found that levels of this hormone varied substantially over time. No woman was found to have consistently low or high levels.[13]

A DVANTAGES
Implants have many advantages for many women:

1. **High efficacy.** See above.

2. **Ease of use.** Once implants are inserted, no attention is required on the part of the user until the time of removal. Implants are thus an excellent contraceptive option for women who have difficulty using a contraceptive at the time of intercourse or adhering to a regular schedule independent of intercourse.

3. **Discreetness.** Implant users need keep no contraceptive supplies at home and do not require resupply or follow-up clinical care until removal. In most users, the rods are not visible under the skin. These features may be attractive to women who desire privacy about their use of contraception. However, insertion leaves a small scar, and subdermal implants can usually be detected by palpation. In some cases, side effects such as irregular vaginal bleeding may be a clue that a woman is using reproductive hormones.

4. **No adverse effect on acne.** In one study of women using Implanon for up to 2 years, 61% of those with acne at baseline reported decreased acne, whereas only 16% of those with no acne at baseline developed acne.[5]

5. **Relief of dysmenorrhea.** In one analysis of 315 women, 48% reported decreased dysmenorrhea after Implanon insertion, whereas only 8% reported increased dysmenorrhea.[5] This change is likely related to the reduction in ovulatory bleeding induced by Implanon.

6. **Relief of endometriosis symptoms.** Implanon, like other hormonal contraceptives, may be effective in reducing pelvic pain associated with endometriosis.[16]

7. **Few known clinically significant metabolic effects.** Implanon appears not to be associated with any clinically important ad-

verse changes in blood pressure, liver function, hemostasis, carbohydrate metabolism, lipid levels, or thyroid function.[17,18] Data conflict about effects on bone mineral density.[19,20] Studies are limited, however, and were conducted mostly in healthy women.

8. **Reduced risk of ectopic pregnancy.** Because implants, like all contraceptives, prevent pregnancy, they also prevent ectopic pregnancy. No ectopic pregnancies have been reported in users of Implanon.[2]

9. **No estrogen.** Implants do not contain estrogen and thus may not be associated with rare but serious complications attributable to estrogenic agents, such as thrombophlebitis, pulmonary embolism, and cardiovascular effects. Women with certain medical conditions that may be exacerbated by estrogen-containing methods (see Chapter 11 on Combined Oral Contraceptives) may be eligible to use implants.

10. **Reversibility.** After Implanon removal, etonorgestrel becomes undetectable in most users within a week, and most users ovulate within 6 weeks.[13,15] Data on pregnancy rates in women after removal of Implanon are scant. In one study of 46 women who discontinued Implanon and did not subsequently use any contraception, 11 (24%) became pregnant within 4 months.[5] This proportion is considerably lower than that expected among women who had never used contraception. However, this difference could have explanations other than a prolonged effect of Implanon on fertility after removal.

11. **High acceptability and continuation rates.** The most common complaints about implants are menstrual disturbances and other perceived side effects, high up-front cost, and in some societies, difficulty in obtaining access to removal. In general, however, satisfaction with this method is very high.[21,22] Clinical trials and observational studies have shown continuation rates of 51% to 87% through 2 years.[5–7,9–11]

DISADVANTAGES AND CAUTIONS

Implants also have disadvantages:

1. **Uterine bleeding abnormalities.** Like all progestin-only methods, implants cause bleeding changes in a large proportion of women. These changes are unpredictable and may include prolonged bleeding, frequent bleeding, irregular bleeding, infrequent bleeding, and amenorrhea. Some studies suggest that the incidence of prolonged bleeding episodes declines after the first 3 months of use, although some women may experience this pat-

tern even in the third year after insertion. Many women may consider amenorrhea, if it occurs, to be a benefit. After Implanon removal, menses returned to normal in the vast majority of women within 3 months, irrespective of the duration of Implanon use. Bleeding abnormalities have been the most common single reason for discontinuing progestin implants; forewarn women about this side effect, emphasizing that it is generally not dangerous.[5–10,23]

2. **Rare insertion complications.** Infection and other serious complications of implant insertion are very rare, occurring in less than 1% of patients in most studies. Delayed infection has occasionally been reported more than a month after insertion.[11] More minor side effects, such as bruising, skin irritation, or pain are more common, but they almost always resolve without treatment. Expulsion of implants has been reported rarely, usually associated with infection.[24] Possibly the most problematic complication of Implanon insertion is provider failure to insert the rods: a case series of pregnancies from Australia included 84 that resulted from "non-insertion." In some cases, the implant was left in the inserter; for most, the circumstances of the non-insertion were not documented.[12]

3. **Possible weight gain.** Several studies have reported that Implanon users experience a small increase in weight over several years. However, none of these studies included a comparison group of women not using Implanon. The mean increase in body mass index in the US study was 0.7 kg/m² over up to 2 years (less than 5 pounds for a woman 5.5 feet tall weighing 120 pounds).[5,9,10]

4. **Ovarian cysts.** Progestin implants do not totally suppress ovarian activity, and persistent follicles or "ovarian cysts" have been reported in a small proportion of users of Implanon, Norplant, and Jadelle. Some studies have suggested that the incidence of ovarian cysts is higher among implant users than among users of non-hormonal contraceptives. Implant-associated cysts or follicles usually resolve without treatment. Intervention is not indicated unless a cyst becomes symptomatic or fails to regress.[24]

5. **Other adverse symptoms.** Headache, emotional lability, abdominal pain, nausea, loss of libido, vaginal dryness, and other symptoms have been reported by women in trials of Implanon and other implants. Whether these symptoms are actually caused by the implants is unknown.[5,7]

6. **Clinician-dependency.** Implants must be inserted and removed by a clinician. Compared with other methods, they may

thus be less available and offer women less control over their contraceptive. Removal of implants requires a minor surgical procedure.

7. **Lack of protection against sexually transmitted infections.** Like other hormonal contraceptives, implants offer no protection from sexually transmitted infections, including HIV. (See Chapter 21 on Reproductive Tract Infections.) Some but not all studies have suggested an increased risk of infection among users of other progestin-containing contraceptives, but no association has been proven. (See Chapter 9 on Injectable Contraceptives.) No specific data are available about implants.

8. **Drug interactions.** Specific information on interactions of other drugs with Implanon is not available. Inferences may be made from data on other hormonal contraceptives. (See Chapter 11 on Combined Oral Contraceptives.) Because etonogestrel levels in Implanon users are so low, drug interactions may be more of a problem with this method than with other hormonal methods.

9. **Possible increased risk of thromboembolic conditions.** Etonogestrel, the progestin in Implanon, is a metabolite of desogestrel, which has been implicated in an increased risk of thromboembolic conditions in users of combined oral contraceptives containing desogestrel.[25] (See Chapter 11 on Combined Oral Contraceptives.) Currently available data offer no suggestion that Implanon itself may increase this risk, but no study of sufficient size to detect a significant increase in such rare conditions has yet been conducted. Serum etonogestrel levels in Implanon users are substantially lower than those in users of desogestrel-containing oral contraceptives,[26] and Implanon does not contain estrogen. Whether these differences might affect the risk of thromboembolic events is unknown. The World Health Organization's *Medical Eligibility Criteria for Contraceptive Use* (Chapter 4) makes no distinction between etonogestrel implants and progestin-only methods containing other progestins with respect to risk for thromboembolic conditions.

10. **Relatively new method.** Although worldwide experience with hormonal contraceptives, including pills containing desogestrel, is substantial, Implanon itself has been marketed only since 1998. It is possible that this particular product could be associated with rare but serious conditions that have not yet been identified.

Special Issues

Effect on pregnancy if inadvertently inserted during pregnancy. In general, hormonal contraceptives are not dangerous for either a pregnant woman or a developing fetus. No information is available specifically about Implanon in pregnancy. If a woman using Implanon is found to be pregnant and wishes to continue the pregnancy, Implanon should be removed, but no other special evaluation or care is needed.

Effect on lactogenesis. In general, progestin-releasing implants have no known clinically important effect on breastfeeding or infant development.[27] However, only one study of Implanon in breastfeeding has thus far been published. This study compared 42 Implanon users to 38 users of nonhormonal contraception for 4 months postpartum and found no differences in the volume or quantity of breast milk or in infant development.[28] Etonogestrel does transfer to breast milk in low concentrations and is orally active; this concern has led to a recommendation to withhold use until 6 to 8 weeks postpartum.[27] The Implanon package guidelines recommend a shorter delay—4 weeks.

Providing the Method

The World Health Organization's *Medical Eligibility Criteria for Contraceptive Use* lists only a few medical conditions that contraindicate use of implants:

- Breastfeeding women less than 6 weeks postpartum (Category 3)

- Current deep venous thrombosis or pulmonary embolus (Category 3)

- Active viral hepatitis or severe (decompensated) cirrhosis, benign or malignant liver tumors (Category 3)

- Unexplained, unevaluated abnormal vaginal bleeding (Category 3)

- Current breast cancer (Category 4)

- Past breast cancer without evidence of current disease within 5 years (Category 3)

In addition, the WHO criteria note that the rods should be removed if a user develops ischemic heart disease, stroke, or migraine with aura while using implants (Category 3).

Notably, the criteria do not include restrictions based on age, smoking, hypertension, migraine without aura, uterine fibroids, diabetes, gall bladder disease, or sickle cell disease. Implants are not a good choice for women who cannot tolerate irregular bleeding or amenorrhea.

Table 8–1 When to insert implants

Previous Method	When to Insert Implants
None	Days 1–5 of menstrual cycle
Combined oral contraceptive pills	While taking active pills or within 7 days after the last active pill
Progestin-only pills	While taking active pills
Injectables	Day next injection is due
Implants or IUD	Day of removal of device
First trimester abortion	Within 5 days after procedure
Second trimester abortion or delivery, if not breastfeeding	Day 21–28 after end of pregnancy
Postpartum, breastfeeding	At least 4 weeks after delivery; must meet other criteria, above

No examinations or laboratory tests are needed to determine whether a woman is eligible to receive implants.

Counseling. Women considering implants should be advised about their advantages and disadvantages, described above. Experience with Norplant particularly suggests that the quality of counseling before insertion can improve a patient's satisfaction with implants and reduce the likelihood she will discontinue them because of side effects.[29]

Timing of insertion. Implant insertion should be timed to minimize the possibility that a woman is pregnant or that she might become pregnant between insertion and the initiation of the implant's contraceptive effect. Exactly when the contraceptive effect begins is unknown. The recommendations provided in Table 8–1 are conservative; insertion may be acceptable at other times if reasonable evidence exists that the patient is not pregnant. Backup contraception (such as condoms) after insertion is not needed if Implanon is inserted as in Table 8–1.

Insertion procedure. Because it consists of only one rod, Implanon is easier to insert and remove than Norplant. It is distributed in a specially designed, preloaded applicator. Insertion is usually quite simple; two studies found that the mean time for insertion was 0.5 to 1 minute.[5,7] Insert Implanon at the inner side of the upper arm in the groove between the biceps and triceps muscles. If a patient has had implants previously, place the new implants in the opposite arm. Inject a local anesthetic along the intended insertion track, and then insert the implant in the subdermal tissue. Insertion deeper than that can hamper removal later. The Implanon inserter works like an IUD inserter: the obturator is held stable while the cannula is withdrawn. After insertion, confirm the presence of the implant in the arm. Palpate the area or, if necessary, use other means such as ultrasound or magnetic resonance imaging (MRI). Insertion failure that is unrecognized by the clinician or the patient is a leading cause of pregnancy among Implanon users.[12]

M ANAGING PROBLEMS AND FOLLOW-UP

No specific clinical follow-up is needed after insertion as long as the patient is not having any problem.

Abnormal vaginal bleeding. Implant users can almost always be reassured that bleeding due to implants is not dangerous. If the implants are in place, were inserted at the recommended time of the woman's cycle, and are not outdated, pregnancy is so unlikely that a pregnancy test or evaluation for pregnancy is not mandatory unless the patient has other signs of an abnormal pregnancy (such as abdominal or pelvic pain) or risk factors for ectopic pregnancy. Prostaglandin inhibitors and supplemental estrogen have been effective treatments for abnormal bleeding caused by other hormonal contraceptives and may be worth trying in implant users. Remove the implants if the patient so desires.

Removal. Implant removal is usually accomplished easily through a minor surgical procedure. Inject a local anesthesia under the distal end of the implant (to avoid skin swelling over the implant, which might cause difficulty locating the implant). Make a small longitudinal incision in the skin. If a fibrous sheath has formed around the implant, the sheath must be incised. Locate and grasp the implant, then remove it with forceps. In two studies, the mean time for removal was 3 and 3.5 minutes.[5,7] Removal may be more difficult if the implant is deeply placed. Migration of implants after insertion is exceedingly rare; it was reported in two women whose implants were inserted through the same skin incision used for removal of previously inserted implants.[30] Rods that are not palpable may be located through ultrasound or magnetic resonance imaging. Breakage of implants in situ or during removal occurs rarely.[7,31] No data are available on the risks of leaving implants in place for longer than the recommended duration of efficacy; if a woman does not desire pregnancy and is not planning to use another hormonal method of contraception, removal may not be necessary.

Detailed instructions and training is expected to be offered by the distributor once Implanon becomes commercially available.

U SER INSTRUCTIONS

1. **Contact a clinician** if you develop symptoms of infection at the insertion site (tenderness, redness, swelling, discharge).

2. **Record the date** when the implant(s) should be removed. After that date, do not rely on the implant(s) for contraception.

REFERENCES

1. Meirik O, Fraser IS, d'Arcangues C. Implantable contraceptives for women. Hum Reprod Update 2003;9:49–59.
2. Sivin I. Risks and benefits, advantages and disadvantages of levonorgestrel-releasing contraceptive implants. Drug Saf 2003;26:303–35.
3. Rekers H, Affandi B. Implanon studies conducted in Indonesia. Contraception 2004; 70:433.
4. Steiner MJ. Contraceptive effectiveness: what should the counseling message be? JAMA 1999;282: 1405–7.
5. Funk S, Miller MM, Mishell DR Jr, et al. Safety and efficacy of Implanon, a single-rod implantable contraceptive containing etonogestrel. Contraception 2005;71:319–26.
6. Rai K, Gupta S, Cotter S. Experience with Implanon in a northeast London family planning clinic. Eur J Contracept Reprod Health Care 2004;9:39–46.
7. Flores JB, Balderas ML, Bonilla MC, Vazquez-Estrada L. Clinical experience and acceptability of the etonogestrel subdermal contraceptive implant. Int J Gynaecol Obstet 2005;90:228–33.
8. Booranabunyat S, Taneepanichskul S. Implanon use in Thai women above the age of 35 years. Contraception 2004;69:489–91.
9. Kiriwat O, Patanayindee A, Koetsawang S, Korver T, Bennink HJ. A 4-year pilot study on the efficacy and safety of Implanon, a single-rod hormonal contraceptive implant, in healthy women in Thailand. Eur J Contracept Reprod Health Care 1998; 3:85–91.
10. Zheng SR, Zheng HM, Qian SZ, Sang GW, Kaper RF. A long-term study of the efficacy and acceptability of a single-rod hormonal contraceptive implant (Implanon) in healthy women in China. Eur J Contracept Reprod Health Care 1999;4:85–93.
11. Smith A, Reuter S. An assessment of the use of Implanon in three community services. J Fam Plann Reprod Health Care 2002;28:193–6.
12. Harrison-Woolrych M, Hill R. Unintended pregnancies with the etonogestrel implant (Implanon): a case series from postmarketing experience in Australia. Contraception 2005;71:306–8.
13. Makarainen L, van Beek A, Tuomivaara L, Asplund B, Coelingh Bennink H. Ovarian function during the use of a single contraceptive implant: Implanon compared with Norplant. Fertil Steril 1998;69:714–21.
14. Van den Bosch T, Donders GG, Riphagen I, et al. Ultrasonographic features of the endometrium and the ovaries in women on etonogestrel implant. Ultrasound Obstet Gynecol 2002;20:377–80.
15. Davies GC, Feng LX, Newton JR, Van Beek A, Coelingh-Bennink HJ. Release characteristics, ovarian activity and menstrual bleeding pattern with a single contraceptive implant releasing 3-ketodesogestrel. Contraception 1993;47:251–61.
16. Yisa SB, Okenwa AA, Husemeyer RP. Treatment of pelvic endometriosis with etonogestrel subdermal implant (Implanon). J Fam Plann Reprod Health Care 2005; 31:67–70.
17. Dorflinger LJ. Metabolic effects of implantable steroid contraceptives for women. Contraception 2002;65:47–62.
18. Biswas A, Viegas OA, Roy AC. Effect of Implanon and Norplant subdermal contraceptive implants on serum lipids–a randomized comparative study. Contraception 2003;68:189–93.

19. Beerthuizen R, van Beek A, Massai R, Makarainen L, Hout J, Bennink HC. Bone mineral density during long-term use of the progestagen contraceptive implant Implanon compared to a non-hormonal method of contraception. Hum Reprod 2000; 15:118–22.
20. Bahamondes L, Monteiro-Dantas C, Espejo-Arce X, et al. A prospective study of the forearm bone density of users of etonorgestrel- and levonorgestrel-releasing contraceptive implants. Hum Reprod 2006;21:466–70.
21. Ortayli N. Users' perspectives on implantable contraceptives for women. Contraception 2002;65:107–11.
22. Weisberg E, Fraser I. Australian women's experience with Implanon. Aust Fam Physician 2005;34:694–6.
23. Bitzer J, Tschudin S, Alder J. Acceptability and side-effects of Implanon in Switzerland: a retrospective study by the Implanon Swiss Study Group. Eur J Contracept Reprod Health Care 2004;9:278–84.
24. Brache V, Faundes A, Alvarez F, Cochon L. Nonmenstrual adverse events during use of implantable contraceptives for women: data from clinical trials. Contraception 2002;65:63–74.
25. Farley TM, Collins J, Schlesselman JJ. Hormonal contraception and risk of cardiovascular disease. An international perspective. Contraception 1998;57:211–30.
26. Bennink HJ. The pharmacokinetics and pharmacodynamics of Implanon, a single-rod etonogestrel contraceptive implant. Eur J Contracept Reprod Health Care 2000;5 Suppl 2:12–20.
27. Diaz S. Contraceptive implants and lactation. Contraception 2002;65:39–46.
28. Reinprayoon D, Taneepanichskul S, Bunyavejchevin S, et al. Effects of the etonogestrel-releasing contraceptive implant (Implanon on parameters of breastfeeding compared to those of an intrauterine device. Contraception 2000;62:239–46.
29. Chikamata DM, Miller S. Health services at the clinic level and implantable contraceptives for women. Contraception 2002;65:97–106.
30. Evans R, Holman R, Lindsay E. Migration of implanon: two case reports. J Fam Plann Reprod Health Care 2005;31:71–2.
31. Agrawal A, Robinson C. Spontaneous snapping of an Implanon in two halves in situ. J Fam Plann Reprod Health Care 2003;29:238.

Injectable Contraceptives

Alisa B. Goldberg, MD, MPH
David A. Grimes, MD

- Injectable contraceptives rank in the top tier of contraceptive effectiveness.

- Progestin-only injections can be an important contraceptive option for women who cannot use estrogen.

- Injections provide a highly private method of contraception.

- Counseling women about the menstrual cycle changes associated with injectable contraceptives can substantially lower discontinuation rates.

- Lactating women may use progestin-only injections, but how soon after delivery they should start remains controversial.

Depo-Provera (DMPA-IM 150 mg/1 ml). The most commonly used injectable contraceptive is depot medroxyprogesterone acetate (DMPA-IM), marketed as Depo-Provera, given in a deep intramuscular injection of 150 milligrams (mg) every 12 weeks (or 3 months). DMPA is extremely effective, in part because it is forgiving for some women who return late for an injection.[1]

Depo-subQ provera 104 (DMPA-SC 104 mg/0.65 ml). This new formulation of DMPA has been dose-adjusted to be given subcutaneously every 12 weeks (or 3 months). Its efficacy and side effect profile are similar to DMPA-IM.[2,3]

Lunelle (Medroxyprogesterone acetate 25 mg and estradiol cypionate 5 mg). This combined injectable, given monthly, is highly effective and is associated with better bleeding patterns than progestin-only injectables. It is no longer available in the United States but is available in other countries. It will not be discussed in this chapter.

EFFECTIVENESS

DMPA IM (150 mg)

DMPA-IM ranks among the top tier of contraceptive effectiveness (see Table 27–1). With correct and consistent use, the probability of pregnancy is only 0.3%. With typical use the failure rate is 3%. These estimates apply to an 11–13 week regimen, with each injection providing 150 mg of DMPA per 1 cc. (For a comparative view of first-year contraceptive failure rates, see Table 27–1 in Chapter 27 on Contraceptive Efficacy.)

DMPA SC (104 mg)

In two large, open-label, phase 3 studies of DMPA-SC there were no reported pregnancies in a total of 16,023 woman-cycles of use.[2] The probability of pregnancy outside of a clinical trial setting is not yet available, but it is likely to be similar to DMPA-IM.

CONTINUATION RATES

In the largest U.S. study of DMPA use, reported in 1973, continuation rates were 59.4% at 1 year, 41.5% at 2 years, 30.2% at 3 years, and 24.1% at 4 years.[4] More recent studies report lower continuation rates: from 26% to 53% at 1 year.[5-7] Counseling about the expected hormonal effects can improve DMPA continuation rates.[8,9] In rural Mexico, 175 women received detailed, structured counseling at both pre-treatment and each injection visit about the hormonal effects of DMPA, while 175 received routine counseling and information. Over 12 months, only 8% of women receiving structured counseling discontinued use due to amenorrhea or irregular or heavy bleeding, compared to 32% of women receiving routine counseling. The total discontinuation rate was 17% among women receiving structured counseling *vs.* 43% among women receiving routine counseling.[9] Simply encouraging women to come in for a visit if they are having a problem with DMPA can also improve continuation rates.[8]

Upon discontinuing DMPA, many women do not switch to another highly effective contraceptive method. Two studies of low-income, urban women reported unintended pregnancy rates of 20% to 22% within 9 months of stopping DMPA.[10,11]

MECHANISM OF ACTION

DMPA primarily prevents pregnancy by inhibiting ovulation.[12] The dose of DMPA provided in each injection suppresses levels of FSH and LH and eliminates the LH surge. The pituitary gland remains responsive to gonadotropin-releasing hormone, which suggests that the site of action of DMPA is the hypothalamus and the primary mechanism of action is inhibition of GnRH pulsatility.[13]

DMPA also prevents pregnancy by thickening and decreasing the quality of cervical mucus, an anti-estrogen effect that prevents sperm penetration.[14,15]

DMPA alters the endometrium, making it atrophic and not receptive to implantation; however, given the effectiveness of DMPA at inhibiting ovulation and thickening the cervical mucous, it is unclear if this contributes to the contraceptive effect of DMPA at all.[15,16]

ADVANTAGES

Advantages of DMPA Injectables

1. **No estrogen.** Because DMPA injections contain no estrogen, they do not appear to cause the rare but serious complications attributable to exogenous estrogen (including deep vein thrombosis and pulmonary embolism). Studies thus far have not shown that serious cardiovascular effects are associated with use of progestin-only contraceptives.[16–18]

2. **Reversibility.** DMPA is reversible once the effect of the last injection wears off. DMPA does not cause long-term loss of fertility; however, ovulation may not return until 9 to 10 months after the last dose.[1]

3. **Intermediate-term effective contraception, even for obese women.** DMPA provides 3 months of highly effective contraception per injection. There is no decrease in the efficacy of DMPA among overweight or obese women.[2]

4. **Reduced risk of ectopic pregnancy.** Compared with women using no contraceptive at all, women who use DMPA have a reduced risk for having an ectopic pregnancy. Although the overall risk of ectopic pregnancy is lowered by DMPA, the possibility of an ectopic pregnancy should be ruled out if a woman using DMPA becomes pregnant. One study showed that 1.5% of women who got pregnant on DMPA had an ectopic pregnancy.[19] There is no increased proportion of ectopic pregnancy among women who conceive while using DMPA.[19]

5. **Absence of menstrual bleeding.** DMPA causes women to have very light periods or to miss periods entirely. These patterns of bleeding are considered by many women to be advantages, pro-

vided they have an opportunity to discuss these changes at counseling sessions. During the first year of DMPA use, approximately 10 to 30% of women are amenorrheic after one injection and 40% to 50% are amenorrheic after the fourth injection.[4,20] By the end of the fifth year of use, approximately 80% of women are amenorrheic.[4] In a study of teenagers, nearly two-thirds of DMPA users reported amenorrhea at 6 months.[21] Although clinicians and some women may consider the absence of menstrual bleeding an advantage of using DMPA, others do not. Decreased bleeding is associated with less anemia.

6. **Improvement of menstrual symptoms.** DMPA is associated with a decrease in ovulation pain, cyclic menstrual cramps, mood changes, headaches, breast tenderness and nausea.[22]

7. **Culturally acceptable.** In some cultures, a woman may consider medication by injection desirable. Some women wish to use a contraceptive without the knowledge of their partner. Many couples find DMPA use attractive because it is not intrusive in a relationship. Disrupted menstrual bleeding patterns may also have positive or negative cultural implications for some women depending on the bleeding pattern.[23] This again stresses the importance of informing women of the expected hormonal effects of DMPA.

8. **Minimal drug interactions.** There has been no demonstrated interaction between DMPA and antibiotics or enzyme-inducing drugs.[24] The only drug that decreases the effectiveness of DMPA is aminoglutethimide, which is usually used to suppress adrenal function in selected cases of Cushing's disease.[25]

9. **Fewer seizures.** DMPA has been found to decrease the frequency of grand mal seizures.[26,27] Improvement in seizure control is probably due to the sedative properties of progestins and this effect may be mediated through gamma-aminobutyric acid (GABA) receptors in the hippocampus.[28] Taking anti-seizure medicine has no impact on the efficacy of DMPA.

10. **Fewer sickle cell crises.**[29] In a randomized trial, DMPA use was associated with a greater reduction in the frequency of sickle cell crises than COC use or no intervention. After one year of DMPA use 70% of women were pain-free (compared to 50% of women not using hormones) and of the women who had continuing crises, only 16% reported the ongoing pain as intense.[29]

11. **Less pain from endometriosis.** A recent randomized, blinded trial compared DMPA-SC to luprolide for management of the pain associated with endometriosis. This trial found equivalent pain reduction with both treatment options and less bone min-

eral density loss with DMPA-SC.[30] In March 2005, DMPA-SC was approved by the FDA for this indication.

12. **Benefits for women with myomas.** DMPA has been used effectively to decrease the bleeding associated with myomas and improve hemoglobin levels.[32,33] DMPA use may also shrink myomas[32]; however, the evidence on this is conflicting.[33] Studies have shown that DMPA use is associated with a lower risk of recurrent myomas after myomectomy.[31]

13. **Decreased risk of pelvic inflammatory disease.**[34] Thickened cervical mucous may prevent ascent of pathogens to the upper genital tract.

Potential Additional Advantages of DMPA-SC

1. Subcutaneous injections may be less painful than IM injections.

2. Subcutaneous injections can be self-administered. Self-administration of DMPA may be acceptable to many women.[35] Self-injection may improve compliance with the method by making it easier for women to receive repeat injections. Whether DMPA continuation rates improve with self-administration remains to be seen.

DISADVANTAGES AND CAUTIONS

Adverse Effects of DMPA

1. **Menstrual cycle disturbances.** Bleeding patterns with DMPA use are unpredictable, with the majority of women experiencing infrequent but prolonged episodes of bleeding or spotting.[20] Many women experience either an increased number of days of light bleeding or amenorrhea. Amenorrhea becomes more common over time among DMPA users. Approximately 40% to 50% of users experience amenorrhea after 1 year of use and 80% after 5 years of use.[4,20] Similar patterns have been observed with DMPA-SC, with 55% of women achieving amenorrhea after 1 year of use.[2] Rarely do women using DMPA experience an increased number of days of heavy bleeding. Menstrual irregularity is the most common reason for discontinuation of DMPA. Approximately 20% to 25% of women will discontinue DMPA within the first year because of menstrual disturbances.[5-7] Of those who discontinue for menstrual disturbances, the majority discontinue for either prolonged bleeding or amenorrhea.[36] The irregular bleeding associated with progestin-only contraception

has been associated with an increased fragility of endometrial capillaries.[37]

2. **Weight gain.** Weight gain is common in many women using DMPA, however this effect is not consistent for all women. In one study of adults, Brazilian women using DMPA for 5 years gained an average of approximately 9 pounds, significantly more than the 5 pounds gained by IUD users over the same time interval.[38] Another large study of DMPA use in Chinese women showed no weight gain over one year of use.[39] A study of teens showed approximately 9 pounds of weight gain in the first year of DMPA use, significantly more than the 5 pounds gained by COC users in the same interval.[40] However, the only randomized trial of DMPA use did not show any significant weight gain compared to placebo.[41] This trial randomly assigned women to DMPA vs. placebo and then measured food intake, energy expenditure and weight gain over 3 months and found no difference between groups.[41] All women in this trial were of normal weight. It is likely that certain women are more likely to gain weight with DMPA use than others. One study showed that 56% of teen DMPA users either lost weight or gained less than 5% of their baseline weight and 25% gained more than 10% their baseline weight. The teens who gained more than 5% of their baseline weight in the first 3 months of use were highly likely to gain more weight with continued use.[42] Women and girls with a higher baseline weight may gain more weight on DMPA,[40,43] but this finding has not been consistent.[42] One study found greater weight gain among black adolescents on DMPA compared to white adolescents on DMPA.[43] In the trials of DMPA-SC, the median weight gain over 1 year of use was approximately 3.5 pounds and 4% to 8% of women reported weight gain as an adverse effect.[2]

Among women who gain weight while on DMPA, the weight gain has been demonstrated to be due to increases in fat deposition, not fluid retention.[43,44] It had been presumed that the observed increase in fat deposition was probably due to increased appetite,[44] however a recent study of adolescent DMPA users that measured appetite in a standardized fashion, found DMPA to be associated with decreased appetite, despite increases in total body fat.[43] Weight gain is commonly cited as a reason for discontinuation of DMPA, with 12% to 19% discontinuing for this reason.[5,7]

3. **Depression.** Individual women may experience an increase in depression when they use DMPA. However data evaluating the impact of DMPA on mood are limited and conflicting. One

recent study showed a slight increase in the likelihood of depression in DMPA users and other studies have shown no association.[45-47] A history of depression is not a contraindication to DMPA use. The WHO medical eligibility criteria rate DMPA use in women with a history of depression a category 2 (benefits usually outweigh the risks). If depression occurs or worsens in a woman following a DMPA injection, her symptoms may persist for the duration of the injection because it is not possible to discontinue DMPA immediately.[48] Clinical management of depression must take this into account. Use caution in providing DMPA postpartum for a woman with a history of severe postpartum depression and consider waiting until 6 weeks postpartum for the first injection. If prescribing DMPA for a woman with current depression, ensure that she has adequate mental health care and follow up.

4. **Bone density decrease.** Long-term DMPA users may develop temporary and usually reversible decreased bone density. (See section on bone density in Special Issues.)

5. **Allergic reactions.** Although rare, severe allergic reactions may occur.[49] Some programs encourage women to remain in the vicinity of the clinic for 20 minutes after an injection. To prevent severe allergic reactions, ask women if they have experienced significant itching or redness at the site of previous DMPA injections and do not repeat DMPA dosing if allergic reaction is suspected.

6. **Other adverse effects.** In one of the largest studies of DMPA users, 17% of the 3,875 women complained of headaches, 11% of nervousness, 5% of decreased libido, 3% of breast discomfort.[4]

Disadvantages of DMPA

1. **Not possible to discontinue immediately.** Weight gain, depression, breast tenderness, allergic reactions, and menstrual irregularities may continue until DMPA is cleared from a woman's body, about 6 to 8 months after her last injection. After discontinuing DMPA, women may also have a 6- to 12-month delay in return of fertility.[1,4]

2. **Return visits are required every 3 months.** For some women, visits for repeated injections of DMPA are unacceptable. Approximately 20% to 50% of women continue to use DMPA at 1 year and many who discontinue do so because of the difficulty in returning for injections.[5,6,8] Home visits for injections have been scheduled for some wheelchair-bound patients. Convenient access to DMPA injections through flexible and expanded clinic

hours or pharmacist-administered injections may improve continuation rates.[50] With DMPA-SC, self-injection may be possible, which may decrease the need for return visits.

PRECAUTIONS

The 2004 World Health Organization's (WHO) *Medical Eligibility Criteria for Contraceptive Use* guide health care providers in determining who can safely use various contraceptive methods. (See Chapter 4 for a full discussion) Compared to estrogen-containing methods, DMPA has only one absolute contraindication. The only condition listed as a category 4, absolute contraindication, for DMPA is current breast cancer.[51] There are several conditions listed as category 3 (risks usually outweigh benefits), generally these conditions include evidence of current cardiovascular disease, women with abnormal liver function or liver tumors, women with a history of breast cancer and women with unexplained vaginal bleeding prior to evaluation (Chapter 4). Providing DMPA in these circumstances "requires careful clinical judgment and access to clinical services".[51]

SPECIAL ISSUES

Breastfeeding Women

Some experts have voiced concern that progestin-only methods may thwart lactation if they are initiated before the post-delivery decline in natural progesterone, which functions as the trigger for milk synthesis.[52] However clinical experience in humans has not substantiated that hypothesis.[53] A prudent approach may be to wait until the flow of breastmilk is established. Unlike the use of combined OCs, use of progestin-only contraceptives once breastfeeding has been established has not been shown to have an adverse effect on breast milk volume; in some studies, milk production has been enhanced. The quality of breast milk is not affected. Because of theoretical concerns over early neonatal exposure to exogenous steroids, several international organizations have urged that progestin-only methods not be initiated until at least 6 weeks postpartum.[51,54] Studies of DMPA initiated within 1 to 3 days postpartum,[53] 7 days postpartum,[55] or within 6 weeks postpartum[56] have found no adverse effects. It is unlikely that a lactating woman will conceive during this time. (See Chapter 18 on Lactational Amenorrhea and Postpartum Contraception.)

Cancer Risk and DMPA

Breast cancer. There is no increase in the risk of breast cancer with DMPA use. In a pooled international study including 1,768 women with breast cancer and more than 13,000 controls, the overall relative risk associated with the use of DMPA was 1.1 (95% CI=0.97–1.4). There was no increased risk with longer use of DMPA, however women who had used DMPA within the past 5 years had an increased risk of breast cancer (RR=2.0; 95%CI=1.5–2.8).[57] This increased risk may reflect either increased detection of breast cancer in DMPA users or accelerated growth of preexisting tumors. Two more recent studies have also shown no association between DMPA use and breast cancer and these studies did not find any increased risk with recent or current use either.[58,59]

Reproductive tract cancers. There does not appear to be any association between invasive cervical cancer and DMPA use. A WHO Collaborative Study of 2,009 women with invasive cervical cancer and more than 9,000 controls failed to demonstrate a significantly increased risk (RR=1.1; 95% CI=1.0–1.3).[60] Another large case control study, similarly found no association between adenocarcinoma or adenosquamous carcinoma of the cervix and DMPA use.[61] Large WHO case-control studies have similarly demonstrated that DMPA use is not associated with ovarian cancer (RR=1.1; 95% CI=0.6, 1.8) and is associated with a significantly decreased risk of endometrial cancer (RR=0.2; 95% CI=0.1, 0.8).[62,63]

Bone Density and DMPA

DMPA is associated with a decrease in bone mineral density[64–68] that is generally temporary and reversible.[69–71] Data suggest that the loss in bone mineral density is rapid within the first 2 years of use, but after approximately 2 years of use, loss of bone density slows dramatically.[69] Although women have a decrease in bone density while using DMPA, studies have consistently demonstrated that bone mineral density is regained when DMPA is discontinued.[69–71] For women over age 21 years, by 30 months after discontinuation of DMPA, bone mineral density values are similar among previous DMPA users as never-users.[71] Other studies comparing past-users of DMPA to never-users have similarly shown no difference in bone mineral density.[72]

Since the effects of contraceptives on bone mass may be particularly important for adolescents who have not yet reached peak bone mass, it is important to know if teenagers who have used DMPA regain bone mass after discontinuing DMPA.[73] A recent study suggests they do.[69] A study of 170 adolescents (80 DMPA users and 90 controls) ages 14 to 18 years were followed with bone mineral density testing every 6 months for 24 to 36 months, even after discontinuation of DMPA. The investigators found that DMPA use was associated with significant declines in bone density but upon discontinuation DMPA users had a rapid and significant gain in bone density beyond the bone gain observed in control women. This is reassuring and suggests that the bone loss associated with DMPA use is transient. Whether adolescents who use DMPA ultimately reach the same peak bone mass as they would have had they not used DMPA remains unknown. Similarly, we do not know the impact of prolonged DMPA use during adolescence on the risk of fracture later in life. Estrogen add-back therapy increases bone mineral density in both adult and adolescent DMPA users, which suggests that DMPA-associated loss of bone density is due to hypoestrogenism.[74,75] A similar pattern of decline in bone mineral density followed by recovery is observed with the hypoestrogenism that occurs with lactation.[76,77] Epidemiological evidence has not demonstrated any negative effect on fracture risk associated with pregnancy and lactation.[78]

Although declines in bone mineral density are concerning and recoveries reassuring, the most important question is whether DMPA use increases the risk of fracture. Low-trauma fractures are rare in healthy premenopausal women and a Medline search identified only one case report of a low-trauma fracture in a long-term DMPA user.[79] Another study of female military recruits evaluated risk factors for stress fractures during basic training and found that age, race, alcohol and tobacco use, weight-bearing exercise, lowest adult weight and corticosteroid use were associated with stress fractures. They also found an increased risk of fractures in white women using depo-medroxyprogesterone acetate (DMPA).[80]

A separate, important question is whether prolonged DMPA use during the premenopausal years is associated with an increased risk of fracture in the menopause. Limited data address this question. One study from New Zealand, where DMPA has been in use for a long time and many previous users are menopausal, did not demonstrate an association between prior DMPA use and post-menopausal fractures, although the study had limited statistical power to detect differences in fracture risk.[81] This study did have adequate power to compare small differences in bone mineral densities between previous users of DMPA and never-users, and found no difference. This study also found no difference in postmenopausal bone mineral densities between women who used DMPA right up until the menopause and those who had discontinued earlier.[81] Another study found similar levels of bone density among women entering the menopause naturally (off hormones) and women with a history of prolonged DMPA use who continued use until they became menopausal. Those entering menopause naturally had a rapid decline in bone density and those on DMPA had little additional loss with the transition to menopause, suggesting that they had already "lost the estrogen-sensitive component of bone."[82]

In November 2004 the FDA added a black box warning to the label of DMPA. It states: "Women who use Depo-Provera Contraceptive Injection may lose significant bone mineral density. Bone loss is greater with increasing duration of use and may not be completely reversible. It is unknown if use of Depo-Provera Contraceptive Injection during adolescence or early adulthood, a critical period of bone accretion, will reduce peak bone mass and increase the risk for osteoporotic fracture in later life. Depo-Provera Contraceptive Injection should be used as a long-term birth control method (e.g. longer than 2 years) only if other birth control methods are inadequate."[83]

In June 2005, the World Health Organization reviewed the evidence on this subject. They concluded, "there should be no restriction on the use of DMPA, including no restriction on duration of use, among women aged 18 to 45 who are otherwise eligible to use the method." They further recommended that: "Among adolescents (menarche to < 18) and women over 45, the advantages of using DMPA usually outweigh the theoretical safety concerns regarding fracture risk. Since data are insufficient to determine if this is the case with long-term use among these age groups, the overall risks and benefits for continuing use of the method should be reconsidered over time with the individual user."[84]

Clinical management should be dictated by evidence that measures outcomes of interest (like fracture-risk), not by surrogate markers of questionable clinical significance (like bone densitometry in healthy premenopausal women).[85] Despite product labeling, bone mineral density testing should play no role in the routine management of healthy DMPA users, because in premenopausal women there is no good correlation between bone densitometry results and fracture risk.[86,87] Similarly, using amenorrhea or serum estradiol levels to guide management is not helpful, since these factors have not consistently been associated with lower bone mineral density or higher fracture risk among DMPA users.[65,68,88]

According to the WHO, "since the effect of DMPA on bone mineral density is largely reversible, any lifetime increase in fracture risk is likely to be small."[84] However, women with medical co-morbidities that place them at high risk for osteoporosis and fracture, such as chronic corticosteroid use, disorders of bone metabolism, a strong family history of osteoporosis (that may represent a genetic mutation associated with fracture) or women with anorexia nervosa—may not be well suited for long-term DMPA use.

Risk of Sexually Transmitted Infections and DMPA

DMPA provides no protection against sexually transmitted infections (STIs), including HIV. Several observational studies have shown an association between DMPA use and acquisition of chlamydia.[34,89,90] In these studies, DMPA use has been inconsistently associated with acquisition of gonorrhea.[34,90] While cervical ectopy may increase the presence of or the identification of chlamydia, ectopy is not an important mediator of the association between DMPA use and chlamydia infection.[34,90] It has been proposed that DMPA might increase the risk of chlamydia because progestins may enhance the growth of chlamydia or impact host immune factors that enable growth.[34,90] Alternatively, the observed relationship between DMPA use and chlamydia may be due to bias inherent in observational studies; women who choose DMPA may be at an increased risk of chlamydia because they are more likely to be a part of social-sexual circles where chlamydia has a higher prevalence.[91] No randomized controlled trial has addressed this question. Despite the association between DMPA use and chlamydia acquisition, DMPA use is associated with a decreased risk of pelvic inflammatory disease.[34,90] Presumably, the progestin-induced thickening of the cervical mucous inhibits ascent of bacteria to the upper genital tract.

Several studies in high risk populations, including sex workers in Kenya and Thailand, have demonstrated an association between DMPA and HIV acquisition,[92,93] while others studies have not observed an association.[94] It is possible that these differences are due to study methodology, or they could be the result of variable levels of risk in different populations (i.e. commercial sex workers with exposure to multiple strains of HIV versus family planning clients).[95] Whether DMPA use causes an increased risk of acquiring HIV in exposed women is unknown. All women at risk of acquiring a sexually transmitted infection should be counseled to use condoms consistently and correctly.

PROVIDING DMPA

DMPA is provided in either 1 cc vials or prefilled syringes containing 150 mg. The label states a 2-year shelf-life. Using a sterile needle and syringe, inject the DMPA deeply into the deltoid or the gluteus maximus muscle. Injections into the deltoid are less embarrassing but may be slightly more painful. The 21- to 23-gauge needle should be 2.5 to 4 cm long.[24] Immediately after injection do not massage the area over the injection, because it could lower the effectiveness of DMPA. DMPA-SC is available in prefilled, single-use syringes. Subcutaneous DMPA injections can be given in the anterior thigh or abdominal wall.

If a DMPA injection is given within 5 to 7 days of a normal last menstrual period, no backup contraception is needed. The WHO states that DMPA can be given at any time in a menstrual cycle if the woman can be reasonably certain that she is not pregnant. If DMPA is given later than the seventh day in the menstrual cycle, it is important that women use backup contraception for 7 days and receive a follow-up pregnancy test several weeks later to diagnose pregnancy in a timely fashion. A recent study of immediate initiation of DMPA among 149 women who presented on cycle day 8 or later, found that 47% of women continued to a second dose of DMPA, 92% returned for their follow up pregnancy test (half required many reminders) and 3 women were pregnant (2%).[96]

Schedule injections for every 3 months. After a single IM or SC DMPA injection, ovulation does not occur for at least 14 weeks (98 days).[3] Repeat DMPA IM or SC injections may be given as late as 14 weeks (98 days) after a previous injection. Women who return more than 14 weeks after a previous injection should have pregnancy excluded before re-injection and need to use backup contraception for 7 days after re-initiating DMPA. Giving DMPA injections in early pregnancy should be avoided if possible, since exposure has been associated with low-birth weight infants.[98] There is no increased risk of birth defects in pregnancies exposed to DMPA.[99,100] The manufacturer recommends re-injection of DMPA-IM between 11 and 13 weeks after a previous injection and re-injection of DMPA-SC 12 to 14 weeks after a previous injection. The manufacturer recommends excluding pregnancy before proceeding with re-injection in women who return more than 13 weeks (91 days) after a previous DMPA-IM injection and more than 14 weeks (98 days) after a previous DMPA-SC injection.

At each re-injection follow-up visit ask about any problems or concerns, the date of the last menstrual period, and any changes in contraceptive or STI prevention needs. Record the patient's weight and blood pressure. If the client is not having any unacceptable symptoms or problems, she may continue getting DMPA injections. If she has had unprotected intercourse, offer emergency contraception. Advise her that after 2 years of continuous use you will have to discuss with her the impact of DMPA on bone mineral density, the unknown effect this may have on fracture risk, reassess any underlying risk factors for bone fragility or fractures and re-evaluate whether DMPA continues to be the best contraceptive option for her. If it is, she may continue to get injections.

MANAGING DMPA PROBLEMS AND FOLLOW-UP

Menstrual changes. Inform women in advance that changes will occur in their menstrual cycles. Do not dismiss the impact of bleeding changes: they are the major reason that women discontinue this method. Spotting or breakthrough bleeding may be managed most easily in a family planning clinic by offering women one or more cycles of combined OCs, although the efficacy of this intervention has not been formally studied. Other options include short courses of exogenous estrogen[101] or a prostaglandin synthetase inhibitor.[101,102] Each of these interventions has been shown to decrease bleeding in the short term; however, when these interventions are discontinued, irregular bleeding patterns resume.[101,102] Counseling helps continuation rates (see section on Effectiveness). Inform women that the irregular bleeding may return, but that over time the likelihood of amenorrhea will increase and amenorrhea in the setting of DMPA use is not harmful and does not require treatment.

Allergic reactions. Fortunately, severe anaphylactic reactions are rare. However, because DMPA is irretrievable once injected, have on hand emergency supportive measures such as epinephrine and diphenhydramine. Encourage patients to stay in the clinic/office area for 20 minutes following their first few injections. Those considering self-injection of DMPA-SC should probably receive their first one or two injections in a clinical setting both to monitor for an allergic reaction and learn self-injection technique.

Weight gain. DMPA is associated with weight gain in some women. In the one randomized study where DMPA was compared to a placebo injection, there was no difference in weight gain between the groups.[41] On average, the weight gain observed with DMPA use has been modest.[2,42,103] Women who gain a modest amount of weight should be encouraged to be careful about food intake and to exercise regularly. However, some women using DMPA have excessive weight gain. If the excessive weight gain is troublesome, cannot be controlled with diet and exercise, or has health consequences, these individual women should consider alternative methods of contraception.

INSTRUCTIONS FOR USING DMPA

1. DMPA injections are very effective if you return on time for a repeat injection. Of 1,000 women who consistently get repeat injections on time, only 3 will become pregnant over a year's time.

2. DMPA injections have many *noncontraceptive benefits.* DMPA injections decrease:
   — Menstrual blood flow
   — Menstrual cramping
   — Risk of anemia
   — Risk of fibroids and bleeding from fibroids
   — Risk of endometrial cancer
   — Risk of pelvic infection
   — Risk of ectopic pregnancy (a pregnancy outside of your uterus)

— Risk of a sickle cell crisis

— Frequency of grand mal seizures

3. **To use DMPA you must be willing to accept unpredictable, frequent, or absent bleeding.** About 50% of women using DMPA will stop having any bleeding after a year of injections. This is to be expected and is not harmful.

4. **Have on hand a backup contraceptive method** such as foam, spermicidal tablets or suppositories, condoms, or a diaphragm. You will need to use your backup method for 1 week after your first injection. (This precaution may not be necessary if the first shot is given during the first 5 days after the beginning of a normal menstrual period.) Ask your clinician to give you a package of the emergency contraceptive pill, Plan B, or a prescription for Plan B as a backup in case you have unprotected sex in the first week after injection or if you are late for your next injection.

5. **Have a latex or plastic condom ready if you:**

— Are late for your injection

— May be at risk for a sexually transmitted infection, including infection with the virus that causes AIDS

6. Because of the rare possibility of an *allergic reaction*, some programs ask that women remain in the vicinity of the clinic for 20 minutes after having their DMPA injections.

7. **Return to the clinic on time** for another injection. Mark your calendar for your next DMPA shot to be sure you will be on time. You may want to get your partner to mark his calendar too. Some programs are beginning to offer women (who have been using DMPA successfully) the opportunity to take home enough DMPA and syringes to last for a full year. If you would like to learn to give yourself your injections of DMPA, ask your clinician.

8. Depression and premenstrual symptoms may improve or become worse. If you become severely depressed, see your clinician immediately.

9. DMPA can decrease estrogen levels, which can cause a decrease in the density of bones. In women who are postmenopausal, decreased bone density can be associated with an increased risk of fractures. There is no evidence that DMPA use in young women increases the risk of fractures later in life. However, given the theoretical risk of fractures, let your clinician know if you frequently take corticosteroids, if you have fractured bones with minimal trauma, if you have a bone me-

tabolism disease, if you have a strong family history of osteoporosis and fractures or if you have (or had) anorexia nervosa. Also, discuss bone health with your clinician if you plan to use DMPA for more than 2 years and are less than 18 years old or over 45.[84]

10. DMPA users may gain weight. Be sure to eat a healthy balanced diet and exercise regularly. If you continue to gain weight excessively despite diet and exercise, discuss this with your clinician.

LATE FOR INJECTION

1. **If you realize after intercourse that you have missed your injection or are late for it,** use emergency contraception right away. Use another method until you are protected by another injection. If you realize you are late for your injection before you have intercourse, use another contraceptive method or abstain. Return as soon as possible for your shot.

2. If you are afraid you will forget your appointment, the company that makes DepoProvera can email you reminders (www.depoprovera.com). Your doctor's office or clinic may also be able to call you or email you with reminders.

DMPA and Your Periods

1. DMPA makes a woman's periods less regular, and spotting between periods is fairly common. Eventually most women stop having periods completely. This is not harmful. Do *not* choose DMPA unless you do not mind having your periods change.

2. If your pattern of bleeding concerns you contact your clinician. She may recommend that you return to the clinic for an evaluation to rule out the possibility of pregnancy or infection. If your bleeding is frequent or heavy, she may want to rule out anemia and there are medications you can use to decrease your bleeding.

3. When you discontinue taking DMPA, it may be a number of months before your periods return to normal after your last DMPA injection. However, there are medications, such as birth control pills that can give you monthly withdrawal bleeding once you have stopped using DMPA.

Discontinuing DMPA

1. If you are more than 1 week late for your injection, use a backup method of contraception as soon as you realize that you are going to be late. Use emergency contraception if you had unprotected intercourse. Visit your clinician as soon as possible for your injection. You will need to continue using a backup method until you get your injection and for a week after your next injection. Many clinicians will give you a pregnancy test to make sure you are not pregnant. If you have any questions about whether intercourse may have been unprotected, use emergency contraception.

2. If you discontinue DMPA and do not want to become pregnant, start using a new contraceptive 13 weeks after your last shot. You may start pills or another contraceptive *before* it is time for your next injection.

3. If you are discontinuing DMPA because you want to become pregnant, remember that the contraceptive effect may take a number of months to go away. Start taking prenatal vitamins as soon as you decide to attempt pregnancy. Be patient.

DMPA and Pregnancy

1. DMPA injections may keep you from getting pregnant for more than 12 weeks (3 months) after your last shot. The average delay in return of fertility is about 10 months from the last injection. DMPA does not decrease your fertility in the long run.

2. If you are over age 35 and want to become pregnant in the near future, you may want to use an alternative contraceptive that has minimal or no delay in return of fertility after you stop using that other method.

3. If you get pregnant while using DMPA, there is no increased risk of birth defects.[99,100]

DMPA WARNING SIGNALS

Serious health problems are very rare with DMPA use. Although DMPA is a highly effective contraceptive method, pregnancies do occur. If you feel pregnant, or think you might be pregnant, check a pregnancy test. See your clinician if you develop any of the following warning signals or if any other symptoms concern you.

- Repeated, very painful headaches
- Heavy bleeding

- Depression

- Severe, lower abdominal pain (may be a sign of pregnancy)

- Pus, prolonged pain, redness, itching or bleeding at injection site (may be a sign of infection)

REFERENCES

1. Mishell DR, Jr. Pharmacokinetics of depot medroxyprogesterone acetate contraception. J Reprod Med 1996;41(5 Suppl):381–390.
2. Jain J, Jakimiuk A, Bode F, Ross D, Kaunitz A. Contraceptive efficacy and safety of DMPA-SC. Contraception 2004;70:269–275.
3. Jain J, Dutton C, Nicosia A, Wajszczuk C, Bode F, Mishell D. Pharmacokinetics, ovulation suppression and return to ovulation follwoing a lower dose subcutaneous formulation of Depo-Provera. Contraception 2004;70:11–18.
4. Schwallie PC, Assenzo JR. Contraceptive use–efficacy study utilizing medroxyprogesterone acetate administered as an intramuscular injection once every 90 days. Fertil Steril 1973;24:331–339.
5. Polaneczky M, Liblanc M. Long-term depot medroxyprogesterone acetate (Depo-Provera) use in inner-city adolescents. J Adolesc Health 1998;23:81–88.
6. Potter LS, Dalberth BT, Canamar R, Betz M. Depot medroxyprogesterone acetate pioneers. A retrospective study at a North Carolina Health Department. Contraception 1997;56:305–312.
7. Paul C, Skegg DC, Williams S. Depot medroxyprogesterone acetate. Patterns of use and reasons for discontinuation. Contraception 1997;56:209–214.
8. Hubacher D, Goco N, Gonzalez B, Taylor D. Factors affecting continuation rates of DMPA. Contraception 1999;60:345–351.
9. Canto De Cetina TE, Canto P, Ordonez Luna M. Effect of counseling to improve compliance in Mexican women receiving depot-medroxyprogesterone acetate. Contraception 2001;63:143–146.
10. Goldberg AB, Cardenas LH, Hubbard AE, Darney PD. Post-abortion depot medroxyprogesterone acetate continuation rates: a randomized trial of cyclic estradiol. Contraception 2002;66:215–220.
11. Davidson AR, Kalmuss D, Cushman LF, Romero D, Heartwell S, Rulin M. Injectable contraceptive discontinuation and subsequent unintended pregnancy among low-income women. Am J Public Health 1997;87:1532–1534.
12. Petta CA, Faundes A, Dunson TR, et al. Timing of onset of contraceptive effectiveness in Depo-Provera users. II. Effects on ovarian function. Fertil Steril 1998;70:817–820.
13. Ismail AA, el-Faras A, Rocca M, el-Sibai FA, Toppozada M. Pituitary response to LHRH in long-term users of injectable contraceptives. Contraception 1987;35:487–495.
14. Petta CA, Faundes A, Dunson TR, et al. Timing of onset of contraceptive effectiveness in Depo-Provera users: Part I. Changes in cervical mucus. Fertil Steril 1998;69:252–257.
15. Croxatto HB. Mechanisms that explain the contraceptive action of progestin implants for women. Contraception 2002;65:21–27.
16. Mishell DR, Jr. Long-acting contraceptive steroids. Postcoital contraceptives and anti-progestins. In: Mishell DR, Jr., Davajan V, Lobo R, eds. Infertility, contraception and reproductive endocrinology. Cambridge: Blackwell Scientific Publications; 1991.
17. McCann MF, Potter LS. Progestin-only oral contraception: a comprehensive review. Contraception 1994;50(6 Suppl 1):S1–195.

18. Speroff L, Darney PD. A clinical guide for contraception. Third ed. Philadelphia: Lippincott Williams & Wilkins; 2001.
19. Borgatta L, Murthy A, Chuang C, Beardsley L, Burnhill MS. Pregnancies diagnosed during Depo-Provera use. Contraception 2002;66:169–172.
20. Belsey EM. Vaginal bleeding patterns among women using one natural and eight hormonal methods of contraception. Contraception 1988;38:181–206.
21. Cromer BA, Smith RD, Blair JM, Dwyer J, Brown RT. A prospective study of adolescents who choose among levonorgestrel implant (Norplant), medroxyprogesterone acetate (Depo-Provera), or the combined oral contraceptive pill as contraception. Pediatrics 1994;94:687–694.
22. Kaunitz AM. Injectable depot medroxyprogesterone acetate contraception: an update for U.S. clinicians. Int J Fertil Womens Med 1998;43:73–83.
23. Dahan MH, Coffler MS, Patel KS. Oral contraceptives for inducing ovulation delay in orthodox Jewish women: a report of 2 cases. J Reprod Med 2005;50:284–286.
24. Injectable contraceptives: their role in family planning. Geneva: World Health Organization; 1990.
25. Hatcher RA, Schnare S. Ask the experts: progestin-only contraceptives. Contracept Technol Update 1993;14:114 115.
26. Mattson RH, Cramer JA, Darney PD, Naftolin F. Use of oral contraceptives by women with epilepsy. JAMA 1986;256:238–240.
27. Mattson RH, Rebar RW. Contraceptive methods for women with neurologic disorders. Am J Obstet Gynecol 1993;168(6 Pt 2):2027–2032.
28. Rhodes ME, Frye CA. Actions at GABA(A) receptors in the hippocampus may mediate some antiseizure effects of progestins. Epilepsy Behav 2005;6:320–327.
29. de Abood M, de Castillo Z, Guerrero F, Espino M, Austin KL. Effect of Depo-Provera or Microgynon on the painful crises of sickle cell anemia patients. Contraception 1997;56:313–316.
30. Crosignani PG, Luciano A, Ray A, Bergqvist A. Subcutaneous depot medroxyprogesterone acetate versus leuprolide acetate in the treatment of endometriosis-associated pain. Hum Reprod 2006;21:248–256.
31. Lumbiganon P, Rugpao S, Phandhu-fung S, Laopaiboon M, Vudhikamraksa N, Werawatakul Y. Protective effect of depot-medroxyprogesterone acetate on surgically treated uterine leiomyomas: a multicentre case–control study. Br J Obstet Gynaecol 1996;103:909–914.
32. Venkatachalam S, Bagratee JS, Moodley J. Medical management of uterine fibroids with medroxyprogesterone acetate (Depo Provera): a pilot study. J Obstet Gynaecol 2004;24:798–800.
33. Johnson N, Fletcher H, Reid M. Depo medroxyprogesterone acetate (DMPA) therapy for uterine myomata prior to surgery. Int J Gynaecol Obstet 2004;85:174–176.
34. Baeten J, Nyange P, Richardson B, et al. Hormonal contraception and risk of sexually transmitted disease acquisition: results from a prospective study. Am J Obstet Gynecol 2001;185:380–385.
35. Lakha F, Henderson C, Glasier A. The acceptability of self-administration of subcutaneous Depo-Provera. Contraception 2005;72:14–18.
36. Gray RH, Parker RA, Diethelm P. Vaginal bleeding disturbances associated with the discontinuation of long-acting injectable contraceptives. From the World Health Organization Special Programme for Research, Development, and Research Training in Human Reproduction; Task Force on Long-acting Systemic Agents for the Regulation of Fertility. Br J Obstet Gynaecol 1981;88:317–321.
37. Hickey M, Dwarte D, Fraser IS. Superficial endometrial vascular fragility in Norplant users and in women with ovulatory dysfunctional uterine bleeding. Hum Reprod 2000;15:1509–1514.
38. Bahamondes L, Del Castillo S, Tabares G, Arce XE, Perrotti M, Petta C. Comparison of weight increase in users of depot medroxyprogesterone acetate and copper IUD up to 5 years. Contraception 2001;64:223–225.

39. Danli S, Qingxiang S, Guowei S. A multicentered clinical trial of the long-acting injectable contraceptive Depo Provera in Chinese women. Contraception 2000;62:15–18.
40. Mangan SA, Larsen PG, Hudson S. Overweight teens at increased risk for weight gain while using depot medroxyprogesterone acetate. J Pediatr Adolesc Gynecol 2002;15:79–82.
41. Pelkman CL, Chow M, Heinbach RA, Rolls BJ. Short-term effects of a progestational contraceptive drug on food intake, resting energy expenditure, and body weight in young women. Am J Clin Nutr 2001;73:19–26.
42. Risser WL, Gefter LR, Barratt MS, Risser JM. Weight change in adolescents who used hormonal contraception. J Adolesc Health 1999;24:433–436.
43. Bonny A, Britto M, Huang B, Succop P, Slap G. Weight gain, adiposity, and eating behaviors among adolescent females on depot medroxyprogesterone acetate (DMPA). J Pediatr Adolesc Gynecol;17:109–115.
44. Amatayakul K, Sivasomboon B, Thanangkul O. A study of the mechanism of weight gain in medroxyprogesterone acetate users. Contraception 1980;22:605–622.
45. Gupta N, O'Brien R, Jacobsen LJ, et al. Mood changes in adolescents using depot-medroxyprogesterone acetate for contraception: a prospective study. J Pediatr Adolesc Gynecol 2001;14:71–76.
46. Civic D, Scholes D, Ichikawa L, et al. Depressive symptoms in users and non-users of depot medroxyprogesterone acetate. Contraception 2000;61:385–390.
47. Westhoff C, Truman C, Kalmuss D, et al. Depressive symptoms and Depo-Provera. Contraception 1998;57(4):237–240.
48. Archer B, Irwin D, Jensen K, Johnson ME, Rorie J. Depot medroxyprogesterone. Management of side-effects commonly associated with its contraceptive use. J Nurse Midwifery 1997;42:104–111.
49. Selo-Ojeme DO, Tillisi A, Welch CC. Anaphylaxis from medroxyprogesterone acetate. Obstet Gynecol 2004;103(5 Pt 2):1045–1046.
50. Picardo C. Pharmacist-administered depot medroxyprogesterone acetate. Contraception 2006;73:559–561.
51. Medical eligibility criteria for contraceptive use, third edition. Geneva: World Health Organization; 2004.
52. Kennedy KI, Short RV, Tully MR. Premature introduction of progestin-only contraceptive methods during lactation. Contraception 1997;55:347–350.
53. Halderman LD, Nelson AL. Impact of early postpartum administration of progestin-only hormonal contraceptives compared with nonhormonal contraceptives on short-term breast-feeding patterns. Am J Obstet Gynecol 2002;186:1250–1256; discussion 1256–1258.
54. International Planned Parenthood Federation. IMAP statement on breast feeding, fertility and postpartum contraception. IPPF Med Bull 1996;30:1–3.
55. McCann MF, Liskin LS, Piotrow PT, Rinehart W, Fox G. Breast-feeding, fertility, and family planning. Popul Rep J 1981;J525–575.
56. Effects of hormonal contraceptives on breast milk composition and infant growth. World Health Organization (WHO) Task Force on Oral Contraceptives. Stud Fam Plann 1988;19(6 Pt 1):361–369.
57. Skegg DC, Noonan EA, Paul C, Spears GF, Meirik O, Thomas DB. Depot medroxyprogesterone acetate and breast cancer. A pooled analysis of the World Health Organization and New Zealand studies. JAMA 1995;273:799–804.
58. Strom BL, Berlin JA, Weber AL, et al. Absence of an effect of injectable and implantable progestin-only contraceptives on subsequent risk of breast cancer. Contraception 2004;69:353–360.
59. Shapiro S, Rosenberg L, Hoffman M, et al. Risk of breast cancer in relation to the use of injectable progestogen contraceptives and combined estrogen/progestogen contraceptives. Am J Epidemiol 2000;151:396–403.

60. Depot-medroxyprogesterone acetate (DMPA) and risk of invasive squamous cell cervical cancer. The WHO Collaborative Study of Neoplasia and Steroid Contraceptives. Contraception 1992;45:299–312.

61. Thomas DB, Ray RM. Depot-medroxyprogesterone acetate (DMPA) and risk of invasive adenocarcinomas and adenosquamous carcinomas of the uterine cervix. WHO Collaborative Study of Neoplasia and Steroid Contraceptives. Contraception 1995; 52:307–312.

62. Depot-medroxyprogesterone acetate (DMPA) and risk of epithelial ovarian cancer. The WHO Collaborative Study of Neoplasia and Steroid Contraceptives. Int J Cancer 1991;49:191–195.

63. Depot-medroxyprogesterone acetate (DMPA) and risk of endometrial cancer. The WHO Collaborative Study of Neoplasia and Steroid Contraceptives. Int J Cancer 1991;49:186–190.

64. Berenson A, Breitkopf C, Grady J, Rickert V, Thomas A. Effects of hormonal contraception use on bone mineral density after 24 months of use. Obstet Gynecol 2004;103: 899–906.

65. Clark M, Sowers M, Nichols S, Levy B. Bone mineral density changes over two years in first-time users of depot medroxyprogesterone acetate. Fertil Steril 2004;82: 1580–1586.

66. Cromer B, Stager M, Bonny A, et al. Depot medroxyprogesterone acetate, oral contraceptives and bone mineral density in a cohort of adolescent girls. J Adol Health 2004; 35:434–441.

67. Cundy T, Cornish J, Roberts H, Elder H, Reid I. Spinal bone density in women using depot medroxyprogesterone contraception. Obstet Gynecol 1998;92:569–573.

68. Paiva L, Pinto-Neto A, Faundes A. Bone density among long-term users of medroxyprogesterone acetate as a contraceptive. Contraception 1998;58:351–355.

69. Scholes D, Lacroix A, Ichikawa L, Barlow W, Ott S. Change in bone mineral density among adolescent women using and discontinuing depot medroxyprogesterone acetate contraception. Arch Ped Adol Med 2005;159:139–144.

70. Cundy T, Cornish J, Evans MC, Roberts H, Reid IR. Recovery of bone density in women who stop using medroxyprogesterone acetate. BMJ 1994;308:247–248.

71. Scholes D, Lacroix A, Ichikawa L, Barlow W, Ott S. Injectable hormone contraception and bone density: results from a prospective study. Epidemiology 2002;13:581–587.

72. Petitti DB, Piaggio G, Mehta S, Cravioto MC, Meirik O. Steroid hormone contraception and bone mineral density: a cross-sectional study in an international population. The WHO Study of Hormonal Contraception and Bone Health. Obstet Gynecol 2000; 95:736–744.

73. Curtis KM, Chrisman CE, Peterson HB. Contraception for women in selected circumstances. Obstet Gynecol 2002;99:1100–1112.

74. Cundy T, Ames R, Horne A, et al. A randomized controlled trial of estrogen replacement therapy in long-term users of depot medroxyprogesterone acetate. J Clin Endocrinol Metab 2003;88:78–81.

75. Cromer B, Lazebnik R, Rome E, et al. Double-blinded randomized controlled trial of estrogen supplementation in adolescent girls who receive depot medroxyprogesterone acetate for contraception. Am J Obstet Gynecol 2005;192:42–47.

76. Sowers M, Corton G, Shapiro B, et al. Changes in bone density with lactation. JAMA 1993;269:3130–3135.

77. Chantry CJ, Auinger P, Byrd RS. Lactation among adolescent mothers and subsequent bone mineral density. Arch Pediatr Adolesc Med 2004;158:650–656.

78. Karlsson MK, Ahlborg HG, Karlsson C. Maternity and bone mineral density. Acta Orthop 2005;76:2–13.

79. Harkins GJ, Davis GD, Dettori J, Hibbert ML, Hoyt RA. Decline in bone mineral density with stress fractures in a woman on depot medroxyprogesterone acetate. A case report. J Reprod Med 1999;44:309–312.

80. Lappe JM, Stegman MR, Recker RR. The impact of lifestyle factors on stress fractures in female Army recruits. Osteoporos Int 2001;12:35–42.
81. Orr-Walker BJ, Evans MC, Ames RW, Clearwater JM, Cundy T, Reid IR. The effect of past use of the injectable contraceptive depot medroxyprogesterone acetate on bone mineral density in normal post-menopausal women. Clin Endocrinol (Oxf) 1998; 49:615–618.
82. Cundy T, Cornish J, Roberts H, Reid I. Menopausal bone loss in long-term users of depot medroxyprogesterone acetate contraception. Am J Obstet Gynecol 2002; 186:978–983.
83. Depo-Provera label. Pharmacia & Upjohn. October 2004. Available at: www.fda.gov/medwatch/SAFETY/2004/nov_PI/Depo-Provera_PI.pdf. Accessed November 21, 2005.
84. WHO statement on hormonal contraception and bone health. Wkly Epidemiol Rec 2005;80:302–304.
85. Grimes DA, Schulz KF. Surrogate end points in clinical research: hazardous to your health. Obstet Gynecol 2005;105(5 Pt 1):1114–1118.
86. Diagnosis of osteoporosis in men, premenopausal women, and children. J Clin Densitom 2004;7:17–26.
87. Lewiecki EM. Premenopausal bone health assessment. Curr Rheumatol Rep 2005; 7:46–52.
88. Gbolade B, Ellis S, Murby B, Randall S, Kirkman R. Bone density in long term users of depot medroxyprogesterone acetate. Brit J Obstet Gynaecol 1998;105:790–794.
89. Jacobson D, Peralta L, Farmer M, Graham N, Gaydos C, Zenilman J. Relationship of hormonal contraception and cervical ectopy as measured by computerized planimetry to chlamydial infection in adolescents. Sex Transm Dis 1999;27:313–319.
90. Morrison C, Bright P, Wong E, et al. Hormonal contraceptive use, cervical ectopy, and the acquisition of cervical infections. Sex Transm Dis 2004;31:561–567.
91. Dayan L, Donovan B. Chlamydia, gonorrhoea, and injectable progesterone. Lancet. Oct 16–22 2004;364:1387–1388.
92. Martin HL, Jr., Nyange PM, Richardson BA, et al. Hormonal contraception, sexually transmitted diseases, and risk of heterosexual transmission of human immunodeficiency virus type 1. J Infect Dis 1998;178:1053–1059.
93. Ungchusak K, Rehle T, Thammapornpilap P, Spiegelman D, Brinkmann U, Siraprapasiri T. Determinants of HIV infection among female commercial sex workers in northeastern Thailand: results from a longitudinal study. J Acquir Immune Defic Syndr Hum Retrovirol 1996;12:500–507.
94. Bulterys M, Chao A, Habimana P, Dushimimana A, Nawrocki P, Saah A. Incident HIV-1 infection in a cohort of young women in Butare, Rwanda. Aids 1994; 8:1585–1591.
95. Martin HL, Jr., Richardson BA, Mandaliya K, Achola JO, Overbaugh J, Kreiss JK. The early work on hormonal contraceptive use and HIV acquisition. J Acquir Immune Defic Syndr 2005;38 Suppl 1:S12–14.
96. Sneed R, Westhoff C, Morroni C, Tiezzi L. A prospective study of immediate initiation of depo medroxyprogesterone acetate contraceptive injection. Contraception 2005;71:99–103.
97. Fotherby K, Koetsawang S, Mathrubutham M. Pharmacokinetic study of different doses of Depo Provera. Contraception 1980;22:527–536.
98. Pardthaisong T, Gray RH. In utero exposure to steroid contraceptives and outcome of pregnancy. Am J Epidemiol 15 1991;134:795–803.
99. Katz Z, Lancet M, Skornik J, Chemke J, Mogilner BM, Klinberg M. Teratogenicity of progestogens given during the first trimester of pregnancy. Obstet Gynecol 1985; 65:775–780.
100. Dahlberg K. Some effects of depo-medroxyprogesterone acetate (DMPA): observations in the nursing infant and in the long-term user. Int J Gynaecol Obstet 1982; 20:43–48.

101. Said S, Sadek W, Rocca M, et al. Clinical evaluation of the therapeutic effectiveness of ethinyl oestradiol and oestrone sulphate on prolonged bleeding in women using depot medroxyprogesterone acetate for contraception. World Health Organization, Special Programme of Research, Development and Research Training in Human Reproduction, Task Force on Long-acting Systemic Agents for Fertility Regulation. Hum Reprod 1996;11 Suppl 2:1–13.
102. Tantiwattanakul P, Taneepanichskul S. Effect of mefenamic acid on controlling irregular uterine bleeding in DMPA users. Contraception 2004;70:277–279.
103. Mainwaring R, Hales HA, Stevenson K, et al. Metabolic parameter, bleeding, and weight changes in U.S. women using progestin only contraceptives. Contraception 1995;51:149–153.

Progestin-Only Pills

10

Elizabeth G. Raymond, MD, MPH

- Progestin-only pills contain a progestin hormone and no estrogen. A woman using progestin-only pills takes one tablet every day.

- Progestin-only pills are highly effective if taken as directed, although they are possibly less effective in typical use than combined oral contraceptive pills.

- Progestin-only pills are safe for almost all women, including many women with contraindications to using combined oral contraceptive pills.

- The most common complaint of progestin-only pill users is irregular bleeding.

Progestin-only pills (POPs), sometimes called "minipills," contain a progestin hormone. One pill is taken every day with no hormone-free days. POPs containing norethindrone are currently available in the United States. POPs containing levonorgestrel, desogestrel, or other progestins are available in other countries. The amount of progestin in POPs is lower than the amount in combined oral contraceptive pills (COCs) containing the same compounds.

EFFECTIVENESS

POPs can be a highly effective contraceptive method when taken properly by motivated users. In studies reviewed in Chapter 27 on Contraceptive Efficacy and in another comprehensive review,[1] The proportion of women becoming pregnant in the first year of use was between 1% and 13%. Pearl indices in these studies ranged up to 3 pregnancies per 100 woman-years. However, effectiveness among typical users outside of trials who are not receiving close counseling and monitoring may be lower than these figures suggest. Several studies showed that the absolute pregnancy risk among women using POPs is strongly influenced by age, coital frequency, lactation, possibly body weight, and other characteristics of the user.[2,3]

Scant data are available comparing efficacy of different POP products. One randomized trial found no significant difference in efficacy between POPs containing norethindrone and POPs containing levonorgestrel.[4] Pregnancy rates in both POP groups in this trial were greater than 9% at one year, higher than in many other studies. Another small randomized trial found fewer pregnancies among women using POPs containing desogestrel than among women using POPs containing levonorgestrel, although the difference was not statistically significant.[5]

POPs are widely believed to be less effective than COCs. This belief probably stems largely (and reasonably) from the fact that the dose of hormone is lower in POPs than in COCs. However, data directly comparing actual pregnancy rates in users of the two methods are limited. One randomized trial comparing two COC and two POP preparations found that the pregnancy rate was significantly lower in one group of COC users than the rates in the other three groups. However, losses from the study for reasons other than pregnancy were very high in all the groups, which seriously compromised the comparisons.[4] In typical use, factors such as compliance may influence pregnancy rates more than relatively minor differences in inherent method efficacy.

Guidelines on use of POPs emphasize that for maximum efficacy, the pills must be taken within several hours of the same time every day. This recommendation is based primarily on data about serum progestin levels, which peak shortly after pill ingestion and then decline to nearly undetectable levels 24 hours later. In this respect, POPs differ from COCs, which produce higher and longer-lasting serum progestin levels. No clinical data are available that correlate pregnancy rates with timeliness in taking POPs.[1] One study suggests that POPs containing desogestrel 75 mg may inhibit ovulation reliably even when pills are occasionally taken 12 hours late.[6]

MECHANISM OF ACTION
POPs may prevent pregnancy by the following mechanisms:

- Ovulation is inhibited in a variable proportion of cycles.

- Cervical mucus is thickened and decreased in amount, which may prevent sperm penetration.

- The activity of the cilia in the fallopian tube is reduced, which may prevent the sperm and the egg from meeting.

- The endometrium is altered, which may inhibit implantation of a fertilized egg.

The specific mechanism active in a particular cycle may vary among women and, in any single woman, between cycles.[1] POPs containing desogestrel 75 mg may inhibit ovulation more consistently than POPs containing levonorgestrel 30 mg.[7]

ADVANTAGES

POPs have many advantages for many women, as described below.

1. **Safety.** Because POPs contain lower doses of progestin than COCs and do not contain estrogen, they are presumably at least as safe as COCs (see Chapter 11 on Combined Oral Contraceptives) and are quite likely safer. However, rigorous data on safety of POPs as distinct from or in comparison to COCs are relatively scant; therefore, it is not always possible to determine for certain which of the concerns related to COCs are not relevant to POP users. In general, data suggest that POPs containing norgestrel or norethindrone appear not to be associated with an overall clinically important increase in risk of hypertension,[8] cardiovascular disease,[9] breast cancer,[10] coagulation factors, or birth defects in women who accidentally take POPs during pregnancy.[1,11]

2. **Few contraindications.** According to the World Health Organization's *Medical Eligibility Criteria for Contraceptive Users*, POPs can safely be used by almost all women (see section below on Providing the Method. These criteria list many fewer contraindications to POPs than to COCs (Chapter 4 on Medical Eligibility Criteria). This difference is partly rationalized by the absence of estrogen in POPs, which suggests that conditions that may be exacerbated by estrogen are not a contraindication to POP use. POPs are frequently recommended instead of COCs to breastfeeding women between 6 weeks and 6 months postpartum.

3. **Acceptable efficacy,** especially if the pills are taken as directed. See above.

4. **Improved menstrual symptoms for some women.** POPs cause menstrual cycle changes that are welcome to some women (see below under Disadvantages.) They may also reduce the severity of menstrual cramps and premenstrual tension symptoms.

5. **Simple, fixed daily regimen.** POP users take the same type of pill every day (same color and hormone content). In POP packages, every pill contains hormone; there is no pill-free week or hormone-free week.

6. **Immediate reversibility.** Limited data suggest that fertility is normal immediately after stopping use of POPs, regardless of the duration of POP use.[1]

7. **Non-contraceptive health benefits.** POPs may reduce the incidence of painful crises in women with sickle cell disease[12] and may be used to treat estrogen dermatitis related to the menstrual cycle.[13] Other non-contraceptive health benefits of POPs have not been rigorously studied. However, it seems reasonable to postulate that POPs might confer some of the same benefits as COCs, such as a reduced risk of uterine and ovarian cancers.

DISADVANTAGES AND CAUTIONS
POPs also have disadvantages, as described below.

1. **Menstrual cycle disturbances.** POPs cause bleeding changes in many or most users. The abnormal menstrual patterns are unpredictable and may include short cycles, irregular periods, intermenstrual bleeding and spotting, and less commonly, prolonged bleeding or amenorrhea. Analysis of bleeding patterns of women in six clinical trials studying various methods of contraception showed that POP users had less regular bleeding patterns and more total bleeding/spotting days over time than users of COCs. Whether or not bleeding patterns tend to become more regular with increased duration of POP use is unclear. Menstrual cycle disturbances are a common reason for discontinuing POPs, although some women consider the altered bleeding pattern, particularly if it constitutes less total bleeding than expected, to be a benefit of the method. One expert has suggested that POP users who have bleeding irregularities may be better protected from pregnancy than those who do not, because the irregularities indicate that the pills are disrupting the normal ovulatory hormonal cycles.[1,14-16]

2. **Other side effects.** Complaints by POP users include headaches, nausea, weight gain or loss, breast tenderness, depression, fatigue, decreased libido, androgenic symptoms such as hirsuitism and acne, and other side effects. However, the precise extent to which these common symptoms are actually caused by the pills cannot be determined from available data.[1]

3. **Vulnerable efficacy.** To maximize contraceptive efficacy, POP users should be especially careful (more careful than users of COCs) to take the pills at the same time each day and to use backup methods such as condoms when taking drugs that may interact with the hormones in the pills or during periods of vomiting or diarrhea. This disadvantage may be less relevant to users

of POPs containing desogestrel than to users of POPs containing norgestrel or norethindrone.

4. **Lower efficacy than some other methods in preventing ectopic pregnancy.** Rigorous data are not available about the effect of POPs on the absolute risk of ectopic pregnancy. One early report suggested that POP users may be at higher risk than users of no method or of other methods[19], but other data seem to refute that contention.[1] However, up to 10% of pregnancies that occur among POP users may be ectopic, a proportion higher than is seen in users of COCs or women who use no method at all. Thus, POPs appear not to prevent ectopic pregnancy as well as they prevent intrauterine pregnancy.[1]

5. **Possible increased risk of diabetes.** One study suggested that use of POPs during breastfeeding after a pregnancy complicated by gestational diabetes may increase the subsequent long-term risk of type II diabetes mellitus.[17] However, POPs are generally felt to be safe for use by diabetic women.

6. **Ovarian cysts.** Unlike COCs, which substantially inhibit ovarian activity and reduce the risk of functional ovarian cysts, POPs may be associated with an increased incidence of functional ovarian cysts or persistent follicles.[18] Most ovarian cysts cause minor or no symptoms and resolve without treatment.

7. **Lack of protection against sexually transmitted infections (STIs).** Progestin-only contraceptives provide no known substantial protection against STIs, including HIV. A full discussion of the data regarding potential associations between progestin use and HIV acquisition may be found in Chapter 9 on Injectable Contraceptives.

8. **Possible increased risk of thromboembolic conditions in users of POPs containing desogestrel.** A full discussion of the potential association between COCs containing desogestrel and thromboembolic phenomena may be found in Chapter 11 on Combined Oral Contraceptives. Whether an association may exist with POPs containing this progestin is unknown. At this time (March, 2006), POPs containing desogestrel are not marketed in the United States.

9. **Limited availability.** In the United States, POPs are much less popular than COCs and may be more difficult for some women to obtain on short notice.

SPECIAL ISSUES

Breastfeeding

The physiologic effects of contraceptive steroids could, in theory, impair lactation. In addition, a small amount of the progestin in the pills passes into breast milk, which exposes a breastfeeding baby to the hormone.[20] A review of five randomized trials evaluating the use of hormonal contraceptives during breastfeeding found no clear evidence that POPs have a clinically important effect on milk volume or on infant growth and development. However, the quality of all the trials was poor, and the conclusions are therefore suspect.[21] Despite the paucity of evidence, the WHO Medical Eligibility Criteria assert that for breastfeeding women the risks of using POPs within the first 6 weeks postpartum generally outweigh the advantages. After 6 weeks, the Criteria indicate no restriction on POP use. The Criteria do recommend against use of COCs during breastfeeding between 6 weeks and 6 months postpartum and thus imply that POPs are a better choice during this time; the controversy over that recommendation is discussed further in Chapter 11 on Combined Oral Contraceptives. One study conducted in Kenya found that the timing of initiation of POPs (6 weeks or 6 months postpartum) did not affect method continuation.[22]

Drug Interactions

Interactions between POPs and other drugs have not been well studied. Because POPs produce relatively low progestin levels even in the absence of other drugs, POPs may not be an especially good hormonal contraceptive option for women who are taking certain drugs on a chronic basis. These drugs include rifampicin, certain anticonvulsants, and some anti-retroviral drugs, and Saint John's Wort, which appear to affect metabolism of COCs (see Chapter 11 on Combined Oral Contraceptives). However, even for women on these drugs, POPs may be more effective than some other contraceptive methods, particularly barriers or natural family planning. Combined use of a barrier method and POPs might be the best choice for women taking potentially interacting drugs if they cannot use other highly effective contraceptive methods. Advise POP users to use a backup method while temporarily taking a potentially interacting drug, and possibly for some period of time after stopping it.

PROVIDING THE METHOD

POPs can be used safely by almost all women, including most women who are not eligible to take COCs and breastfeeding women at least 6 weeks postpartum. The WHO's *Medical Eligibility Criteria* for

POPs include no restriction based on age, smoking, hypertension, migraine without aura, uterine fibroids, diabetes, gall bladder disease, or sickle cell disease. No examination or laboratory test is needed to determine whether a woman is eligible to receive POPs.

The WHO criteria (Chapter 4) list only a few contraindications to POPs:

- Breastfeeding women less than 6 weeks postpartum (Category 3)
- Current deep venous thrombosis or pulmonary embolus (Category 3)
- Active viral hepatitis or severe (decompensated) cirrhosis, benign or malignant liver tumors (Category 3)
- Current breast cancer (Category 4)
- Past breast cancer with no evidence of disease for 5 years (Category 3)

In addition, the WHO criteria note that POPs should be stopped if the user develops ischemic heart disease, stroke, or migraine with aura while using POPs (Category 3).

POPs are not a good choice for women who cannot tolerate irregular bleeding or amenorrhea. Because they should be taken at close to the same hour each day, they may not be suitable for women whose schedules do not allow such consistency.

Counseling. Women considering POPs should be advised about their advantages and disadvantages, described above.

Timing of initiation. A woman may start taking POPs at any time when it is reasonably certain that she is not pregnant (Quick Start). The WHO recommends that no backup method is needed if she starts POPs at any of the following times:

- During the first five days of her menstrual cycle
- Between 6 weeks and 6 months postpartum if she is fully or nearly fully breastfeeding and amenorrheic
- Within the first 21 days postpartum if she is not breastfeeding
- Immediately after an abortion
- The day after she stops another hormonal method (i.e., she is switching to POPs from another hormonal method with no break in between)

However, the WHO recommends that if she starts POPs at any time other than these listed, she should use a backup method such as male condoms for the first two days of taking POPs. Another, simpler, approach is to tell *all* POP users to use a backup method (or abstain from vaginal sex) for the first two days after starting POPs.

Provide or prescribe as many packs of POPs as the patient wants.

MANAGING PROBLEMS AND FOLLOW-UP

Abnormal bleeding in women using POPs can be managed by a number of approaches, including reassurance, prostaglandin inhibitors, estrogen supplementation, or switching methods.

If a woman becomes pregnant while using POPs, be vigilant for the possibility of ectopic pregnancy.

USER INSTRUCTIONS

To use POPs, follow these instructions:

1. Start taking the pills during the first 5 days of your normal menstrual period or on any day you are reasonably sure that you are not pregnant. If you are switching from estrogen-containing oral contraceptive pills (regular birth control pills), skip the 7 inactive pills at the end of the pack, and instead start the POPs the day after the last active pill.

2. Use a backup method such as male condoms every time you have sex or abstain from vaginal sex for the first 48 hours (2 days) after starting POPs.

3. Take 1 pill every day. Choose a time and take the pill at that time or within 3 hours after that time.

4. Start the next pack the day after the last pack is finished. Do not take any break or days off between packs. Always have your next pack ready *before* you finish each pack.

5. If you miss taking a pill during the 3-hour window, take it as soon as you remember, even if that means you will take 2 pills in one day. Use a backup method such as male condoms or abstain from vaginal sex during the next 48 hours. Take further pills at the usual time If you vomit within 4 hours after taking a pill, or if you have diarrhea, your body might not properly absorb the medicine in the POPs. Keep taking the pills on schedule, but use a backup method such as male condoms every time you have sex through 48 hours after the vomiting or diarrhea are over.

6. If you have already had intercourse without adequate protection because you missed pills, call your clinician or another family planning provider such as Planned Parenthood immediately. You may be able to use an emergency contraceptive.

7. Get a pregnancy test if—

   — Your menstrual period is late, and you have not taken all your pills on time, and you had sex without a condom or other backup method

   — You miss two periods in a row, even if you took all your POPs on time

   — You are concerned about pregnancy for any reason

   Do not stop taking the pills until you know the pregnancy test result. If the result is positive, then stop taking the pills and consult your clinician about your options. If the result is negative, then the late or missed periods are probably due to the pills and are not dangerous. Consult your clinician about other possible causes and your options.

8. Certain medicines and some over-the-counter preparations can reduce the effectiveness of POPs. If you take any other drug while using POPs, ask your clinician whether it might interact with POPs. If so, you should use a backup method (such as male condoms) during the entire time you are taking the other drug and possibly for some time after you stop taking it. If you are planning to take the other drug for a long period of time, consult with your clinician about whether a contraceptive method other than POPs might be appropriate for you.

9. Changes in your menstrual periods (frequency and length and bleeding between periods) are common in women taking POPs. These changes are usually not dangerous. If you have unusual bleeding, keep taking the POPs. If the bleeding lasts for more than 8 days or is particularly heavy, or if you want to switch to another contraceptive method that is less likely to cause bleeding irregularities, consult your clinician.

10. If you have other problems or questions while taking POPs, keep taking the pills according to schedule while you figure out what to do.

11. If you stop taking POPs and do not want to become pregnant, start using another contraceptive immediately, or abstain from vaginal sex. Your ability to become pregnant returns right away after you stop POPs.

12. Ask your clinician to provide you with a package of emergency contraceptive pills or a prescription for them. You can use emergency contraception if you have had sex that was not properly protected by POPs or another contraceptive method (that is, if you did not follow the instructions above).

REFERENCES

1. McCann MF, Potter LS. Progestin-only oral contraception: a comprehensive review. Contraception 1994;50:S1–195.
2. Vessey M, Lawless M, Yeates D, McPherson K. Progestogen-only oral contraception. Findings in a large prospective study with special reference to effectiveness. Br J Fam Plan 1985;10:117–21.
3. Steiner M, Dominik R, Trussell J, Hertz-Picciott I. Measuring contraceptive effectiveness: a conceptual framework. Obstet Gynecol 1996;88:24S-30S.
4. Sheth A, Jain U, Sharma S, et al. A randomized, double-blind study of two combined and two progestogen-only oral contraceptives. Contraception 1982;25:243–52.
5. A double-blind study comparing the contraceptive efficacy, acceptability and safety of two progestogen-only pills containing desogestrel 75 micrograms/day or levonorgestrel 30 micrograms/day. Collaborative Study Group on the Desogestrel-containing Progestogen-only Pill. Eur J Contracept Reprod Health Care 1998;3:169–78.
6. Korver T, Klipping C, Heger-Mahn D, Duijkers I, van Osta G, Dieben T. Maintenance of ovulation inhibition with the 75-microg desogestrel-only contraceptive pill (Cerazette) after scheduled 12-h delays in tablet intake. Contraception 2005;71:8–13.
7. Rice CF, Killick SR, Dieben T, Coelingh Bennink H. A comparison of the inhibition of ovulation achieved by desogestrel 75 micrograms and levonorgestrel 30 micrograms daily. Hum Reprod 1999;14:982–5.
8. Hussain SF. Progestogen-only pills and high blood pressure: is there an association? A literature review. Contraception 2004;69:89–97.
9. Heinemann LA, Assmann A, DoMinh T, Garbe E. Oral progestogen-only contraceptives and cardiovascular risk: results from the Transnational Study on Oral Contraceptives and the Health of Young Women. Eur J Contracept Reprod Health Care 1999;4:67–73.
10. Skegg DC, Paul C, Spears GF, Williams SM. Progestogen-only oral contraceptives and risk of breast cancer in New Zealand. Cancer Causes Control 1996;7:513–9.
11. Simpson JL, Phillips OP. Spermicides, hormonal contraception and congenital malformations. Adv Contracept 1990;6:141–67.
12. de Abood M, de Castillo Z, Guerrero F, Espino M, Austin KL. Effect of Depo-Provera or Microgynon on the painful crises of sickle cell anemia patients. Contraception 1997;56:313–6.
13. Randall K, Steele R. Estrogen dermatitis: treatment with progestin-only pill. Arch Dermatol 2005;141:792–3.
14. Broome M, Fotherby K. Clinical experience with the progestogen-only pill. Contraception 1990;42:489–95.
15. Belsey EM. Vaginal bleeding patterns among women using one natural and eight hormonal methods of contraception. Contraception 1988;38:181–206.
16. Guillebaud, J. Contraception - Your Questions Answered. 2nd. London: Churchill Livingstone, 1993.
17. Kjos SL, Peters RK, Xiang A, Thomas D, Schaefer U, Buchanan TA. Contraception and the risk of type 2 diabetes mellitus in Latina women with prior gestational diabetes mellitus. JAMA 1998;280:533–8.
18. Tayob Y, Adams J, Jacobs HS, Guillebaud J. Ultrasound demonstration of increased frequency of functional ovarian cysts in women using progestogen-only oral contraception. Br J Obstet Gynaecol 1985;92:1003–9.
19. Bergsjo P, Langengen H, Aas J. Tubal pregnancies in women using progestagen-only contraception. Acta Obstet Gynecol Scand 1974;53:377–8.
20. Betrabet SS, Shikary ZK, Toddywalla VS, Toddywalla SP, Patel D, Saxena BN. ICMR Task Force Study on hormonal contraception. Transfer of norethisterone (NET) and levonorgestrel (LNG) from a single tablet into the infant's circulation through the mother's milk. Contraception 1987;35:517–22.

21. Truitt ST, Fraser AB, Grimes DA, Gallo MF, Schulz KF. Hormonal contraception during lactation. Systematic review of randomized controlled trials. Contraception 2003;68:233–8.
22. Were EO, Kendall JZ, Nyongesa P. Randomised clinical trial to determine optimum initiation time of norgestrel-progestin only contraception in Eldoret Teaching Hospital, Kenya. East Afr Med J 1997;74:103–7.

Combined Oral Contraceptives

Anita L. Nelson, MD

- More than 75 million women throughout the world currently rely on combined oral contraceptives (COCs). In the United States, 4 out of 5 women born since 1945 have used COCs at some time in their lives.

- COCs effectively prevent pregnancy. Of 1,000 women taking pills correctly and consistently, only 3 will become pregnant during their first year. However, because of inconsistent use in the real world, 8% of women become pregnant in the first year of typical use.

- COCs are safe for healthy reproductive aged women, especially non-smokers. COCs are often safer than pregnancy for women with selected medical problems.

- Dual protection with both condoms and COCs will provide important protection against sexually transmitted infections as well as excellent protection against an unintended pregnancy.

- The new ways of using oral contraceptive that should be encouraged include Quick Start, extended cycle use and shortened pill-free intervals.

- Prescribing/providing generous supplies of pill packets will help reduce barriers to access and encourage consistent pill use.

The introduction of "the pill" in the United States, in May 1960, transformed family planning. For the first time in history, women were able to control their own fertility effectively. Family planning was recognized by the CDC as one of the 10 greatest public health achievements of the 20th century.[1] In the United States, pills and condoms made the greatest contributions to family planning. The first pill, called Enovid, had 150 mcg mestranol and 9.85 mg norethynodrel.[2] These high doses of hormones were utilized because they were found to be effective. In those days, studies were not done to identify the lowest effective dose. Another interesting historical note is that the clinical trials of that first pill were conducted in Puerto Rico, because contraception was outlawed in both Massachusetts and Pennsylvania where the pill investigators worked. Fortunately, one of the original pill pioneers also had an academic appointment in Puerto Rico and was able to conduct very comprehensive and advanced trials of the safety and efficacy of Enovid in Spanish. It is important to be familiar with the highlights of the history of the pill to understand better the issues surrounding its evolution over time and women's perceptions about the pill. Since that first pill, the doses of the sex steroids in combined oral contraceptive (COC) preparations have decreased dramatically, which has both increased their safety and reduced their side effects. In addition, with time, numerous noncontraceptive benefits have been identified with both short- and long-term COC use.

HORMONES IN COMBINED ORAL CONTRACEPTIVES

COCs are safe and effective for the vast majority of reproductive-aged women. They are the most extensively studied medications in the history of medicine. Over 80% of U.S. women born after 1945 have used the pill at some time.[3] In the United States, COCs are available only by prescription; in some other countries, they are available over-the-counter. The keys to successful and safe COC use include selection of appropriate COC candidates, patient motivation, and effective counseling that is responsive to women's concerns about pill safety and side effects. Familiarity with the general classes of hormones found in pills can provide clinicians with a basis to successfully select initial pills for women with different issues and to more productively treat side effects that women may develop with pill use.

Pills have been made of only a limited number of compounds over the decades. All COCs contain an estrogen and a progestin; progestin-only pills (POPs) are discussed in Chapter 10. The properties of each pill formulation, including its side effects, depend upon its constituent hormones, as well as the doses of each of these hormones. There are interactions between the hormones. The progestins with higher androgenic activity can cancel some of the metabolic impacts the estrogen would normally have; estrogen can blunt some of the androgen's impacts.

Estrogens

Two estrogenic compounds are used in the oral contraceptives available in the United States: mestranol and ethinyl estradiol (EE). Mestranol, which was the estrogen in the original pills, is a prodrug (a precursor of a drug) that must be metabolized by the liver into EE to have biological activity. Today mestranol is found only in a few 50 mcg pills. Since 50 mcg of mestranol is equivalent to 35 to 40 mcg of EE, avoid using 50 mcg mestranol-containing pills when high-dose estrogen pills are needed.

Ethinyl estradiol is much more potent and long-acting than the ovarian steroid estradiol. This potency allows once-a-day dosing, but also means that the metabolic impacts of EE are greater than those of estradiol. Doses of ethinyl estradiol in U.S. pills vary from 20 to 50 mcg per pill. In other countries lower doses of EE (15 mcg) are used.

Progestins

Since progestins provide the majority of the pill's contraceptive activity, it is critical that therapeutic serum levels be maintained for at least 24 hours, with an adequate margin of drug to allow for variations in the way different women absorb and metabolize the pill's hormones, and to allow for some inconsistent pill use. The power of a particular progestin results not only from its intrinsic potency, but also from the dose that is used. Each compound has a different potency and different metabolic effects.

Natural progesterone is poorly absorbed from the gastrointestinal tract and is rapidly metabolized. At high doses, progesterone is sedating. For all these reasons, the original developers of the pill turned to more long-lasting compounds (C-19 androgens) to use as a basis of the pill's progestin.

Eight different progestins have been used in the COCs sold in the United States. Several different classification systems for the progestins exist, but the one most commonly used system recapitulates the history of the pill in the United States by categorizing the progestins into the so-called "generations of progestins" that were introduced over time. The first three generations of progestins are derived from C-19 androgens.

The first generation progestins (norethindrone, norethindrone acetate and ethynodiol diacetate in the United States and lynestrenol and norethynodrel elsewhere) have excellent potency and are well tolerated. Formulations with low doses of norethindrone are often used when low levels of progestins are desirable. However, as the dose of progestin in the pills was reduced over time, some women experienced more problems with unscheduled bleeding and spotting with these first generation progestins.

In response, the second generation progestins (norgestrel and levonorgestrel) were developed. These norgestrel-related compounds are significantly more potent and have longer half lives than the norethindrone-related progestins. Levonorgestrel is so potent that it has been the progestin used in most situations where progestin needs to last for years—such as in the Norplant capsules and the Mirena Intrauterine System (IUS). The typical dose of levonorgestrel used in birth control pills is 0.15 mg compared to the 0.5 to 1.0 mg doses needed with norethindrone. Norgestrel is a racemic mixture of the biologically active conformation of levonorgestrel (the left-handed version) and the inactive dextronorgestrel (the right-handed version). Therefore, pills with norgestrel (LoOvral) have twice the amount of progestin as do the equivalent levonorgestrel pills (Nordette). The second generation progestins have more androgenic activity than the first generation progestins. While the extra androgenic activity may be theoretically appealing for the libido, there are clinical situations where it is not helpful, especially in women with hirsutism, acne or dyslipidemia.

Therefore, the third generation progestins (desogestrel, norgestimate and, elsewhere, gestodene) were introduced to maintain increased progestational activity and to reduce androgenic activity. Because these third generation formulations have less androgenic activity, they allow a more full metabolic expression of the pill's estrogens. This has some beneficial impacts. One particular product (Ortho TriCyclen) with the third generation progestin (norgestimate) received FDA labeling indicating that it is an effective treatment for mild to moderate cystic acne primarily because the estrogen induced a significant increase in sex hormone binding globulin (SHBG). (See General Health Benefits discussion below). On the other hand, concern arose that this increased expression of estrogen may have adverse effects—that pills with these progestins might be associated with a slightly higher risk of thrombotic events than the second generation progestins with greater androgenic activity. (See VTE discussion below).

The fourth generation progestin (drospirenone) has different origins. The parent compound of drospirenone is spironolactone, a potassium-sparing diuretic used to treat hypertension. Drospirenone retains some anti-mineralocorticoid and anti-androgenic properties of spironolactone.

A more functional categorization of the progestins is based on the metabolites of the progestins. Under this system, there are three groups of progestins. The *estranes* include norethindrone and other progestin prodrugs that metabolize to norethindrone (norethindrone acetate and ethynodiol diacetate). The *gonanes* include levonorgestrel, norgestrel, desogestrel, and norgestimate in the United States and gestodene elsewhere. Drospirenone is the third group.

Even within their respective groups, progestins vary greatly in their properties of bioavailability, binding affinity, and half-life. *Bioavailability* reflects the percent of drug that is absorbed into the bloodstream. Much of a drug can be metabolized by the liver after it is first absorbed from the intestine and before it reaches the bloodstream. This "first pass" metabolism is discussed in more detail in the drug-drug interaction section.

Different individuals differ significantly in their "first pass" metabolisms. Lower doses of a drug are needed if its bioavailability is higher. A compound with greater bioavailability will also have less inter- and intra-individual variation. *Relative binding affinity* reflects how well a drug binds to its target receptor. Greater binding affinity means that a smaller dose is needed to achieve a clinical affect. Both bioavailability and relative binding affinity are considered when the dose of progestin is selected. These differences can help explain why the dose of norethindrone in pills needs to be many times greater than that of levonorgestrel. The final property that can have significant clinical implications is the half-life of a progestin. *Half-life* is the time necessary for the blood level of a drug to fall to 50% of its maximum. The greater the serum half-life, the longer it stays in the patient's circulation. Longer half-lives of sex steroids in the pills are helpful in reducing the incidence of unscheduled spotting and bleeding. Longer half-lives also reduce the chance that missed pills will permit escape ovulation and, therefore, may be more forgiving when pills are missed.

MECHANISMS OF ACTION

Birth control pills work as contraceptives, acting to prevent fertilization. The progestins in all COCs provide most of the contraceptive effect, although the estrogens also contribute to ovulation suppression. Cycle control is enhanced by estrogen.

The mechanisms of action for birth control pills that have been repeatedly *proven* include

- Thickening of the cervical mucus to prevent sperm entry into the upper genital tract
- Suppression of ovulation by providing negative feedback to the hypothalamic-pituitary system:
  - Decreased GnRH pulsatility
  - Decreased pituitary responsiveness to GnRH stimulation
  - Suppression of LH and FSH production
  - Inhibition of mid-cycle LH surge

EE and progestins have other effects on the reproductive system, but the contributions these effects make to the efficacy of the birth control pill have never been substantiated:

- Slowing of tubal motility and disruption of transport of the ova (interfere with fertilization)
- Endometrial atrophy, changes in function of endometrial vessels, alterations in the metalloproteinase content in the endometrium (progestin effects that might inhibit implantation)

- Localized edema of the endometrium (an estrogen effect that might inhibit implantation)

The incidence of "escape ovulation" in oral contraceptive users in earlier higher dose pills was estimated to be around 2%.[4] Breakthrough ovulation is probably higher in current lower dose pills. In a study of 20 mcg pills, progesterone levels indicative of luteinization and ovulation were found in 2 of 24 women (8.3%).[5] In these situations, the impenetrability of the cervical mucus is a backup mechanism that prevents fertilization from occurring.

EFFECTIVENESS

In general, COCs belong in the second tier of contraceptive effectiveness, having higher failure rates than IUDs, implants, and injections but lower failure rates than the barrier and behavioral methods.

Among women who use COCs correctly and consistently, not missing any pills and following instructions perfectly, only about 3 in 1,000 (0.3%) are expected to become pregnant within the first year. However, the first-year failure rates with *typical* use as observed in real world use are estimated to be 8% (see Chapter 3 on Choosing a Contraceptive). This means that 1 woman in 12 will become pregnant in the first year of typical COC use. Studies with computer chips embedded in the pill bottle showed that over 50% of women missed 3 or more pills in the third cycle of use.[6] Pill-taking mistakes that increase the length of the hormone-free interval are likely to lead to failures. The conventional 7-day pill-free interval with the low-dose pills may also play an important role in their failure. Ultrasound studies have demonstrated that by the 7th placebo pill day, 23% of women can have ovarian follicles that measure at least 10 mm in diameter.[7] If a woman misses pills early in her pack of pills, it may be much more difficult to suppress ovulation and protect against pregnancy during that cycle. Thus, COCs may be made more effective by eliminating or shortening the pill-free interval (see Choosing a Pattern of Pill Use section).

Many pregnancies that are credited to the pill occur in the month when women discontinue COCs and do not use another method of contraception. Studies show that 11% of women discontinue their pills in the first month of use, and 19% of those who discontinue fail to adopt a new method.[8] By 6 months, 28% of pill users have stopped the pill; by 1 year, that percentage approaches 33% to 50%.[9] Quite disturbingly, 42% of women who discontinued COC use did so *without* consulting their clinicians. Because of these concerns, women starting the pill should also be given a second method (such as condoms) they can implement on their own in case they discontinue pill use before returning for follow-up. Provide each new start COC patient with a packet of or prescription for emergency contraception (Plan B) or, at a minimum, inform her about its availability.

IMPACT OF WEIGHT ON COC EFFICACY

Two retrospective studies reported by the same author have suggested that heavier women may experience higher COC failure rates than do lighter women. The first study found that failures were highest in women weighing more than 154 pounds who used the lower dose formulations.[10] However, the follow-up report, which did substantiate the overall higher failure rates in heavier women, did not claim any dose-dependent relationship.[11]

A retrospective analysis of the 1997 National Health Interview survey and the 1995 National Survey of Family Growth found that the higher pregnancy rates seen in COC-users with a BMI over 30 was not statistically significant after adjustments were made for age, marital status, education, poverty level, ethnic/race, parity, dual method use, and fecundity status.[12] The hypothesis that a woman's weight may directly reduce pill efficacy was also recently challenged by the findings of a national telephone survey; compared to normal-weight pill users, obese pill users were more likely to report nonuse of their pills.[13] In the clinical trials, heavier women who used extended cycles of COCs had no increase in pregnancy risk.[14] Given this information, it would *not* be prudent to routinely prescribe high-dose COCs to heavier women, especially in view of the fact those patients are clearly at higher risk of thrombosis.[15] It may be better to decrease (or eliminate) the pill free interval for heavier women rather than to prescribe them pills with the higher dose of hormones.

COST

The cost of brand-named COCs may easily exceed $50 per month. Generic brands are typically less expensive, but may also cost $30 or more per month. Many insurance companies do not cover the costs of contraceptives as a benefit. For the systems that do provide "coverage," there is often a high co-payment, especially for the more expensive formulations. Some women are bypassing the medical system and ordering birth control pills over the internet. Researchers report that women (even higher risk patients) are able to get oral contraceptives without a prescription and conclude that the internet is "rapidly breaking down the safety barriers" between prescriber and patient.[16]

ORAL CONTRACEPTIVE FORMULATIONS

In recent years, several innovations have been introduced in pill formulations and packaging. A recent count found 71 different oral contraceptive brand names. Formulations vary not only by the type and amounts of their constituent hormones, but also by the patterns of those amounts within the pill packet. Formulations also differ in the numbers of active pills in a packet.

COCs are available in either monophasic or multiphasic packaging:

- **Monophasic formulations.** Each active (hormone-containing) pill contains the same doses of the estrogen and progestin as every other active pill.

- **Multiphasic formulations.** The amounts of hormones in the active pills vary.

  — *Biphasic* formulations have two different combinations of estrogen and progestin in the packet of pills

  — *Triphasic* formulations have three different combinations. Sometimes the progestin content increases in stepwise progression during the cycle, but some other formulations may also alter the amounts of estrogen given during the cycle. One formulation holds the progestin dose constant while increasing the estrogen content in tablets later in the cycle.

COCs are also available with different mixtures of active and placebo pills. Most pill packs contain 21 active (hormone containing) pills with or without 7 placebo pills (28-pill packs versus 21-pill packs). This pattern of 3 weeks of active pills followed by 1 week without hormones was adopted for very valid reasons early in the history of the pill. The monthly withdrawal bleed was built into pill taking to reassure women on an ongoing basis that they were not pregnant and that their reproductive systems were still working. It must be remembered that in the 1950s and early 1960s, there were no rapid or early pregnancy tests. *Seven* days without hormones were needed because with the very high dose pills of the 1960's, it took 4 to 5 days for a woman to metabolize the pill hormones and reduce her serum levels low enough to initiate endometrial shedding. In the decades following the introduction of Enovid, the doses of estrogen and progestin have been reduced to a fraction of the original doses; now serum levels drop low enough for endometrial sloughing to start 2 to 3 days after the last active pill is taken. That also means that ovarian follicle stimulation starts early during that placebo-pill week. Reducing the number of placebo pills in low dose formulations is needed to prevent recruitment of follicles.[17] There are two formulations with 24 active pills and 4 placebo pills and one formulation with 21 active pills, 2 placebo pills and 5 pills with 10 mcg EE.

Table 11–1 Common Myths that make women hesitate to use COCs

The most important **myth** to confront is that pregnancy is safe because it is "natural." The facts speak for themselves:

- 500,000 women die each year from pregnancy and pregnancy-related causes worldwide.

- Another 3 million women are severely disabled each year by pregnancy and delivery.

Other **myths** are more specific to pills:

- Pills reduce a woman's fertility even after she stops using them.

- Pills cause cancer, depression, weight gain, acne, headaches, diminished libido. . .

- Withdrawal bleeding is needed every month when using pills.

- Pills should not be used by women with any medical problems.

- Pills should not be used by any woman who smokes.

- Pills should not be used by young teens because it will stunt their growth, make them want to have sex, make them not use condoms. . .

A DVANTAGES AND INDICATIONS

Oral contraceptives provide women with safe and effective control of their fertility; they also decrease many of the menstrually-related problems that women suffer, and they provide women many general health benefits. As important as those benefits are to improving the quality of women's lives, it is astonishing that most women are unaware of them.[18] In fact, myths abound that make women hesitate to use COCs (See Table 11–1), but the demonstrated health advantages are taken for granted or go largely unnoticed.

General Advantages

1. **Effectiveness.** When taken correctly and consistently, COCs are very effective contraceptives that give women control over their own fertility.

2. **Safety.** Through prudent selection of users (see below), COCs are safer for a woman's health than are pregnancy and delivery. Recent large-scale studies show that COC use does not increase the risk of death among non-smokers.[19] Furthermore, solid evidence demonstrates that fetuses inadvertently exposed in utero to COCs are not at any increased risk for birth defects.[20,21]

3. **An option throughout the reproductive years.** Pregnancy prevention is a priority for women of all ages. Healthy women can safely use COCs throughout their reproductive lives. Age itself is not a reason to avoid COCs. Moreover, the non-contraceptive benefits of the pill address specific issues for women in different age groups. Young women benefit from reduction in severe dys-

menorrhea, primary menorrhagia, and acne, while at the other end of reproductive life, perimenopausal women often benefit from the cycle control and hot flash reduction provided by COCs.

4. **Rapid reversibility.** On average, women who stop taking COCs have only a 2-week delay in return of ovulation. Women also need to understand that COC use neither hastens nor delays the onset of menopause.

Contraceptive Health Benefits

1. **Reduction of maternal deaths.** The CDC calculated that in the United States there were 11.8 pregnancy-related deaths per 100,000 live births in the 1990s, but the CDC also recognized that there was significant under-reporting.[22] Embolism, hemorrhage, and pregnancy-induced hypertension were the three leading causes of maternal death. Considering that nearly half the pregnancies in this country are unintended, preventing those pregnancies could significantly decrease maternal deaths.

2. **Reduction of ectopic pregnancies.** COCs reduce the risk of ectopic pregnancy by over 90%.[23-25] The ectopic pregnancy rate in the United States is now estimated to be about 2% of all pregnancies; ectopic pregnancy is the leading cause of maternal death in the first trimester.

Menstrually-Related Health Benefits

1. **Decreased dysmenorrhea.** COCs significantly decrease menstrual cramps and pain. Although the original studies that demonstrated this benefit were based on high-dose formulations, low-dose formulations have also been shown to help when given in the conventional cyclic fashion.[26] COC use reduces the incidence of all degrees of dysmenorrhea by 60%.[27] The worse a woman's problems are, the more effective the pill is in reducing her symptoms. Severe dysmenorrhea is reduced by almost 90%.[28] In a randomized clinical trial, low-dose COC users reported fewer absences from school and work and used less pain relief medicine than placebo users. Even more significant relief from dysmenorrhea can be achieved by continuous or extended cycle COC use, which eliminates withdrawal periods for months.

2. **Decreased menstrual blood loss.** COCs decrease the number of days of bleeding and the amount of blood women lose each

cycle. In women with menorrhagia, high-dose COC use reduced blood loss by 53%.[29] In studies with low-dose COCs (30 mcg EE), menstrual blood loss and duration of flow were also decreased.[30] Overall, a 38% to 49% reduction in menstrual blood loss was seen in another study with a 30 mcg EE preparation.[31,32] In addition, nearly 50% of women experienced a reduction in duration of menstrual bleeding with COC use.[33] Women who use any of the extended cycle options reduce their numbers of withdrawal bleeds each year and further decrease their total menstrual blood loss. These features are particularly important for women with idiopathic menorrhagia, adenomyosis, and coagulation defects. Hormonal methods, including COCs, are also first-line therapies for treatment of menorrhagia due to fibroids.

3. **Regulations of menses**. For women using COCs cyclically, the birth control pill produces very predictable withdrawal bleeding. This predictability allows women to plan their lives around their menses, rather than having to make last minute adjustments in their schedules when their menstrual flow starts.

4. **Reduction in premenstrual syndrome (PMS) symptoms.** COCs can reduce menstruation-associated PMS symptoms such as mastalgia, cramping, and pain. Drospirenone-containing pills have also been shown to improve symptoms of water retention, bloating, negative affect, and increased appetite associated with menstruation.[34,35] Extended-cycle low-dose levonorgestrel formulations may also be more effective in reducing symptoms of PMS than is reported with selective serotonin reuptake inhibitors (SSRIs).[36]

5. **Reduction of premenstrual dysphoric disorder (PMDD).** In a randomized double-blind placebo-controlled study, one low-dose drospirenone-containing birth control pill with 24 active pills and 4 placebo pills has been shown to significantly reduce the severity and frequency symptoms of PMDD. Both physical symptoms (P< 0.001 scores) and behavioral symptoms (P=0.015) were reduced significantly more by the active treatment groups than by placebos.[37]

6. **Decreased anovulatory bleeding.** Low-dose COC use was associated with a more than 80% improvement in dysfunctional uterine bleeding in a randomized, double-blind, placebo-controlled study.[38] Anovulatory bleeding is a significant challenge for women with polycystic ovarian syndrome (PCOS), for women in the perimenopause, and for growing numbers of women with anovulatory cycles due to obesity.

7. **Mittelschmerz relief.** By preventing ovulation, COCs can eliminate the midcycle pain some women experience with ovarian follicle swelling and oocyte extrusion.

8. **Reduced risk of post-ovulatory ovarian cysts.** Because COCs suppress ovulation, women who use COCs of any dose have less risk of developing post-ovulatory luteal cysts,[39,40] including hemorrhagic corpus luteum cysts, a condition which can require emergency surgery if the cyst ruptures. However, low-dose pills taken cyclically (21/7) do not protect against follicular cyst formation,[41,42] since they do not sufficiently suppress FSH levels.[43] It is quite likely that shortening the placebo period or extending use of low-dose pills will more effectively reduce follicular ovarian cyst formation.

9. **Improvement in menstrual migraines.** Menstrual migraines are caused by estrogen withdrawal. Cyclic COC use may worsen the intensity of a woman's migraine during her menses; on the other hand, menstrual migraine symptoms may be prevented if she takes active pills every day continuously and reduces her number of withdrawal bleeds. (See the section on Headaches, in Managing Side Effects.)

General Health Benefits

1. **Ovarian cancer risk reduction.** Ovarian cancer is the most lethal gynecologic cancer because most of the 26,000 cases diagnosed each year in the United States are not detected until the women have advanced disease.[44] When compared with women who have never used COCs, COC users are 34% less likely to develop epithelial ovarian cancer. Use of monophasic formulations for at least 10 years reduces a woman's risk of developing such cancers by 80%.[45] This protection lasts for up to two decades beyond the time the woman takes her last COC.[45,46] Some studies that focus on the newer lower-dose formulations (< 35 mcg EE) have found that the lower-dose formulations protect as well as higher-dose formulations,[46] but other studies report less protection with a lower dose of progestins.[47]

A compelling argument can be made that COCs can be used to prevent cancer in high-risk women even if they do not need contraception.[48] Women with a family history of ovarian cancer enjoy a greater benefit of ovarian cancer risk reduction than do women with no family history.[49] Women with first-degree relatives with ovarian cancer who used COCs for 4 years had a 90% reduction in ovarian cancer risk.[50] Most studies have found that women with BRCA1 mutations have similar protection from ovarian cancer with COC use,[46,51] although one study found that increased duration of COC use did not reduce further the risk of ovarian cancer in BRCA1 or BRCA2 mutation carriers and cautioned against routine use of COCs for chemoprevention.[52] Longer term experience will be needed to resolve this issue.

2. **Endometrial cancer risk reduction.** COC use for at least 12 months reduces a woman's risk of developing endometrial cancer by about 40%.[53] In women who use COCs for at least a decade, the risk of developing endometrial cancer is only one fifth of that of non-pill users (an 80% reduction).[42] The protection that pills offer against endometrial cancer protection also endures for up to 20 years after COC discontinuation.[54] This feature is particularly important in women who have risk factors for developing endometrial hyperplasia and carcinoma, such as anovulatory cycling due to PCOS or obesity. The incidence of endometrial cancer is increasing in the United States because of an increasing lifespan among women and an epidemic of obesity. Over 40,000 women develop this cancer each year. Women who are 50 pounds or more overweight have almost a 10-fold increased risk of developing endometrial cancer compared to normal weight controls.

3. **Decreased risk of benign breast conditions.** COC users are less likely to develop fibrocystic breast changes, cysts, or fibroadenoma and are less likely to experience progression of those breast conditions.[55] In one case-control study with over 500 women, the risk of benign breast conditions was lower in the COC users, and markedly lower in women who started COC use before their first full-term pregnancy.[56] COC use does not reduce the risk of developing hyperplasia with atypia, but it does not increase that risk.[57]

4. **Improvement of acne and hirsutism.** Dutch surveys reported that COC use reduced the prevalence of acne by over two-thirds.[58] In prospective, randomized, placebo-controlled, double-blind trials, women who used COCs had a reduction in the numbers and size of acne lesions.[59,60] Only two formulations have received formal FDA approval for treatment of mild to moderate acne (Ortho Tri-Cyclen and Estrostep), but other formulations can be effective.[61-63] In a randomized comparative trial, women receiving a drospirenone-containing formulation for 6 cycles more effectively reduced total lesion count compared to norgestimate-containing pills.[64] A recent Cochrane review concluded that COCs in clinical trials are effective in reducing inflammatory and non-inflammatory facial acne lesions. Few differences were found in acne effectiveness between COC types.[65]

COCs reduce acne by suppressing ovarian production of testosterone, by blocking conversion of testosterone to dihydrotestosterone, and most significantly, by inducing hepatic production of sex hormone binding globulin (SHBG). SHBG binds circulating testosterone and, thereby, reduces serum concentrations of free (biologically active) testosterone by up to 50%. This decreases androgen stimulation of sebum production and reduces the substrate for acne formation. Because this action is indirect, COCs do not have an immediate impact on acne; women need to be advised that maximal effect may not be seen for up to 6 months.[59,60] There is some residual beneficial effect of COCs; SHBG levels may remain elevated for several months after discontinuation of COCs.[66]

Just as estrogen in COCs helps reduce androgen activation of sebum production, it also helps reduce that hormone's stimulation of androgen-sensitive (sexual) hair growth. Women with excessive facial or body hair (hirsutism) have a reduction in the hair shaft diameter with COC use.[67,68] The time course of this beneficial impact is also slow; it generally takes 1 to 2 years to see the maximal beneficial effect of COCs on hirsutism. In these situations, the most appropriate formations will be those with progestins with low androgen impact and high-dose estrogens.

5. **Reduced risk of hospitalization for gonorrheal pelvic inflammatory disease (PID).** COCs may reduce the risk that a gonorrheal infection in a woman's cervix will ascend into the cavity of the uterus (endometritis), fallopian tubes (salpingitis), or other pelvic organs (PID). In studies conducted in the 1980s (when fewer women with PID were treated on an outpatient basis), the risk of hospitalization for PID was reduced by 50% to 60% in current users after 12 months of COC use.[69] The exact mechanism of this protection is not known. It may be due to thickened cervical mucus blocking sperm penetration or to atrophy of the endometrium (fewer days of bleeding). Alternatively, COCs may suppress expression of inflammatory symptoms, thus creating a higher proportion of "silent" PID. COCs do not reduce the risk of chlamydial PID.[70]

6. **Reducing symptoms of endometriosis.** Current or recent COC use is associated with a lower incidence of symptomatic endometriosis, especially among parous women (see Chapter 20, Menstrual Problems and Common Gynecologic Concerns).[71] The risk of developing endometriomas has also been found to be significantly reduced in current COC users over the age of 25.[72] COCs reduce menstrual flow and presumably decrease the volume of retrograde menses, which is generally believed to be the primary

cause of endometriosis. Extended or continuous use of progestogenic COCs induces pseudo-decidualization of the endometriotic implants and reduces symptoms during use.[73] Such treatment is not curative, however; the implants undergo atrophy during treatment but remain ready for reactivation whenever COCs are stopped.[74]

7. **Decrease risk of iron deficiency anemia.** By reducing menstrual blood loss, each cycle of COC use conserves women's hemoglobin and ferritin levels.[75] This benefit is especially important for women with sickle cell anemia or Von Willebrand disease, women using anticoagulants or anticonvulsants, and women with fibroids or other causes of primary or secondary menorrhagia (see Chapter 20, Menstrual Problems). Obviously, this benefit is maximized by extended-cycle use of COCs.

8. **Treatment of hot flashes and other hormonal fluctuation symptoms** in perimenopausal women.[76,77] (See Chapter 26 on Menopause for more discussion.)

Other Potential Health Benefits

1. **Reduced risk of uterine fibroids.** COC users have fewer fibroids, especially with long-term use,[78] but COC use early in life may increase risk of fibroid formation.[79] COCs are often prescribed to help women control the excess menstrual blood loss that leiomyomas can cause. In fact, many insurance carriers require that women with moderate-sized fibroids must fail a trial of medical management (usually with COCs) for menorrhagia before they can be considered for surgical therapies.

2. **Favorable impact on bone for high-risk women.** Women who have hypothalamic amenorrhea have low levels of circulating estrogens and are at risk for osteoporosis and, possibly, for fractures later in life. COC use increases bone mineral density (BMD) in young women with hypothalamic amenorrhea[80] and in anorexic teenagers.[81] COC use by women with osteopenia due to anorexia nervosa is not sufficient to completely protect bone, but when added to anabolic agents such as insulin growth factor (IGF), COC use significantly improves that agent's effectiveness.[82] COC use also modulates the negative impact of smoking in young women and improves BMD in young women with irregular menses.[83]

For women with normal estrogen levels, the effect of COCs on bone density is less clear. Studies in postmenopausal women who previously had used high dose COC have shown a lower risk for postmenopausal hip fractures,[84] increased BMD especially in the lumbar spine,[85] and a slight reduction in osteoporosis.[86] In contrast, one prospective study of euestrogenic COC users reported an increased risk of fracture.[86] However, a comprehensive review of 13 studies of low-dose COCs use found that 9 studies showed favorable impact on BMD, and 4 were neutral.[87] Review of self reports of participants in the Women's Health Initiative revealed that past COC use for less than 5 years was associated with a slight increase in the adjusted risk for fracture, but women who had 5 years or more of COC use had no statistically significant difference in fractures from newer users.[88] Newer data from a study of nearly 65,000 women with fractures found that low-dose COC use was not associated with an increase or a decrease in fracture risk.[89]

The WHO concluded that adolescent COC users may gain less BMD than adolescent non-users while perimenopausal COC users generally have higher BMD compared to age-matched non-users.[90]

3. **Fewer episodes of sickle cell crises and catamenial seizures, porphyria, and asthma.**   Sickle cell crises are cut in half by COC use.[91] Extended cycle and continuous use of COCs can significantly reduce menstrual exacerbations of seizure disorders, porphyria, and asthma attacks.

4. **Influence on sexual enjoyment.**   There is considerable controversy about the impact of COCs on sexual enjoyment, because sexuality is complex. Sexual appetite and enjoyment are affected by virtually everything in a woman's life. Reducing a woman's risk of pregnancy can permit her to enjoy the encounter. However, some have suggested that the same mechanism by which COCs decrease a woman's acne and hirsutism—increased SHBG and reduced circulating levels of biologically active testosterone—might decrease COC users' desire for sexual activity. One study, which found that SHBG remained elevated for several months after women discontinued COCs, concluded that pills have a persistent negative effect on sexual pleasure.[66] This study made headlines for months in women's magazines. Interestingly, a study that directly measured sexual satisfaction of users of the least androgenic COC formulation found that, compared to their baseline, women using that COC had significant improvement in sexual enjoyment, sexual satisfaction, and orgasm frequency. Longer term use also was associated with significant increases in arousal and frequency of sexual activity. Sexual desire (libido) remained unchanged.[92]

5. **Other Benefits.**   Although early studies suggested that COC use was associated with a reduced risk of rheumatoid arthritis

(RA), controversy still exists about this benefit. One meta-analysis suggested that instead of protecting against the condition, COC use slowed progression of RA,[93] and a later metaanalysis found no protective effect.[94] Some studies have shown that COC use may improve lung mechanics.[95] Some have shown that women who have used COCs may have a reduced risk for developing colorectal cancer later in life.[95] Some formulations have added vitamins to their placebo pills: Iron has been added to reduce anemia, and folate has been added to the placebo pills in other COC formulations to reduce the risk of neural tube defects in offspring.

NON-CONTRACEPTIVE APPLICATIONS FOR COCS

After underlying pathology has been ruled out, oral contraceptives are first line therapy for otherwise healthy women who suffer from the following conditions, even if they are not at risk for pregnancy:

- Menorrhagia (heavy bleeding), dysmenorrhea (painful menses), or oligomenorrhea (few periods)
- Dysfunctional uterine bleeding
- Recurrent luteal phase ovarian cysts
- Family history of ovarian cancer
- Personal risk factors for endometrial cancer
- Acne or hirsutism
- Polycystic ovary syndrome (PCOS)

In addition, *extended use* COC may be particularly helpful for women with

- Dysmenorrhea
- Menstrually related PMS symptoms
- PMDD
- Pain from endometriosis
- Anemia due to menorrhagia
- Mentally challenged women whose monthly menstruations terrify them and present a hygiene challenge to their caregivers
- Hypothalamic amenorrhea from athletic triad or isolated eating disorders
- Personal preference

Finally, if Plan B is not available for emergency contraception, COCs with levonorgestrel or norgestrel may be used. Some studies suggest that COCs with norethindrone may be used for emergency contraception if norgestrel-related compounds are not available, but they have slightly higher pregnancy rates (see Chapter 6 on Emergency Contraception).[96]

DISADVANTAGES AND HEALTH COMPLICATIONS

Even for healthy women, COC use can impose certain demands, cause rare complications, or result in side effects. Counsel women about these possibilities before they decide to use COCs.

GENERAL DISADVANTAGES

1. **Daily administration.** Inconsistent or incorrect use of COCs reduces protection from pregnancy and increases the incidence of side effects, such as unscheduled bleeding and spotting.

2. **Expense and access.** In most states, insurance plans are not required to cover contraception, so women must pay out of pocket for their COCs. Often, the number of packets provided is severely restricted, so women are required to return to pharmacies each month to purchase another package. The mismatch between calendar months with 30 to 31 days and pill packs with only 28 pills can present challenges in use. Women who desire to use extended cycles of pills are faced with more difficulties in obtaining adequate pill supplies if they cannot get extended-cycle, brand-named products with adequate numbers of active pills.

3. **Need for storage and ready access.** Adolescent women and older women whose partners do not want them to use contraception may not have a place to store their pills. Practitioners need to confirm that the woman's plans for storage are realistic (school lockers are not an answer) and guide them to more private contraceptive methods, if needed. Homeless women and women who travel extensively may have difficulty storing their pill packs.

4. **No protection against sexually transmitted infections (STIs).** Women at risk for STIs may use COCs, but they should be advised that birth control pills do not provide them protection from those infections. They need to reduce their risk for STIs by confining their sexual activity to mutually monogamous,

uninfected partners, or by using condoms with every act of coitus.

HEALTH COMPLICATIONS

Despite the wide range of health benefits associated with pill use, much attention has been focused in the public eye on possible health risks associated with COC use. To put the pill's potential relative risks into perspective, remind women that pregnancy carries with it considerable health risks, especially for women with health problems. Always compare the risks associated with pill use with the risks associated with pregnancy. Add non-contraceptive benefits into the equation before deciding if a woman is a candidate for a birth control pill.

In counseling women about potential risks associated with COC use, it is important to understand some fundamental statistical concepts.

- *Relative risk* represents the ratio of the probability that a complication will arise with pill use compared to the probability that the complication will arise without pill use. Mathematically, this is written:

$$RR = \frac{\text{Probability of developing condition X with pill use}}{\text{Probability of developing condition X without pill use}}$$

A relative risk of 1 means that pill use does not affect the risk one way (increase) or the other (decrease). Because pill use has no effect on eye color, the relative risk of having blue eyes with pill use would be 1.0. However, if some event happens more often in pill users than in non pill users, the relative risk will be greater than 1. If pill use reduces the risk of an event, the relative risk will be less than one. For example, the relative risk of developing ovarian cancer after 10 years of COC use is 0.2, which means that long-term COC users have an 80% reduction in their risk of getting ovarian cancer. If there is only a slight increase in risk (RR=1.10 (a 10% increase)), the clinical significance is generally small unless the problem is very common or very serious. The odds ratio (OR) and the hazard ratio (HR) represent similar calculations and should be interpreted as a relative risk in clinical settings.

- *The absolute risk* of an event happening is also important to note. Even if the relative risk is very high, the absolute risk of a complication may still be low if the background risk in the population is low. For example, the relative risk of developing benign liver tumors with COC use is 500. This risk appears to be enormous until you understand that this is such a rare tumor that the chance that a COC user will develop liver tumors (the absolute risk) is only 1 in 50,000. A large multiple of a rare event is still a rare event.

- The *attributable* risk reflects how much using pills changes a woman's risk from her background risk. Health problems (like headaches) happen to women whether or not they take pills. The attributable risk is what a woman needs to know—how much more or less often she is apt to have headaches because she is using the pill.

Putting this all together, one study of breast cancer risk reported that young women faced a doubling of the risk of breast cancer if they used birth control pills before their first pregnancy.[97] In statistical terms, the *relative* risk for young women using COCs was 2.0. This sounds very frightening. However, breast cancer in women under age 35 is very rare; the background risk is 1 in 1,000.[98] Therefore, the *absolute* risk of developing breast cancer with COC use would be 1 in 500 (2 times 1:1,000). However, not all of that risk is due to the pill; half of it is the baseline risk a woman faces even if she does not take the pill. The *attributable* risk (the risk due to taking the pills) is only 1 in 1,000. When women understand that the risk they face from taking the pill is that rare, pill use seems far less frightening.

- One final statistical principle is useful: the confidence interval. Studies will report both a relative risk and the confidence interval. This is important because the relative risk calculated in a study is only an estimate. Studies are based on samples of women. No one study ever reflects the experience of every woman in the world. So when researchers calculate the relative risk for the women in their study, they also calculate (based on how many subjects were involved in the study and how similar the experiences of those women were) the limits in which the true answer could fall if all the women in the world were studied. The 95% Confidence Interval (95% CI) says that 95 times out of 100, the real answer lies between the 2 numbers quoted. For example, when a study of pills reports that RR = 1.5 (95% CI = 1.2 – 1.7), the reader would know that the event among the study's participants is 50% more likely to occur with pills than without them. However, the study also calculates with 95% confidence that the real risk lies somewhere between a 20% to 70% increase. There is one important rule to remember when interpreting the confidence interval: a relative risk is significant only if both confidence interval numbers reflect the same answer, either an increase or a decrease in risk. Mathematically, if the confidence interval includes the number 1, the relative risk is not significant and should not change practice. For example, if a study reports RR = 2.5 (95% CI = 0.7 – 4.8), the researchers are saying that the women in their study were 2.5 times more likely to have this complication when they used pills compared to women who did not use pills. However, they estimate that the real answer is that the complication may occur 30% less often with pills or 4.8 times more frequently. Obviously, since the study could not determine whether the complication increased or decreased with pill use, it should not alter anyone's clinical practice.

1. **Pregnancy.** COC users have no higher rates of spontaneous abortion, preterm delivery, birth defects, or compromise of fertility in their offspring than non-users.[99-104] The risk of significant congenital anomalies with in utero exposure to COCs is no higher than in the general population. No extra testing during prenatal care is needed because of early pregnancy exposure to steroidal hormones. Women should consider all their pregnancy options (keeping the baby, adoption, foster care, and abortion) based on their own personal situations; fetal exposure to COC hormones should not influence that decision process.

2. **Myocardial infarction (MI).** Early pills with higher doses of estrogen were associated with an increased risk of arterial thrombosis and heart attacks, but lower dose formulations have a different effect. A pivotal U.S. study showed that low-dose COCs (< 50mcg EE) do not significantly increase the risk of MI or stroke in healthy, non-smoking women.[105] Compared to never-users, current users as a group had a relative risk of 1.3 for MI; however, most of the increased risk was seen in women with known risk factors. Two other subsequent studies supported those findings.[106,107] A 2003 meta-analysis demonstrated that current use of all doses of COCs increased the overall risk of MI by 2.48 times, but that risk dropped to 1.97 for preparations with 30 to 49 mcg EE while pills with 20 mcg EE did not increase the risk of MI.[108] The risks for MI increase with age, but are greatly magnified by the combination of age, smoking, and hypertension (see Table 11–2). COC use in women with uncontrolled hypertension increased the risk of MI and ischemic stroke significantly, especially if the women also smoked.[109,110] The attributable risk of death from MI with COC use is very low; estimates are that it occurs in only 4 women per million among non-smoking women age 20 to 24, and 10 women per million among same age smokers who use COCs.[111]

The increased risk of MI in COC users who smoke has been reaffirmed by every study. However, these risks are reversible. Once women over 40 have stopped smoking or using nicotine-containing products for 3 to 12 months, they may be candidates for

Table 11–2 Age-specific estimates of attributable MI deaths due to low-dose COC use per 1 million users in international studies: the effect of smoking and hypertension

| | MI Risk per 1 Million Users | | |
| | Age Range (years) | | |
Risk Category	20–24	30–34	4–44
Healthy nonsmokers	4	6	20
With smoking	10	20	200
With hypertension	100	120	450

Modified from Farley TM, et al. (1998).[113]

COC use. The older the woman, the more cigarettes she smoked, the longer the wash out period must be.

The risk of COC-related MI posed by controlled hypertension is more controversial. International studies have demonstrated marked increases in rate of MI in women with hypertension (Table 11–2), but most of the women in those studies had blood pressures that were not well controlled. Carefully monitor blood pressure in hypertensive women using COCs, because one study found that COC users being treated for hypertension had poor control of their blood pressure.[112]

There was early evidence that third generation progestins might be associated with a lower risk of myocardial infarction compared to second generation formulations.[108] However, those conclusions were based on limited numbers of cases, which makes their interpretation difficult. This is particularly true in light of the convincing evidence that there is *no* increase in the incidence of MIs in healthy young COC users.

Several other findings about COC use and cardiovascular disease are reassuring. There is no increase in the risk of MI with increasing duration of use.[114] Past COC users have no increased risk of MI due to their prior COC use.

The increase in heart attacks seen with use of COCs is due to arterial thrombosis caused by estrogen. Therefore, women with serious risk factors for MI who may not be able to use COCs may still be candidates for progestin-only methods.

3. **Stroke.** Cerebrovascular disease is rare in young reproductive-age women, but becomes more common in women in their 40s. There are two different types of stroke—ischemic and hemorrhagic. Each type has a different etiology and somewhat different risk factors to consider when prescribing COCs. Older higher dose pill formulations consistently reported increases in

the risk of both types of strokes. However, lower dose formulations have significantly less risk. A study of the Kaiser membership found that low-dose COC use by healthy women did not affect their risk of stroke.[115]

Women with risk factors including smoking, hypertension, diabetes, overweight/obesity, and lower socioeconomic status, are at higher baseline risk for *ischemic stroke*. The U.S. and European WHO reports from studies with sub-50 mcg EE formulations found no increase risk for ischemic stroke. However, in studies in developing countries where women are *not* screened for hypertension, there was a 3-fold increased risk of ischemic stroke, regardless of the dose of estrogen. Smoking more than 10 cigarettes a day raised the stroke risk to about the same levels as hypertension and COC use. The risk for ischemic stroke was greatest in women over age 35, which was also thought to be due to undiagnosed hypertension. Women with hypertension who use COCs have three times the risk of ischemic stroke as do COC users without hypertension.[116,117] Similarly, the risk of ischemic stroke is about 15 to 20 times higher in smokers compared to nonsmokers.[116] WHO studies also found a significant increase in the risk of ischemic stroke, but not hemorrhagic stroke, among COC users who experienced migraine with aura (odds ratio 3.0, 95% CI 1.3–11.3) and a nonsignificant increase in COC users who reported migraine without aura (OR 3.0, 95% CI 0.7–14.8) (see Headache section in Managing Side Effects, below).[118] A typical aura lasts 5 to 60 minutes before the headache and is visual. The WHO panel stated that migraineurs with aura have a higher risk of stroke than those without aura, but no study had sufficient proof to examine risk of stroke by type of migraine.[119]

The important risk factors for *hemorrhagic stroke* are aging, hypertension, and smoking, but other factors such as obesity and heavy alcohol use are also important. The risk of hemorrhagic stroke increases 10-fold in COC users with hypertension compared to non-hypertensive users.[120] The WHO study on hemorrhagic stroke found that current use of COCs raised the risk of hemorrhagic stroke only in developing countries, where blood pressure could not be monitored. The risk of hemorrhagic stroke in women who smoke is about double that of nonsmokers.[120] Smokers who use COCs may have up to triple the risk of stroke compared to nonsmoking non users.

COC package inserts state, "The relative risk of hemorrhagic stroke is reported to be 1.2 for nonsmokers who used oral contraceptives, 2.6 for smokers who did not use oral contraceptives, 7.6 for smokers who used oral contraceptives, 1.8 for normotensive users, and 25.7 for users with severe hypertension. The attributable risk is also greater in older women."[121] There is no apparent increase in the risk of either type of stroke with increasing duration of COC use[122] or with past use of COCs.[120] There are insufficient data to make conclusions about how the type or dose of progestin might influence the risk of stroke.[123] COC use does not affect the risk of subarachnoid hemorrhage.[124]

4. **Venous thromboembolism** (VTE). VTE can be a life-threatening condition; 200,000 new cases are diagnosed in the United States each year. Two thirds of VTE cases are deep vein thromboses (DVTs); DVT carries a 6% mortality rate. One third of VTEs events involve pulmonary embolism (PE), which has a 12% mortality rate. Although frequently treated after surgery, 70% to 80% of fatal PE's occur in nonsurgical patients. Risk factors for venous thrombosis include obesity, previous venous compromise, and immobilization. VTE can develop in a variety of organs and present with different symptoms as listed on Table 11–3.

Older estimates of VTE prevalence are listed in Table 11–4. The risk of VTE varies greatly by age. In a Swedish study of women undergoing venography, the incidence of thrombosis per 10,000 women was 0.5 for women under 20; 1.1 for women 20 to 29 years; 2.6 for women 30 to 39 and 9.7 for women 40 to 49.[125] In addition, obesity increases the risk of thrombosis. For these reasons, ACOG advises caution in the use of estrogen-containing

Table 11–3 Thrombotic diseases attributable to COCs (See ACHES below)

ACHES	Diagnosis	Location of Pathology	Symptoms
A (Abdominal pain)	Mesenteric vein thrombosis	Intestines	Abdominal pain, vomiting, weakness
	Pelvic vein thrombosis	Pelvis	Lower abdominal pain, cramps
C (Chest pain)	Pulmonary embolism	Lung	Cough (including coughing up blood), chest pain, shortness of breath
	Myocardial infarction	Heart	Crushing chest pain, left arm and shoulder pain, shortness of breath, weakness
H (Headaches)	Stroke	Brain	Headache, weakness or numbness, visual problem, sudden intellectual impairment
E (Eye problems)	Retinal vein thrombosis	Eye	Headache, complete or partial loss of vision
S (Severe leg pain)	Thrombophlebitis	Leg	Swelling, heat or redness, tenderness in thigh or lower leg; calf pains

Table 11–4 Classic estimates of venous thromboembolism per 100,000 women years

	Incidence	Relative Risk
Young women—general population	4–5	1
Pregnant women	48–60	12
COC *with* 50 or more mcg EE	24–60	6–10
COC with less than 50 mcg EE	12–20	3–4

Speroff L, Fritz M. (2005).[128]

methods in obese women (BMI>30) who are over age 35.[241] High-dose COCs were associated with VTE risks that were 6 to 15 times higher (24 to 60 events per 100,000) than general population.[126,127] VTE risks with COC use consistently decreased with every drop in the estrogen content of COCs until the introduction of sub-50 mcg EE formulations, when the incidence of VTE dropped to 12 to 20 cases per 100,000 women years. There is no validated proof that EE doses lower than 35 mcg a day have less VTE risk than 35 mcg formulations.

Even though the relative risk of thrombosis with COCs is increased, COC users face a low absolute risk of thrombosis because VTE is a rare event. The risk of thrombosis is greatest in the first year of COC use, but a slightly elevated risk persists with continued COC use. The risk of VTE associated with COC use does not change with tobacco use,[129] varicose veins, or hypertension. Past COC users have no increased risk of VTE; the risk of thrombosis usually disappears 30 days after COC discontinuation.

VTE risks have been greatly diminished by both the significant reduction in estrogen dose in pills and more careful evaluation of potential COC candidates. Offsetting these safety measures, however, has been a steady increase in obesity in the United States, use of COCs by older women, and frequent use of noninvasive imaging studies to diagnose VTE in mildly symptomatic women. The impact of obesity is significant. In one large U.S. study comparing the risk of VTE in COC users with a BMI less than 25, it was found that the relative risk was 1.78 in COC users with BMIs between 25 and 30 and the relative risk was 3.47 with a BMI greater than 30.[130] All of these factors have increased the occurrence and detection of VTEs in COC users (see Table 11–5). Recent analyses have also been done to update the estimates of the risk of thrombosis in pregnancy (see Table 11–6).

Progestins alone have virtually no impact on the clotting system, but when combined with estrogen they can modulate estrogen's

Table 11–5 Rates of non-fatal VTEs per 100,000 women-years with low dose (sub 50 mcg EE) COCs: 2006 estimates

Types of Progestins	% of Rise in Pregnancy*	Rates (95% CI)
Levonorgestrel-containing COCs	22.0%	27.1 (21.1–34.3)
Norgestrel-containing COCs	24.9%	30.6 (25.3–36.5)
Desogestrel-containing COCs	43,5%	53.5 (42.9–66.0)

Source: Jick SS, et al. (2006).[131]

* Based on pregnancy rates of 123/100,000 woman-years

actions. In the mid 1990s, international studies indicated that pills containing the progestins desogestrel and gestodene (not available in the United States) may be associated with higher rates of thrombosis (up to 2-fold increase) compared to formulations containing levonorgestrel and norgestrel.[133–135] U.S. labeling reflects these findings. There has been controversy about the validity of those findings since it has been shown that there were confounding factors such as duration of use, selection bias (healthy user effect), and detection biases that may have accounted for the observed increase in VTE risk. Cerebral venous sinus thrombosis, which is a very rare event with an etiology similar to DVT, has been reported to occur at rates in the third-generation progestins that have no statistically significant difference from rates in second-generation progestins.[242] The fourth-generation progestin, drospirenone, has antiandrogenic effects; therefore, it may also allow fuller expression of estrogen's thrombotic impact.[136]

Norgestimate was not included in the early international studies, but was implicated in a subsequent transnational study.[137] As part of the evaluation of the impact the transdermal patch may have on VTE risk, an epidemiologic study of a database for managed care systems was conducted which compared the rates of nonfatal VTE with 30 mcg EE with levonorgestrel, 30 mcg EE with desogestrel (monophasic and triphasic formulations) and a 35 mcg EE with norgestimate between the years 2000 and 2005.

Table 11–6 Rates of VTE per 100,000 women-years in pregnancy: 2005 estimates

Pregnancy	123
Postpartum	320
Pregnancy in thrombophilia	4,000
Pregnancy with prior VTE	11,000

Romero A, et al. (2005).[132]

The rates shown on Table 11–5 support the findings that desogestrel was associated with higher thrombosis, but was still lower than rates in pregnancy.[131]

To understand the mechanisms by which estrogen-rich states, such as COC use and pregnancy increase the risk of VTE, it is helpful to understand the basic balance that maintains the body's ability to form clots when needed but to avoid inappropriate clot formation. Schematically, this is a four-way balance between clot forming factors (fibrinogen, Factors VII, IX and X) and factors that block clot formation (antithrombin III, Protein C and Protein S) as well as the balance between factors that organize the clot (plasminogen, plasminogen activator inhibitor-1) and those that lyse clots (tissue plasminogen activator, antiplasmin). Clinically significant VTE occurs when there is imbalance between these opposing forces. Estrogen increases hepatic production of elements that promote clot formation by the extrinsic clotting system (Factor VII, Factor VIII, Factor X) and elements that promote clot lysis. COC users also develop an increased resistance to anticoagulant effect of activated protein C. The net result is a prothrombotic effect.

The increase in VTE risk seen with COC use is greatly magnified in the face of genetic thrombogenic mutation disorders such as factor V Leiden mutation or Protein S and C synthesis disorders, in which the factors that inhibit thrombosis are deficient. The factor V Leiden mutation alone explains 30% of all deep venous thromboses. In the United States, it is estimated that 5.3% of Caucasians, 2.2% of Hispanics, 1.2% of Blacks and Native Americans, and 0.5% of Asians carry this factor V mutation. The WHO review of literature reported that COC users with factor V Leiden mutations were 6.4 to 99.0 times more likely to form venous blood clots than were nonusers without the mutation.[138] Genetic mutations in prothrombin also increase VTE risks. When a carrier uses COCs, her VTE risk rises 100 times higher than non-affected non COC users.[139] The relative risks for VTE with deficiencies in antithrombin, protein C, and protein S are 8 to 10, with an absolute risk of 120 to 150/100,000 a year.[140] (For further discussion, see section on Patient Selection.)

5. **Hypertension.** COCs increase circulating levels of angiotensinogen. Some women are very sensitive to angiotensinogen metabolites (angiotensin II), which can increase both their diastolic and systolic blood pressures. Most women compensate for the increase in angiotensinogen by decreasing plasma renin concentrations. Both estrogen and progestin enhance aldosterone activity, which results in fluid retention, which, in turn also contributes to

an increase in blood pressure. Most studies find no increase in clinically significant hypertension with the use of low-dose pills, although a 3 to 5 mm rise is not uncommon.[141,142] However, one study found that elevated blood pressured occurred in 41.5 cases per 10,000 COC users.[141] Women who experience hypertension attributable to COC use will normalize their blood pressures within 3 to 6 months of stopping estrogen-containing contraceptives. The women whose readings do not return to normal should undergo a standard work-up; most will be found to have essential hypertension. Women with significantly elevated hypertension may need to begin antihypertensive agents as well as to discontinue COCs immediately.

6. **Glucose intolerance and diabetes.** COCs currently available in the United States do not have any clinically significant adverse affect on carbohydrate metabolism and do not produce an increase in diabetes.[143,144] Older COC formulations with high doses of sex steroids had a more profound impact on glucose tolerance and in some instances resulted in hyperglycemia with hyperinsulinemia. By contrast, in the CARDIA study, current use of modern COCs was associated with lower glucose levels and with a lower odds ratio of diabetes.[145] Concerns have been raised about COC use in women at risk for developing diabetes because progesterone is a competitive inhibitor of the insulin receptor and estrogen influences the release of insulin from the pancreatic islet cells and decreases insulin sensitivity.[146] However, women with a history of gestational diabetes who used COCs with low progestin content had no higher risk of developing glucose intolerance or overt diabetes compared to controls who used non-hormonal methods when both groups were studied for up to 7 years.[147]

7. **Gallbladder disease.** Recent studies of low-dose COCs are not associated with the increased risk of cholelithiasis and cholecystitis that had been seen earlier with high-dose COCs. However, it may still be possible that low-dose COCs accelerate the development of symptomatic gallbladder disease in women with pre-existing gallstones or sludge. COCs do not increase the risk of gallbladder cancer.[148]

8. **Cholestatic jaundice.** Active transport of bile can be impaired by high-dose COCs, resulting in cholestatic jaundice with pruritus. This condition reverses with discontinuation of hormones. The incidence in the general population using low-dose formulations is not known but is assumed to be very rare.

9. **Hepatic neoplasms.** Benign liver tumors have been associated with the use of high-dose COCs, especially with long-term use.

Focal nodular hyperplasia may be increased nearly 3-fold in COC users.[149] Adenomas are the most clinically significant neoplasia, since they can cause rupture of the liver capsule, extensive intraperitoneal hemorrhage, and even death. Women may or may not have abdominal pain with adenomas; their liver function tests are usually normal. Palpate the liver edge as part of the annual physical exam. If the liver is enlarged or tender, discontinue COCs and evaluate with MRI or CT tests; ultrasound is not reliable. Tumor regression is expected after stopping COCs.

Hepatocellular carcinoma risk is not increased with low-dose COC use.[150] Use of hormonal contraception by high-risk women (with chronic hepatitis B virus) does not appear to increase the risk of hepatocellular carcinoma, but use may increase the risk in a low-risk population.

10. **Risks for acquiring STIs.**   The recent WHO review of the literature concluded that women who use COCs are at increased risk for acquiring Chlamydia cervicitis, although the authors noted that nearly all the studies failed to adjust for confounders, had relatively small sample sizes, and were given a "poor" quality rating. The pooled odds ratio was 2.9 (95% CI, 1.86 – 4.55).[151] A previous meta-analysis had concluded that women using oral contraceptives maybe more likely to have cervical ectopy and that women with cervical ectopy may be more likely to acquire chlamydial infection.[152] However, a prospective study found that cervical ectopy is a risk factor for cervicitis, but the presence of cervical ectopy did not change the association between COC use and cervicitis.[153] This suggests that cervical ectopy may make the detection of chlamydial infection easier.[154]

COC use does not increase a woman's risk for infection with gonorrhea, trichomoniasis, herpes, or syphilis.[151] The data on HPV susceptibility is less certain. Review of cross-sectional studies found no evidence for a strong association between ever using COCs and having HPV infection.[155] Two subsequent prospective studies had conflicting results. One study of college students found a slight increase in HPV infection risk (HR = 1.4; 95% CI 1.01 – 1.8),[156] while a study of a broader age group (18 to 49 years) found no such association, (OR = 0.7; 95% CI 0.2 – 2.0) after adjusting for risky sexual behavior.[157]

Theoretical concerns have previously been raised about COC use increasing the consequences of STIs. COCs influence transcription of natural antimicrobials in the human endometrium, which might increase a woman's vulnerability to upper-tract chlamydia or HIV infection.[158] The question of HIV susceptibility and COC use has now been answered by carefully designed clinical trials. HIV-uninfected women who used either COCs or injectable progestins for contraception were not at any significantly increased risk of acquiring HIV compared to women who used other methods. After reviewing the data, neither the WHO nor the International Planned Parenthood Federation (IPPF) has changed its current recommendations regarding hormonal contraceptive use.[159]

To reduce risks for STIs, women should choose to be sexually active with one uninfected, monogamous partner or, at a minimum, use latex or polyurethane condoms with every act of vaginal or rectal intercourse and should consider condom use with oral-genital contact too.

11. **Melanoma.** A pooled analysis of 10 case-control studies involving nearly 2,400 cases of melanoma revealed no correlation between COC use and the development of melanoma. No effect of duration of use or current use was observed.[160] However, it is recommended that women with a history of melanoma refrain from getting pregnant or using hormonal contraception for at least 3 years after their original therapy, since the risk of recurrence is highest at this time.

12. **Leiomyoma** (uterine fibroids) contain both estrogen and progesterone receptors. Since fibroids often shrink after menopause, when estrogen levels decrease, it has been suggested that estrogen-containing contraceptives might increase the growth of these benign uterine tumors. However, clinical studies with low-dose COCs have found no impact on the risk of developing new fibroids or increasing the size of pre-existing fibroids[161–163] except in women who used COCs early in life.[79] In fact, COCs are often used to control excessive menstrual bleeding caused by fibroids.

13. **Cervical dysplasia and cervical carcinoma.** Cervical dysplasia and cervical carcinoma are caused by the human papillomavirus (HPV), especially the subtypes HPV 16 and 18. In one study, women who used COCs for more than 5 years and who were infected with HPV had a 3- to 4-fold increased risk for in situ and invasive squamous cell cervical carcinoma.[164] A large meta-analysis of 28 studies including 12,531 women with cervical cancer found RR 1.1 after 5 years of COC use, RR 1.6 after 5 to 10 years, and RR 2.2 more than 10 years (see Table 11–7).[165] However, this COC-associated risk is lower than with high parity. For example, women with HPV infection who had 7 or more pregnancies had higher RR (8.29) for cervical cancer. Pregnancy before 18 years of age increases the relative risk (RR) for cervical cancer to 10.71.[166] Studies demonstrate that COC use may in-

Table 11–7 COC Use and Cancer Risk

Cancer Type	# of Cases in US—2006	Impact of COC Use on Risk of Carcinoma				
		Significant Decrease	Some Decrease	Neutral	Some Increase	Significant Increase
Ovarian	20,180					
COC users < 5 yrs			X			
COC use ≥ 5 yrs		X				
Endometrial	41,200					
COC use < 1 yr			X			
COC use ≥ 1 yr		X				
Cervical	7,916					
COC use < 5 yrs				X		
COC use ≥ 5 yrs[1]					X	
Breast	212,920					
Age < 35					X	
Age ≥ 35				X		
Hepatic[2]	5,910			X		
Gallbladder	4,850			X		
Melanoma	27,930			X		

[1] No increased risk unless patient persistently infected with HR-HPV

[2] Increased risk, even in Hepatitis B virus carriers

crease the risk of cervical adenocarcinoma (cancer of the "glandular" cells of the cervix).[167] COC use may be associated with artifacts that mimic ASC-US (glycogen vacuoles create perinuclear halos in COC users) on liquid-based cytology tests. Reflex high-risk HPV testing will demonstrate that two-thirds of those women have no virus.[168]

Despite this slight increase in risk, even long-term COC users do not need to have cervical cytology testing performed more frequently than required by their other risk factors. Similarly, women do not need to be screened with more sensitive tests just because they use COCs.

14. **Breast cancer.** The risk of breast cancer in current users of COCs was evaluated by a meta-analysis in 1996 by the Collaborative Group on Hormone Factor in Breast Cancer, which found a 24% increased risk. The cancers diagnosed in COC users were more localized and, therefore, more curable. This same study confirmed that this increased risk was transient and reversible; after COCs were discontinued, the risk declined steadily and re-

turned to baseline within 10 years.[169] Subsequent studies have shed more light on the role age and hormone dose may have had on this estimate. Studies of daughters and granddaughters of women diagnosed with breast cancer found that women who took pills before 1978 (higher dose formulations) were at a modestly increased risk for developing breast cancer; however, those who had pills after 1978 (lower dose formulations) were at no higher risk.[170] Age is also an important factor. The CDC study found that among high-dose COC users, only women who used high potency progestin pills and started using COCs at a young age before their first pregnancy were at any higher risk for developing breast cancer.[97] Long-term findings published after the 1996 metaanalysis found that current and past COC users age 35 to 64 were at no higher risk for developing breast cancer than non-users.[171] Subsequent meta-analyses and subgroup analyses have caught media attention but add little to change our counseling of women using modern low-dose COCs.[243] Even if there were a slight increase in risk in women under age 35, breast cancer is so rare in women in that age group that these are very reassuring findings about the safety of low dose COCs. Several studies of high-risk women (BRCA1 or BRCA2 mutations or a strong family history of breast cancer) showed no increased risk of breast cancer if they used COCs.[244,245]

15. **Decreased libido.** Studies have reported conflicting results. Some women have reported reduced libido,[172] while others have reported enhanced enjoyment.[173,174] See 'Influence on sexual enjoyment section,' above, for more details.

16. **Hyperkalemia for drospirenone-containing COCs.** Drospirenone has antimineralocorticoid activity, which introduces the potential for hyperkalemia in high-risk patients; the 3 mg of drospirenone found in Yasmin has the same impact on electrolytes as a 25 mg dose of spironolactone. Chronic use of ACE inhibitors, angiotensin-II receptor antagonists, potassium-sparing diuretics, heparin, aldosterone antagonists, and NSAIDs may increase serum potassium. Note that *intermittent* use of NSAIDs does not pose any problems.

PROVIDING ORAL CONTRACEPTIVES

Patient selection is the key to safe COC use. The benefits of COCs generally far outweigh any significant adverse events. However, some women have medical conditions or personal habits that increase their risk of developing serious complications with use of COCs. In addition to issues of medical safety, be aware that some women may not be good candidates for COCs because they are uncomfortable with COCs due to underlying beliefs about the nature of hormones in contraceptives, "natural" menses, or a lack of belief in the importance of avoiding pregnancy.[175] Women who are seeking the most effective protection from pregnancy may be better served by IUDs, implants, injections or sterilization. Those who have difficulty with daily pill administration should consider all of those methods as well as the longer-acting combined hormonal methods, such as the transdermal patch or the vaginal ring.

Explore the patient's medical and reproductive health history and her family history to ensure that she has no conditions that would preclude her using birth control pills. The contraindications listed in product labeling for COCs differ greatly from the WHO evidence-based list of conditions in which the risks associated with COC use outweigh the benefits (See Table 11–8). The labeling contraindications are listed for completeness only; package labeling for many drugs has been shown to be 20 to 30 years obsolete.[176] For a complete list of WHO's *Medical Eligibility Criteria for Contraceptive Use* upon which to make your clinical decisions, see Chapter 4.

Discuss the potential non-contraceptive benefits and examine all the patient's lifestyle issues to ensure that she can realistically expect to take a pill each day. Anticipatory counseling about safety concerns can reduce later discontinuation. Determine if she wants to have monthly withdrawal bleeding or if she would prefer less frequent bleeding episodes. Ask if she has any other complaints that need to be addressed at this visit. In particular, find out if she needs any STI testing or if she needs emergency contraception now or if she may need it in the future. If she is at risk for STIs, advise her to follow safer sex practices.

Measure the woman's blood pressure. It may be prudent to do a breast examination, but a pelvic examination is *not* needed before initiating COCs in an asymptomatic woman.[177,178] A Pap smear is not needed prior to starting COCs. STI screening, if needed, can be urine-based. No other screening tests are routinely needed unless her history or blood pressure indicates a need for further assessment.[179] In particular, routine screening for thrombotic mutations is *not* recommended prior to prescribing estrogen-containing contraceptives.[180] However, it may be very appropriate to test (not screen) women who have a strong family history of multiple, unexplained clots in many family members at a young age. Remember, many women discontinue pills without consulting their clinicians. Prescribe/provide condoms and emergency contraception for all new start COC users. Invest time teaching her to use her condoms and emergency contraception (EC) so she knows how to use them as well as she knows how to use her COCs.

Table 11–8 Medical conditions precluding COC use, as listed in COC prescribing information compared to the WHO *Eligibility Criteria for Contraceptive Use*

There are specific medical conditions that are not compatible with COC use. The FDA-approved prescribing information lists a set of medical conditions that preclude COC use. This list is often not in agreement with the more up-to-date, evidence-based WHO medical eligibility criteria. Below is the FDA-approved prescribing information list of medical conditions that indicate COCs "should not be used." The category assigned in the WHO medical eligibility criteria is included in the adjacent column. Only a WHO rating of 4 would preclude COC use.

Medical Conditions Precluding COC Use from COC Prescribing Information	WHO Category
Thrombophlebitis or thromboembolic disorder	4
Past history of deep vein thrombophlebitis or thromboembolic disorders	4
Cerebrovascular or coronary artery disease	4
Valvular heart disease with complications	4
Severe hypertension	4
Diabetes with vascular involvement	3/4
Headaches with focal neurological symptoms	4
Major surgery with prolonged immobilization	4
Breast cancer	4
Carcinoma of the endometrium	1
Other known or suspected estrogen-dependent neoplasia	Not discussed
Undiagnosed abnormal genital bleeding	2
Cholestatic jaundice of pregnancy	2
Jaundice with prior pill use	3
Hepatic adenomas or carcinomas	4
Known or suspected pregnancy	"Not applicable"
Hypersensitivity to any component of the product	Not discussed

CHOICES FOR PILL INITIATION

Quick Start

For the Quick Start or Same-Day Start method, the woman is told to take the *first* pill in the pill pack on the day of her office visit, as long as it is reasonably certain that she is not pregnant and not in need of emergency contraception. If she needs emergency contraception, she should take both tablets of Plan B at once or an equivalent EC on the visit day, and start her pills no later than the next day. Tell her to use a backup method with her pills for at least 7 days. Her next menses will be delayed until she completes the active pills in her pack and starts the placebo pills. If she has concern about an undetectable early pregnancy, she can start her pills and be instructed to return for a urine pregnancy test in 2 to 3 weeks, or to do a home pregnancy test at that time. The hormones in the pills will not adversely affect an early pregnancy (see Pregnancy section above) and the prompt repeat pregnancy testing will detect the pregnancy early enough to begin the pregnancy care she chooses. Quick Start is an off-label practice supported by good clinical research.

Quick Start is preferred because other approaches generally leave a time gap between the time the patient is prescribed her pills and the time she is intended to start taking them. As many as 25% of young women given pills to start using one of the conventional start methods (see below) fail to begin taking the pills as instructed because they conceive in the interim, forget the pill-taking instructions, fail to fill the prescription, or are worried about taking the pill after their visit.[181,182] The Quick Start approach has not only been more successful at getting women started on the pill than were the two methods discussed below, but more women were still using pills by the third cycle, especially if they had menstrual-related problems.[183] The WHO endorses the Quick Start method.[184] Quick Start does not increase irregular spotting or bleeding.[185]

First-day Start

The first-day start was introduced to gain early control of ovarian follicles during the first cycle. In this approach, a woman takes her first pill on the first day of her next period. It is important to have the woman determine that her period is normal—that it occurs at the predicted time and is preceded by symptoms that are usual for her. If there is any question that the menses is not normal, she may want to rule out pregnancy before she starts her pills. No backup contraception is needed when pills are started on the first day of menses.

Sunday Start

The Sunday start was the most common method for starting pills for decades. Women were told to start their first active pill on the first Sunday of their menses. For example, if a woman were to start bleeding on Friday, she should take her first pill two days later on Sunday. If her period were to start on Sunday, she should start on that day. Make sure the patient understands that she should not wait to start the first pill on the Sunday after her menses *ends*. Today, the Sunday start is not generally recommended because it is often difficult for women to get refills when they need them on weekends. In addition, many women are working outside the home and prefer not to menstruate during their work week. However, some of the generic pill packages still direct a woman to use a Sunday start, so familiarly with this approach is still needed. If women start their menses more than 5 days before starting their pills, they should use a backup method for 7 days.

SWITCHING FROM OTHER METHODS

Women who switch from other methods can start COCs immediately, using the guidelines for the Quick Start initiation. For example, women who have contraceptive implants or IUDs removed can start their COCs that same day and be told to use a backup contraceptive method for the next 7 days. Women who have had recent unprotected intercourse can be given emergency contraception (EC) immediately and told to start their COCs no later than the next day and to use a backup method for at least the first 7 days of COC use. A urine pregnancy test in 2 to 3 weeks may be offered to detect any EC failures. Women using injectable methods generally start their COCs at the end of the effective period of the injection. However, if a woman is amenorrheic as a result of the injection and is late for reinjection, she can start the COCs the same day with a 7-day use of a backup method. Add EC and follow-up pregnancy testing if she has had recent unprotected sex.

CHOOSING A PATTERN OF PILL USE

1. **Monthly cycling 21/7.** Conventional pill packaging contains 3 weeks of active pills followed by 7 placebo pills to provide a predictable, coordinated withdrawal bleed that women will interpret to be a normal (although lighter) menses. The pill's inventors touted this feature as a distinct benefit for women,[186] which it was at the time.

2. **Shortened pill-free interval.** It is possible that with low dose pill formulations, the 7-day pill-free interval allows too much time for follicular development and offers the opportunity to increase the failure rate. Shortening the pill-free interval with 20 mcg EE pills from 7 to 5 days suppressed ovarian activity more effectively,[187] although data from shortening the pill-free interval with 30 mcg EE formulations is not as impressive.[188] One way to implement this approach is to have the woman use the "first-day start" for every cycle; she should begin a new pill pack on the first day of her withdrawal bleeding. If she has no menses by the 5th placebo pill day, she should start her new pack that day. If a woman has no withdrawal bleeding, a pregnancy test is not necessary, but may reassure her. Three brands currently have reduced the numbers of placebo pills in the monthly cycling packets. Mircette has 21 active pills, 2 placebo pills, and 5 pills with 10 mcg EE. Yaz has 24 active pills and 4

placebo pills. Loestrin 24-Fe has 24 active pills and 4 placebo pills containing iron. Other brands are expected to follow suit. Other benefits from shortening the pill-free interval may also be possible. In a trial comparing a 23-day regimen to the traditional 21-day regimen of 20 mcg EE pills, the withdrawal bleeding was shorter in the group using more active pills.[189]

3. **Extended cycle use.** Studies have clearly documented that the majority of the pill's "side effects" (such as headache, cramping, breast tenderness, bloating and/or swelling) occur during the week women are taking their placebo pills, not when they are not taking hormone pills.[190] Because recent surveys have shown that many women would prefer to bleed less frequently than once a month,[191] it is time to re-evaluate the need for monthly withdrawal bleeding.[192] Fifty percent of Italian women without menstruation-related symptoms said they wanted to lessen the frequency of menstrual periods; half of them wanted amenorrhea.[193]

The purpose of menstruation in spontaneously cycling women is to end the prior unsuccessful cycle (no pregnancy) and to prepare for the next cycle (which may result in pregnancy). COC users are trying to avoid pregnancy. They have no biological need to endure artificial pill-induced withdrawal bleeding on a monthly basis. Unless the patient wants to use bleeding as a reassurance that she is not pregnant, monthly cycling is *not* necessary; it is not healthy and may be avoided by extended COC use.[194]

In clinical studies, women with prolonged flow had fewer menstrual-related problems with extended cycle use,[195] and the majority of those women continued to use the extended cycle.[196] A recent Cochrane review reported that five out of six studies found that women's bleeding patterns were equivalent or improved with continuous-dosing regimens.[197] A regimen of extended pill use with extra packs of pills is cost-effective for women with menorrhagia.[198] Trials with extended cycles with levonorgestrel, norethindrone, and drospirenone have all demonstrated safety and efficacy.[199-201] Other women for whom extended use would be particularly attractive are those with dysmenorrhea or menstrual migraines, and those on active military duty or who have other types of demanding jobs.

Options for extended use include the following:

- *Brief manipulation of a cycle for convenience* such as for a honeymoon, trip, athletic event, camping experience, business meetings, exams or presentations.

- *"Bi-cycling"*, which is the back-to-back use of 2 packs of active pills by taking the first pack of 21 active pills, throwing away the 7 placebo pills in that first pack and immediately starting the second pack of 21 active pills followed by the 7 placebo pills at the end of the second package.

- *"Tri-cycling"*, meaning taking the 21 active pills from 3 packages followed by the 7 placebo pills from the third package.

- *Taking FDA-approved products for extended cycle use.* Two products are now available to reduce the number of withdrawal bleeds to 4 times per year. Another product that provides 12 months (13 cycles) of active pills is also FDA-approved.

- *No-cycling*, meaning taking active pills indefinitely (for many months or years) with no placebo pills as long as the woman has no troublesome spotting. Any strong progestin monophasic pills may be used in this off-label manner, but extra prescriptions are needed.

CHOOSING A FORMULATION

Clinicians in the United States have more than 70 COCs from which to choose. (See the color insert for photographs and formulations of pills available in the United States). Select a COC based on the hormonal dose and on the woman's clinical picture, her preferences, her past experiences with COCs, and cost. Both the World Health Organization and the Food and Drug Administration recommend using the *lowest dose pill* that is effective. When recommending a formulation, remember to consider potential side effects. Women who have hormone sensitivity may benefit from lower dose formulations. However, studies have shown that several COCs containing 20 mcg EE are associated with higher rates of bleeding pattern and higher rates of discontinuation due to those problems than are higher-dose formulations.[202] Figure 11–1 gives an algorithm to help clinicians.

Oral Contraceptive Supplies

The WHO recommends providing up to 1 year's supply of oral contraceptives to women initiating the pill and at every subsequent annual exam to reduce women's barriers to access to contraception.[204] Today in the US, many third-party payers limit women to fewer cycles of COCs; some plans provide only one pack of pills (28 tablets) a month. This places considerable (and unwarranted) burden on a woman's ability to continue uninterrupted use. Payers adopt this approach for many

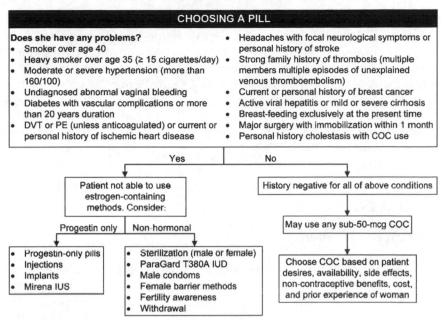

Source: Modified from Hatcher RA, et al. (2003),[203] with permission.

Figure 11–1 Choosing a Pill

reasons. They claim that women often discontinue or switch their pill formulations early on; when this happens, the previously dispensed cycles are wasted. Payers also may lose dispensing fees (or co-pays) if women are able to collect all their packets at once. Finally, with annual reassignments to insurance carriers, plans may pay to cover women's contraceptive needs beyond the time that they are actual plan members.

Other Issues

Remember to instruct new COC users in condom use and to provide them with condoms and EC in case they discontinue COC use or miss pills before returning.

Women should be reminded that COCs are intended for oral administration only. Vaginal placement of the tablets results in slower absorption of the hormones and sub-therapeutic serum levels.[205]

FOLLOW-UP

Because side effects can appear in the first few months of COC use, a follow-up visit at 3 or 6 months is quite commonly recommended but dispensing policies should not be linked to follow-up visits. Encourage women to return if problems develop. Assess how well they are able to take their tablets each day. Recognize how difficult it may be for patients to take pills daily,[206] but that such administration is critical for COC efficacy. As former Surgeon General C. Everett Koop said, "Drugs don't work in patients who don't take them." Responsiveness to patient concerns increases patient continuation of COCs. Remind women that if they are scheduled for major surgery requiring prolonged immobilization they should discontinue COCs 1 month prior to surgery. Similarly, women being treated with short-term anticoagulants for thrombotic disorders should stop their COCs 1 month prior to stopping their anticoagulant therapy.

SPECIAL POPULATIONS

Adolescent Women

Menstruating teenage women who are sexually active and those who are contemplating becoming sexually active are usually healthy; therefore, for young women, the medical and social risks of pregnancy far outweigh the small health risks associated with COC use. Explore the teen's decision to become (or stay) sexually active. Is she comfortable with that decision or would she prefer to delay sexual intercourse? (See Chapter 5, Abstinence and the Range of Sexual Expression.)

Many teens can benefit from taking COCs to treat primary dysmenorrhea, anovulatory cycling, or acne. A pelvic examination is not needed prior to COC initiation for an asymptomatic woman (see the section on Pill Initiation). Reassure anxious parents that COC use for non-contraceptive indications has not been shown to encourage young women to become sexually active. A teenager who has had irregular periods or oligomenorrhea will have regular menses while taking COCs; however, when she stops taking her COCs, her periods may again become irregular. Estrogen in the current low-dose COCs does not stunt a young woman's height due to premature closure of the epiphyses. Teens may be more likely to abandon COCs because of minor side effects such as nausea or spotting, so take all minor side effects in teenagers seriously.

Provide concrete counseling to adolescents, who may find it more challenging to use COCs correctly and consistently than do older women. Instruct each teen who wants to use COCs about condom use, both for reducing the risk of acquiring STIs and for backup in case she discontinues taking the pill. Provide emergency contraception and instructions on how to use it if she needs it. Studies have shown that women of all ages are more able to successfully use the once-a-week or once-a-month methods than they are able to remember to take a pill once a day, but teens benefit most.[207] For this reason, offer the vaginal ring and patch to teens who desire combined hormonal contraception.

Perimenopausal Women

The balance between benefits and risks changes with the woman's age, as the health risks of pregnancy increase and women develop more medical problems.

Healthy, nonobese and nonsmoking women in their 40s are candidates for COCs. COCs can help regulate menstrual bleeding and reduce the risks of irregular bleeding and endometrial hyperplasia associated with anovulatory cycling during the perimenopausal years. Women in their 40s are at highest risk for menorrhagia due to leiomyoma and adenomyosis; COCs can provide a medical alternative to surgical therapies, such as endometrial ablation or hysterectomy. COCs also help reduce the risk of ovarian and endometrial cancers. ACOG has raised concerns about obese women over age 35 using estrogen-containing contraceptives.[241] ACOG's rationale is that both age and obesity are independent risk factors for venous thromboembolism; adding estrogen increases that risk. However, since pregnancy presents an even greater risk of DVT, use in these women when they cannot use other effective methods is not absolutely contraindicated.

No special testing is required prior to prescribing COCs for women in their 40s, except for blood pressure measurements. Screening measures such as clinical breast exams, mammograms, serum lipids, and pelvic exam with Pap smears are important elements of well-woman care, but do not need to be performed in apparently healthy women of any age prior to COC initiation.

COC users in their late 40s or early 50s may not experience traditional symptoms of menopause while taking COCs. They will not experience menstrual irregularities or hot flashes, especially if the COCs are used on an extended basis. In this context, it may be difficult to detect when menopause occurs. Do not rely on blood tests to diagnose menopause in perimenopausal women. (See Chapter 26 on Menopause.)

Smokers

Heavy smoking by women older than 35 precludes the use of estrogen-containing hormonal methods. *Any* smoking by women older than 40 prohibits the use of estrogen-containing contraceptive on an ongoing basis. Light smoking by women age 35 to 40 merits caution (WHO category 3). For example, smoking increases a COC user's risk of heart attack nearly 13- to 14-fold.[208] Indeed, women who smoke as few as 1 to 4 cigarettes a day have a 2.5 fold increased risk of coronary heart disease.[209] The older the smoker, the more cigarettes she smokes, and the more comorbid cardiovascular risk factors she faces, the less likely she is to be a candidate for COCs. In otherwise healthy young women, the absolute risk of cardiovascular disease is low, so that use of COCs by women who smoke is still safer than the risks of pregnancy. The first priority in caring for a woman who smokes is to encourage and aid her to stop smoking, or to significantly reduce the number of cigarettes she smokes each day. Three to 12 months after stopping smoking, past smokers have the same COC-related cardiovascular risks as nonsmokers.

In selecting a pill for smokers, the clinician is conflicted. On the one hand, the ideal pill would have the lowest estrogen content (to reduce arterial thrombosis) and the lowest androgenic activity (to minimize any adverse impacts on lipids). On the other hand, smokers tend to metabolize estrogen more rapidly and to increase SHBG levels more than nonsmokers do, so that a 20-mcg EE dose pill may not provide as much contraceptive efficacy for a smoker. There are no clinical trials to provide guidance. It may be prudent to start smokers and nicotine patch/gum/etc. users on 20 mcg EE formulation with a strong (low androgenic) progestin, advise them to use a backup method during the first 2 to 3 months, and monitor breakthrough bleeding as a marker of adequate serum levels. If she has persistent breakthrough bleeding on a 20-mcg EE pill, use of a 25 to 30 mcg EE formulation or a different delivery system may be advisable. Consider shortening the pill-free interval for smokers.

Postpartum Women

Pregnancy is a hypercoagulable state. Estrogen increases the risk of venous thrombosis and embolism (VTE). As a result, it is generally recommended that postpartum women delay use of estrogen-containing contraception until 3 to 4 weeks postpartum, when those pregnancy-induced changes in the coagulation system start to resolve.

Breastfeeding Women

Although many progestin-only methods may be used immediately postpartum, there has been concern that estrogen may adversely affect breast milk. A thorough review of the world literature found that existing trials are insufficient to establish any effect of hormonal contraception on milk quality or its nutrients.[210] (see Chapter 18 on Postpartum Contraception and Lactation). However, the American Academy of Pediatrics advises against use of estrogen-containing pills as long as the woman is exclusively breast-feeding, but agrees that COCs can be used as soon as supplemental sources of nutrition are introduced into the infant's diet (if the mother is at least 3 to 4 weeks postpartum).

Women With Medical Problems

The WHO criteria for providing COCs to women with medical problems are listed in Chapter 4 on Medical Eligibility Criteria.

DRUG-DRUG INTERACTIONS: GENERAL PRINCIPLES

There are many ways one drug can alter the effectiveness of another drug. In order to evaluate possible drug-drug interactions, a clinician must first understand how the COC's estrogen and progestin are absorbed, distributed, metabolized, and eliminated.

Sex steroids are absorbed from the small intestine and shunted primarily through the liver (so called "first pass"). About 60% of the absorbed EE is conjugated by the intestinal mucosa and the liver to form glucuronic and sulfate conjugates; these conjugated estrogens are excreted through the gallbladder back into the small intestines without entering the bloodstream.[211] These conjugates cannot be absorbed from the small intestines. However, bacteria in the large intestine can enzymatically unconjugate the estrogen metabolites. The newly freed estrogen metabolites are then absorbed from the colon and delivered to the liver via the enterohepatic circulation for additional hepatic "passes" for either absorption into the bloodstream or conjugation and excretion through the gallbladder. Sex steroids that enter the circulation are also ultimately conjugated hepatically and excreted in the urine.

When the ethinyl estradiol (EE) is in contact with the liver, it induces profound changes in hepatic enzyme activity and protein synthesis. EE is much more potent than estradiol and it induces greater production of carrier proteins (e.g., sex hormone binding globulin, thyroxin binding globulin, and albumin). It also induces production of clotting factors of the extrinsic pathway and (generally) balancing fibrinolytic factors (See section on thrombosis risk). EE results in increased HDL and triglyceride levels and diminished LDL levels. Importantly, the cytochrome P-450 enzymes are activated, increasing the rate at which many drugs are cleared from the bloodstream.

Theoretically, interactions between COCs and other drugs could result from production of binding protein, influences on enterohepatic circulation, or changes in cytochrome P-450 activity. The only significant influence on binding proteins caused by EE are changes in hormone levels. For example, with COC use total thyroxine levels increase, but free thyroxine levels remain constant. On the other hand, free testosterone levels drop with COC use, because much of the testosterone binds to the SHBG that is induced by EE. COC-induced binding globulins do not affect the efficacy of any drugs. Other drugs do not induce binding globulins at rates that can affect COC efficacy.

The role that the enterohepatic circulation has on COC efficacy remains controversial. At the heart of the matter is concern that use of broad spectrum antibiotics, such as tetracycline and ampicillin, might destroy the colonic bacteria needed to unconjugate the estrogen conjugates to permit reabsorption ("second pass") of the estrogens. Studies have shown that peak levels of serum EE are *not* altered when women take tetracycline,[212] doxycycline,[213] ampicillin, metronidazole[214] or quinoline antibiotics.[215] There is no enterohepatic recirculation of progestins. Therefore, antibiotics that destroy colonic bacteria do not affect serum levels of progestins—the hormone which provides most of the contraceptive effect of the COC. Most convincingly, women who have had colectomy and have no enterohepatic circulation do not experience any reduction in the efficacy of COCs.[216] Therefore, it is generally agreed that women who use these broad-spectrum antibiotics do not need to use a backup method, contrary to the instructions in product labeling.

The most important cause of drug-drug interactions with COCs is mediated through cytochrome P-450 enzyme activity. Cytochrome P-450 is a family of enzymes that regulate hepatic clearance of drugs and other elements in the bloodstream. Cytochrome P-450 enzyme activity may be stimulated or inhibited by drugs. Some drugs, such as rifampin and griseofulvin, *activate* hepatic clearance of sex steroids so significantly that COC use is contraindicated with use of these drugs until 1 month after those medications are discontinued. Other drugs may more mildly affect the levels of EE. For example, carbamazepine, phenytoin, and St. John's Wort reduce serum EE to sub-therapeutic levels, though this effect may be offset by administering higher dose COCs.

On the other hand, drugs that *decrease* cytochrome P-450 activity raise circulating levels of drugs that require cytochrome P-450 clearance. Therefore, doses of those drugs must be reduced. For example, fluconazole slows the metabolism of warfarin; chronic use of fluconazole may lead to bleeding if the dose of the anti-coagulant is not decreased. Some of the antiretroviral agents slow cytochrome P-450 clearance; lower dose lower COC formulations may be preferred.

The other side of the equation must also be considered. It must be remembered that EE itself significantly induces cytochrome P-450 activity. One month after initiating COCs, patients using phenobarbital or other similar anticonvulsants should have their serum anticonvulsant levels tested to ensure that they are still in the therapeutic range. Lamotrigine levels decrease by 25% to 70% during COC use; therefore, dosing adjustments of lamotrigine as a single agent may be necessary for women while they are taking the active pills. Levels return almost to baseline during the pill-free week. In general, cytochrome P-450 activity normalizes within 1 month of discontinuing the activating or inhibiting agent.

Complicating these recognized potential drug-drug interactions is the fact that there is a great inter-individual variation in drug processing. Some women absorb less hormone from their intestines than others. Some individuals' cytochrome P-450 enzyme activity changes in response to drugs more dramatically than others do. In addition, the drugs themselves may complicate the situation by being pro-drugs that require hepatic metabolism to transform them into their active forms. For example, mestranol must be metabolized in the liver to form the biologically active ethinyl estradiol and desogestrel is metabolized into the active etonogestrel; the extent of that transformation again varies from person to person. On top of all of these biologic considerations is the concern that inconsistent use of COCs creates an opportunity for higher failure rates.

SPECIFIC GROUPS OF DRUG-DRUG INTERACTIONS INVOLVING COCS

Anti-HIV protease inhibitors. Several of the anti-HIV protease inhibitors can change (either increase or decrease) serum levels of estrogen and progestins. Consult the labeling for specific anti-HIV protease inhibitors to see if COC users require additional backup methods, if different contraceptives may need to be considered, or if lower dose COC formulations are preferred.

Broad-spectrum antibiotics. Broad-spectrum antibiotics such as amoxicillin and tetracycline, which alter the intestinal flora thought to be instrumental in promoting reabsorption of the sex steroids, do *not* reduce the efficacy of COCs. Women using the antibiotics do have statistically significant lower serum levels of estrogen and progestins. However, virtually every woman taking these antibiotics has remained well within the therapeutic range for the sex steroids.[217-219] As a result, backup methods should not be necessary unless the patient has problems taking her pills, e.g., if her underlying medical condition interferes with pill-taking or absorption. Long-term use of broad-spectrum antibiotics (such as erythromycin or tetracycline for acne) is compatible with COC use; backup methods are not routinely needed for pregnancy prevention.[220] On the other hand, estrogen stimulates the clearance of some antibiotics; serum levels of fluoroquinolones, such as moxifloxacin and trovafloxacin, are significantly lower in COC users.[221]

Other prescription drug interactions. COCs may increase the effect of theophylline (used to treat asthma), the antipsychotic drugs diazepam (Valium), chlordiazepoxide (Librium), and tricyclic antidepressants. Doses of these drugs may need to be lowered with COC use.

Drospirenone acts as an antimineralocorticoid and can interact with other potassium-sparing drugs to cause hyperkalemia. Women using ACE inhibitors, angiotensin-II receptor antagonists, potassium-sparing diuretics, heparin, aldosterone antagonists, and NSAIDS on a daily basis to treat chronic conditions or diseases should have their serum potassium checked during the first cycle of drospirenone use.

Over-the-counter drugs. St. John's Wort is taken by many women to treat mild depression. Since this botanical agent does not require a prescription, women sometimes neglect to tell their health care providers that they are using it. St. John's Wort greatly increases hepatic metabolism of exogenous estrogen and progestin. In one study of women using 35 mcg EE pills, St. John's Wort use was associated with a significant increase in the oral clearance of norethindrone and a significant reduction in the half-life of EE.[222] The FDA has alerted providers that St. John's Wort may decrease the therapeutic effect of COCs.[223]

Women who use orlistat to block fat absorption may also reduce intestinal absorption of COC hormones. This concern is magnified if the woman experiences diarrhea from orlistat use.

On a lighter note, the German National Chemists Association has advised women who use COCs to avoid eating too much licorice. Eating more than 10 to 50 gm a day of black licorice may trigger edema or elevate blood pressure.

MANAGING MISSED PILLS

After having taken at least 7 pills at the correct time, women are at little risk for ovulation until they have missed 7 consecutive pills. The traditional pill-free interval provides these 7 days. Escape ovulation is much more likely to occur if pills early in the packet are missed and if the patient is using a lower dose (20 mcg EE) pill versus a higher dose (50 mcg EE) pill. Therefore, the recommendations for coping with missed pills vary not only with the number of pills missed, but also with the strength of the pill and the week in which the pills were missed. Management recommendations must include instructions about 3 items: when to take the missed (and subsequent) pills; the need for backup method; and the need for EC. The instructions for EC are covered in Chapter 6.

Currently accepted recommendations for missed pill management do not provide explicit guidance for 25 mcg EE formulations. We have included the 25 mcg EE formulations with the 20 mcg EE formulations in a group we call sub-30 mcg EE formulations

For a woman using pills with at least 30 mcg EE who—

- Missed 1 to 2 pills. Have her take 1 active pill as soon as possible, and then continue taking pills daily (including pill for this day). No backup contraception is needed. Emergency contraception should be considered if pills were missed in the first week and intercourse was unprotected.

- Missed 3 or more pills during the first 2 weeks of the pack. Have her take one active pill as soon as possible, and then continue taking pills daily, 1 each day (including the pill for this day). She should use condoms or abstain from vaginal intercourse until she has taken active pills for 7 days in a row. Consider EC if COCs were missed during the first week and intercourse was unprotected.

- Missed 3 or more pills during the 3rd week of the pack (of a traditional 4 week pack). Have her finish the active pills in the current pack and start a new pack the next day without using any placebo pills.

For a woman using sub-30 mcg EE formulations who

- Missed 1 active pill, have her take 1 active pill as soon as possible, and then continue taking pills daily (including the pill for this day). No backup contraception is needed. Consider EC if pills were missed during the first week and intercourse was unprotected.

- Missed ≥ 2 active pills. Treat her as if 3 or more pills of 30 mcg EE formulations were missed.[204]

These recommendations have not been universally adopted. Some clinicians have pointed out that they are too complicated for women who are given EC by advance prescription, especially women with low literacy skills. Furthermore, the recommendations are based on trials in which women took all their earlier pills as directed. More than half of women miss more than 2 pills each cycle.[6] Finally, some of the recommendations may not be feasible. Women who are told to skip the placebo pills and start the next packet may not be able to get another packet of pills until the usual refill time due to restrictive dispensing protocols imposed by third party payers.

To answer these concerns, a simplified approach may be adopted to provide women guidance when they are prescribed their pills in case they can not call for instructions at the time of the missed pills. This simplified approach admittedly overuses EC and backup methods. Women who miss any pills are encouraged to use EC (2 tablets at once) if they have had any unprotected intercourse in the last 5 days, to take one COC tablet twice the following day and to return to daily use for the rest of the pack, while using condoms for the first 7 days of renewed COC use. Women who do not need EC should take 2 tablets of COC the first day they recognize that they have missed any pills and use condoms for the following 7 days.

Women who vomit a pill within 2 hours of taking it or who have severe vomiting and diarrhea for 2 or more days should be treated as if they had missed pills.

MANAGING SIDE EFFECTS

A double-blind trial showed no difference in the incidence of any of the traditionally "hormonally-related" side effects during the 6-month comparison of COC users and placebo pills users. Similar percentages of women in each group developed headaches, nausea, vomiting, mastalgia, weight gain, etc.[224] This finding differs from the impression given by the pill package labeling. Interestingly, when women with "pill side effects" such as nausea, headache, mood changes, fatigue, weight gain, breast tenderness, and breakthrough bleeding were treated in another study with either Vitamin B6 or sugar pill, both groups improved in all symptoms.[225]

However, 59% to 81% of women who discontinued COC use in one study reported that they stopped due to side effects. Some researchers have noted significant differences in rates of discontinuation among different groups of women; discontinuation rates are higher in women in developing countries where women may have lower endogenous hormone levels than do U.S. women.[226] Acknowledgement and management of side effects are crucial to successful use of COCs. Counsel all potential hormonal contraceptive users that side effects are possible, but not necessarily to be expected. Advise women that side effects are usually transient and often respond to changes in pill formulation. Familiarity with the hormones theoretically implicated in the different side effects can aid clinicians in selecting new formulations for patients (see Table 11–9). The side effects discussed below are grouped by system: menstrually-related side effects, symptomatic complaints, and metabolic impacts.

MENSTRUALLY-RELATED SIDE EFFECTS

Absence of Withdrawal Bleeding

Advise women that the amount of withdrawal bleeding with COCs may be significantly lower than with spontaneous cycling menses. Even scant bleeding or spotting on the placebo pills counts as withdrawal bleeding. The incidence of a complete lack of withdrawal bleeding varies with different formulations and increases with duration of use. Some women deliberately extend the number of active pills they use to achieve prolonged amenorrhea. For women using cyclic regimens of COCs who fail to have withdrawal bleeding, obvious causes of amenorrhea (such as

Table 11–9 Estrogenic, progestogenic, and combined effects of oral contraceptive pills

Estrogen Related	Progesterone Related	Androgen Related
Weight gain in breast, hips, and thighs	Hypoglycemic headaches	Acne
Cervical eversion or ectopy	Cyclic weight gain	Hirsutism
Increased blood pressure	Constipation, bloating	Elevated LDL-C
Rise in gallbladder cholesterol	Fatigue	Slow, steady weight gain
Skin changes	Depressive symptoms	
Melasma	Increased insulin resistance	
Telangiectasia		
Hepatocellular adenoma		
Arterial thrombosis		
Stroke		
Myocardial infarction		
Venous thromboembolism		
Headaches		
Increased HDL-C triglycerides		
Nausea		

pregnancy and new medications) must be excluded. Other specific conditions, such as cervical stenosis, need to be evaluated, particularly if the patient has recently had cervical surgery (e.g., D&C, cone biopsy, LEEP, etc). When women use COCs, it is far less likely that other common causes of amenorrhea are responsible for her lack of bleeding. Thyroid problems, prolactinoma, and hypothalamic amenorrhea (due to stress or excessive exercise) or anovulatory states (such as PCOS or obesity) are important considerations when a woman not using COCs develops amenorrhea. However, COCs restore predictable menstrual cycling in women with these problems.

Women who enjoy the lack of withdrawal bleeding but just want to reassure themselves periodically that they are not pregnant may use home pregnancy tests or may want to monitor their basal body temperature (BBT) during 3 sequential days of placebo pills. If that BBT is lower than 98°F, the likelihood of pregnancy is very low. If a woman desires to have cyclic withdrawal bleeding, switch her to a more estrogenic formulation or to a triphasic formulation with lower levels of progestin in the early pills to increase endometrial proliferation.

Unscheduled Vaginal Spotting or Bleeding

Unscheduled spotting and bleeding are common (30% to 50%) in the first few months of COC use. Progestins administered early in the cycle reduce estrogen's proliferative influence and induce atrophy (thinning) of the uterine lining over time. By the third pack of pills, 70% to 90% of women (depending upon the formulation) have no further unscheduled bleeding or spotting.

Before changing COC type, rule out more likely and more serious causes of unscheduled bleeding, such as pregnancy, infection (vaginitis and cervicitis), medications that block hormone absorption (olestin) or increase their metabolism by the liver (anticonvulsants, cigarette smoking, St. John's Wort, rifampin, griseofulvin), and gastrointestinal problems (vomiting and diarrhea that may prevent adequate hormone absorption to sustain the uterine lining). *Remember that one of the most common causes of pill-associated spotting and bleeding is missed pills.*

For women with persistent irregular bleeding after 2 to 3 months of use, and for those who will stop COC use early, consider changing to other formulations. No research indicates that any specific COC is best at eliminating unscheduled spotting or bleeding, because the data reported on different formulations are not comparable.[227]

- Women who report spotting or bleeding before they complete their active pills probably need more endometrial support. Increase the progestin content of their pills, either by changing to a different monophasic formulation or by switching to a triphasic formulation that increases progestin levels in the last active pills.

- Women with continued spotting after the withdrawal bleed may need more estrogen support. Increase the estrogen in the first tablets in the pack or decrease the progestin in those pills.

- The cause of mid-cycle spotting/bleeding is not clear. One approach to this relatively uncommon bleeding pattern is to use triphasic formulations that increase both estrogen and progestin in the middle pills.

- Extended cycle users tend to experience unscheduled spotting and bleeding, especially after week 5 in the first cycle. Inform users that, as with all other pills, they will have more spotting initially when they begin taking pills. This spotting will decrease rapidly over time. However, women who find this spotting bothersome after they have completed the first 21 days of pills, can stop taking pills for 2 to 3 days to allow a withdrawal bleed to start. Then they should restart the active pills, taking at least 3 weeks of active pills each time before they stop again. As they take pills in this pattern, the length of time between unscheduled spotting and bleeding episodes will increase, and they eventually will be able to take pills for 3 to 12 months at a time.

Symptomatic Side Effects

Weight Changes

Three placebo-controlled, randomized clinical trials have demonstrated that women do not experience weight gain due to low-dose COC use.[224,228] A prospective trial of women using triphasic COCs with daily weight measurements for 4 months showed no change in mean weight at the end of the trial compared to baseline, although some weight fluctuations were noted during the cycle.[229] Oral contraceptive use by adolescent women has been shown not to be associated with either weight gain or increased body fat in a 9-year study.[230] In clinical trials, women who use COCs do not typically gain any more weight than other women living in the United States typically gain in the same time interval. A Cochrane review confirmed that available evidence is insufficient to determine the effect of combination contraceptives on weight, but no large effect was evident.[231] However, it is important for clinicians to understand that what troubles patients is their *perception* of weight changes and that women's opinions about weight change in clinical trials are not correlated with measured changes.[232]

In addition, individual women may respond robustly to any of the pill's hormones. Increased measurements in the breasts, hips, and thighs reflect estrogen's impact on adipose cells (hypertrophy). Decreasing estrogen in the pill can reduce this impact. Weight gain similar to premenstrual fluid retention is due to increased aldosterone release and results from estrogen activity augmented by progesterone. In this situation, switch to a pill with both lower estrogen and progestin levels. Drospirenone-containing COCs, which have an antimineralocorticoid activity (mild diuretic effect), may also be an appropriate choice to deal with this problem. Steadily increasing weight may be attributed to the nitrogen retention and an increase in muscle mass stimulated by androgens. Although it is unlikely that the pill would be responsible for this type of weight gain, switching to a pill with low or no androgenic activity may address that patient's concerns. Every woman should be encouraged to adopt a healthy diet and to exercise routinely to achieve and maintain a healthy weight.

Headaches

Headaches occur commonly. Randomized, placebo-controlled trials have found that women using placebo pills experienced headaches as frequently as did COC users.[224] Nonetheless, new onset or worsening headaches in a COC user should be investigated because those symptoms can be an indication of serious medical problems, such as hypertension, or transient ischemic attacks or impending stroke. Approximately 4% of COC users discontinue pill use because of headaches.[233] Some women do appear to have higher risk of headache exacerbation of or new onset headaches attributable to COC use. This risk is highest among women with a strong personal or family history of headache, especially migraine. The incidence increases with age, peaking in the late 40s.

Headache complaints decrease with continued use. Women experiencing headaches the first cycle have only a 1 in 3 chance of having those headaches the second month. That risk drops to 1 in 10 by the third cycle. A systematic review of the literature found that there is no scientific evidence to support the common clinical practice of switching formulations to treat headache. However, the authors suggested that manipulation of the extent or duration of estrogen withdrawal may be beneficial.[234] Stepwise evaluation of the headache is necessary.

- Confirm that the headaches started or worsened in frequency or severity with the onset of COC use.

- **Rule out other causes.** Measure the patient's blood pressure. Obtain a history of medication use, caffeine intake, and other prescription, nonprescription, and recreational drug use. Inquire about recent trauma. Note if there are other associated problems with vision, sensation, or other functions. Evaluate for signs and symptoms of transient ischemic attacks, cerebrovascular accidents, temporal arteritis, sinusitis, viremia, sepsis, allergy, temporomandibular joint (TMJ) disorders, dental problems, drug use, alcohol or caffeine withdrawal, or central nervous system tumor.

- **Characterize the type of headache.** The consequences are different for different types of headaches. If a woman claims she is having "migraines," obtain information about how the diagnosis was made; many women use the word "migraine" to describe a severe headache. Ask about the severity of the headache, aura, duration, character (throbbing or constant), cyclicity, and location (including asymmetry). Ask about associated symptoms, such as photophobia, nausea, vomiting, dizziness, scotomata, blurred vision, watering of the eyes, loss of vision or speech, weakness, or numbness. Can the patient function when the headaches are most severe? What medication provides relief? Also, determine when in her cycle the woman has her headaches—during the active pills or placebo pills.

  — *Tension headache.* The most common headache is the tension headache, which usually starts as a neck pain late in the day and radiates through the occipital area over the scalp to involve the forehead. There are no associated neurologic sensations, but women with tension headaches may experience nausea or vomiting from the intensity of the pain. These headaches usually respond to over-the-counter analgesics and/or rest. Tension headaches that do start with COC use tend to improve with continued use. Rarely is it necessary to change pill formulations.

— *Migraine headache.* The headache that causes most medical concern is the migraine headache, which tends to occur in the temporal region and is more frequently unilateral. Since the word "migraine" has become almost synonymous with severe headaches, it is important to identify true migraine. If a woman develops new-onset migraine or a worsening in the severity or frequency of her migraine headaches during her active pill days, she may no longer be a candidate for COCs. If she has any associated neurological auras (flashing lights, tingling sensation, paresthesias, etc), stop the COCs immediately and provide contraception without estrogen. On the other hand, if her symptoms develop or worsen only on the days she takes placebo pills (when her estrogen levels drop), it may be possible to offer her extended-use, low-dose COCs to reduce her menstrual migraines.

— *Stroke.* Strokes are often preceded for weeks or months by either visual symptoms or headaches or both. Discontinue COCs and refer the patient for immediate evaluation if she has experienced transient, total, or partial loss of vision; elevated blood pressure; or other neurologic symptoms.

If the headaches are not serious and are related to COC use, consider the following approaches:

- **Headaches during active pills.** There is no evidence to support the common clinical practice of switching oral contraceptive formulations to treat these headaches,[234] but Figure 11–2 outlines some empiric recommendations.

- **Headaches during placebo pills.** Shorten or eliminate the placebo pills. Menstrual migraine was one of the earliest indications for extended cycle COC use.

Mood swings and depression

Multiple studies have demonstrated that there is no increase in the risk of clinical depression in women using COCs. Both estrogen and progestin in high-dose pills interact with tryptophans and serotonin; however, low-dose pills have not been implicated in any of these complaints.[59,235] Women on COCs remain solidly within normal ranges for all

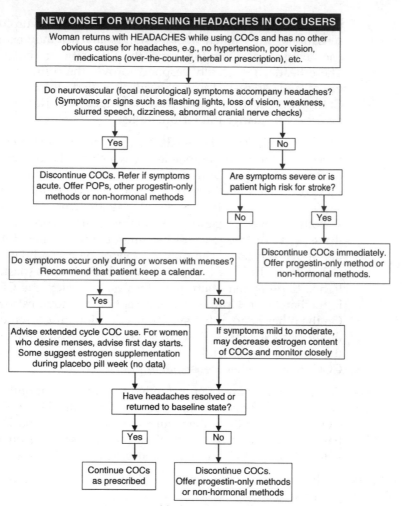

NEW ONSET OR WORSENING HEADACHES IN COC USERS

Woman returns with HEADACHES while using COCs and has no other obvious cause for headaches, e.g., no hypertension, poor vision, medications (over-the-counter, herbal or prescription), etc.

↓

Do neurovascular (focal neurological) symptoms accompany headaches? (Symptoms or signs such as flashing lights, loss of vision, weakness, slurred speech, dizziness, abnormal cranial nerve checks)

Yes → Discontinue COCs. Refer if symptoms acute. Offer POPs, other progestin-only methods or non-hormonal methods

No → Are symptoms severe or is patient high risk for stroke?

No → Do symptoms occur only during or worsen with menses? Recommend that patient keep a calendar.

Yes → Discontinue COCs immediately. Offer progestin-only method or non-hormonal methods.

Yes → Advise extended cycle COC use. For women who desire menses, advise first day starts. Some suggest estrogen supplementation during placebo pill week (no data)

No → If symptoms mild to moderate, may decrease estrogen content of COCs and monitor closely

Have headaches resolved or returned to baseline state?

Yes → Continue COCs as prescribed

No → Discontinue COCs. Offer progestin-only methods or non-hormonal methods

Source: Modified from Hatcher RA, et al. (2003),[203] with permission.

Figure 11–2 New onset or worsening headaches in COC users

vitamins and do not require vitamin B supplementation.[236] Some women do report an increase in depressive symptoms, moodiness, and other emotional states when on COCs. This may represent an idiosyncratic response to hormones, which may warrant a decrease in hormone doses or pill cessation. However, it is important to identify when in a woman's cycle these symptoms develop. If the symptoms appear just before the menses, then extended or continuous use of active pills may dampen her hormonal swings.[196] If the woman desires withdrawal bleeding, have her start her active pills from the next pack on the first day of her menses. The low dose drospirenone-containing formulation that has FDA approval for treatment of premenstrual dysphoric disorder (PMDD) may be helpful in this situation.[37] If there is any concern about an underlying depressive or anxiety disorder, these conditions deserve an explicit evaluation and treatment; cessation of COCs is not adequate therapy. Suicidal women need emergency treatment by specialists. Less acutely ill women may be managed locally with close follow-up.

Changes in libido

Decreased libido is occasionally a problem and may be the reason a woman seeks a different pill or a different contraceptive. When a patient complains of a decrease in libido, evaluate depression and other life stresses. Ask about thyroid-related symptoms. In some women, the pill alters vaginal secretions.[172] Progestin may reduce cervical secretions, which can decrease vaginal lubrication and make sexual intercourse less comfortable and occasionally painful. Consider using a more estrogenic COC or the vaginal ring to increase lubrication. A link has been suggested between suppressed free testosterone with COC use and decreased libido.[172] However, randomized clinical trials found no change in libido in women using drospirenone-containing COCs, which are antiandrogenic.[92] Despite this evidence, women who complain of decreased libido with COC use, an empiric trial with a more androgenic formulation; this change is not contraindicated and may please the patient.

Skin changes

Every COC increases sex hormone binding globulin. Progestin inhibits LH release, which decreases ovarian androgen production. In clinical trials, less than 5% of women typically report worsening or new onset of *acne, oily skin,* or *hirsutism.* Consider other causes of androgen exposure (other medications, ovarian tumors, etc.) if her symptoms are severe. If it appears her COC may be contributing to her problem, switch to a formulation with less androgenic activity. Two formulations have FDA approval for treatment of acne (Ortho TriCyclen and Estrostep). One clinical trial demonstrated that a drospirenone-containing COC was superior to the norgestimate formulation.[64]

Estrogen stimulates the production of melanocytes and can cause darkening of pigmented areas (linea nigra). Dark patches on the face, often called the "mask of pregnancy," *melasma* or *chloasma* can also develop. Women with darker skin pigment are more susceptible. The melasma fades slowly and, often, incompletely after discontinuation of estrogen. Progestin-only methods may be preferable for at-risk women. Recommend consistent use of sunscreen and hats.

Estrogen can also stimulate the formation of telangiectasias, which are fine, dilated intracutaneous veins that are not clinically significant, but may be cosmetically disturbing to a woman. Avoid the use of estrogen-containing hormonal methods in women troubled by telangiectasias.

Mastalgia

Both estrogen and progestin affect the breast. Ovulating women routinely experience up to a 20% increase in breast volume during the luteal phase due to venous and lymphatic engorgement. Estrogen causes hypertrophy of the adipose cells in the breast and can cause increase in breast size. In addition, both hormones stimulate the terminal ductal lobular tuft growth especially in nulliparous women. Nearly 30% of women experience mastalgia or breast tenderness after they start taking COCs. A proper fitting bra is the first recommendation. Reduction of the doses of both steroids may be necessary if symptoms do not resolve rapidly enough to satisfy the patient. Lower dose pills (20 mcg EE) produced less mastalgia than higher dose (35 mcg EE) pills in one comparative trial.[235] If the symptoms develop just before menses, extended cycle COC use can help.

Gastrointestinal complaints

Working at the level of the central nervous system, estrogen can induce nausea or vomiting. Sex steroid hormones do not directly affect the gastric lining, although new research has demonstrated a hormonal impact on the intrinsic firing rate of the gastric pacemaker cells. Progesterone slows peristalsis and can increase constipation and sensations of bloating and distention. Most affected women acclimate to the hormones, and nausea resolves within 1 to 3 months of use. If a woman complains of nausea, she can try taking her pills with food or at night. Avoid double dosing. Counsel the patient to "catch up" any pills she forgets by taking pills at 12-hour intervals, rather than taking 2 pills at one time. In addition, advise more fluids and fresh fruits and vegetables. Women with recent onset of severe gastrointestinal symptoms should be evaluated promptly to rule out acute, serious problems, such as cholecystitis, appendicitis and diverticulitis, and more chronic, intermittent problems, such as inflammatory bowel syndrome (IBS).

If vomiting or diarrhea is related to taking the pill, try the following approaches:

- Decrease hormone dose. A 20 mcg COC dramatically decreases nausea for many women, although it may also lead to more unscheduled spotting and bleeding.

- Bloating and constipation may be helped with a reduction in the progestin component in the pill. Bloating associated with menses can be diminished by extended cycle or continuous active pill use or use of a formulation with drospirenone for its antimineralocorticoid activity.

- Try progestin-only formulations to control nausea and other symptoms.

Contact lens effects

Women who wear contact lenses may note some visual changes or change in lens tolerance with COC use. Normal saline eye drops often provide adequate treatment, but consultation with an ophthalmologist may be helpful.

Metabolic Effects

Hyperlipidemia

Routine screening for lipids is not necessary before prescribing COCs unless a patient has pre-existing hyperlipidemia or a very strong family history of premature cardiovascular disease. Estrogen is known to increase HDL-C, triglycerides, and total cholesterol levels and to decrease LDL-C. The androgen-derived progestins may be neutral or may reverse some of estrogen's stimulatory effects on HDL-C and triglycerides and may increase LDL-C. The net effect depends upon the dose, potency, and estrogen/androgen balance of each formulation. If LDL levels rise or HDL levels drop significantly with COC use, change to a formulation with more estrogenic activity and less androgenic activity.

Hypertriglyceridemia is an independent risk factor for early cardiovascular disease in women. Although most modern COC formulations increase triglycerides by about 30%, these estrogen-induced triglycerides are different in size than endogenously produced triglycerides. COC-induced triglycerides do not appear to increase a woman's risk for atherosclerosis.[247] However, excessively high serum triglycerides (greater than 500 mg/dl) can cause pancreatitis. Therefore, women with triglycerides levels greater than 350 mg/dl should use COCs only with caution. Lower dose pills (20 to 25 mcg EE) would be preferred to higher dose ones; progestin-only formulations may be necessary.

Vaginal discharge

Some women notice an increase in vaginal secretions with estrogen-containing contraceptives. These secretions generally are not an indication of infection. Women who use low-dose COCs are not at any increased risk for developing uncomplicated candidal infections or bacterial vaginosis (BV). Reassurance is generally the only intervention needed once infection has been ruled out. Point out to the woman that these secretions are healthy and serve as lubricant during coitus.

INSTRUCTIONS FOR USING ORAL CONTRACEPTIVES

Pills work primarily by stopping ovulation (release of an egg), and they thicken a woman's mucus in her cervix to keep sperm out of the upper genital track. Pills have less than a 1% rate of failure if they are taken every day on schedule. In addition to preventing pregnancy, pills lower your risk of ovarian cancer, cancer of the lining of the uterus (endometrium), benign breast masses, and some kinds of ovarian cysts. Pills decrease menstrual blood loss, cramps, and pain. Pills tend to make acne and oily skin better. Pills also decrease your chance of having a dangerous ectopic pregnancy—a pregnancy outside of the uterus.

Remember: pills do not protect you from AIDS (acquired immunodeficiency syndrome) or other sexually transmitted infections. Use a latex or polyurethane male condom or a female condom every time you have sexual intercourse that could expose you or your partner to infection.

Be sure you know your clinician's telephone number in case of questions or problems.

GETTING STARTED

Your clinician will suggest one of three ways to begin taking pills:

- *Quick Start.* Take your first pill the day you visit your clinician. This is the preferred method. Use a backup contraceptive method for 7 days. You will not get your period until you finish taking the active pills. You may also need to take emergency contraception (EC) if you have recently had unprotected intercourse.

- *First-day start.* Take your first pill on the first day of your next period.

- *Sunday start.* Take your first pill on the first Sunday, during your period. Use a backup method for 7 days.

- Be sure to ask your clinician about Plan B, so that you will have it on hand in case you forget to take your pills on time.

DAILY PILL ROUTINE

1. Each day at the same time of day, take 1 pill from your pill pack.

2. Check your pack of pills each morning to make sure you took your pill the day before.

3. Use a backup contraceptive method if any of the following occurs:

   — Missed taking pills

   — Were late starting your new pill pack

   — Had severe vomiting or diarrhea

— Started taking medications that lower the ability of your body to absorb contraceptive hormones (see the instructions on these specific problems).

If you think you may have had sexual intercourse that was not adequately protected, consider emergency contraception. Call 1–888-NOT-2-LATE for more information.

4. Use condoms every time you have intercourse if you suspect, even a little, that you or your partner may be exposed to a sexually transmitted infection or if you are late taking a pill.

5. If you see a clinician for any reason or are hospitalized, be sure to mention that you are taking birth control pills.

6. If you are using pills to have monthly bleeding and you have

— 21 pills in your pill packet, stop taking pills for 7 days after you finish your current packet, and then start a new packet.

— 28 pills in your pill packet, start a new packet the day after you finish your packet.

Note: your clinician may give you special instructions on doing a first-day start each month. You would begin a new packet of pills when your withdrawal bleeding starts.

7. If you are using pills to avoid having monthly bleeding, you will take an active pill each day at the same time for months at a time.

— If you have a product that has pills packaged for long term use, take one pill each day.

— If you are using conventional 28-day packets, take the 1 active pill each day until you get to the placebo pills. Discard the rest of the packet, open a new packet, and take the first active pill in that packet in place of the discarded placebo. Talk to your clinician about how many active pill packets you can take in a row.

8. Mark your calendar to remind yourself of the days you will begin a new pack of pills. Some women mark their calendar each day as they take their pills.

9. You do *not* need to take a "rest" from taking pills. If you stop taking your pills, you risk becoming pregnant.

Missed Pills

COC pills should be taken every day at about the same time. Missing a pill means taking it after an interval of more than 24 hours or not at all (completely missing a pill). What you need to do if you miss pills depends upon what kind of pill you are taking, how many tablets you missed, and where in your packet you are. These are the current recommendations. If you missed only one pill in your packet, follow these directions in Figure 11–3.

While these instructions are very complete, they are also complicated. The odds are that if you miss a pill late in the pack, you may have missed a pill or took it late sometime earlier in the pill pack. For this reason, it has been suggested that if you miss active pills, think about whether you had intercourse in the last 5 days:

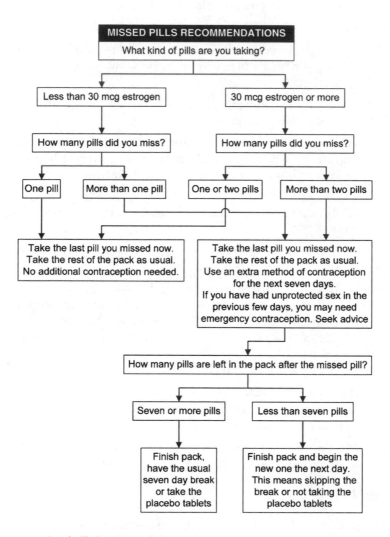

Figure 11–3 Missed pills recommendations

- *If you had no unprotected intercourse in the last 5 days,*
  - take 2 active COCs all at once, and
  - use a backup method for 7 days, and
  - finish the pill pack by taking 1 pill daily. (If you missed more than 4 pills, you can skip the placebo pills in this pack and start a new pack immediately.)
- *If you had unprotected intercourse in the last 5 days,*
  - use emergency contraception today (call your clinician to get some if you do not have any on hand) and
  - restart daily COCs the next day to finish the pack, and
  - use a backup method for 7 days. (If you missed more than 4 pills, you can skip the placebo pills of this pack and start a new pack immediately.)

Vomiting or Diarrhea

Repeated vomiting or severe diarrhea can decrease the absorption of the hormones in pills. The longer you have vomiting or diarrhea, the more important it would be to avoid intercourse, use condoms as a backup contraceptive, and/or use emergency contraceptive pills.

Pills and Your Periods

1. *Short and scanty.* A drop of blood or a brown stain on your panty liner, pad, or underwear during the week you are taking no hormonal pills counts as a period when you are on the pills.

2. *Spotting.* You may have very light bleeding between periods for the first few months you are on pills. If you have bleeding between periods, take your pills at the same time every day. Spotting is generally not a sign of any serious problem. However, if you have bleeding between periods (especially after intercourse) and have not missed pills or taken pills late, have your clinician check you for an infection or other problems. Spotting between periods may also be a sign that your pills may not work as well for you. *Start each new package of pills on time.* Some clinicians recommend a backup contraceptive when you have spotting, especially if you are taking a medication that may make the pill less effective.

3. *Missed period.* If you have not missed any pills and you miss one period without having any other signs of pregnancy, you are probably not pregnant, but you may wish to get a pregnancy test if you are worried. Many women miss one period now and then.

Call your clinician if you are worried or take your temperature with a basal body temperature (BBT) thermometer. The BBT thermometer measures your lowest temperature, generally in the morning before you get out of bed. If your BBT is less than 98° F for 3 days in a row during the pill-free week, you are probably not pregnant. You are fairly safe and can start a new pack of pills on your regular day.

Pills and Pregnancy

If you decide that you want to become pregnant, take prenatal vitamins for at least 3 months before you try to get pregnant. Stop the pills after you have had your preconception care visit with your clinician. It is safe to become pregnant immediately after you stop the pill. You may wish to use another contraceptive method until you have at least 1 normal menstrual period off the pill. That way, when you become pregnant, your date of delivery can be calculated more easily.

Getting pregnant while you are using the pill does not increase your risk of having a baby with birth defects or of having a spontaneous abortion.

PILL WARNING SIGNS

Call your clinician if you have any of the Pill Warning Signs (Figure 11–4) or if you develop depression, jaundice (a yellowing of the skin), a breast lump, a fainting attack or collapse, a seizure (epilepsy), difficulty speaking, a blood pressure above 160/95 mm Hg, a severe allergic skin rash, or if you are immobilized (in a wheelchair or bedridden) after an accident or major surgery. If you are planning to have major surgery, stop using an estrogen containing contraceptive method 4 weeks before your operation and start another method. The risk of a blood clot in a vein is greatest if any of the following conditions are present: if you are overweight, immobile, have severe varicose veins, or if several members of your family have had a blood clot in a vein before age 45. Usually these warning signs have an explanation other than pills; get checked to be sure. *Do not ignore these problems or wait to see if they disappear.*

Pills have been studied extensively and are very safe. However, very rarely, pills can lead to serious problems. Here are the warning signals to watch out for while using pills. These warning signs spell out the word **ACHES**. If you have one of these symptoms, it may or may not be related to pill use. You need to check with your clinician as soon as possible.

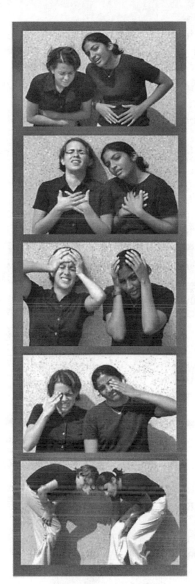

ABDOMINAL PAIN

- Blood clot in the pelvis or liver
- Benign liver tumor or gallbladder disease
- Pregnancy in your tubes

CHEST PAIN

- Blood clot in the lungs
- Heart attack
- Angina (heart pain)
- Breast lump

HEADACHES

- Stroke
- Migraine headache, blurred vision, spots, zigzag lines, weakness, difficulty speaking
- High blood pressure

EYE PROBLEMS

- Stroke
- Blurred vision, double vision, or loss of vision
- Migraine headache with blurred vision, spots, zigzag lines
- Blood clots in the eyes
- Change in shape of cornea (contacts don't fit)

SEVERE LEG PAIN

- Inflammation and blood clots of a vein in the leg

You should also return to the office if you develop severe mood swings or depression, become jaundiced (yellow-colored skin), miss 2 periods or have signs of pregnancy.

Source: Hatcher RA, et al. (2003),[203] with permission.

Figure 11–4 Pill warning signs—ACHES

Pills and Future Fertility

1. Pills are a good option for women who want to become pregnant in the future.

2. By reducing the risk of causes of infertility such as pelvic infections, uterine fibroids, ectopic pregnancies, ovarian cysts, ovarian cancer, endometrial cancer, and endometriosis, pills may improve your future ability to become pregnant.

3. If your periods are irregular before you start taking pills, your periods will probably return to being irregular after you stop taking them.

4. Your long-term fertility is not improved by taking a break from pills.

5. You may experience some delay (about 1 month) in becoming pregnant compared with the amount of time it would have taken if you had not taken the pills. Do *not* count on this; if you do not want to become pregnant now, start using another contraceptive method right after you stop taking pills.

6. Taking pills will not save your eggs for future pregnancies and will not change the age you enter into menopause.

Pills and Smoking

If you smoke, stop. This is the single most important thing you can do for your health. If you cannot stop, try to cut back on the number of cigarettes you smoke. It is all the more important that you watch for the pill warning signals. If you smoke, your clinician will not give you birth control pills if you are over age 35.

Pills and Mood Changes

Usually, the pill has no effect on a woman's mood. However, if you notice mood changes—depression, irritability, or a change in sex drive—see your clinician. You may have another problem. If your clinician believes that your problem may be due to the pills, switching brands may help you. Depression, premenstrual symptoms (PMS), and sexual pleasure can improve on pills, but in some women, they become worse. Newer ways of using pills have been found to help women eliminate these problems if they occur during the week when you take the placebo pills.

Pills and Drug Interactions

A few drugs you may need to take for medical conditions may interfere with the pill. Be sure to tell all your clinicians that you are using COCs. Also, tell the clinician giving you your birth control pills all of the drugs (prescription, over-the-counter, and street drugs) that you are using. If you are using drugs such as rifampin, griseofulvin, phenytoin, phenobarbital, topiramate, carbamazepine, or St. John's Wort, tell your clinician, because you may need to use different pills or another method of contraception. Women using HIV drugs may need lower or higher dose COCs.

DO BIRTH CONTROL PILLS CAUSE BREAST CANCER?

WHO has concluded that long-term use of COCs causes a small and temporary increase in breast cancer risk. A decade after stopping COCs, users return to their baseline risk. The Woman's Care Study found no increased risk for breast cancer among women currently using pills and a decreased risk of breast cancer for those women who had previously used pills. Use of pills by women with a family history of breast cancer was not associated with an increased risk for breast cancer, nor was the initiation of pill use at a young age.[171]

A recent summary of studies suggested that current users of pills are slightly more likely to be *diagnosed* with breast cancer.[169] Two factors may explain the increased risk of breast cancer being diagnosed in women currently taking pills: 1) a *detection bias,* meaning that pill users are simply more likely to have existing breast cancer identified because they have more breast exams or more mammography, or 2) *promotion* of an existing lesion that is nearly cancer into one that is cancer, usually an early cancer. Most authorities think the first explanation is most likely because the duration of pill use has no effect on risk and the excess risk seen in current users is restricted to breast cancers that are localized. Breast cancers diagnosed in women currently on pills or women who have taken pills in the past are more likely to be localized.[169] *By the age of 55,* the risk of having had breast cancer diagnosed is the *same* for women who have used pills and those who have not.

The conclusion of several studies of the risk for breast cancer in women on pills is that women with a strong family history of breast cancer do not further increase their risk for breast cancer risk by taking pills.[169,171,237-240]

While there are still unanswered questions about pills and breast cancer, today, four decades after their arrival on the contraceptive scene, the overall conclusion is that pills have little or no effect on breast cancer. *"Many years after stopping oral contraceptive use, the main effect may be protection against metastatic disease."*[169]

REFERENCES

1. Centers for Disease Control and Prevention. Ten great public health achievements—United States, 1900–1999. JAMA 1999;281(16):1481.
2. Djerassi C. Chemical birth of the pill. 1992. Am J Obstet Gynecol 2006;194(1):290–298.

3. Blackburn RD, Cunkelman A, Zlidar VM. Oral contraceptives—an update. Popul Rep A 2000;28(1):1–16, 25–32.
4. Bronson RA. Oral contraception: mechanism of action. Clin Obstet Gynecol 1981; 24(3):869–877.
5. Killick SR, Fitzgerald C, Davis A. Ovarian activity in women taking an oral contraceptive containing 20 microg ethinyl estradiol and 150 microg desogestrel: effects of low estrogen doses during the hormone-free interval. Am J Obstet Gynecol 1998; 179(1):S18–24.
6. Potter L, Oakley D, de Leon-Wong E, Canamar R. Measuring compliance among oral contraceptive users. Fam Plann Perspect 1996;28(4):154–158.
7. Tayob Y, Robinson G, Adams J, Nye M, Whitelaw N, Shaw RW, et al. Ultrasound appearance of the ovaries during the pill-free interval. Br J Family Planning 1990; 16:94–96.
8. Rosenberg MJ, Waugh MS. Oral contraceptive discontinuation: a prospective evaluation of frequency and reasons. Am J Obstet Gynecol 1998;179(3 Pt 1):577–582.
9. Potter LS. Oral contraceptive compliance and its role in the effectiveness of the method. In Cramer JA, Spilker B, eds. Patient Compliance In Medical Practice And Clinical Trials. New York: Raven Press, 1991 pp 195–207.
10. Holt VL, Cushing-Haugen KL, Daling JR. Body weight and risk of oral contraceptive failure. Obstet Gynecol 2002;99(5 Pt 1):820–827.
11. Holt VL, Scholes D, Wicklund KG, Cushing-Haugen KL, Daling JR. Body mass index, weight, and oral contraceptive failure risk. Obstet Gynecol 2005;105(1):46–52.
12. Brunner LR, Hogue CJ. The role of body weight in oral contraceptive failure: results from the 1995 national survey of family growth. Ann Epidemiol 2005;15(7):492–499.
13. Chuang CH, Chase GA, Bensyl DM, Weisman CS. Contraceptive use by diabetic and obese women. Womens Health Issues 2005;15(4):167–173.
14. Anderson FD, Hait H; The Seasonale-301 Study Group. A multicenter, randomized study of an extended cycle oral contraceptive. Contraception 2003;68:89–96.
15. Zieman M, Nelson AL. Contraceptive efficacy and body weight. Female Patient 2002; 27(10):36–38.
16. Memmel LM, Miller L, Gardner J. Over-the-internet availability of hormonal contraceptives regardless of risk factors. Contraception 2006;73(4):372–375.
17. Mishell DR Jr. Rationale for decreasing the number of days of the hormone-free interval with use of low-dose oral contraceptive formulations. Contraception 2005; 71(4):304–5.
18. American College of Obstetricians and Gynecologists. The pill at 40: Women say it's safer, has extra benefits, but not covered by insurance. Press release. Washington DC: ACOG, May 2, 2001.
19. Vessey M, Painter R, Yeates D. Mortality in relation to oral contraceptive use and cigarette smoking. Lancet 2003;362(9379):185–191.
20. Brent RL. Nongenital malformations following exposure to progestational drugs: the last chapter of an erroneous allegation. Birth Defects Res A Clin Mol Teratol 2005; 73(11):906–918.
21. Ahn HK, Poster presentation at annual meeting of Teratology Society, ObGyn News 2005;40(18):7.
22. Chang J, Elam-Evans LD, Berg CJ, Herndon J, et al. Pregnancy-related mortality surveillance-United States, 1991–1999. MMWR Surveill Summ 2003;52(2):1–8.
23. Franks AL, Beral V, Cates W Jr, Hogue CJ. Contraception and ectopic pregnancy risk. Am J Obstet Gynecol 1990;163(4 Pt 1):1120–1123.
24. Sivin I. Dose- and age-dependent ectopic pregnancy risks with intrauterine contraception. Obstet Gynecol 1991;78(2):291–298.
25. Marchbanks PA, Annegers JF, Coulam CB, Strathy JH, Kurland LT. Risk factors for ectopic pregnancy. A population-based study. JAMA 1988;259(12):1823–1827.

26. Milsom I, Sundell G, Andersch B. The influence of different combined oral contraceptives on the prevalence and severity of dysmenorrhea. Contraception 1990; 42(5):497–506.
27. Mishell DR Jr. Noncontraceptive health benefits of oral steroidal contraceptives. Am J Obstet Gynecol 1982;142(6 Pt 2):809–816.
28. Robinson JC, Plichta S, Weisman CS, Nathanson CA, Ensminger M. Dysmenorrhea and use of oral contraceptives in adolescent women attending a family planning clinic. Am J Obstet Gynecol 1992;166(2):578–583.
29. Nilsson L, Rybo G. Treatment of menorrhagia. Am J Obstet Gynecol 1971; 110(5):713–720.
30. Larsson G, Milsom I, Lindstedt G, Rybo G. The influence of a low-dose combined oral contraceptive on menstrual blood loss and iron status. Contraception 1992; 46(4):327–334.
31. Fraser IS, McCarron G. Randomized trial of 2 hormonal and 2 prostaglandin-inhibiting agents in women with a complaint of menorrhagia. Aust N Z J Obstet Gynaecol 1991;31(1):66–70.
32. Iyer V, Farquhar C, Jepson R. Oral contraceptive pills for heavy menstrual bleeding. Cochrane Database Syst Rev 2000;(2):CD000154.
33. Runnebaum B, Grunwald K, Rabe T. The efficacy and tolerability of norgestimate/ ethinyl estradiol (250 micrograms of norgestimate/35 micrograms of ethinyl estradiol): results of an open, multicenter study of 59,701 women. Am J Obstet Gynecol 1992;166(6 Pt 2):1963–1968.
34. Parsey KS, Pong A. An open-label, multicenter study to evaluate Yasmin, a low-dose combination oral contraceptive containing drospirenone, a new progestogen. Contraception 2000;61(2):105–111.
35. Borenstein J, Yu HT, Wade S, Chiou CF, Rapkin A. Effect of an oral contraceptive containing ethinyl estradiol and drospirenone on premenstrual symptomatology and health-related quality of life. J Reprod Med 2003;48(2):79–85.
36. Freeman EW, Borisute H, Deal L, Smith L, Grubb GS, Constantine GD. A Continuous-Use Regimen of Levonorgestrel/Ethinyl Estradiol Significantly Alleviates Cycle-Related Symptoms: Results of a Phase 3 Study. Fertil Steril 2005;84 Suppl 1):S25.
37. Yonkers KA, Brown C, Pearlstein TB, Foegh M, Sampson-Landers C, Rapkin A. Efficacy of a new low-dose oral contraceptive with drospirenone in premenstrual dysphoric disorder. Obstet Gynecol 2005;106(3):492–501.
38. Davis A, Godwin A, Lippman J, Olson W, Kafrissen M. Triphasic norgestimateethinyl estradiol for treating dysfunctional uterine bleeding. Obstet Gynecol 2000;96(6):913–920.
39. Lanes SF, Birmann B, Walker AM, Singer S. Oral contraceptive type and functional ovarian cysts. Am J Obstet Gynecol 1992;166(3):956–961.
40. Vessey M, Metcalfe A, Wells C, McPherson K, et al. Ovarian neoplasms, functional ovarian cysts, and oral contraceptives. Br Med J (Clin Res Ed) 1987; 294(6586):1518–1520.
41. Young RL, Snabes MC, Frank ML, Reilly M. A randomized, double-blind, placebo-controlled comparison of the impact of low-dose and triphasic oral contraceptives on follicular development. Am J Obstet Gynecol 1992;167(3):678–682.
42. Chiaffarino F, Parazzini F, La Vecchia C, Ricci E, Crosignani PG. Oral contraceptive use and benign gynecologic conditions. A review. Contraception 1998;57(1):11–18.
43. Holt VL, Cushing-Haugen KL, Daling JR. Oral contraceptives, tubal sterilization, and functional ovarian cyst risk. Obstet Gynecol 2003;102(2):252–258.
44. Vessey MP, Painter R. Endometrial and ovarian cancer and oral contraceptives—findings in a large cohort study. Br J Cancer 1995;71(6):1340–1342.
45. Rosenberg L, Palmer JR, Zauber AG, Warshauer ME, et al. A case-control study of oral contraceptive use and invasive epithelial ovarian cancer. Am J Epidemiol 1994; 139(7):654–661.

46. Ness RB, Grisso JA, Klapper J, Schlesselman JJ, et al. Risk of ovarian cancer in relation to estrogen and progestin dose and use characteristics of oral contraceptives. SHARE Study Group. Steroid Hormones and Reproductions. Am J Epidemiol 2000; 152(3):233–241.
47. Schildkraut JM, Calingaert B, Marchbanks PA, Moorman PG, Rodriguez GC. Impact of progestin and estrogen potency in oral contraceptives on ovarian cancer risk. J Natl Cancer Inst 2002;94(1):32–38.
48. Jensen JT, Speroff L. Health benefits of oral contraceptives. Obstet Gynecol Clin North Am 2000;27(4):705–721.
49. Gross TP, Schlesselman JJ. The estimated effect of oral contraceptive use on the cumulative risk of epithelial ovarian cancer. Obstet Gynecol 1994;83(3):419–424.
50. Walker GR, Schlesselman JJ, Ness RB. Family history of cancer, oral contraceptive use, and ovarian cancer risk. Am J Obstet Gynecol 2002;186(1):8–14.
51. Narod SA, Risch H, Moslehi R, Dorum A, et al. Oral contraceptives and the risk of hereditary ovarian cancer. Hereditary Ovarian Cancer Clinical Study Group. N Engl J Med 1998;339(7):424–428.
52. Modan B, Hartge P, Hirsh-Yechezkel G, Chetrit A, et al; National Israel Ovarian Cancer Study Group. Parity, oral contraceptives, and the risk of ovarian cancer among carriers and noncarriers of a BRCA1 or BRCA2 mutation. N Engl J Med 2001; 345(4):235–240.
53. Combination oral contraceptive use and the risk of endometrial cancer. The Cancer and Steroid Hormone Study of the Centers for Disease Control and the National Institute of Child Health and Human Development. JAMA 1987;257(6):796–800.
54. Schlesselman JJ. Risk of endometrial cancer in relation to use of combined oral contraceptives. A practitioner's guide to meta-analysis. Hum Reprod 1997; 12(9):1851–1863.
55. Brinton LA, Vessey MP, Flavel R, Yeates D. Risk factors for benign breast disease. Am J Epidemiol 1981;113(3):203–214.
56. Charreau I, Plu-Bureau G, Bachelot A, Contesso G, et al. Oral contraceptive use and risk of benign breast disease in a French case-control study of young women. Eur J Cancer Prev 1993;2(2):147–154.
57. Rohan TE, Miller AB. A cohort study of oral contraceptive use and risk of benign breast disease. Int J Cancer 1999;82(2):191–196.
58. Jemec GB, Linneberg A, Nielsen NH, Frolund L, et al. Have oral contraceptives reduced the prevalence of acne? A population-based study of acne vulgaris, tobacco smoking and oral contraceptives. Dermatology 2002;204(3):179–184.
59. Redmond GP, Olson WH, Lippman JS, Kafrissen ME, et al. Norgestimate and ethinyl estradiol in the treatment of acne vulgaris: a randomized, placebo-controlled trial. Obstet Gynecol 1997;89(4):615–622.
60. Lucky AW, Henderson TA, Olson WH, Robisch DM, et al. Effectiveness of norgestimate and ethinyl estradiol in treating moderate acne vulgaris. J Am Acad Dermatol 1997;37(5 Pt 1):746–754.
61. Palatsi R, Hirvensalo E, Liukko P, Malmiharju T, Mattila L, Riihiluoma P, Ylostalo P. Serum total and unbound testosterone and sex hormone binding globulin (SHBG) in female acne patients treated with two different oral contraceptives. Acta Derm Venereol 1984;64(6):517–523.
62. Palatsi R. Delayed hypersensitivity and febrile acne conglobata. Acta Derm Venereol 1977;57(1):51–53.
63. Wishart JM. An open study of Triphasil and Diane 50 in the treatment of acne. Australas J Dermatol 1991;32(1):51–54.
64. Thorneycroft H, Gollnick H, Schellschmidt I. Superiority of a combined contraceptive containing drospirenone to a triphasic preparation containing norgestimate in acne treatment. Cutis 2004;74(2):123–130.
65. Arowojolu AO, Gallo MF, Grimes DA, Garner SE. Combined oral contraceptive pills for treatment of acne. Cochrane Database Syst Rev 2004;(3):CD004425.

66. Panzer C, Wise S, Fantini G, Kang D, Munarriz R, Guay A, Goldstein I. Impact of oral contraceptives on sex hormone-binding globulin and androgen levels: a retrospective study in women with sexual dysfunction. J Sex Med 2006;3(1):104–113.

67. Dewis P, Petsos P, Newman M, Anderson DC. The treatment of hirsutism with a combination of desogestrel and ethinyl oestradiol. Clin Endocrinol (Oxf) 1985; 22(1):29–36.

68. Lobo RA. The androgenicity of progestational agents. Int J Fertil 1988;33 Suppl:6-12.

69. Panser LA, Phipps WR. Type of oral contraceptive in relation to acute, initial episodes of pelvic inflammatory disease. Contraception 1991;43(1):91–99.

70. Washington AE, Gove S, Schachter J, Sweet RL. Oral contraceptives, Chlamydia trachomatis infection, and pelvic inflammatory disease. A word of caution about protection. JAMA 1985;253(15):2246–2250.

71. Sangi-Haghpeykar H, Poindexter AN 3rd. Epidemiology of endometriosis among parous women. Obstet Gynecol 1995;85(6):983–992.

72. Westhoff C, Britton JA, Gammon MD, Wright T, Kelsey JL. Oral contraceptive and benign ovarian tumors. Am J Epidemiol 2000;152(3):242–246.

73. Parazzini F, Ferraroni M, Bocciolone L, Tozzi L, Rubessa S, La Vecchia C. Contraceptive methods and risk of pelvic endometriosis. Contraception 1994;49(1):47–55.

74. Nisolle Pochet M, Casanas-Roux F, Donnez J. Histologic study of ovarian endometriosis after hormonal therapy. Fertil Steril 1988;49(3):423–426. Erratum in: Fertil Steril 1988 Jul;50(1):184.

75. Task Force for Epidemiological Research on Reproductive Health, United Nations Development Programme/United Nations Population Fund/World Health Organization/World Bank Special Programme of Research, Development and Research Training in Human Reproduction, World Health Organization, Geneva, Switzerland. Effects of contraceptives on hemoglobin and ferritin. Contraception 1998; 58(5):262–273.

76. Shargil AA. Hormone replacement therapy in perimenopausal women with a triphasic contraceptive compound: a three-year prospective study. Int J Fertil 1985; 30(1):15, 18–28.

77. Casper RF, Dodin S, Reid RL, Study Investigators. The effect of 20 g ethinyl estradiol/1 mg norethindrone acetate (Minestrin®), a low-dose oral contraceptive, on vaginal bleeding patterns, hot flashes, and quality of life in symptomatic perimenopausal women. Menopause 1997;4(3):139–147.

78. Chiaffarino F, Parazzini F, La Vecchia C, Marsico S, Surace M, Ricci E. Use of oral contraceptives and uterine fibroids: results from a case-control study. Br J Obstet Gynaecol 1999;106(8):857–860.

79. Marshall LM, Spiegelman D, Goldman MB, Manson JE, Colditz GA, Barbieri R, et al. A prospective study of reproductive factors and oral contraceptive use in relation to the risk of uterine leiomyomata. Fertil Steril 1998;70(3):432–439.

80. Hergenroeder AC, Smith EO, Shypailo R, Jones LA, Klish WJ, Ellis K. Bone mineral changes in young women with hypothalamic amenorrhea treated with oral contraceptives, medroxyprogesterone, or placebo over 12 months. Am J Obstet Gynecol 1997;176(5):1017–1025.

81. MacNeil JS. COC counters bone loss in anorexic teenagers. Ob.Gyn News 2005 July 1.

82. Grinspoon S, Thomas L, Miller K, Herzog D, Klibanski A. Effects of recombinant human IGF-I and oral contraceptive administration on bone density in anorexia nervosa. J Clin Endocrinol Metab 2002;87(6):2883–2891.

83. Elgan C, Samsioe G, Dykes AK. Influence of smoking and oral contraceptives on bone mineral density and bone remodeling in young women: a 2-year study. Contraception 2003;67(6):439–447.

84. Seeman E, Szmukler GI, Formica C, Tsalamandris C, Mestrovic R. Osteoporosis in anorexia nervosa: the influence of peak bone density, bone loss, oral contraceptive use, and exercise. J Bone Miner Res 1992;7(12):1467–1474.

85. Pasco JA, Kotowicz MA, Henry MJ, Panahi S, Seeman E, Nicholson GC. Oral contraceptives and bone mineral density: A population-based study. Am J Obstet Gynecol 2000;182(2):265–269.
86. Cooper C, Hannaford P, Croft P, Kay CR. Oral contraceptive pill use and fractures in women: a prospective study. Bone 1993;14(1):41–45.
87. Kuohung W, Borgatta L, Stubblefield P. Low-dose oral contraceptives and bone mineral density: an evidence-based analysis. Contraception 2000;61(2):77–82.
88. Barad D, Kooperberg C, Wactawski-Wende J, Liu J, Hendrix SL, Watts NB. Prior oral contraception and postmenopausal fracture: a Women's Health Initiative observational cohort study. Fertil Steril 2005;84(2):374–383.
89. Vestergaard P, Rejnmark L, Mosekilde L. Oral contraceptive use and risk of fractures. Contraception Epub 2006 March 13.
90. d'Arcangues C. WHO statement on hormonal contraception and bone health. Contraception 2006;73(5):443–444.
91. de Abood M, de Castillo Z, Guerrero F, Espino M, Austin KL. Effect of Depo-Provera or Microgynon on the painful crises of sickle cell anemia patients. Contraception 1997;56(5):313–316.
92. Caruso S, Agnello C, Intelisano G, Farina M, Di Mari L, Sparacino L, Cianci A. Prospective study on sexual behavior of women using 30 microg ethinylestradiol and 3 mg drospirenone oral contraceptive. Contraception 2005;72(1):19–23.
93. Spector TD, Hochberg MC. The protective effect of the oral contraceptive pill on rheumatoid arthritis: an overview of the analytic epidemiological studies using meta-analysis. J Clin Epidemiol 1990;43(11):1221–1230.
94. Pladevall-Vila M, Delclos GL, Varas C, Guyer H, Brugues-Tarradellas J, Anglada-Arisa A. Controversy of oral contraceptives and risk of rheumatoid arthritis: meta-analysis of conflicting studies and review of conflicting meta-analyses with special emphasis on analysis of heterogeneity. Am J Epidemiol 1996;144(1):1–14.
95. Strinic T, Eterovic D. Oral contraceptives improve lung mechanics. Fertil Steril 2003;79(5):1070–1073.
96. Ellertson C, Webb A, Blanchard K, Bigrigg A, Haskell S, Shochet T, Trussell J. Modifying the Yuzpe regimen of emergency contraception: a multicenter randomized controlled trial. Obstet Gynecol 2003;101(6):1160–1167.
97. The Cancer and Steroid Hormone Study of the Centers for Disease Control and the National Institute of Child Health and Human Development. Oral-contraceptive use and the risk of breast cancer. N Engl J Med 1986 14;315(7):405–411.
98. Ries LAG, Eisner MP, Kosary CL, Hankey BF, Miller BA, Clegg L, Mariotto A, Feuer EJ, Edwards BK (eds). SEER Cancer Statistics Review, 1975–2002, National Cancer Institute. Bethesda, MD, http /seer.cancer.gov/csr/1975_2002/, based on November 2004 SEER data submission, posted to the SEER web site 2005.
99. Raman-Wilms L, Tseng AL, Wighardt S, Einarson TR, Koren G. Fetal genital effects of first-trimester sex hormone exposure: a meta-analysis. Obstet Gynecol 1995;85(1):141–149.
100. Lammer EJ, Cordero JF. Exogenous sex hormone exposure and the risk for major malformations. JAMA 1986;255(22):3128–3132.
101. Contraceptives and congenital anomalies. ACOG Committee Opinion: Committee on Gynecologic Practice. Number 124-July 1993. Int J Gynaecol Obstet 1993; 42(3):316–317.
102. Bracken MB. Oral contraception and congenital malformations in offspring: a review and meta-analysis of the prospective studies. Obstet Gynecol 1990;76(3 Pt 2):552–557.
103. Cardy GC. Outcome of pregnancies after failed hormonal postcoital contraception-an interim report. Br J Fam Plann 1995;21(3):112–115.
104. Hemminki E, Gissler M, Merilainen J. Reproductive effects of in utero exposure to estrogen and progestin drugs. Fertil Steril 1999;71(6):1092–1098.

105. Tanis BC, van den Bosch MA, Kemmeren JM, Cats VM, Helmerhorst FM, Algra A, et al. Oral contraceptives and the risk of myocardial infarction. N Engl J Med 2001; 345(25):1787–1793.
106. Rosenberg L, Palmer JR, Rao RS, Shapiro S. Low-dose oral contraceptive use and the risk of myocardial infarction. Arch Intern Med 2001;161:1065–1070.
107. Dunn N, Thorogood M, Faragher B, de Caestecker L, MacDonald TM, McCollum C, Thomas S, Mann R. Oral contraceptives and myocardial infarction: results of the MICA case-control study. BMJ 1999;318(7198):1579–1583.
108. Khader YS, Rice J, John L, Abueita O. Oral contraceptives use and the risk of myocardial infarction: a meta-analysis. Contraception 2003;68(1):11–17.
109. Petitti DB. Combination estrogen-progestin oral contraceptives. N Engl J Med 2003; 349:1443–1450.
110. Schwingl PJ, Ory HW, Visness CM. Estimates of the risk of cardiovascular death attributable to low-dose oral contraceptives in the United States. Am J Obstet Gynecol 1999;180(1 Pt 1):241–249.
111. WHO Scientific Group. Cardiovascular disease and steroid hormone contraception. WHO Technical Report Series, No. 877. Geneva, World Health Organization, 1998.
112. Lubianca JN, Faccin CS, Fuchs FD. Oral contraceptives: a risk factor for uncontrolled blood pressure among hypertensive women. Contraception 2003;67(1):19–24.
113. Farley TM, Collins J, Schlesselman JJ. Hormonal contraception and risk of cardiovascular disease. An international perspective. Contraception 1998;57(3):211–30.
114. WHO Collaborative Study of Cardiovascular Disease and Steroid Hormone Contraception. Acute myocardial infarction and combined oral contraceptives: results of an international multicentre case-control study. Lancet 1997;349(9060):1202–1209.
115. Petitti DB, Sidney S, Bernstein A, Wolf S, Quesenberry C, Ziel HK. Stroke in users of low-dose oral contraceptives. N Engl J Med 1996;335(1):8–15.
116. WHO Collaborative Study of Cardiovascular Disease and Steroid Hormone Contraception. Ischaemic stroke and combined oral contraceptives: results of an international, multicentre, case-control study. Lancet 1996;348(9026):498–505.
117. Heinemann LA, Lewis MA, Thorogood M, Spitzer WO, Guggenmoos-Holzmann I, Bruppacher R. Case-control study of oral contraceptives and risk of thromboembolic stroke: results from International Study on Oral Contraceptives and Health of Young Women. BMJ 1997;315(7121):1502–1504.
118. Chang CL, Donaghy M, Poulter N. Migraine and stroke in young women: case-control study. The World Health Organisation Collaborative Study of Cardiovascular Disease and Steroid Hormone Contraception. BMJ 1999;318(7175):13–18.
119. Curtis KM, Chrisman CE, Peterson HB, WHO Programme for Mapping Best Practices in Reproductive Health. Contraception for women in selected circumstances. Obstet Gynecol 2002;99(6):1100–1112.
120. WHO Collaborative Study of Cardiovascular Disease and Steroid Hormone Contraception.Haemorrhagic stroke, overall stroke risk, and combined oral contraceptives: results of an international, multicentre, case-control study. Lancet 1996; 348(9026):505–510.
121. Patient package inserts for Alesse, Ortho TriCyclen, and Yasmin. April 2006.
122. Hannaford PC, Croft PR, Kay CR. Oral contraception and stroke. Evidence from the Royal College of General Practitioners' Oral Contraception Study. Stroke 1994; 25(5):935–942.
123. Kemmeren JM, Tanis BC, van den Bosch MA, Bollen EL, Helmerhorst FM, van der Graaf Y, et al. Risk of Arterial Thrombosis in Relation to Oral Contraceptives (RATIO) study: oral contraceptives and the risk of ischemic stroke. Stroke 2002; 33(5):1202–1208.
124. Feigin VL, Rinkel GJ, Lawes CM, Algra A, Bennett DA, van Gijn J, Anderson CS. Risk factors for subarachnoid hemorrhage: an updated systematic review of epidemiological studies. Stroke 2005;36(12):2773–2780.

125. Nordstrom M, Lindblad B, Bergqvist D, Kjellstrom T. A prospective study of the incidence of deep-vein thrombosis within a defined urban population. J Intern Med 1992; 232(2):155–160.
126. Stolley PD, Tonascia JA, Tockman MS, Sartwell PE, Rutledge AH, Jacobs MP. Thrombosis with low-estrogen oral contraceptives. Am J Epidemiol 1975;102(3):197–208.
127. Royal College of General Practitioners' Oral Contraception Study. Oral contraceptives, venous thrombosis, and varicose veins. J R Coll Gen Pract 1978; 28(192):393–399.
128. Speroff L, Fritz MA. Oral contraception. In: Clinical Gynecologic Endocrinology and Infertility, 7th ed., Baltimore: Lippincott Williams & Wilkins, 2005:861–942.
129. World Health Organization Collaborative Study of Cardiovascular Disease and Steroid Hormone Contraception. Venous thromboembolic disease and combined oral contraceptives: results of international multicentre case-control study. Lancet 1995; 346(8990):1575–1582.
130. Sidney S, Petitti DB, Soff GA, Cundiff DL, Tolan KK, Quesenberry CP Jr. Venous thromboembolic disease in users of low-estrogen combined estrogen-progestin oral contraceptives. Contraception 2004;70(1):3–10.
131. Jick SS, Kaye JA, Russmann S, Jick H. Risk of nonfatal venous thromboembolism with oral contraceptives containing levonorgestrel. Contraception Epub 2006 Mar 29.
132. Romero A, Alonso C, Rincon M, Medrano J, Santos JM, Calderon E, Marin I, Gonzalez MA. Risk of venous thromboembolic disease in women A qualitative systematic review. Eur J Obstet Gynecol Reprod Biol 2005;121(1):8–17.
133. World Health Organization Collaborative Study of Cardiovascular Disease and Steroid Hormone Contraception. Effect of different progestagens in low oestrogen oral contraceptives on venous thromboembolic disease. Lancet 1995;346(8990):1582–1588.
134. Spitzer WO, Lewis MA, Heinemann LA, Thorogood M, MacRae KD. Third generation oral contraceptives and risk of venous thromboembolic disorders: an international case-control study. Transnational Research Group on Oral Contraceptives and the Health of Young Women. BMJ 1996;312(7023):83–88.
135. Jick H, Jick SS, Gurewich V, Myers MW, Vasilakis C. Risk of idiopathic cardiovascular death and nonfatal venous thromboembolism in women using oral contraceptives with differing progestagen components. Lancet 1995;346(8990):1589–1593.
136. Sheldon T. Dutch GPs warned against new contraceptive pill. BMJ 2002; 324(7342):869.
137. Lewis MA, Heinemann LA, MacRae KD, Bruppacher R, Spitzer WO. The increased risk of venous thromboembolism and the use of third generation progestagens: role of bias in observational research. The Transnational Research Group on Oral Contraceptives and the Health of Young Women. Contraception 1996 Jul;54(1):5–13. Erratum in: Contraception 1996 Aug;54(2):121.
138. Mohllajee AP, Curtis KM, Martins SL, Peterson HB. Does use of hormonal contraceptives among women with thrombogenic mutations increase their risk of venous thromboembolism? A systematic review. Contraception 2006;73(2):166–178.
139. Vandenbroucke JP, Koster T, Briet E, Reitsma PH, Bertina RM, Rosendaal FR. Increased risk of venous thrombosis in oral-contraceptive users who are carriers of factor V Leiden mutation. Lancet 1994;344(8935):1453–1457.
140. Vandenbroucke JP, van der Meer FJ, Helmerhorst FM, Rosendaal FR. Factor V Leiden: should we screen oral contraceptive users and pregnant women? BMJ 1996; 313(7065):1127–1130.
141. Chasan-Taber L, Willett WC, Manson JE, Spiegelman D, Hunter DJ, Curhan G, Colditz GA, Stampfer MJ. Prospective study of oral contraceptives and hypertension among women in the United States. Circulation 1996;94(3):483–489.
142. Darney P. Safety and efficacy of a triphasic oral contraceptive containing desogestrel: results of three multicenter trials. Contraception 1993;48(4):323–337.

143. Chasan-Taber L, Willett WC, Stampfer MJ, Hunter DJ, Colditz GA, Spiegelman D, Manson JE. A prospective study of oral contraceptives and NIDDM among U.S. women. Diabetes Care 1997;20(3):330–335.

144. Troisi RJ, Cowie CC, Harris MI. Oral contraceptive use and glucose metabolism in a national sample of women in the United States. Am J Obstet Gynecol 2000; 183(2):389–395.

145. Kim C, Siscovick DS, Sidney S, Lewis CE, Kiefe CI, Koepsell TD; CARDIA Study. Oral contraceptive use and association with glucose, insulin, and diabetes in young adult women: the CARDIA Study. Coronary Artery Risk Development in Young Adults. Diabetes Care 2002;25(6):1027–1032.

146. Kojima T, Lindheim SR, Duffy DM, Vijod MA, Stanczyk FZ, Lobo RA. Insulin sensitivity is decreased in normal women by doses of ethinyl estradiol used in oral contraceptives. Am J Obstet Gynecol 1993;169(6):1540–1544.

147. Kjos SL, Peters RK, Xiang A, Thomas D, Schaefer U, Buchanan TA. Contraception and the risk of type 2 diabetes mellitus in Latina women with prior gestational diabetes mellitus. JAMA 1998;280(6):533–538.

148. Milne R, Vessey M. The association of oral contraception with kidney cancer, colon cancer, gallbladder cancer (including extrahepatic bile duct cancer) and pituitary tumours. Contraception 1991;43(6):667–693.

149. Scalori A, Tavani A, Gallus S, La Vecchia C, Colombo M. Oral contraceptives and the risk of focal nodular hyperplasia of the liver: a case-control study. Am J Obstet Gynecol 2002;186(2):195–197.

150. The WHO Collaborative Study of Neoplasia and Steroid Contraceptives. Combined oral contraceptives and liver cancer. Int J Cancer 1989;43(2):254–259.

151. Mohllajee AP, Curtis KM, Martins SL, Peterson HB. Hormonal contraceptive use and risk of sexually transmitted infections: a systematic review. Contraception 2006; 73(2):154–165.

152. Cottingham J, Hunter D. Chlamydia trachomatis and oral contraceptive use: a quantitative review. Genitourin Med 1992;68(4):209–216.

153. Morrison CS, Bright P, Wong EL, Kwok C, Yacobson I, Gaydos CA, Tucker HT, Blumenthal PD. Hormonal contraceptive use, cervical ectopy, and the acquisition of cervical infections. Sex Transm Dis 2004;31(9):561–567.

154. Rahm VA, Odlind V, Gnarpe H. Chlamydia trachomatis among sexually active teenage girls: influence of sampling location and clinical signs on the detection rate. Genitourin Med 1990;66(2):66–69.

155. Green J, Berrington de Gonzalez A, Smith JS, Franceschi S, Appleby P, Plummer M, Beral V. Human papillomavirus infection and use of oral contraceptives. Br J Cancer 2003;88(11):1713–1720.

156. Winer RL, Lee SK, Hughes JP, Adam DE, Kiviat NB, Koutsky LA. Genital human papillomavirus infection: incidence and risk factors in a cohort of female university students. Am J Epidemiol 2003;157(3):218–226. Erratum in: Am J Epidemiol 2003; 157(9):858.

157. Sellors JW, Karwalajtys TL, Kaczorowski J, Mahony JB, Lytwyn A, Chong S, Sparrow J, Lorincz A; Survey of HPV in Ontario Women Group. Incidence, clearance and predictors of human papillomavirus infection in women. CMAJ 2003;168(4):421–425.

158. Fleming DC, King AE, Williams AR, Critchley HO, Kelly RW. Hormonal contraception can suppress natural antimicrobial gene transcription in human endometrium. Fertil Steril 2003;79(4):856–863.

159. Morrison CS, Richardson BA, Celentano DD, Chipato T, Mmiro F, Padian NS, Rugpao S, Cornelisse PGA, Salata RA. Hormonal Contraception and Risk of HIV-1 Acquisition (HC-HIV) study: background, results and discussion. Presented at the 16th biennial meeting of the International Society for Sexually Transmitted Diseases Research (ISSTDR), Amsterdam, July 12, 2005.

160. Karagas MR, Stukel TA, Dykes J, Miglionico J, Greene MA, Carey M, et al. A pooled analysis of 10 case-control studies of melanoma and oral contraceptive use. Br J Cancer 2002;86(7):1085–1092.

161. Ross RK, Pike MC, Vessey MP, Bull D, Yeates D, Casagrande JT. Risk factors for uterine fibroids: reduced risk associated with oral contraceptives. Br Med J (Clin Res Ed). 1986;293(6543):359–362. Erratum in: Br Med J (Clin Res Ed) 1986;293(6553):1027.

162. Parazzini F, Negri E, La Vecchia C, Fedele L, Rabaiotti M, Luchini L. Oral contraceptive use and risk of uterine fibroids. Obstet Gynecol 1992;79(3):430–433.

163. Marshall LM, Spiegelman D, Goldman MB, Manson JE, Colditz GA, Barbieri RL, Stampfer MJ, Hunter DJ. A prospective study of reproductive factors and oral contraceptive use in relation to the risk of uterine leiomyomata. Fertil Steril 1998; 70(3):432–439.

164. Moreno V, Bosch FX, Munoz N, Meijer CJ, Shah KV, et al.; International Agency for Research on Cancer. Multicentric Cervical Cancer Study Group. Effect of oral contraceptives on risk of cervical cancer in women with human papillomavirus infection: the IARC multicentric case-control study. Lancet 2002;359(9312):1085–1092.

165. Smith JS, Green J, Berrington de Gonzalez A, Appleby P, Peto J, Plummer M, et al. Cervical cancer and use of hormonal contraceptives: a systematic review. Lancet 2003;361(9364):1159–1167.

166. Munoz N, Franceschi S, Bosetti C, Moreno V, et al.; International Agency for Research on Cancer. Multicentric Cervical Cancer Study Group. Role of parity and human papillomavirus in cervical cancer: the IARC multicentric case-control study. Lancet 2002;359(9312):1093–1101.

167. Ursin G, Peters RK, Henderson BE, d'Ablaing G 3rd, et al. Oral contraceptive use and adenocarcinoma of cervix. Lancet 1994;344(8934):1390–1394.

168. Morrison C, Prokorym P, Piquero C, Wakely PE Jr, Nuovo GJ. Oral contraceptive pills are associated with artifacts in ThinPrep Pap smears that mimic low-grade squamous intraepithelial lesions. Cancer 2003;99(2):75–82.

169. Collaborative Group on Hormonal Factors in Breast Cancer. Breast cancer and hormonal contraceptives: collaborative reanalysis of individual data on 53,297 women with breast cancer and 100,239 women without breast cancer from 54 epidemiological studies. Lancet 1996;347:1713–1727.

170. Grabrick DM, Hartmann LC, Cerhan JR, Vierkant RA, Therneau TM, Vachon CM, Olson JE, Couch FJ, Anderson KE, Pankratz VS, Sellers TA. Related Risk of breast cancer with oral contraceptive use in women with a family history of breast cancer. JAMA 2000;284(14):1791–1798.

171. Marchbanks PA, McDonald JA, Wilson HG, Folger SG, et al. Oral contraceptives and the risk of breast cancer. N Engl J Med 2002;346(26):2025–2032.

172. Graham CA, Ramos R, Bancroft J, Maglaya C, Farley TMM. The effects of steroidal contraceptives on the well-being and sexuality of women: A double-blind, placebo-controlled, two-centre study of combined and progestogen-only methods. Contraception 1995;52:363–369.

173. Egarter C, Putz M, Strohmer H, Speiser P, Wenzl R, Huber J. Ovarian function during low-dose oral contraceptive use. Contraception 1995;51(6):329–333.

174. Ernst U, Baumgartner L, Bauer U, Janssen G. Improvement of quality of life in women using a low-dose desogestrel-containing contraceptive: results of an observational clinical evaluation. Eur J Contracept Reprod Health Care 2002;7(4):238–243.

175. Cheung E, Free C. Factors influencing young women's decision making regarding hormonal contraceptives: a qualitative study. Contraception 2005;71(6):426–431.

176. Mullen WH, Anderson IB, Kim SY, Blanc PD, Olson KR. Incorrect overdose management advice in the Physicians' Desk Reference. Ann Emerg Med 1997;29(2):255–261.

177. Stewart FH, Harper CC, Ellertson CE, Grimes DA, Sawaya GF, Trussell J. Clinical breast and pelvic examination requirements for hormonal contraception: Current practice vs evidence. JAMA 2001;285(17):2232–2239.

178. Harper C, Balistreri E, Boggess J, Leon K, Darney P. Provision of hormonal contraceptives without a mandatory pelvic examination: the first stop demonstration project. Fam Plann Perspect 2001;33(1):13–18.

179. Hannaford PC, Webb AM. Evidence-guided prescribing of combined oral contraceptives: consensus statement. An International Workshop at Mottram Hall, Wilmslow, U.K., March, 1996. Contraception 1996;54(3):125–129.

180. Comp PC. Should coagulation tests be used to determine which oral contraceptive users have an increased risk of thrombophlebitis? Contraception 2006;73(1):4–5.

181. Oakley D, Sereika S, Bogue EL. Oral contraceptive pill use after an initial visit to a family planning clinic. Fam Plann Perspect 1991;23(4):150–154.

182. Polaneczky M, Slap G, Forke C, Rappaport A, Sondheimer S. The use of levonorgestrel implants (Norplant) for contraception in adolescent mothers. N Engl J Med 1994;331(18):1201–1206.

183. Lara-Torre E, Schroeder B. Adolescent compliance and side effects with Quick Start initiation of oral contraceptive pills. Contraception 2002;66(2):81–85.

184. Curtis KM, Chrisman CE, Mohllajee AP, Peterson HB. Effective use of hormonal contraceptives: Part I: Combined oral contraceptive pills. Contraception 2006; 73(2):115–124.

185. Westhoff C, Morroni C, Kerns J, Murphy PA. Bleeding patterns after immediate vs. conventional oral contraceptive initiation: a randomized, controlled trial. Fertil Steril 2003;79(2):322–329.

186. Gladwell M. John Rock's Error: What the co-inventor of the Pill didn't know about menstruation can endanger women's health. New Yorker Magazine 2000 Mar 10:52–63.

187. Spona J, Elstein M, Feichtinger W, Sullivan H, et al. Shorter pill-free interval in combined oral contraceptives decreases follicular development. Contraception 1996; 54(2):71–77.

188. Schwartz JL, Creinin MD, Pymar HC, Reid L. Predicting risk of ovulation in new start oral contraceptive users. Obstet Gynecol 2002;99(2):177–182.

189. Endrikat J, Cronin M, Gerlinger C, Ruebig A, et al. Open, multicenter comparison of efficacy, cycle control, and tolerability of a 23-day oral contraceptive regimen with 20 microg ethinyl estradiol and 75 microg gestodene and a 21-day regimen with 20 microg ethinyl estradiol and 150 microg desogestrel. Contraception 2001;64(3):201–207.

190. Sulak PJ, Scow RD, Preece C, Riggs MW, Kuehl TJ. Hormone withdrawal symptoms in oral contraceptive users. Obstet Gynecol 2000;95(2):261–266.

191. Extended Regimen Contraception Clinical Proceedings. ARHP Clinical Proceedings. 2003 May 2. Available at: www.arhp.org/healthcareproviders/cme/onlinecme/extendedregimencp/index.cfm?ID=328.

192. Coutinho E, Segal S. Is menstruation obsolete? New York: Oxford University Press; 1999.

193. Ferrero S, Abbamonte LH, Giordano M, Alessandri F, Anserini P, Remorgida V, Ragni N. What is the desired menstrual frequency of women without menstruation-related symptoms? Contraception 2006;73(5):537–541.

194. Miller L, Notter KM. Menstrual reduction with extended use of combination oral contraceptive pills: randomized controlled trial. Obstet Gynecol 2001;98(5 Pt 1):771–778.

195. Edelman A, Gallo MF, Nichols MD, Jensen JT, Schulz KF, Grimes DA. Continuous versus cyclic use of combined oral contraceptives for contraception: systematic Cochrane review of randomized controlled trials. Hum Reprod 2006;21(3):573–578.

196. Sulak PJ, Kuehl TJ, Ortiz M, Shull BL. Acceptance of altering the standard 21-day/7-day oral contraceptive regimen to delay menses and reduce hormone withdrawal symptoms. Am J Obstet Gynecol 2002;186(6):1142–1149.

197. Edelman AB, Gallo MF, Jensen JT, Nichols MD, Schulz KF, Grimes DA. Continuous or extended cycle vs. cyclic use of combined oral contraceptives for contraception. Cochrane Database Syst Rev 2005;(3):CD004695.

198. Schwartz JL, Creinin MD, Pymar HC. The trimonthly combination oral contraceptive regimen: is it cost effective? Contraception 1999;60(5):263–267.
199. Anderson FD, Hait H. A multicenter, randomized study of an extended cycle oral contraceptive. Contraception 2003;68(2):89–96. Erratum in: Contraception 2004; 69(2):175.
200. Foidart JM, Sulak PJ, Schellschmidt I, Zimmermann D; Yasmin Extended Regimen Study Group. The use of an oral contraceptive containing ethinylestradiol and drospirenone in an extended regimen over 126 days. Contraception 2006;73(1):34–40.
201. Edelman AB, Koontz SL, Nichols MD, Jensen JT. Continuous oral contraceptives: are bleeding patterns dependent on the hormones given? Obstet Gynecol 2006; 107(3):657–665.
202. Gallo MF, Nanda K, Grimes DA, Schulz KF. 20 mcg versus > 20 mcg estrogen combined oral contraceptives for contraception. Cochrane Database Syst Rev 2005; (2):CD003989.
203. Hatcher RA, Nelson AL, Zieman M, et al. Managing contraception. Tiger, GA: Bridging the Gap Foundation, 2003.
204. Faculty of Family Planning and Reproductive Health Care Clinical Effectiveness Unit. Faculty statement from the CEU on a new publication: WHO Selected Practice Recommendations for Contraceptive Use Update. Missed pills: new recommendations. J Fam Plann Reprod Health Care 2005;31(2):153–155.
205. Coutinho EM, Silva AR, Carreira C, Barbosa I. Ovulation inhibition following vaginal administration of pills containing norethindrone and mestranol. Contraception 1984; 29(2):197–202.
206. Osterberg L, Blaschke T. Adherence to medication. N Engl J Med 2005;353(5): 487–497.
207. Archer DF, Cullins V, Creasy GW, Fisher AC. The impact of improved compliance with a weekly contraceptive transdermal system (Ortho Evra) on contraceptive efficacy. Contraception 2004;69(3):189–195.
208. Chasan-Taber L, Stampfer M. Oral contraceptives and myocardial infarction—the search for the smoking gun. N Engl J Med 2001;345(25):1841–1842.
209. Willett WC, Green A, Stampfer MJ, Speizer FE, Colditz GA, Rosner B, et al. Relative and absolute excess risks of coronary heart disease among women who smoke cigarettes. N Engl J Med 1987;317(21):1303–1309.
210. Truitt ST, Fraser AB, Grimes DA, Gallo MF, Schulz KF. Combined hormonal versus nonhormonal versus progestin-only contraception in lactation. Cochrane Database Syst Rev 2003;(2):CD003988.
211. Faculty of Family Planning and Reproductive Health Care Clinical Effectiveness Unit. FFPRHC Guidance (April 2005). Drug interactions with hormonal contraception. J Fam Plann Reprod Health Care 2005;31(2):139–151.
212. Murphy AA, Zacur HA, Charache P, Burkman RT. The effect of tetracycline on levels of oral contraceptives. Am J Obstet Gynecol 1991;164(1 Pt 1):28–33.
213. Neely JL, Abate M, Swinker M, D'Angio R. The effect of doxycycline on serum levels of ethinyl estradiol, norethindrone, and endogenous progesterone. Obstet Gynecol 1991;77(3):416–420.
214. Joshi JV, Joshi UM, Sankholi GM, Krishna U, Mandlekar A, Chowdhury V, Hazari K, Gupta K, Sheth UK, Saxena BN. A study of interaction of low-dose combination oral contraceptive with Ampicillin and Metronidazole. Contraception 1980;22(6):643–652.
215. Maggiolo F, Puricelli G, Dottorini M, Caprioli S, Bianchi W, Suter F. The effect of ciprofloxacin on oral contraceptive steroid treatments. Drugs Exp Clin Res 1991; 17(9):451–454.
216. Grimmer SF, Back DJ, Orme ML, Cowie A, Gilmore I, Tjia J. The bioavailability of ethinyloestradiol and levonorgestrel in patients with an ileostomy. Contraception 1986;33(1):51–59.
217. Murphy AA, Zacur HA, Charache P, Burkman RT. The effect of tetracycline on levels of oral contraceptives. Am J Obstet Gynecol 1991;164(1 Pt 1):28–33.

218. Neely JL, Abate M, Swinker M, D'Angio R. The effect of doxycycline on serum levels of ethinyl estradiol, norethindrone, and endogenous progesterone. Obstet Gynecol 1991;77(3):416–420.
219. Friedman CI, Huneke AL, Kim MH, Powell J. The effect of ampicillin on oral contraceptive effectiveness. Obstet Gynecol 1980;55(1):33–37.
220. Helms SE, Bredle DL, Zajic J, Jarjoura D, et al. Oral contraceptive failure rates and oral antibiotics. J Am Acad Dermatol 1997;36(5 Pt 1):705–710.
221. Amsden GW, Mohamed MA, Menhinick AM. Effect of hormonal contraceptives on the pharmacokinetics of trovafloxacin in women. Clin Drug Invest. 2001; 21(4):281–286. (Available at www.medscape.com/viewarticle/406222).
222. Hall SD, Wang Z, Huang SM, Hamman MA, Vasavada N, Adigun AQ, Hilligoss JK, Miller M, Gorski JC. The interaction between St John's wort and an oral contraceptive. Clin Pharmacol Ther 2003;74(6):525–35.
223. Henney JE. From the Food and Drug Administration. Risk of drug interactions with St. John's wort. JAMA. 2000;283(13):1679. (Also available at www.fda.gov/cder/drug/advisory/stjwort.htm).
224. Redmond G, Godwin AJ, Olson W, Lippman JS. Use of placebo controls in an oral contraceptive trial: methodological issues and adverse event incidence. Contraception 1999;60(2):81–85.
225. Villegas-Salas E, Ponce de Leon R, Juarez-Perez MA, Grubb GS. Effect of vitamin B6 on the side effects of a low-dose combined oral contraceptive. Contraception 1997; 55(4):245–248.
226. Vitzthum VJ, Ringheim K. Hormonal contraception and physiology: a research-based theory of discontinuation due to side effects. Stud Fam Plann 2005;36(1):13–32.
227. Thorneycroft IH. Cycle control with oral contraceptives: A review of the literature. Am J Obstet Gynecol 1999;180(2 Pt 2):S280-S287.
228. Coney P, Washenik K, Langley RG, DiGiovanna JJ, Harrison DD. Weight change and adverse event incidence with a low-dose oral contraceptive: two randomized, placebo-controlled trials. Contraception 2001;63(6):297–302.
229. Rosenberg M. Weight change with oral contraceptive use and during the menstrual cycle. Results of daily measurements. Contraception 1998;58(6):345–349.
230. Lloyd T, Lin HM, Matthews AE, Bentley CM, Legro RS. Oral contraceptive use by teenage women does not affect body composition. Obstet Gynecol 2002;100(2): 235–239.
231. Gallo MF, Lopez LM, Grimes DA, Schulz KF, Helmerhorst FM. Combination contraceptives: effects on weight. Cochrane Database Syst Rev 2006;(1):CD003987.
232. O'Connell KJ, Osborne LM, Westhoff C. Measured and reported weight change for women using a vaginal contraceptive ring vs. a low-dose oral contraceptive. Contraception 2005;72(5):323–327.
233. Scher AI, Stewart WF, Liberman J, Lipton RB. Prevalence of frequent headache in a population sample. Headache 1998;38(7):497–506.
234. Loder EW, Buse DC, Golub JR. Headache as a side effect of combination estrogen-progestin oral contraceptives: a systematic review. Am J Obstet Gynecol 2005;193(3 Pt 1):636–649.
235. Rosenberg MJ, Meyers A, Roy V. Efficacy, cycle control, and side effects of low- and lower-dose oral contraceptives: a randomized trial of 20 micrograms and 35 micrograms estrogen preparations. Contraception 1999;60(6):321–329.
236. Mooij PN, Thomas CM, Doesburg WH, Eskes TK. Multivitamin supplementation in oral contraceptive users. Contraception 1991;44(3):277–288.
237. Lipnick RJ, Buring JE, Hennekens CH, et al. Oral contraceptives and breast cancer: a prospective cohort study. JAMA 1986;255:58–61.
238. Colditz GA, Rosner BA, Speizer FE. Risk factors for breast cancer according to family history of breast cancer.For the Nurses' Health Study Research Group. J Natl Cancer Inst 1996;88(6):365–371.

239. Murray PP, Stadel BV, Schlesselman JJ. Oral contraceptive use in women with a family history of breast cancer. Obstet Gynecol 1989;73:977–983.
240. The Centers for Disease Control Cancer and Steroid Hormone Study. Long-term oral contraceptive use and the risk of breast cancer. JAMA 1983;249:1591–1595.

LATE REFERENCES

241. ACOG Committee on Practice Bulletins-Gynecology. ACOG practice bulletin. No. 73: Use of hormonal contraception in women with coexisting medical conditions. Obstet Gynecol 2006;107(6):1453–1472.
242. Jick SS, Jick H. Cerebral venous sinus thrombosis in users of four hormonal contraceptives: levonorgestrel-containing oral contraceptives, norgestimate-containing oral contraceptives, desogestrel-containing oral contraceptives and the contraceptive patch. Contraception 2006;74(4):290–292.
243. Kahlenborn C, Modugno F, Potter DM, Severs WB. Oral contraceptive use as a risk factor for premenopausal breast cancer: a meta-analysis. Mayo Clin Proc 2006;81(10): 1290–1302.
244. Milne RL, Knight JA, John EM, et al. Oral contraceptive use and risk of early-onset breast cancer in carriers and noncarriers of BRCA1 and BRCA2 mutations. Cancer Epidemiol Biomarkers Prev 2005;14(2):350–356.
245. Silvera SA, Miller AB, Rohan TE. Oral contraceptive use and risk of breast cancer among women with a family history of breast cancer: a prospective cohort study. Cancer Causes Control 2005;16(9):1059–1063.
246. Walsh BW, Sacks FM. Effects of low dose oral contraceptives on very low density and low density lipoprotein metabolism. J Clin Invest 1993;91(5):2126–2132.

Contraceptive Patch and Vaginal Contraceptive Ring

Kavita Nanda, MD, MHS

- Both the weekly contraceptive patch and the monthly vaginal contraceptive ring are highly effective in clinical trials: of 1,000 women using the patch or the ring, only 12 will become pregnant within a year.

- Both the contraceptive patch and the vaginal contraceptive ring do not require daily use, which could facilitate consistent and correct use and might improve typical-use failure rates compared with COCs.

- Hormone levels with the patch may be higher than with COCs, while levels are lower with the vaginal ring. Whether these differences lead to clinically significant differences in adverse outcomes is unknown.

CONTRACEPTIVE PATCH

DESCRIPTION OF METHOD

A transdermal contraceptive patch (Ortho Evra™) was approved by the Food and Drug Administration in 2002. It is a thin, flexible, beige, 20 cm² patch with three layers: an outer protective polyester layer; a middle medicated adhesive layer; and a clear liner. Each patch contains 6 milligrams (mg) of norelgestromin (the primary active metabolite of norgestimate) and 0.75 mg of ethinyl estradiol (EE), and releases 150 micrograms (µg) of norelgestromin and 20 µg of EE daily. The patch can be applied to the buttocks, upper arm, lower abdomen, or upper torso (excluding the breasts). It is designed to mimic the 28-day dosing schedule of combined oral contraceptives (COCs), with 21 days of active hormones. Women use three 7-day patches for 1 week each, and then have a

7-day patch-free interval. Ortho Evra is dispensed in packages of three patches for the monthly cycle of use. Packages of a single replacement patch are also available.

Another weekly combined contraceptive patch, containing 1.9 mg gestodene and 0.9 mg EE, is being developed by Schering AG, and is currently in phase III clinical trials. The patch reviewed in this chapter will be the Ortho Evra patch, however, because it is the only contraceptive patch currently approved and marketed.

EFFECTIVENESS

In general, patches belong in the second tier of contraceptive effectiveness, with higher failure rates than those of IUDs, implants, and injections (see Chapter 27). In clinical trials, the failure rates for patches were low and similar to those with COCs. Pearl indices with the patch range from 0.71 to 1.24 with overall use, to 0.59 to 0.99 with perfect use.[1,2] In a pooled analysis of the three pivotal clinical trials (two comparative and one non-comparative), 15 pregnancies occurred in 22,160 treatment cycles, with an overall life-table failure rate of 0.8% (95% CI, 0.3%–1.3%) and overall Pearl index of 0.88 (95% CI, 0.44–1.33).[3] In this analysis the contraceptive patch was less effective in obese women (See section on Special issues).

Because the contraceptive patch is new, typical-use failure rates have not yet been published. In clinical trials, however, correct and consistent use is higher with the patch than with daily COCs.[2,4] Moreover it appears that breakthrough ovulation is less with errors in patch dosing then with errors in contraceptive pill dosing.[5] Thus, in routine practice, the contraceptive patch might be associated with typical-use pregnancy rates lower than those associated with COCs.

MECHANISM OF ACTION

The patch, like other combined hormonal contraceptives, works mainly by suppressing gonadotropins, thus preventing ovulation.[5] Other likely mechanisms of action include thickening of the cervical mucus to prevent sperm penetration and endometrial changes that could affect implantation.

ADVANTAGES

1. **Weekly regimen.** The weekly regimen appears to enhance consistent and correct use of the patch compared with daily COCs. In the pivotal clinical trials, perfect use of the patch and COCs was defined as 21 days of consecutive therapy followed

by a 7-day drug-free interval. Additionally patch users could not wear any patch for more than 7 days. Perfect use of the patch ranged from 88.7% to 96.5% compared with perfect use of COCs which ranged from 79.2% to 90.6%.[1,2,4] In contrast to compliance with COCs, which was worse in younger women, patch users of all age groups, including younger women (age 18 to 24), had consistently improved compliance.[4] Another 3-month study in 50 adolescents found that 87.1% of participants reported perfect compliance. Ease of use and the fact that the patch does not require daily attention were among the main reported advantages.[6]

2. **Forgiving.** Hormone levels remain therapeutic for at least 9 days after application of the second patch, suggesting that ovulation inhibition would be maintained even if a scheduled patch change was missed for as long as 2 days.[7] Additionally, missed patches (either forgetting to start a new patch or forgetting to change a patch) are less likely to lead to follicular growth or ovulation than would COCs. In a randomized comparative study, healthy ovulating women using the contraceptive patch or COCs intentionally made dosing errors, such as taking the patch for only 7 dosing days, followed by 3 drug-free days, or wearing one patch for 10 consecutive days to simulate a missed patch change. The contraceptive patch group had significantly lower follicular sizes than did the COC groups, even after the dosing errors; a 3-day dosing error had no impact on the patch's ability to suppress ovarian activity.[5] Follicular size and ovulation are only surrogate markers, however, and no studies have evaluated risk of pregnancy among patch wearers who make dosing errors.

3. **Adheres well under a variety of conditions.** In clinical trials very few patches (< 5%) needed replacement because of complete or partial detachment. Heat, humidity, and exercise do not affect patch adhesion or pharmacokinetics.[7,8]

4. **Verifiable.** The user can easily verify the presence of the patch. This reassurance about continued protection reduces the anxiety many women report with COCs—questioning if they remembered to take their daily pills and worrying that they might forget to take it.

5. **Cycle control comparable to COCs.** Although patch users may experience higher breakthrough bleeding and spotting in the first 2 cycles, cycle control in subsequent cycles is comparable to that seen with COCs.[1,2]

6. **Does not cause significant weight gain.** In a randomized placebo-controlled trial, the contraceptive patch was not associated with weight gain,[9] and the mean change in body weight from baseline to the end of treatment was an increase of 0.3 kg in a pooled analysis of the clinical trials, with 79% of participants remaining within 5% of their baseline weight.[9]

7. **Rapidly reversible.** Women discontinuing the patch have a rapid return to fertility, with FSH and LH levels returned to nearly baseline levels and 86% of women ovulating in the month following patch discontinuation.[5]

8. **Safe in women with latex allergies.** Because Ortho Evra is made from polyester, it is safe for use in women with latex allergies.

9. **No clinically significant metabolic effects.** Although there are no studies in women with cardiovascular or other diseases, studies in healthy women have shown no clinically meaningful changes in hematology or blood chemistry. Clinicians should remember, however, that surrogate markers such as cholesterol and triglyceride levels may not truly reflect any possible effect of treatment on the true outcomes (e.g., myocardial infarction, stroke).[10]

10. **Non-contraceptive benefits.** Because the hormonal levels and mechanisms of action are similar to those of COCs, the contraceptive patch may provide many of the same advantages and non-contraceptive health benefits (see Chapter 11 on Combined Oral Contraceptives). Data about long-term health benefits are not yet available.

11. **No need for oral administration.** Patches can be used by women who cannot take a pill orally or who have abnormal intestinal drug absorption.

DISADVANTAGES AND CAUTIONS

Potentially serious health effects.

1. **Possible increased risk of venous thromboembolic conditions.** Media reports of 17 deaths in healthy patch users have received great attention. These events were allegedly from cardiovascular events, primarily pulmonary emboli. However, the manufacturer was informed of only 6 deaths: several deaths were reported multiple times, thus 17 is likely an erroneous number.[11] Two of the 6 deaths reported by the manufacturer were unlikely

to be related to the use of the patch: 1 was due to myocardial infarction in a woman with Down syndrome and Eisenmenger syndrome; another was from suicide.[11] Concern has arisen because hormone levels associated with Ortho Evra use may be higher than those associated with use of a COC containing 35 μg EE.[12] However, pharmacokinetic parameters are surrogate endpoints only. They do not necessarily reflect an increased risk of rare estrogen-related complications such as pulmonary embolism, deep vein thrombosis, ischemic stroke, or myocardial infarction. In a recent case control study, the risk of venous thromboembolism with patch use was similar to that with use of a COC containing 35 μg EE and norgestimate (OR 0.9, 95% CI 0.5–1.6).[13]

2. **Other health complications.** In pivotal studies, other serious related adverse events included migraine, cholecystitis, parasthesia at the patch site, cervical adenocarcinoma in situ, and menorrhagia.[9] Although data are scarce, the contraceptive patch may also be associated with some of the rare but serious health complications associated with COCs, such as myocardial infarction, stroke, cholestatic jaundice, hepatic adenomas, or other conditions. It is possible that the patch could also be associated with rare but serious conditions that have not yet been identified.

Side effects

1. **Skin reactions.** One side effect unique experienced by up to half of patch users is a transient skin reaction, such as irritation, redness or rash, at the site of patch application. These reactions lead to patch discontinuation less than 3% of the time, however. Most application-site reactions are mild to moderate, and the reactions do not appear more frequently over time.[9,14]

2. **Breast symptoms.** In a pooled analysis of the 3 pivotal clinical trials, 22.0% of patch users experienced breast discomfort, engorgement, or pain, mainly in cycles 1 and 2. Breast symptoms were generally mild or moderate, decreased with continued use, and rarely led to patch discontinuation.[9] Compared to women using COCs, women using the patch were more likely to experience breast symptoms in the first two cycles.

3. **Headache.** In one study, 22% of women using either the patch or COCs reported headaches. Headaches led to patch discontinuation in 1.1% of patch users and were more likely to lead to discontinuation among patch users than among COC users.[9]

4. **Nausea.** Nausea is another frequent complaint, reported by approximately one-fifth of both patch and COC users in a pooled

study.[9] In the clinical trials, nausea led to patch discontinuation in 1.7% of women.

SPECIAL ISSUES

Obesity

One group of potential patch users deserves special counseling. Higher body weight is associated with lower serum levels of EE and norelgestromin in contraceptive patch users.[3] Furthermore, limited evidence suggests that heavier women, weighing more than 90 kg (198 lbs), may be at higher risk of pregnancy when using the contraceptive patch. In a pooled analysis of the three pivotal trials, 5 of the 15 pregnancies that occurred in patch users were in women weighing more than 90 kg, though such women comprised only 3% of the study populations.[3] This decrease in effectiveness does not preclude use of the patch by heavier women, because such women are at risk for adverse outcomes from unplanned pregnancies. However, obese women may benefit from additional counseling regarding use of the patch. Obesity may also decrease the effectiveness of COCs, though the relationship has not been fully studied.

Adolescence

Adolescents are more likely than older women to experience problems with pill compliance and unintended pregnancy with COCs. They are more likely to use the contraceptive patch consistently and correctly than COCs, making it a method particularly appropriate for this age group.[4,6] However, they also are more likely than older women to experience application site reactions and patch detachment, and need to be counseled adequately.[6] Ease of use, the fact that use does not require daily attention, and the ease of concealment were among the main advantages reported by adolescents in a study.[6]

Postpartum

Recommendations for use of the contraceptive patch postpartum, in both breastfeeding and non-breastfeeding women are the same as for COCs (see Chapter 4 and Chapter 11).

PROVIDING THE METHOD

Explore the patient's medical, reproductive, and social history and conduct a review of systems to ensure that she does not have contraindications to using the contraceptive patch. Generally, women who have medical or other contraindications to COC use (except for those related to intestinal absorption) also have contraindications to initiation and continuation of patch use. To identify such situations, please refer to Chapter 4 on Medical Eligibility Criteria, and Chapter 11 on COCs. Although not absolute contraindications, women with skin conditions such as psoriasis, eczema, or sunburn, may not be able to use the patch.

Measure the woman's blood pressure, if possible. No other screening tests are routinely needed before starting the contraceptive patch unless her history, review of systems, or blood pressure indicates a need for further assessment.[15]

WHEN CAN A WOMAN START USING THE METHOD?

Patch use should be timed to minimize the possibility that a woman is already pregnant and the risk that she might become pregnant between patch placement and the initiation of the patch's contraceptive effectiveness. With Ortho Evra, serum levels of norelgestromin reach levels within the reference range in 24 to 48 hours.[5,7] The contraceptive patch also provides higher and more consistent estrogen levels than do COCs, and it is associated with less breakthrough ovulation.[5,22] However, because the exact timing of contraceptive effectiveness is unknown, recommendations, based on the package insert, are conservative.

If a woman is having menses and not using hormonal contraception or an IUD, advise her that she can start her patch on the first day of her menstrual period or on the Sunday following the first day of her menses. If she starts on the first day, she does not need additional contraceptive protection, but if she begins the patch after the first day of her period, the package insert recommends that she use an additional method of contraception for 7 days. The calendar reminders that accompany the patches can accommodate either approach. Alternatively, women do not need to wait for a menstrual period if it is reasonably certain they are not pregnant. A recent small randomized trial showed that immediate start of Ortho Evra on any cycle day was acceptable, although it did not lead to greater compliance or continuation rates compared with starting with menses.[16] Seven days of additional contraception is also recommended with the immediate start approach.

Switching from other methods. Instruct a woman switching to the Ortho Evra from COCs that she can start the first patch on the day her withdrawal period starts; she does not need additional contraception. Alternatively, she can start on the Sunday following the start of her withdrawal bleed. If she begins the patch after the first day of her withdrawal bleed, she will need 7 days of additional contraception. She can also switch to the patch immediately and not wait until her next menstrual period; if she chooses this method she will not have a withdrawal bleed that month, and she will not need to use additional contraception.

If a woman is switching from injectables, she should place the patch on the day she is due for her next injection. The Ortho Evra package insert does not provide instructions for women switching from other methods such as IUDs or implants; however, it is reasonable to follow the recommendations for COCs, because the hormonal mechanisms of action are similar (see Chapter 11).

After abortion or miscarriage.   After an abortion or miscarriage that occurs in the first trimester, women can start Ortho Evra immediately; additional contraception is not needed. If the patch is not started within 5 days following a first-trimester abortion, the woman should follow the instructions for a woman who is having her menses and is not using hormonal contraception or an IUD. Postpartum women who are not breastfeeding or women who have second trimester losses may start using the patch 3 to 4 weeks after delivery.[5]

Helping a woman choose a pattern of patch use.   Conventional use of the Ortho Evra patch follows a 28-day cycle. A woman places a new patch weekly for 3 weeks, then has a patch-free week to allow withdrawal bleeding, placing a new patch a week later. Recently, extended use of combined hormonal contraceptives has been studied in healthy women who wish to avoid estrogen-withdrawal side effects during the hormone-free week or to avoid withdrawal bleeding.[17] In a recent study, extended (84 day) use of the Ortho Evra patch resulted in fewer bleeding days and bleeding or spotting episodes compared with cyclic use.[18] Women in both groups reported more headache days during the patch-off weeks compared with patch-on weeks, but women in the extended group also reported more headache days per week while wearing the patch. Both regimens led to decreased headache frequency over time, and women in both groups were highly satisfied.[18]

COUNSELING

Advise women of the advantages, potential risks, and side effects. Quality of counseling has been shown to improve satisfaction with some contraceptive methods.[19] If women express concerns about the reports of fatalities with the patch, counsel them that the overall risk of death with patch use is extremely low, and that many more years of use by many women will be needed to determine their exact frequency.[11] Remind them that no studies have shown a higher risk of thromboembolic complications associated with the patch, and that pregnancy carries higher risks of death due to thromboembolic complications than do hormonal contraceptive methods.

Advise women to confirm periodically that the patch is firmly adherent and to avoid using any creams, lotions, or oils near or at the patch site.

If multiple patches are given, advise women to store them at 25°C (77°F) in their protective pouches, and not to put them in the refrigerator or freezer.

MANAGING PROBLEMS AND FOLLOW UP

As with COCs, it is reasonable to prescribe or give a woman a full year's supply of patches at the very first visit and then encourage a re-visit or two only if needed due to problems or side effects. If only a few patches are given at a time, then also prescribe or give a single replacement patch.

Dislodged or detached patches. If the patch is partially or completely detached for less than 24 hours, instruct the woman to try to reapply it firmly, holding pressure for 10 seconds, and confirm that the edges are sticking well. If they do not stick well, tell her to remove the patch and apply a replacement. She should not use other adhesives or wraps to hold the patch in place. No additional contraception is needed, and the day she should change her patch will be the same. If the edges stick well, she can continue to use the patch for the full 7 days.

If the patch has been partially or completely detached for more than 24 hours or if the woman does not know how long it has been unstuck, instruct her to use start a new patch cycle immediately and use additional contraceptive protection for 7 days. She will now have a new patch-change day. If she has had unprotected intercourse she may need emergency contraception.

Missed or forgotten patches. Missed or forgotten patches may refer to forgetting to place a patch at all, when referring to the first week of the cycle, or forgetting to remove and replace a patch (when referring to the 2nd or 3rd weeks). Management of forgotten patches depends upon which patch is forgotten and for how long. See Table 12–1.

Application-site reactions. To decrease the risk of skin irritation, instruct women to rotate application sites when new patches are applied, and not to apply the patch to areas of skin that are irritated or cut. If a woman experiences skin reactions at a patch application site, she can remove the patch and apply a new patch in a different location.

Other side effects. If a woman experiences breast symptoms, headache, nausea, or breakthrough bleeding or spotting, advise her that these symptoms usually decrease over time; counsel her to try to continue using the patch.

Drug interactions. Although data are limited, the contraceptive effectiveness of the patch could be reduced by drugs that affect hepatic metabolism, similar to the effect on COCs (see Chapter 4 and Chapter

Table 12–1 Management of missed or forgotten patches

When patch forgotten/missed	Management
1st week	If a patch is forgotten or late the first week, and the woman has had unprotected intercourse, provide emergency contraception.
	Tell her to place a patch immediately.
	She should use an additional contraceptive method or abstain for 7 days.
	Remind her to change her patch each week, from now on, on the day of the week she started the new patch.
2nd—3rd week	*1–2 days late:* If a woman forgets to remove and replace a patch, advise her to remove the old patch and replace it with a new patch immediately. She needs no additional contraceptive method or emergency contraception.
	More than 2 days late: Have her remove the old patch and place a new one on immediately. Provide emergency contraception if she has had unprotected intercourse (especially if she is 4 days or more late in applying her patch). She should use additional contraception or abstain for 7 days. Tell her to change the patch each week on the day of the week that she placed this new patch.
4th week	If she forgets to remove her third patch, tell her to remove the patch.
	She should place a new one on the usual day.
	She needs no additional contraceptive method or emergency contraception.

11). Because the transdermal patch avoids hepatic first-pass metabolism, however, drugs that only affect the enterohepatic recirculation without affecting hepatic metabolism (such as some broad-spectrum antibiotics) are unlikely to interact with the contraceptive patch. In a pharmacokinetic study, a short course of oral tetracycline did not significantly affect the pharmacokinetics of norelgestromin or EE.[7]

USER INSTRUCTIONS

Use one patch for 7 days. Apply a new patch once a week on the same day for 7 weeks in a row. During the fourth week, do not wear a patch. At the end of the week, start another cycle of patches.

Ask your clinician to provide you with a package of or a prescription for emergency contraceptive pills. You can use these pills if you have had sex that was not properly protected by the patch or by another contraceptive method (you forget to place a patch during the first week of the cycle, or you are more than two days late replacing a patch in the second or third week of the cycle).

Applying the Patch

1. Each patch is packaged in an individual foil packet. Open the pouch by tearing along the top edge and one side edge. Peel the foil pouch apart and open it. Using a fingernail to peel the unit off the foil pouch, lift out the patch along with its clear plastic cover—take care not to remove the clear liner as you remove the patch.

2. Fold the patch open. While holding onto one half, peel the plastic off the other half. Avoid touching the adhesive surface after you remove the liner.

3. Apply the sticky side of the opened patch to your skin, and then remove the other half of the clear liner. You can put the patch on your buttocks, abdomen, upper torso (except the breasts), or on the outside of your upper arm. Avoid placing patches in areas of friction, such as under bra straps or thongs. Only apply the patch to clean, dry skin, and never put it over skin that is irritated, sunburned, red, or infected. Make sure there are no creams, oils, powder, sunscreen, or sweat on the skin—or the patch will not stick. Press firmly on the patch for 10 seconds. Run your finger around the edges of the patch to make sure that all parts of the patch are sticking properly.

Wearing the Patch

1. Keep the patch in the same place for 7 days; then remove it. Check the patch every day to make sure it is fully adherent. You can wear the patch while bathing, showering, swimming, and exercising.

2. After a week, apply a new patch in a different spot on your body. Every new patch should be applied on the same day of the week, called the "Patch Change Day." Because the hormone levels remain protective for up to 9 days, you do not need to apply a new patch at exactly the same time. Wear the new patch for 7 days. Repeat the procedure for a third week.

3. During the fourth week, do not wear a patch. You will begin your menstrual period.

4. After a week without wearing a patch, apply a new "first-week" patch on the same day of the week you applied your other patches.

5. Store the patches in their protective pouches at room temperature.

REMOVING THE PATCH

1. To remove the patch, grasp it by an edge and pull it off. Fold it closed on itself on the adhesive side to seal in the medication.

2. Discard the patch in the garbage; do not flush it into the toilet.

3. If any stickiness or adhesive remains on your skin, remove it by using baby oil or lotions.

VAGINAL CONTRACEPTIVE RING

DESCRIPTION OF METHOD

A vaginal contraceptive ring (NuvaRing®) was approved by the FDA in 2001. NuvaRing is a soft, transparent, flexible ring of ethylene vinyl acetate copolymer, with an outer diameter of 54 mm and a cross-sectional diameter of 4 mm. The ring releases 120 μg of etonogestrel (3-keto desogestrel), the major metabolite of desogestrel, and 15 μg of EE daily. Each ring is designed to be placed vaginally once every 28 days; it is kept in place for 21 days and removed for a 7-day ring-free period to allow a withdrawal bleed.[20]

Another combined contraceptive vaginal ring, releasing 150 μg of the progestin nestorone and 15 μg EE daily, is being developed by the Population Council, and is currently in clinical trials.[21] This ring is designed to be effective for 1 year; users keep the ring in place for 3 weeks, and then remove it for 1 week, reinserting the same ring a week later. A nestorone-only ring, available in Chile and Peru, is designed for use by breastfeeding women.[21]

The rest of this chapter will focus on the NuvaRing, because it is the only contraceptive vaginal ring currently approved by the FDA and marketed in the United States.

EFFECTIVENESS

The vaginal contraceptive ring belongs in the second tier of contraceptive effectiveness, with higher failure rates than IUDs, implants, and injectables. Failure rates with the NuvaRing from clinical trials are low and similar to the patch and COCs (see Chapter 27).[22] Pearl indices range from 0.40 to 0.96 with perfect use, to 0.65 to 1.23 overall.[22-23] In one study, more pregnancies occurred in the North America study than in the European arm; the overall Pearl Index was 1.75 for the in North America and 0.65 in Europe;[24] reasons for this difference are unclear.

Because the vaginal contraceptive ring is new, typical use failure rates have not been published. Theoretically, the avoidance of daily pill taking with the ring's regimen could lead to lower typical-use rates than with COCs due to improved compliance. Although a non-comparative trial showed rates of correct and consistent ring use (91%) that were higher than those of COC use in older studies,[25] a randomized comparative trial showed the rates of the two methods to be more similar.[22] The ring has never been directly compared with the patch; however, an ongoing multicenter randomized trial will compare continuation, side effects, acceptability, and sexual functioning in NuvaRing and Ortho Evra patch users.

MECHANISM OF ACTION

The contraceptive mechanism of action of NuvaRing is primarily ovulation suppression. Other likely mechanisms include effects on cervical mucus viscosity and endometrial thinning.[26]

ADVANTAGES

1. **Easy to use.** Women in clinical trials report that the ring is easy to insert, comfortable to use, and easy to remove.[25,23,27] It is also relatively easy for a woman to verify that the device is in place. The ring's effectiveness does not depend on its exact position, because hormonal absorption occurs through the vaginal walls. The ring rests against the vaginal wall, around the cervix. It does not exert pressure on the urethra, and walking and movement do not lead to expulsion.[28] Although up to 28% of women and 42% of their partners reported feeling the ring during intercourse at times, this did not affect acceptability or continuation for most women.[25]

2. **Forgiving.** Hormone levels remain therapeutic for at least 35 days after application of NuvaRing, suggesting that ovulation inhibition would be maintained even if a woman forgets to remove the ring up to 2 weeks late.[29] Additionally, ring use for as few as 3 days has been shown to be sufficient to suppress ovarian follicular growth (compared with 7 days for COCs).[29] Such uses are not recommended by the manufacturer, however. Additionally, follicular size and ovulation are only surrogate markers, and no studies have evaluated the risk of pregnancy due to dosing errors in ring use.

3. **High levels of consistent and correct use.** NuvaRing's dosing schedule is convenient. Because the ring is left in place for 3 weeks at a time, it avoids the inconvenience of both coi-

tally-dependent methods, such as the diaphragm, and daily COCs. In studies, 86 to 91% of ring users are perfectly compliant.[2,25]

4. **Low, steady release of hormones.** The ring has a steady release rate, providing a low and consistent release of hormones. Although the ring users have progestin levels similar to those of COC users, their EE levels are lower: two-fold lower than those in women taking 35 μmg EE COCs and three-fold lower than those in women wearing the patch.[12] One recent study found that, in the first 3 months of use, fewer patients called about side effects from the NuvaRing than they did about the patch or COCs.[30] Pharmacokinetic parameters are only surrogate endpoints, however, and may not necessarily reflect a decreased risk of estrogen-related side effects or long-term risks.

5. **Vaginal hormone delivery.** The vaginal route of delivery increases the bioavailability of hormones, thus enabling the use of a lower total hormone dose, potentially reducing side effects. The ring can be used by women who cannot take a pill orally, and by women with abnormal intestinal absorption.

6. **Rapidly effective and rapidly reversible.** Hormone levels needed to suppress ovulation are achieved within the first day of vaginal ring use,[31] and as few as 3 consecutive days of NuvaRing use interferes with follicular growth.[24] Return to ovulation after ring removal is rapid, occurring in a median of 17 to 19 days.[24]

7. **Excellent cycle control.** Compared with COCs, the ring is less likely to produce irregular bleeding, especially in the first few cycles. Most vaginal ring users experience withdrawal bleeding on schedule.[23,32,33]

8. **Does not cause weight gain.** In clinical studies, women are as likely to lose weight as to gain it when using the ring for a year.[22,23,34]

9. **No adverse effects on cervico-vaginal epithelium.** NuvaRing use does not appear to have adverse effects on the cervico-vaginal epithelium or on cervical cytology.[23,35]

10. **Does not adversely affect the endometrium.** NuvaRing use for up to 2 years has not led to endometrial hyperplasia or other adverse effects on endometrial histology.[36]

11. **Can be used concurrently with tampons.** Occasionally, a user may need to insert a ring while she is still having withdrawal bleeding. A pharmacokinetic study showed that tampons can be used concurrently with the ring without any

effects on hormone absorption.[37] Ring users need to ensure that the ring is not inadvertently withdrawn at the time of tampon removal.

12. **Can be removed for up to 3 hours without compromising effectiveness.** Although most women and their partners do not report discomfort due to the ring during vaginal intercourse, NuvaRing can be removed or left out for up to 3 hours in any 24-hour period without requiring a backup method.[20] The same ring can then be reinserted.

13. **Safe in women with latex allergies.** Because NuvaRing is made from vinyl acetate and not latex, it can be used safely by women with latex allergies.

14. **No clinically significant metabolic effects.** In healthy women, the vaginal ring has had no clinically important adverse effects on surrogate markers of disease such as heart rate, blood pressure, blood chemistries, lipids, adrenal and thyroid function, carbohydrate metabolism, or hematology.[23,38,39] These surrogate markers may not reflect the actual risk of adverse outcome, and no studies exist in women with cardiovascular or other diseases.

15. **Does not affect bone density.** In a recent study, bone mineral density showed no change from baseline after as long as 24 months of NuvaRing use.[40] The study did not include adolescents or perimenopausal women. No study has looked at risk of fractures.

16. **Non-contraceptive benefits.** Because the hormonal levels and mechanisms of action are similar, the vaginal ring may provide many of the same advantages and non-contraceptive health benefits that COCs do, although data about long-term health benefits are not yet available.

D ISADVANTAGES AND CAUTIONS
POTENTIAL SERIOUS HEALTH RISKS

1. **Possible increased risk of thromboembolic conditions.** Etonogestrel, the progestin in NuvaRing, is a metabolite of desogestrel. Women using desogestrel-containing COCs appear to be at an increased risk of thromboembolic conditions in compared with women using COCs containing second-generation progestins.[41,42,43] Although, two cases of deep vein thrombosis (DVT) were reported in the NuvaRing studies,[32,22] current data

are insufficient to detect a significant increase in such rare events.

2. **Other health complications.** Although data are scarce, the vaginal ring may also be associated with other rare but serious health complications associated with COCs, such as myocardial infarction, stroke, cholestatic jaundice, gallbladder disease, hepatic adenomas, or other conditions. Because NuvaRing is a recently developed method, it is possible that this product could also be associated with other rare but serious conditions that have not yet been identified.

3. **Toxic shock syndrome.** Very rare cases of TSS have been reported by NuvaRing users; some of these users were also using tampons.[20] Although causation has not been determined, any ring user with signs or symptoms of TSS should get appropriate medical evaluation and treatment.

SIDE EFFECTS

1. **Headache.** Headache is the most common reported hormonal side-effect occurring in ring users, reported by 6% of users.[23,39]

2. **Vaginal symptoms.** In clinical trials, the most common reason for discontinuation was vaginal symptoms or problems related to ring use, such as ring expulsion, foreign body sensation or coital problems, occurring in 1–2.6% of women.[25] Other self-reported vaginal symptoms include vaginitis, leukorrhea, and vaginal discomfort. In a recent randomized comparative trial, however, the only vaginal symptom significantly associated with NuvaRing use was vaginal wetness; 63% of ring-users reported vaginal wetness compared with 43% of COC users. Microbiological evaluation showed ring use to be associated only with an increase in hydrogen peroxide producing Lactobacillus.[44]

3. **Other side effects.** Other reported side effects include decreased libido, nausea, and breast tenderness.[23,32,39]

SPECIAL ISSUES

Adolescence

The vaginal contraceptive ring may be particularly appropriate for adolescents, because it offers both privacy and the convenience of monthly dosing. Improved consistent and correct use could ultimately lead to improved typical-use effectiveness. There are no studies evaluating acceptability in adolescents; a randomized trial comparing acceptability of the NuvaRing to COCs among college women is ongoing. It is possible that adolescents may feel uncomfortable with a vaginal device; in one study of women aged 18–41, there was a trend towards increased sexual comfort with increasing age, for both the woman and her partner.[45] Clinicians should counsel and reassure adolescents about user and partner satisfaction with the NuvaRing.

Postpartum

Recommendations for use of the vaginal ring postpartum, in both breastfeeding and non-breastfeeding women are the same as for COCs (See Chapter 4 and Chapter 11).

PROVIDING THE METHOD

Explore the patient's medical, reproductive, and social history and conduct a review of systems to ensure that she does not have contraindications to using the vaginal ring. Generally, women who have medical or other contraindications to COC use (except for those related to intestinal absorption) also have contraindications to the initiation and continuation of vaginal ring use. To identify such situations, please refer to Chapter 4 on Medical Eligibility Criteria, and Chapter 11 on COCs. Women may not be suitable candidates for the vaginal ring if they have significant pelvic relaxation, vaginal stenosis or obstruction (if it prevents placement or retention of the ring), conditions that make the vagina more susceptible to irritation or ulceration, or an inability or unwillingness to touch their genitalia.

Measure the woman's blood pressure, if possible. No other screening tests are routinely needed before starting the contraceptive ring unless her history, review of systems, or blood pressure indicates a need for further assessment.[15]

WHEN CAN A WOMAN START USING THE METHOD?

Use of NuvaRing is timed to minimize the possibility that a woman is already pregnant and the risk that she might become pregnant between insertion and the initiation of the ring's effectiveness. NuvaRing inhibits ovulation even when it is started on cycle day 5.[26] Another study showed that 3 days of ring use inhibited ovulation even with a follicle of up to 13 millimeters size.[25] However, because the exact timing of contraceptive effectiveness is unknown, recommendations, based on the package insert, are conservative.

- If a woman is menstruating and not using hormonal contraception, advise her that there are several options for initiating the NuvaRing:

  — On the first day of her cycle (i.e., the first day of her menses); she needs no additional contraception.

  — On cycle days 2 to 5, even if she has not finished her menstrual bleeding. The manufacturer recommends that women inserting the ring between cycle days 2 to 5 should use an additional method of contraception (male or female condom or spermicide, but not diaphragm) for the first 7 days of ring use in the first cycle.[20]

  — On any day, if it is reasonably certain she is not pregnant (also called QuickStart). A recent study showed that immediate insertion of NuvaRing on any cycle day had advantageous bleeding patterns and was acceptable.[46] Seven days of additional contraception is also recommended with the immediate start approach.

Switching from other hormonal methods. Instruct a woman switching to the NuvaRing from COCs that she can insert the first NuvaRing on any day, but no later than the day following her usual hormone-free interval (the day she would start a new pack of pills). If she has used COCs consistently and correctly, no additional back-up contraceptive is needed. If she is switching from progestin-only pills, she may switch on any day, placing the first ring the day after she takes the last pill. Seven days of additional contraception is recommended.

If a woman is switching from an implant or the Mirena intrauterine system (IUS), she should place the first ring on the day that the implant or IUS is removed. If she is switching from injectables, she should insert the ring the day she is due for her next injection. Although ovulation inhibition with progestin injectables is robust, the NuvaRing labeling recommends the use of additional contraception for 7 days for women switching from all progestin-only methods.

After abortion or miscarriage. If a woman has recently had a first-trimester abortion or miscarriage, advise her that the ring may be inserted within 5 days; she needs no additional contraception. If she does not insert the ring within 5 days she will need to follow the recommendations for menstruating women not using hormonal contraception.

A postpartum woman who is not breastfeeding or who has had a second trimester loss may start using the NuvaRing 3 to 4 weeks after delivery (see Chapter 18), if it is reasonably certain she is not pregnant. She should use additional contraception for 7 days. Advise breastfeeding women to use other forms of contraception for at least 6 months.

HELPING A WOMAN CHOOSE A PATTERN OF RING USE

Conventional use of the NuvaRing follows a 28 day cycle. A woman keeps each ring in for 3 weeks, then removes it for a week to allow withdrawal bleeding, placing a new ring every 4 weeks. Recently, extended use of combined hormonal contraceptives has been studied to avoid estrogen-withdrawal side effects during the hormone-free week or to avoid bleeding in women who prefer amenorrhea.[17,18] Extended ring cycles of 49, 91, or 364 days (with women changing the ring every 21 days) are well-tolerated and acceptable. Bleeding days are reduced overall but spotting days may increase and could lead to discontinuation.[47] Although it has not been studied with NuvaRing, and only with the experimental combined nestorone ring, extended use with removal when menstrual bleeding or prolonged spotting occurs may prove the most acceptable.[48]

COUNSELING

Advise women considering the vaginal contraceptive ring about its advantages, potential risks, and side effects.

MANAGING PROBLEMS AND FOLLOW UP

As for COCs and the patch, it is reasonable to prescribe a full year's supply of rings at the first visit. If a year's supply is dispensed at one time, advise the woman to refrigerate the rings at 2–8°C (36–46°F) to extend the shelf-life beyond 4 months. Rings may be stored for up to 4 months at 25°C (77°F).

EXPELLED RING

A woman may accidentally remove or expel her NuvaRing while removing a tampon, engaging in intercourse, or having a bowel movement. If the ring has been out of the vagina for less than 3 hours, no additional contraception is required. Instruct the woman to rinse the ring with lukewarm water and reinsert it as soon as possible. If a woman loses the NuvaRing, have her insert a new ring and then continue the regimen without alteration.

During the first or second week, if the NuvaRing is removed or expelled and has been out of the vagina for more than 3 hours, it may still be reinserted. However, advise her that an additional contraceptive method should be used for the next 7 days, and offer her emergency contraception if she has had unprotected intercourse.

If a women in her third week of ring use reports that NuvaRing has been out of her vagina for more than 3 hours, advise her to discard that ring. She can then choose one of two options:

- Insert a new ring immediately to begin a new 3-week cycle.

- Have a withdrawal bleed and insert a new ring no later than 7 days from when the last ring was removed/expelled. Advise the woman that this is an option only if the ring was used continuously for the preceding 7 days.

For either option, advise her to use an additional method of contraception until the new ring has been used continuously for 7 days.

PROLONGED USE

If a woman reports that the ring was left in the vagina for more than 3 weeks (but less than 4 weeks), advise her that it is still effective in preventing pregnancy. Counsel her to remove the ring and insert a new one after a 1-week interval. If the ring was left in place for more than 4 weeks, contraceptive effectiveness could be compromised. Consider pregnancy testing, and advise the woman to consider emergency contraception if indicated, and to use an additional contraceptive method until a new ring has been in place for at least 7 days.

DISCONNECTED (BROKEN) RING

If a woman calls to report that her NuvaRing has disconnected or broken, counsel her to discard the ring and replace it with a new ring. She does not need additional contraception.

VAGINAL SYMPTOMS

Advise women that they may perceive more vaginal discharge or wetness while using the ring, but that this does not signify infection. Counsel them that there is no increased risk of vaginal infection with NuvaRing use. However, if a woman complains of vulvovaginal itching or a foul odor, she should be evaluated and treated as needed.

OTHER SIDE EFFECTS

If a woman experiences headache, nausea, or breast tenderness, advise her that these symptoms usually decrease over time, and counsel her to try to continue using the ring.

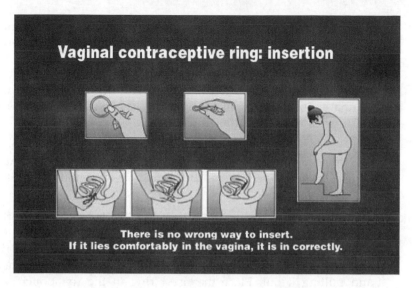

Vaginal contraceptive ring: insertion

There is no wrong way to insert.
If it lies comfortably in the vagina, it is in correctly.

Source: Ballagh SA (2002),[51] with permission courtesy of Organon USA.

Figure 12–1 Inserting the NuvaRing

DRUG INTERACTIONS

Although data are limited, drugs that affect hepatic metabolism could reduce the ring's effectiveness, just as they reduce the effectiveness of COCs (see Chapter 4 and Chapter 11). Because the ring is used vaginally and avoids hepatic first-pass metabolism, drugs that affect the enterohepatic recirculation such as broad-spectrum antibiotics are unlikely to interact with the vaginal ring. In a pharmacokinetic study, co-administration of three antimycotic formulations led to slight increases in etonogestrel and EE levels, with suppositories having the greatest effect.[37] In another study, a single-dose of 100 mg nonoxynol-9 gel did not affect the serum concentrations of etonogestrel or EE.[49] Serum concentrations of etonogestrel and EE were also not affected by concomitant administration of 10 days of oral amoxicillin or doxycycline in standard dosages.[50]

USER INSTRUCTIONS

1. Each NuvaRing comes in a reclosable foil pouch. After washing and drying your hands, remove the ring and keep the foil pouch for ring disposal.

2. Insert the ring into your vagina. Use any position you find most comfortable: standing with one leg up, squatting, or lying down. Squeeze the rim of the ring and put the leading edge into the opening of the vagina. If you feel the ring, just slide it farther into your vagina until it is comfortable; the muscles of your vagina should keep it in place. The exact position of the Nu-vaRing is not critical for its function.

3. Leave the ring in place for 3 weeks. You do not need to remove the ring for intercourse. If you do remove the ring for inter-course, do not leave it out of the vagina for more than 3 hours in any 24-hour period.

4. After 3 weeks of use, remove the ring for 7 days. During this break, you will experience withdrawal bleeding. Remove the NuvaRing by hooking your index finger under the forward rim or by grasping the rim between your index and middle finger and pulling it out. Place the used ring in the foil pouch and throw it away in a trash container out of the reach of children and pets (do not flush it down the toilet).

5. After the 7-day break, insert a new vaginal ring to begin the cycle again. Insert the new NuvaRing on the same day of the week you inserted the previous ring, even if you have not fin-ished your period.

6. If the NuvaRing is out of your vagina for more than 3 hours during the 21-day period, re-insert it and use additional contra-ception for the next 7 days. If you have had unprotected inter-course, consider using emergency contraception. You can ask your clinician to provide you with a package of or a prescription for emergency contraceptive pills.

REFERENCES

1. Audet MC, Moreau M, Koltun WD, et al. Evaluation of contraceptive efficacy and cycle control of a transdermal contraceptive patch vs an oral contraceptive: a ran-domized controlled trial. JAMA 2001;285:2347–54.
2. Urdl W, Apter D, Alperstein A, et al. Contraceptive efficacy, compliance and beyond: factors related to satisfaction with once-weekly transdermal compared with oral con-traception. Eur J Obstet Gynecol Reprod Biol 2005;121:202–10.
3. Zieman M, Guillebaud J, Weisberg E, Shangold GA, Fisher AC, Creasy GW. Contra-ceptive efficacy and cycle control with the Ortho Evra/Evra transdermal system: the analysis of pooled data. Fertil Steril 2002;77:S13–8.
4. Archer DF, Bigrigg A, Smallwood GH, Shangold GA, Creasy GW, Fisher AC. Assess-ment of compliance with a weekly contraceptive patch (Ortho Evra/Evra) among North American women. Fertil Steril 2002;77:S27–31.
5. Pierson RA, Archer DF, Moreau M, Shangold GA, Fisher AC, Creasy GW. Ortho Evra/Evra versus oral contraceptives: follicular development and ovulation in normal cycles and after an intentional dosing error. Fertil Steril 2003;80:34–42.

6. Rubinstein ML, Halpern-Felsher BL, Irwin CE Jr. An evaluation of the use of the transdermal contraceptive patch in adolescents. J Adolesc Health 2004;34:395–401.
7. Abrams LS, Skee D, Natarajan J, Wong FA. Pharmacokinetic overview of Ortho Evra/Evra. Fertil Steril 2002;77:S3–12.
8. Zacur HA, Hedon B, Mansour D, Shangold GA, Fisher AC, Creasy GW. Integrated summary of Ortho Evra/Evra contraceptive patch adhesion in varied climates and conditions. Fertil Steril 2002;77:S32–5.
9. Sibai BM, Odlind V, Meador ML, Shangold GA, Fisher AC, Creasy GW. A comparative and pooled analysis of the safety and tolerability of the contraceptive patch (Ortho Evra/Evra). Fertil Steril 2002;77:S19–26.
10. Grimes DA, Schulz KF. Surrogate end points in clinical research: hazardous to your health. Obstet Gynecol 2005;105:1114–8.
11. Grimes DA, Mishell DR. Assessing rare event reports: a numerator in search of a denominator. Dialogues in Contraception 2004;8:7.
12. van den Heuvel MW, van Bragt AJ, Alnabawy AK, Kaptein MC. Comparison of ethinylestradiol pharmacokinetics in three hormonal contraceptive formulations: the vaginal ring, the transdermal patch and an oral contraceptive. Contraception 2005;72:168–74.
13. Jick SS, Kaye JA, Russmann S, Jick H. Risk of nonfatal venous thromboembolism in women using a contraceptive transdermal patch and oral contraceptives containing norgestimate and 35 microg of ethinyl estradiol. Contraception 2006;73:223–8.
14. Weisberg F, Bouchard C, Moreau M, et al. Preference for and satisfaction of Canadian women with the transdermal contraceptive patch versus previous contraceptive method: an open-label, multicentre study. J Obstet Gynaecol Can 2005;27:350–9.
15. Stewart FH, Harper CC, Ellertson CE, Grimes DA, Sawaya GF, Trussell J. Clinical breast and pelvic examination requirements for hormonal contraception: Current practice vs evidence. JAMA 2001;285:2232 9.
16. Murthy AS, Creinin MD, Harwood B, Schreiber CA. Same-day initiation of the transdermal hormonal delivery system (contraceptive patch) versus traditional initiation methods. Contraception 2005;72:333–6.
17. Miller L, Hughes JP. Continuous combination oral contraceptive pills to eliminate withdrawal bleeding: a randomized trial. Obstet Gynecol 2003;101:653–61.
18. Stewart FH, Kaunitz AM, Laguardia KD, Karvois DL, Fisher AC, Friedman AJ. Extended use of transdermal norelgestromin/ethinyl estradiol: a randomized trial. Obstet Gynecol 2005;105:1389–96.
19. Canto De Cetina TE, Canto P, Ordonez Luna M. Effect of counseling to improve compliance in Mexican women receiving depot-medroxyprogesterone acetate. Contraception 2001;63:143–6.
20. Organon USA I. NuvaRing prescribing information. Roseland, NJ: 2005.
21. Johansson ED, Sitruk-Ware R. New delivery systems in contraception: vaginal rings. Am J Obstet Gynecol 2004;190:S54–9.
22. Oddsson K, Leifels-Fischer B, de Melo NR, et al. Efficacy and safety of a contraceptive vaginal ring (NuvaRing) compared with a combined oral contraceptive: a 1-year randomized trial. Contraception 2005;71:176–82.
23. Dieben TO, Roumen FJ, Apter D. Efficacy, cycle control, and user acceptability of a novel combined contraceptive vaginal ring. Obstet Gynecol 2002;100:585–93.
24. Mulders TM, Dieben TO, Bennink HJ. Ovarian function with a novel combined contraceptive vaginal ring. Hum Reprod 2002;17:2594–9.
25. Roumen FJ, Apter D, Mulders TM, Dieben TO. Efficacy, tolerability and acceptability of a novel contraceptive vaginal ring releasing etonogestrel and ethinyl oestradiol. Hum Reprod 2001;16:469–75.
26. Duijkers IJ, Klipping C, Verhoeven CH, Dieben TO. Ovarian function with the contraceptive vaginal ring or an oral contraceptive: a randomized study. Hum Reprod 2004;19.2668–73.

27. Szarewski A. High acceptability and satisfaction with NuvaRing use. Eur J Contracept Reprod Health Care 2002;7 Suppl 2:31–6.
28. Barnhart KT, Timbers K, Pretorius ES, Lin K, Shaunik A. In vivo assessment of NuvaRing(R) placement. Contraception 2005;72:196–9.
29. Killick S. Complete and robust ovulation inhibition with NuvaRing. Eur J Contracept Reprod Health Care 2002;7 Suppl 2:13–8.
30. Victor, I. Comparing Patient Telephone Callback Rates for Different Hormonal Birth Control Delivery Systems. 42nd Annual Meeting of the Association of Reproductive Health Professionals. St. Petersburg, FL. September 7–10, 2005
31. Timmer CJ, Mulders TM. Pharmacokinetics of etonogestrel and ethinylestradiol released from a combined contraceptive vaginal ring. Clin Pharmacokinet 2000;39:233–42.
32. Bjarnadottir RI, Tuppurainen M, Killick SR. Comparison of cycle control with a combined contraceptive vaginal ring and oral levonorgestrel/ethinyl estradiol. Am J Obstet Gynecol 2002;186:389–95.
33. Oddsson K, Leifels-Fischer B, Wiel-Masson D, et al. Superior cycle control with a contraceptive vaginal ring compared with an oral contraceptive containing 30 microg ethinylestradiol and 150 microg levonorgestrel: a randomized trial. Hum Reprod 2005;20:557–62.
34. O'connell KJ, Osborne LM, Westhoff C. Measured and reported weight change for women using a vaginal contraceptive ring vs. a low-dose oral contraceptive. Contraception 2005;72:323–7.
35. Roumen FJ, Boon ME, van Velzen D, Dieben TO, Coelingh Bennink HJ. The cervicovaginal epithelium during 20 cycles' use of a combined contraceptive vaginal ring. Hum Reprod 1996;11:2443–8.
36. Bulten J, Grefte J, Siebers B, Dieben T. The combined contraceptive vaginal ring (NuvaRing) and endometrial histology. Contraception 2005;72:362–5.
37. Verhoeven CH, Dieben TO. The combined contraceptive vaginal ring, NuvaRing, and tampon co-usage. Contraception 2004;69:197–9.
38. Tuppurainen M, Klimscheffskij R, Venhola M, Dieben TO. The combined contraceptive vaginal ring (NuvaRing) and lipid metabolism: a comparative study. Contraception 2004;69:389–94.
39. Roumen F. Contraceptive efficacy and tolerability with a novel combined contraceptive vaginal ring, NuvaRing. Eur J Contracept Reprod Health Care 2002;7 Suppl 2:19–24.
40. Massai R, Makarainen L, Kuukankorpi A, Klipping C, Duijkers I, Dieben T. The combined contraceptive vaginal ring and bone mineral density in healthy pre-menopausal women. Hum Reprod 2005;20:2764–8.
41. Jick H, Kaye JA, Vasilakis-Scaramozza C, Jick SS. Risk of venous thromboembolism among users of third generation oral contraceptives compared with users of oral contraceptives with levonorgestrel before and after 1995: cohort and case-control analysis. BMJ 2000;321:1190–5.
42. Farmer RD, Lawrenson RA, Todd JC, et al. A comparison of the risks of venous thromboembolic disease in association with different combined oral contraceptives. Br J Clin Pharmacol 2000;49:580–90.
43. Hedenmalm K, Samuelsson E. Fatal venous thromboembolism associated with different combined oral contraceptives: a study of incidences and potential biases in spontaneous reporting. Drug Saf 2005;28:907–16.
44. Veres S, Miller L, Burington B. A comparison between the vaginal ring and oral contraceptives. Obstet Gynecol 2004;104:555–63.
45. Novak A, de la Loge C, Abetz L, van der Meulen EA. The combined contraceptive vaginal ring, NuvaRing: an international study of user acceptability. Contraception 2003;67:187–94.

46. Westhoff C, Osborne LM, Schafer JE, Morroni C. Bleeding patterns after immediate initiation of an oral compared with a vaginal hormonal contraceptive. Obstet Gynecol 2005;106:89–96.
47. Miller L, Verhoeven CH, Hout J. Extended regimens of the contraceptive vaginal ring: a randomized trial. Obstet Gynecol 2005;106:473–82.
48. Weisberg E, Brache V, Alvarez F, et al. Clinical performance and menstrual bleeding patterns with three dosage combinations of a Nestorone progestogen/ethinyl estradiol contraceptive vaginal ring used on a bleeding-signaled regimen. Contraception 2005;72:46–52.
49. Haring T, Mulders TM. The combined contraceptive ring NuvaRing and spermicide co-medication. Contraception 2003;67:271–2.
50. Dogterom P, van den Heuvel MW, Thomsen T. Absence of pharmacokinetic interactions of the combined contraceptive vaginal ring NuvaRing with oral amoxicillin or doxycycline in two randomised trials. Clin Pharmacokinet 2005;44:429–38.
51. Ballagh, SA. NuvaRing® Vaginal Contraceptive Ring. Contraception online slide series. www.contraceptiononline.org/slides/slide01.cfm?tk=20. Accessed December 27, 2005

Male Condoms

13

Lee Warner, PhD, MPH
Markus J. Steiner, PhD, MSPH

- When used consistently and correctly, male latex condoms can reduce the risk of pregnancy and many sexually transmitted infections (STIs), including human immunodeficiency virus (HIV).

- Condoms are inexpensive, available without a prescription, and easy to use.

- By preventing STIs and their long-term sequelae, condoms help protect future fertility.

- Clients at risk for STI should be encouraged to use condoms even if they already rely on more effective methods of contraception.

Male latex condoms remain the most widely available and commonly used barrier method to prevent sexually transmitted infections (STI) in the United States. When used consistently and correctly, male condoms can reduce the risk of pregnancy and most STIs, including human immunodeficiency virus (HIV), based on results from laboratory and clinical studies. Condom use has continued to increase in recent years, according to national surveys of adolescents and adults,[1-3] largely in response to the HIV epidemic. According to the 2002 National Survey of Family Growth (NSFG),[1] more than 13 million reproductive-age women in the United States reported currently using condoms for contraception or protection from STIs, an increase from 9 million in the 1995 survey.[4] Among women using any contraceptive, 18% reported currently using male condoms for prevention of pregnancy, making it the third most popular method. Condom use was highest among women ages 15 to 24, who have the highest incidence of STI. Condom use thus continues to be an important part of public health efforts to prevent new cases of infection with HIV as well as other STIs.

MECHANISM OF ACTION

The male condom acts as a physical barrier by covering the penile glans and shaft. The condom prevents pregnancy by blocking the passage of semen; it prevents infections by covering the major portals of entry and exit for many STI pathogens. Because of their coitally-dependent nature, condoms must be used consistently and correctly with each act of intercourse to be effective. Among barrier contraceptive methods, the condom provides the most protection of the genital tract and effective protection against many STIs (see section on Special Issues).

A sheath worn over the penis can be traced as far back as 1350 B.C., when Egyptian men wore decorative covers for their penises. In 1564 A.D., Fallopius first described linen sheaths used to protect against syphilis.[5] Protective sheaths were made from dried animal intestines in the 18th century, when they were first given the name "condom," presumably after inventor Colonel Cundum.[5] With the advent of vulcanized rubber in 1843 came the mass production of condoms made from natural rubber latex.[6] In the 1990s, manufacturers also began to use synthetic materials (e.g., polyurethane) to develop new condom options.

CONDOM OPTIONS

Condoms are available in a wide variety of shapes, sizes, colors, and thicknesses, as well as with or without lubricants or spermicides, and with or without reservoir-tip or nipple-ends. Condoms can be straight-sided or tapered toward the closed end, textured (e.g., ribbed) or smooth, solid-colored or nearly transparent, and odorless or scented or flavored. Most condoms are about 7 inches (180 mm) long, 2 inches (52 mm) wide, and up to 0.003 inches (0.08 mm) thick. Comprehensive listings of characteristics for some condoms commercially available in the United States can be found in a 2005 article from Consumer Reports.[7]

About 97% of male condoms available in the United States are manufactured from natural rubber latex ("rubber" condoms).[8] A small proportion are made from the intestinal caecum of lambs ("natural skin," "natural membrane," or "lambskin" condoms). Unlike latex condoms, natural membrane condoms contain small pores that may permit the passage of viruses, including hepatitis B virus, herpes simplex virus, and HIV.[9,10] Because of this porosity, natural membrane condoms may not provide the same level of protection against STIs as latex condoms.[11] No clinical data are available on the effectiveness of natural membrane condoms for STI prevention, however. Some condoms are manufactured from polyurethane or other synthetic materials. Compared with latex condoms, synthetic condoms are generally more resistant to deterioration, have a longer shelf-life, and are compatible with use of both oil-based and water-based lubricants.[12] For pregnancy, synthetic male

Table 13–1 Characteristics of latex, natural membrane, and synthetic condoms

Type	Latex	Natural Membrane	Synthetic
Material	Natural rubber	Lamb caecum	Polyurethane*
Lubricant use	Water-based only	Any	Any
Cost	Low	Moderate	Moderate/high
Recommended for prevention of pregnancy	Yes	Yes	Yes**
Recommended for prevention of STIs and HIV	Yes	No	Yes**

Source: Modified from Contraceptive Technology Update (March, 1995).

* Most synthetic condoms are made from polyurethane

** For latex sensitive or allergic persons

condoms have rates of failure similar to their latex counterparts. The effectiveness of synthetic condoms to prevent STI has not been studied, and FDA labeling restricts their recommended use to latex-sensitive or allergic persons; however, synthetic condoms are believed to provide STI and contraception protection similar to latex condoms. See Table 13–1 for a comparison of condom types.

Spermicidal Condoms

Condoms lubricated with a small amount of the spermicide nonoxynol-9 (N-9) have been available in the United States since 1983. However, their use is not recommended, because spermicidal condoms are no more effective than other lubricated condoms despite their higher cost and shorter shelf-life.[13] Concerns have been raised about genital ulceration and irritation resulting from high-frequency use of vaginal spermicidal N-9 products and the potential for facilitating transmission of STIs including HIV.[14] (See Chapter 14 on Vaginal Barriers and Spermicides.) Since the amounts of N-9 contained in a spermicidal condom are much lower than those found in separately applied vaginal products,[15] they are probably less likely to cause adverse effects; however, spermicidal condom use was associated with increased risk of urinary tract infections among young women in one study.[16]

EFFECTIVENESS AGAINST PREGNANCY

Method failure of the male condom resulting in unintended pregnancy is uncommon. Of 100 couples using condoms, 2% are estimated to become pregnant during consistent and correct use during the first 12 months of use (Table 13–2). (A summary of studies of contraceptive failure for the male condom, as well as a detailed discussion of the esti-

Table 13–2 First year probability of pregnancy* for couples using condoms, withdrawal, diaphragm, and pill

Method	% of Women Experiencing an Unintended Pregnancy Within the First Year of Use		% of Women Continuing Use at One Year
	Typical Use	Perfect Use	
Withdrawal	27	4	43
Diaphragm	16	6	57
Condom			
Male	15	2	53
Female (Reality)	21	5	49
Pill	8	0.3	68

* See Table 27–1 for first-year probability of pregnancy for all methods.

Emergency Contraceptive Pills: Treatment initiated within 120 hours after unprotected intercourse reduces the risk of pregnancy by at least 75%. (See Chapter 6 for more information.)

mates used to derive these rates, can be found in Chapter 27 on Contraceptive Efficacy.)

Couples vary widely in their ability to use male condoms consistently and correctly. Among those using condoms for contraception, about 15 of every 100 will become pregnant during the first year of typical use. The marked difference between the condom's probabilities of pregnancy during typical use versus perfect use generally reflects errors in use, most notably the failure of couples to use condoms during every act of sexual intercourse. Several user behaviors, described later, likely contribute to the risk of unintended pregnancy and the transmission of infection despite condom use. Detailed instructions for condom use are provided at the end of this chapter.

CONDOM TESTING

Condoms are regulated as medical devices by the U.S. Food and Drug Administration (FDA), and manufacturing standards have become more stringent in recent years. Every condom is tested electronically for holes and weak spots before it is packaged and released for sale. Samples of condoms also undergo a series of additional laboratory tests for leakage, strength, dimensional requirements, and package integrity.[17] If the sample condoms fail any of these tests, the entire lot is rejected and destroyed to prevent access to the public. Imported condoms are required to comply with the same performance requirements as domestic condoms and should be equally safe. A recent Consumer Reports Survey showed that all condoms tested met industry standards, and that test performance did not vary with price, thickness, or country of manufacture.[7]

ADVANTAGES AND INDICATIONS

Male condoms offer several noncontraceptive benefits to users.

1. **Protection against STIs.** When used consistently and correctly, condoms reduce the risk of many STIs, including HIV (see Special Issues). By preventing STIs and their long-term sequelae, condoms also protect fertility. (See Chapter 25 on Impaired Fertility.)

2. **Accessibility.** Usage does not require medical examination, prescription, or fitting. Condoms can be obtained from many sources, including drug stores, grocery stores, family planning and STI clinics, vending machines, gas stations, bars, and mail-order services.

3. **Low cost.** Condoms are among the most inexpensive and cost-effective contraceptives, especially considering the added protection against STIs. There is no evidence to suggest that less expensive condoms indicate lower quality. Condoms are available at low cost in both the private and public sectors and often for free from publicly funded programs.

4. **Delayed ejaculation.** For some men, condom use may help prolong intercourse and also prevent premature ejaculation.

5. **Portability.** Condoms can be easily and discretely carried by men or women.

6. **Minimal side effects.** Because condoms are non-hormonal, they rarely cause medical problems among users. The most frequent side effect is most likely latex sensitivity; men or women with this condition can be directed to use synthetic condoms if STIs are of concern (see the section on Managing Problems and Follow-up).

DISADVANTAGES AND CAUTIONS

Male condoms also have disadvantages that may result in inconsistent or nonuse of the method.

1. **Reduced sensation.** Many men and their partners complain that condoms reduce sensitivity. Men can try different types of

condoms and add lubricant to the outside of the condom to increase sensation.

2. **Lack of spontaneity.** Some men and their partners dislike interrupting foreplay to put on the condom and may find the coitally-dependent nature of condom use to be inconvenient.

3. **Problems with erection.** Some men cannot consistently maintain an erection during condom use, so condom use becomes unacceptable. Female condom use may be appropriate in these cases.

4. **Embarrassment and mistrust.** Some men and women may be embarrassed to obtain condoms or to suggest or initiate condom use because they perceive condom use implies a lack of trust or intimacy. Counsel clients (and partners, when possible) about their embarrassment and teach clients about condoms and how to negotiate their use. (See section on Providing Condoms—Counseling).

5. **Lack of cooperation.** In some instances, men will not accept responsibility for contraception or prevention of infection, thus making male condom use impossible.

6. **Latex allergy.** Some men and women, especially health care workers repeatedly exposed to latex, may be allergic or sensitive to latex and thus unable to use latex condoms. Synthetic condoms are excellent alternatives. (See section on Managing Problems and Follow-Up.)

S PECIAL ISSUES

Protection Against STIS and HIV

The primary noncontraceptive benefit of condom use is the protection offered against STI. When placed on the penis before any genital contact and used throughout intercourse, condoms prevent direct contact with semen; genital lesions and subclinical viral shedding on the glans and shaft of the penis; and penile, vaginal, or anal discharges or infectious fluids. Condoms thus greatly reduce the risk of STIs that are transmitted primarily to or from the penile urethra (such as gonorrhea, chlamydia, trichomoniasis, hepatitis B infection, and HIV). Condoms also provide protection against STIs that are transmitted primarily through skin-to-skin contact or contact with mucosal surfaces (such as genital herpes, human papillomavirus (HPV), syphilis, and chancroid) to the extent that these areas are covered by the condom. Protection may be less when these STIs involve areas not covered by the condom.[15,18,19] In vitro laboratory studies indicate that latex condoms provide an effective physical barrier against passage of even the smallest sexually transmitted pathogen (hepatitis B).[8–10,20–25]

The levels of protection for condoms are likely to vary for different STIs because STIs differ in their routes of transmission, as well as in their infectivity and prevalence.[26–28] Well-designed clinical studies of discordant couples (where one partner is infected and the other is not) have shown consistent use of latex condoms to be highly effective against sexually acquired HIV infection, the most serious STI; thus, male condoms should be promoted to sexually active clients at risk for STI for this reason alone.[29] Two recent meta-analyses of these studies place the estimated effectiveness of consistent condom use between approximately 80% and 95%.[30–31]

Clinical studies of effectiveness against most other STIs suggest inconsistent protective effects for condoms.[8,18,28,32–35] Much of this inconsistency in condom use effectiveness estimates can be attributed to limitations in study design, as the overall quality of clinical studies for these STIs is considerably weaker than for the HIV studies. Specifically, limitations in measurement of self-reported condom use and exposure to infected partners complicate interpretation of condom effectiveness estimates.[8,18,28,35–44] Recent studies and analyses[38,41,42,45–48] have empirically documented that effectiveness against many STIs is underestimated because of limitations in study design. Despite these limitations, studies and systematic reviews have found condom use to be associated with reduced risk of many STIs in addition to HIV, including gonorrhea, chlamydia, trichomoniasis, syphilis, genital herpes, HPV infection, and HPV-associated conditions.[28,32–35,49–65] For more extensive discussion of condom effectiveness for STI prevention, we refer readers elsewhere.[18,19,28,35,37,65]

Condom Use During Anal and Oral Intercourse

Latex and synthetic condoms also can be used during anogenital and orogenital intercourse to reduce the risk of STI.[15] Latex sheets to be used for cunnilingus and anilingus have also been cleared by the FDA for over-the-counter sales, but no effectiveness data are available. Household plastic wrap (including the microwaveable variety) is another option for cunnilingus and anilingus, although it has not been manufactured or cleared by the FDA for medical applications, and no effectiveness data are available. Dental dams (or oral dams) and condoms adapted to form a barrier sheet have also been proposed as barriers for cunnilingus; however, their limited size may allow potentially infectious fluids to roll onto adjacent tissues, and these products also have not been evaluated or cleared by the FDA for this use.

CONDOM PROMOTION

Though there is general consensus that male condoms must play a central role in any STI/HIV prevention program,[66] the mix of condom promotion versus other prevention strategies (e.g., abstinence and mutual monogamy) remains controversial in many countries, including the United States. Condom promotion has been particularly controversial within specific settings and populations (e.g., adolescents).[3] Concerns also have been raised about the potential negative consequences of condom promotion,[67,102] given that increased availability of condoms may not necessarily translate into sufficient use for effective STI prevention. For example, even among studies of couples discordant for HIV or genital herpes simplex virus (HSV) for whom there is known risk for infection, fewer than half of couples report regular use of condoms.[30,31] Of increasing interest is whether interventions promoting condom use may result in risk compensation[67,118] that facilitates the onset or frequency of high-risk sexual activity, as hypothesized in some studies.[68,69] No randomized controlled trials have evaluated whether a potential disinhibition effect exists or whether it outweighs the protective effects of condom use for persons at risk. However, a review of 174 condom-related prevention approaches concluded that interventions designed to reduce the risk of HIV infection do not increase unsafe sexual behavior.[104]

PROVIDING CONDOMS—COUNSELING

All clients should understand when to use condoms, how to use them most effectively, how to discuss condom use with their partner(s), and how to integrate condom use into intercourse:

STI protection. Emphasize the need for condom use during all sexual activities that can transmit STIs and HIV. Recommend that clients use a new condom for each act of anal, vaginal, or oral intercourse when any risk of infection exists.[15] (See the section on Effectiveness against STIs and HIV).

Dual method use. Encourage clients to use a condom plus another contraceptive, which may dramatically reduce the risk of both pregnancy and STI.[70] Clients potentially at risk for STI who appear amenable to this strategy should be encouraged to use two methods of contraception. Use caution when recommending dual method use to clients, since simultaneous use of multiple methods can be overly complicated for some couples, who may instead opt to use no method of contraception at all. Follow the client's lead and perhaps suggest a brief trial period of dual method use. If this proves difficult for the client, consider recommending consistent and correct use of condoms alone to provide adequate protection against both pregnancy and infection. Emergency contraception can be used as a backup method against pregnancy in case a condom breaks, falls off, or is not used.

Tailored counseling. Adapt counseling messages on condom use to each client's needs. Clients may have formed their own attitudes about condom use and may have had varying experiences with condoms. Tailor the counseling session to each client's risk factors, abilities, needs, and readiness to change.[71] Many clinicians use behavioral change models to assess the ability of their clients to use condoms consistently and to guide the content of the counseling session, a process that makes effective use of time.[72]

Communication of pregnancy rates. Ensure clients choosing contraceptive methods (including condoms) understand the risks and benefits of the range of methods available. Although the ability to prevent pregnancy is often mentioned as the single most important criterion considered when choosing a method,[73-76] clients may have difficulty understanding typical use and perfect use pregnancy rates across methods (see Table 13–2).[75] Because clients may find it difficult to understand contraceptive failure rates, show them a scale of the relative effectiveness of contraceptives, as shown in Figure 3–1 (see Chapter 3 on Choosing a Contraceptive Method). Consider using a similar approach when counseling clients about the ability of condoms to prevent STIs, including HIV (see the section on Protection Against STIs and HIV).

Personal benefits. Make sure clients understand how condom use benefits them personally. Explain that condoms protect future fertility by preventing long-term sequelae of STIs. (See Chapter 21 on Reproductive Tract Infections.) Strongly encourage pregnant women at high risk for STIs to use condoms to protect their fetus, their partner(s), and themselves.

Partner negotiation. Teach clients how to negotiate condom use with partners. Many clients may have contemplated using condoms but may be uncomfortable suggesting condom use to their partners. Teach clients how to negotiate condom use with their partner(s), and help them develop replies they can use when a partner objects to condoms.[77] Assess the likelihood of a partner's negative reaction to the suggestion of condom use; some clients fear that they will be abused or abandoned if they insist on using condoms. Counsel or refer as appropriate if you detect battering or other forms of abuse. It is particularly important that a condom be available and its use agreed upon in advance by both partners.

Effective use. Make sure clients understand how to use condoms effectively. Emphasize that condoms are most effective when used correctly during every act of intercourse. Assessing condom use among clients is a two-tiered process. First ask clients how often they are using condoms (e.g., always, most of the time, sometimes, never). Then, to recognize potential misuse, ask clients to explain (and perhaps demonstrate on an appropriate model of a penis) how they use condoms. (See sections on Increasing Effective Use and Instructions for Condom Use.) Encourage clients to use condoms consistently and correctly with every act of anal, vaginal, and oral intercourse.

Suitability. Offer to help clients select a condom most suitable to their needs, including the female condom. Some clinics now provide a variety of condoms to clients, although a recent study[103] found that providing a choice of condoms increased acceptability but had no impact on levels of use or STI.

Practice. Encourage clients to practice using condoms. Many problems that occur during condom use can be attributed to inexperience[78] and can be overcome with practice. Users who have had negative experiences with condoms may be at risk of discontinuing condom use altogether;[79] encourage them to continue practicing with condoms. When providing instruction on how to use condoms, have the client unroll a condom onto a model of a penis or similarly shaped object (e.g., banana), both with eyes open and then again in the dark.

Provision of condoms. Provide each client a large number of condoms at low or no cost. Providing clients with a few condoms is only a short-term solution for clients who find the health care system inaccessible or who find it embarrassing to return repeatedly for condoms. Selling condoms, even at a low cost, dramatically reduces the number of condoms a client will obtain from a clinic compared with the number of free condoms s/he will take.

STRATEGIES FOR INCREASING EFFECTIVE CONDOM USE

Condom effectiveness depends heavily on the skill level and experience of the user.[19] Studies have documented relatively high levels of problems with condom use that may reduce their effectiveness, many of which can be minimized with appropriate counseling and practice.

Interventions promoting condom use should address user-related behaviors that result in exposure to STIs and pregnancy, including the following:

1. **Failure to use condoms with every act of intercourse.** Nonuse of condoms, rather than poor condom quality or other condom-related problems, is the most common problem.[80,81] The highest single priority for any STI/HIV prevention program should be to address factors that lead to nonuse of condoms, including lack of device acceptability, poor partner negotiation skills for use, and latex allergy or sensitivity. New strategies that emphasize condom use for contraception in addition to disease prevention[70]

may help decrease nonuse. Persons at risk should be provided with an adequate supply of condoms at low or no cost.

2. **Failure to use condoms throughout intercourse.** Recent studies have documented that some men put condoms on after starting intercourse or remove condoms prior to ejaculation.[40,48,82–84] These behaviors represent product misuse and could expose partners to risk of pregnancy or STI despite condom use. Clients should be counseled to use condoms every time throughout intercourse, from beginning to end.

3. **Condom breakage and slippage.** Although users often fear that the condom will break or fall off during use, these events are rare with proper use and tend to be concentrated among a small proportion of users.[78] The majority of studies show that during vaginal sex, condoms break approximately 2 percent of the time during intercourse or withdrawal; a similar proportion slip off completely.[85–89] However, rates of condom breakage and slippage vary widely across studies (0% to 22% for breakage[85,90]; 0–9% for slippage).[85,91] Reviews of studies evaluating breakage and slippage during anal intercourse indicate that the rates may be slightly higher than during vaginal intercourse.[92,93] Because breakage or slippage are possible, advise users to have several condoms available in case a condom is torn or put on incorrectly, or repeated intercourse is desired.

4. **Improper lubricant use with latex condoms.** Unlike water-based lubricants (e.g., K-Y Jelly), oil-based lubricants (e.g., petroleum jelly, baby oil, and hand lotions) reduce latex condom integrity[94] and may facilitate breakage (See Table 13–3). People may use oil-based products as condom lubricants, mistaking

Table 13–3 Examples of lubricant products that should and should not be used with natural rubber latex condoms[a]

Safe	Not safe
Egg whites	Baby oil
Glycerine	Cold creams
Saliva	Edible oils (olive, peanut, corn, sunflower)
Silicone	Hand and body lotions
Spermicides	Massage oil
Water	Petroleum jelly
Water-based lubricants (e.g., K-Y Jelly, Astroglide)	Rubbing alcohol
	Suntan oil and lotions
	Vegetable or mineral oil
	Vaginal infection medications in cream or suppository form

[a] All lubricants, including oil-based products, may be used with polyurethane condoms.

them for water-based lubricants because they readily wash off with water. Because vaginal medications (e.g., for yeast infections) often contain oil-based ingredients that can damage latex condoms, advise clients to remain abstinent or use synthetic condoms until the medication is fully completed and the infection is cured. Note that oil-based products may be safely used as lubricants with polyurethane condoms, although they may not be compatible with all synthetic condoms.

MANAGING PROBLEMS AND FOLLOW-UP

Persons sensitive or allergic to natural rubber latex may experience irritation, allergic contact dermatitis, or systemic anaphylactic symptoms when exposed to latex-containing products.[95,96] While 1% to 6% of the U.S. population are believed to be allergic to latex,[96] the prevalence of latex sensitivity is believed to be much higher among health care workers who have repeated exposure to latex-containing medical devices (e.g., surgical and examination gloves, catheters, intubation tubes, anesthesia masks, and dental dams).[95–97] Proteins in the latex appear to be the primary source of allergic reactions. All patients should be questioned for potential latex allergy.[96,97] Ask whether the client experiences itching, rash, or wheezing after wearing latex gloves or inflating a balloon.[97] If you suspect a client has generalized latex sensitivity, consider recommending synthetic condoms and refer the client for allergy skin testing.[98] While latex condom use is contraindicated for clients with general latex sensitivity, both synthetic and natural membrane condoms can be recommended for prevention of pregnancy, while only synthetic condoms should be recommended for prevention of STIs, including HIV.

Allergic reactions that occur only after exposure to latex condoms and not after exposure to other latex-containing products may be attributable to brand-specific condom attributes such as spermicides, lubricants, perfumes, local anesthetics, or other chemical agents added during the manufacturing process.[99] Advise clients to try different brands of latex and synthetic condoms. In any case, clients should immediately contact their health care provider for follow-up if they or their partner(s) experience a severe allergic reaction while using latex condoms or spermicides. Additional comprehensive information on latex allergy can also be obtained from the American Latex Allergy Association (see www. latexallergyresources.org).

INSTRUCTIONS FOR USING CONDOMS

Instructions for condom use are often overcomplicated and may have no scientific basis.[100] During a World Health Organization Experts Meeting (Geneva, June 22–24, 2005) to develop a Global Handbook for

Family Planning Providers, consensus was reached on five key condom instructions. These five messages, with recent minor modifications,[19] are:

Five Key Instructions for Condom Use
1. Use a new condom for each act of intercourse if any risk of pregnancy or STI exists.
2. Before any genital contact, place the condom on the tip of the erect penis with the rolled side out.
3. Unroll the condom all the way to the base of the erect penis.
4. Immediately after ejaculation, hold the rim of the condom and withdraw the penis while it is still erect.
5. Throw away the used condom safely.

Updated, more detailed instructions for using condoms[77] are included below:

Before Intercourse

1. Have on hand an adequate supply of latex or synthetic condoms and water-based lubricant if you think you may need to use a condom, even if you plan to use another contraceptive. Have extra condoms available in case the first is damaged, torn before use, or put on incorrectly. You will need a new condom if you have repeated intercourse.

2. Discuss condom use with your partner before you have intercourse.

At Time of Intercourse

1. Open the condom package carefully to avoid damaging it with fingernails, teeth, or other sharp objects.

2. Put on the condom before the penis comes in contact with the partner.

3. Unroll the condom a short distance to make sure the condom is being unrolled in the right direction. Then hold the tip of the condom and unroll it down to the base of the erect penis. If the condom does not unroll easily, you probably put it on inside-out. Discard the condom and begin with a new one, because flipping it over and using it could expose your partner to infectious organisms contained in the pre-ejaculate.

4. Adequate lubrication is important. For latex condoms, use only water-based lubricants like water, lubricating jellies (e.g., K-Y Jelly), or spermicidal lubricants, jellies, foam, or suppositories. Avoid oil-based lubricants like cold cream, mineral oil, cooking

oil, petroleum jelly, body lotions, massage oil, or baby oil that can damage latex condoms (see Table 13–3).

5. Keep the condom on the penis until after intercourse. If the condom breaks or falls off during intercourse but before ejaculation, stop and put on a new condom. Use a new condom when you have prolonged intercourse, and when you have different types of intercourse within a single session (e.g., after anal sex, change the condom before having vaginal sex to decrease risk of urinary tract infection).

After Intercourse

1. Soon after ejaculation, withdraw the penis while it is still erect. Hold the condom firmly against the base of the penis to prevent slippage and leakage of semen.

2. Check the condom for visible damage such as holes, then wrap it in tissue and discard. Do not flush condoms down the toilet.

3. If the condom breaks, falls off, leaks, is damaged, or is not used, the following may help:

   — Discuss the possibility of pregnancy or infection with your partner and contact your health care provider as soon as you can. Do not douche. Emergency contraception may be used to prevent pregnancy if it is started within 120 hours of having unprotected intercourse. Call 1–888-NOT-2-LATE to learn more about emergency contraceptives or obtain this information from the World Wide Web at http://ec.princeton.edu. (See Chapter 6 on Emergency Contraception.)

   — Gently wash the penis, vulva, anus, and adjacent areas with soap and water immediately after intercourse to help reduce the risk of acquiring an STI. Then insert an applicator full of spermicide into the vagina as soon as possible.

Repeated Intercourse

1. Use a new condom from "beginning to end" with each act of anal, vaginal, or oral intercourse. Do not reuse condoms.

Taking Care of Supplies

1. Store condoms in a cool and dry place out of direct sunlight (excessive heat will weaken latex). Latex condoms can probably be stored in a wallet for up to 1 month when kept away from heat and sunlight.[101]

2. Check the expiration or manufacture date on the box or individual package of condoms. Expiration dates are marked as "Exp"; otherwise, the date is the manufacture date (MFG). Latex condoms should not be used beyond their expiration date or more than 5 years after the manufacturing date. Condoms in damaged packages or that show obvious signs of deterioration (e.g., brittleness, stickiness, or discoloration) should not be used regardless of their expiration date.

REFERENCES

1. Chandra A, Martinez GM, Mosher WD, Abma JC, Jones J. Fertility, family planning, and reproductive health of U.S. women: data from the 2002 National Survey of Family Growth. Vital Health Stat 2005;Series 23, Number 25:1–160.
2. Centers for Disease Control and Prevention. Trends in sexual risk behaviors among high school students—United States, 1991–2001. MMWR 2002;51:856–9.
3. American Academy of Pediatrics, Committee on Adolescence. Condom use by adolescents. Pediatrics 2001;107:1463–1469.
4. Abma JC, Chandra A, Mosher WD, et al. Fertility, family planning, and women's health: new data from the 1995 National Survey of Family Growth. Vital Health Stat 1997;Series 23, Number 9.
5. Valdiserri RO. Cum hastis sic clypeatis: the turbulent history of the condom. Bull NY Acad Med 1988;64:237–245.
6. Murphy JS. The condom industry in the United States, 1990. Jefferson NC: McFarland & Company, Inc., Publishers, 1990.
7. Consumer Union: Condoms: Extra protection. Consumer Reports 2005; February.
8. National Institute of Allergy and Infectious Diseases. Workshop Summary: Scientific Evidence on Condom Effectiveness for Sexually Transmitted Diseases (STD) Prevention. July 20, 2001. www.niaid.nih.gov/dmid/stds/condomreport.pdf.
9. Carey RF, Lytle CD, Cyr WH. Implications of laboratory tests of condom integrity. Sex Transm Dis 1999;26:216–220.
10. Lytle CD, Routson LB, Seaborn GB, et al. An in vitro evaluation of condoms as barriers to a small virus. Sex Transm Dis 1997;24:161–164.
11. Consumer's Union. Condoms get better: tests of 30 models show far fewer failures than in past years. Consumer Reports 1999; June.
12. Gallo M, Grimes D, Lopez L, Schulz K. Non-latex versus latex male condoms for contraception. Cochrane Database Syst Rev 2006; 1:CD003550.
13. Centers for Disease Control and Prevention. Nonoxynol-9 spermicide contraception use—United States 1999. MMWR 2002;51:389–92.
14. Centers for Disease Control and Prevention. CDC statement on study results of products containing nonoxynol-9. MMWR 2000;49:717–718.
15. Centers for Disease Control and Prevention. Sexually transmitted diseases treatment guidelines 2002. MMWR 2002;51(No. RR-6).
16. Fihn SD, Boyko EJ, Normand EH, et al. Association between use of spermicide-coated condoms and Escherichia coli urinary tract infection in young women. Am J Epidemiol 1996;144:512–20.
17. ASTM (American Society for Testing Materials). Annual book of ASTM standards: Easton MD: ASTM: section 9, rubber. Volume 09.02 Rubber products; standard specifications for rubber contraceptives (male condoms-D3492). West Conshohocken, PA: American Society for Testing Materials, 1996.

18. Stone KM, Thomas E, Timyan J. Barrier methods for the prevention of sexually transmitted diseases. In: Holmes KK, Sparling PF, Mardh P-A, eds. Sexually Transmitted Diseases 1998, 3rd ed., McGraw-Hill, New York.

19. Steiner MJ, Warner L, Stone KM, Cates W Jr. Condoms and other barrier methods for prevention of STD/HIV infection, and pregnancy. In: Holmes KK, Sparling PF, Mardh P-A, eds. Sexually Transmitted Diseases, 4th ed., McGraw-Hill, New York (in press).

20. Carey RF, Herman WA, Retta SM, et al. Effectiveness of latex condoms as a barrier to human immunodeficiency virus-sized particles under conditions of simulated use. Sex Transm Dis 1992;19:230–4.

21. Conant MA, Spicer DW, Smith CD. Herpes simplex virus transmission: condom studies. Sex Transm Dis 1984;11:94–5.

22. Katznelson S, Drew WL, Mintz L. Efficacy of the condom as a barrier to the transmission of cytomegalovirus. J Infect Dis 1984;150:155–7.

23. Rietmeijer CA, Krebs JW, Feorina PM, et al. Condoms as physical and chemical barriers against human immunodeficiency virus. JAMA 1988;259:1851–1853.

24. Van de Perre P, Jacobs D, Sprecher-Goldberger S. The latex condom, an efficient barrier against sexual transmission of AIDS-related viruses. AIDS 1987; 1:49–52.

25. Judson FN, Ehret JM, Bodin GF, Levin MJ, Rietmeijer CA. In vitro evaluations of condoms with and without nonoxynol 9 as physical and chemical barriers against Chlamydia trachomatis, herpes simplex virus type 2, and human immunodeficiency virus. Sex Transm Dis 1989; 16:51–6.

26. Cates W Jr. The condom forgiveness factor: the positive spin. Sex Transm Dis 2002;29:350–2.

27. Mann JR, Stine CC, Vessey J. The role of disease-specific infectivity and number of disease exposures on long-term effectiveness of the latex condom. Sex Transm Dis 2002;29:344–9.

28. Warner L, Stone KM, Macaluso M, Buehler J, Austin HD. A systematic review of design factors assessed in epidemiologic studies of condom effectiveness for preventing gonorrhea and chlamydia. Sex Transm Dis 2006;33:36–51.

29. Cates W Jr. The NIH condom report: the glass is 90% full. Fam Plann Perspect 2001;33:231–3.

30. Weller S, Davis K. Condom effectiveness in reducing heterosexual HIV transmission. Cochrane Database Syst Rev 2001;(3):CD003255.

31. Pinkerton SD, Abramson PR. Effectiveness of condoms in preventing HIV transmission. Soc Sci Med 1997;44:1303–1312.

32. d'oro LC, Parazzini F, Naldi L, et al. Barrier methods of contraception, spermicides, and sexually transmitted diseases: A review. Genitourin Med 1994;70:410.

33. Manhart LE, Koutsky LA. Do condoms prevent genital HPV infection, external genital warts, or cervical neoplasia? A meta-analysis. Sex Transm Dis 2002; 29:725–35.

34. Centers for Disease Control and Prevention. Report to Congress: prevention of genital human papillomavirus infection, January 2004.

35. Holmes KK, Levine R, Weaver M. Effectiveness of condom in preventing sexually transmitted infections. Bull WHO 2004; 84:454–461.

36. Aral SO, Peterman TA. Measuring outcomes of behavioural interventions for STD/HIV prevention. Int J STD AIDS. 1996;7 Suppl 2:30–8.

37. Crosby R, DiClemente RJ, Holtgrave DR, Wingood GM. Design, measurement, and analytical considerations for testing hypotheses relative to condom effectiveness against non-viral STIs. Sex Transm Inf 2002;78:228–31.

38. Devine OJ, Aral SO. The impact of inaccurate reporting of condom use and imperfect diagnosis of sexually transmitted disease infection in studies of condom effectiveness: a simulation-based assessment. Sex Transm Dis 2004;31:588–95.

39. Steiner MJ, Feldblum PJ, Padian N. Invited commentary: condom effectiveness—will Prostate specific antigen shed new light on this perplexing problem: Am J Epidemiol 2003;157:298–300.

40. Warner L, Clay-Warner J, Boles J, Williamson J. Assessing condom use practices. Implications for evaluating method and user effectiveness. Sex Transm Dis 1998; 25:273–7.
41. Warner L, Macaluso M, Austin HD, et al. Application of the case-crossover design to reduce unmeasured confounding in studies of condom effectiveness. Am J Epidemiol 2005;161:765–73.
42. Warner L, Newman DR, Austin HD, et al. Condom effectiveness for reducing transmission of gonorrhea and chlamydia: the importance of assessing partner infection status. Am J Epidemiol 2004;159:242–51.
43. Warner L, Macaluso M, Newman DR, et al. Re: Condom effectiveness for prevention of chlamydia trachomatis infection. Sex Transm Inf 2006;82:265
44. Zenilman JM, Weisman CS, Rompalo AM, et al. Condom use to prevent incident STDs: the validity of self-reported condom use. Sex Transm Dis 1995;22:15–21.
45. Niccolai L, Rowhani-Rahbar A, Jenkins H, et al. Condom effectiveness for prevention of Chlamydia trachomatis infection. Sex Transm Inf 2005;81:323–5.
46. Shlay JC, McClung MW, Patnaik JL, Douglas JM Jr. Comparison of sexually transmitted disease prevalence by reported condom use: errors among consistent condom users seen at an urban sexually transmitted disease clinic. Sex Transm Dis 2004; 31:526 32.
47. Shlay JC, McClung MW, Patnaik JL, Douglas JM Jr. Comparison of sexually transmitted disease prevalence by reported level of condom use among patients attending an urban sexually transmitted disease clinic. Sex Transm Dis 2004;31:154–160.
48. Paz-Bailey G, Koumans EH, Sternberg M, et al. The effect of correct and consistent condom use on chlamydial and gonococcal infection among urban adolescents. Arch Pediatr Adolesc Med 2005;159:536–42.
49. Winer RL, Hughes JP, Feng Q, et al. Condom use and the papillomavirus infection in young women. N Engl J Med 2006;354:2645–2654.
50. Casper C, Wald A. Condom use and the prevention of genital herpes acquisition. Herpes 2002; 9:10–4.
51. Wald A, Langenberg AG, Krantz, et al. The relationship between condom use and herpes simplex virus acquisition. Ann Intern Med 2005;143:707–713.
52. Wald A, Langenberg AG, Link K, et al. Effect of condoms on reducing the transmission of herpes simplex virus type 2 from men to women. JAMA 2001; 285:3100–6.
53. Barlow D. The condom and gonorrhoea. Lancet 1977; 222:811–812.
54. Ramstedt K, Forssman L, Giesecke J, Granath F. Risk factors for Chlamydia trachomatis in 6810 young women attending family planning clinics. Int J STD AIDS 1992;3:117–122.
55. Upchurch DM, Brady WE, Reichart CA, Hook EW III. Behavioral contributions to acquisition of gonorrhea in patients attending an inner-city sexually transmitted disease clinic. J Infect Dis 1990;161:938–941.
56. Fennema JSA, van Ameijden EJC, Coutinho RA, van Den Hoek A. Clinical sexually transmitted diseases among human immunodeficiency virus-infected and noninfected drug-using prostitutes. Associated factors and interpretation of trends, 1986 to 1994. Sex Transm Dis 1997; 24:363–371.
57. Levine WC, Revollo R, Kaune V, et al. Decline in sexually transmitted disease prevalence in female Bolivian sex workers: impact of an HIV prevention project. AIDS 1998;12:1899–1906.
58. Hooper RR, Reynolds GH, Jones OG, et al. Cohort study of venereal disease. I: the risk of gonorrhea transmission from infected women to men. Am J Epidemiol 1978;108:136–144.
59. Baeten JM, Nyange PM, Richardson BA, et al. Hormonal contraception and risk of sexually transmitted disease acquisition: results from a prospective study. Am J Obstet Gynecol 2001;185:380–5.
60. Cates W Jr., Holmes KK. Re: condom efficacy against gonorrhea and nongonococcal urethritis. Am J Epidemiol 1996;143:843–844.

61. Sanchez J, Gutuzzo E, Escamilla J. Sexually transmitted infections in female sex workers: reduced by condom use but not by a limited periodic examination program. Sex Transm Dis 1998;25:82–89.
62. Schwartz MA, Lafferty WE, Hughes JP, Handsfield HH. Risk factors for urethritis in heterosexual men. Sex Transm Dis 1997;24:449–455.
63. Hogewoning CJ, Bleeker MC, van den Brule AJ, et al. Condom use promotes regression of cervical intraepithelial neoplasia and clearance of human papillomavirus: a randomized clinical trial. Int J Cancer 2003;107:811–6.
64. Bleeker MC, Hogewoning CJ, Voorhorst FJ, et al. Condom use promotes regression of human papillomavirus-associated penile lesions in male sexual partners of women with cervical intraepithelial neoplasia. Int J Cancer 2003;107:804–10.
65. Alfonsi GA, Shlay J. The effectiveness of condoms for the prevention of sexually transmitted diseases. Current Women's Health Reviews 2005;1:151–9.
66. Halperin DT, Steiner MJ, Cassell MM, et al. The time has come for common ground on preventing sexual transmission of HIV. Lancet 2004; 364:1913–5.
67. Richens J, Imrie J, Copas A. Condoms and seat belts: the parallels and the lessons. Lancet 2000;355:400–3.
68. Kajubi P, Kamya MR, Kamya S, et al. Increasing condom use without reducing HIV risk: results of a controlled community trial in Uganda. J Acquir Immune Defic Syndr 2005; 40:77–82.
69. Imrie J, Stephenson JM, Cowan FM, et al. A cognitive behavioural intervention to reduce sexually transmitted infections among gay men: randomised trial. BMJ 2001; 322:1451–1456.
70. Cates W Jr., Steiner MJ. Dual protection against unintended pregnancy and sexually transmitted infections: What is the best contraceptive approach? Sex Transm Dis 2002;29:168–174.
71. Centers for Disease Control and Prevention. Revised guidelines for HIV counseling, testing and referral. MMWR 2001;50 (RR-19):1–58.
72. Contraceptive Technology Update. Can't get patients to use condoms? Try mix of staging and counseling. Contraceptive Technology Update 1997;18:1–12.
73. Grady WR, Klepinger DH, Nelson-Wally A. Contraceptive characteristics: the perceptions and priorities of men and women. Fam Plann Perspect 1999;31:168–75.
74. Edwards JE, Oldman A, Smith L, et al. Women's knowledge of, and attitudes to, contraceptive effectiveness and adverse health effects. Br J Fam Plann 2000;26:73–80.
75. Steiner MJ, Dalebout S, Condon S, et al. Understanding risk: a randomized controlled trial of communicating contraceptive effectiveness. Obstet Gynecol 2003;102:709–17.
76. Snow R, Garcia S, Kureshy N, et al. Attributes of contraceptive technology: women's preferences in seven countries. Reproductive Health Matters 1997;(special issue:36–4).
77. Warner L, Hatcher RA, Steiner MJ. Male Condoms. In: Hatcher RA, Trussell J, Stewart F, Nelson A.L., Cates Jr W, Guest F, et al, editors. Contraceptive Technology. 18 ed. New York: Ardent Media Inc., 2004:331–353.
78. Steiner M, Piedrahita C, Glover L, Joanis C. Can condom users likely to experience condom failure be identified? Fam Plann Perspect 1993;25:220–223,226.
79. Norris AE, Ford K. Associations between condom experiences and beliefs, intentions, and use in a sample of urban, low-income, African-American and Hispanic youth. AIDS Educ Prev 1994;6:27–39.
80. Steiner MJ, Cates W Jr, Warner L. The real problem with male condoms is nonuse. Sex Transm Dis 1999;26:459–62.
81. Warner L, Steiner MJ. Condom access does not ensure condom use: you've got to be putting me on. Sex Transm Inf 2002; 78:225.
82. Fishbein M, Pequegnat W. Evaluating AIDS prevention interventions using behavioral and biological outcome measures. Sex Transm Dis 2000; 27:101–10.

83. Calzavara L, Burchell AN, Remis RS, et al. Delayed application of condoms is a risk factor for human immunodeficiency virus infection among homosexual and bisexual men. Am J Epidemiol 2003;157:210–17.

84. Crosby RA, Sanders SA, Yarber WL, et al. Condom use errors and problems among college men. Sex Transm Dis. 2002;29:552–7.

85. Albert AE, Warner DL, Hatcher RA, Trussell J, Bennett C. Condom use among female commercial sex workers in Nevada's legal brothels. Am J Publ Health 1995; 85:1514–1520.

86. Cook L, Nanda K, Taylor D. Randomized crossover trial comparing the eZ.on plastic condom and a latex condom. Contraception 2001; 63:25–31.

87. Valappil T, Kelaghan J, Macaluso M, et al. Female condom and male condom failure among women at high risk of sexually transmitted diseases. Sex Transm Dis 2005;32:35–43.

88. Macaluso M, Kelaghan J, Artz L, et al. Mechanical failure of the latex condom in a cohort of women at high STD risk. Sex Transm Dis 1999;26:450–8.

89. Walsh TL, Frezieres RG, Peacock K, et al. Effectiveness of the male latex condom: combined results for three popular condom brands used as controls in randomized clinical trials. Contraception 2004;70:407–13.

90. Mukenge-Tshibaka L, Alary M, Geraldo N, Lowndes CM. Incorrect condom use and frequent breakage among female sex workers and their clients. Int J STD AIDS 2005;16:345–7.

91. Russell-Brown P, Piedrahita C, Foldesy R, et al. Comparison of condom breakage during human use with performance in laboratory testing. Contraception 1992; 45:429–37.

92. Silverman BG, Gross TP. Use and effectiveness of condoms during anal intercourse. A review. Sex Transm Dis 1997; 24:11–7.

93. Richters J, Kippax S. Condoms for anal sex. In: Mindel A, editor. Condoms. First ed. London: BMJ Publishing Group, 2000, 132–146.

94. Voeller B, Coulson AH, Bernstein GS, Nakamura RM. Mineral oil lubricants cause rapid deterioration of latex condoms. Contraception 1989; 39:(1)95–102. 0010–7824.

95. Zaza S, Reeder JM, Charles LE, Jarvis WR. Latex sensitivity among perioperative nurses. AORN 1994;60:806–812.

96. National Institute for Occupational Safety and Health. Preventing allergic reactions to natural rubber latex in the workplace [NIOSH alert]. National Institute for Occupational Safety and Health, June 1997 [DHHS (NIOSH) publication No. 97–135].

97. Food and Drug Administration. Allergic reactions to latex-containing medical devices [press release]. Rockville MD; Food and Drug Administration, March 29, 1991.

98. Yassin MS, Lierl MB, Fischer TJ, et al. Latex allergy in hospital employees. Ann Allergy 1994;72:245–249.

99. Hamann CP, Kick SA. Update: immediate and delayed hypersensitivity to natural rubber latex. Cutis 1993;52:307–311.

100. Spencer B, Gerofi J. Can we tell them how to do it? In: Mindel A, editor. Condoms. First ed. London: BMJ Publishing Group, 2000, 207–219.

101. Glasser G, Hatcher RA. The effect on condom integrity of carrying a condom in a wallet for three months [abstract]. Proceedings of the American College of Obstetricians and Gynecologists District IV Conference, November 1992. San Juan PR.

102. Cassell MM, Halperin DT, Shelton JD, Stanton, D. Risk compensation: the Achilles' heel of innovations in HIV prevention? BMJ 2006;332:605–7.

103. Steiner MJ, Hylton-Kong T, Figueroa JP, et al. Does a choice of condoms impact sexually transmitted infection incidence? A randomized, controlled trial. Sex Transm Dis 2006;33:31–35.

LATE REFERENCE

104. Smoak ND, Scott-Sheldon LA, Johnson BT, Cary MP. Sexual risk reduction interventions do not inadvertently increase the overall frequency of sexual behavior: A meta-analysis of 174 studies with 116,735 participants. J Acquir Immune Defic Syndro 2006;41:374–384.

Vaginal Barriers and Spermicides

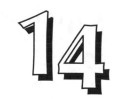

Willard Cates Jr., MD, MPH
Elizabeth G. Raymond, MD, MPH

- Vaginal barriers and spermicides are relatively simple to use and require little advance planning apart from having them accessible.

- Using vaginal barrier methods and spermicides does not require the direct involvement of the male partner and can be timed not to interrupt lovemaking.

- Spermicides are an integral component of most vaginal barrier methods (diaphragm, sponge, and cap).

- Vaginal barriers and spermicides used alone are less effective in typical use than other modern contractive options.

- Consistent and correct use is essential for optimal contraceptive effectiveness; most pregnancies occur because the method is not used.

- Protection against human immunodeficiency virus (HIV) has not been documented either for vaginal barriers with or without spermicide or for spermicides alone.

- Frequent (twice a day or more) spermicide use causes tissue irritation.

Vaginal barriers have a rich contraceptive heritage. In the early 1900s, a wide variety of diaphragm models were being used in Europe. Since then, diaphragm technology has changed little, although new prototypes are currently being tested.

The first female condom, called Reality, was approved by the FDA in 1993 for over-the-counter sale in the United States. Like the diaphragm, new prototypes are under investigation.

Spermicidal products containing nonoxynol-9 (N-9) have also been available for many years. They can be purchased without prescription in pharmacies and supermarkets. They can be used alone, with a vaginal barrier method, or as an adjunct to any of the other contraceptive methods for added protection against pregnancy.

MECHANISM OF ACTION

Vaginal barriers work by blocking and/or killing sperm. The female condom provides a physical barrier that lines the vagina entirely and partially shields the perineum. Diaphragms, caps, and sponges usually combine two contraceptive mechanisms: a physical barrier to shield the cervix and a chemical to kill sperm. These devices also may help to hold spermicide in place against the cervix, and in the case of the sponge, absorb and trap sperm.

Spermicidal preparations consist of two components: 1) a formulation (gel, foam, cream, film, suppository, or tablet), also called a carrier or base; and 2) a chemical that kills the sperm in different doses and concentrations. For some products, the formulation helps disperse the spermicide. In the case of viscous gel and foam, the formulation itself may provide both lubrication and an additional barrier effect. The active chemical agent in spermicide products available in the United States, N-9, is a surfactant that destroys the sperm cell membrane. Other surfactant products, including menfegol and benzalkonium chloride, are widely used in other parts of the world.

VAGINAL BARRIERS

Female condom. The Reality Female Condom is a soft, loose-fitting polyurethane sheath, 7.8 cm in diameter and 17 cm long. It contains two flexible polyurethane rings. One ring lies inside, at the closed end of the sheath, and serves as an insertion mechanism and internal anchor. The other ring forms the external, open edge of the device and remains outside the vagina after insertion (Figure 14–1). The external portion of the device provides some protection to the labia and the base of the penis during intercourse. The sheath is coated with a silicone-based lubricant; additional lubricant for the outside is provided with the device. The lubricant does not contain spermicide. Reality, approved for over-the-counter sale without prescription, is intended for one-time use. Female and male condoms should not be used together; they can adhere to each other, causing slippage or displacement of one or both devices.

The polyurethane used in the sheath is a thin (0.05 mm) but impermeable material with good heat-transfer characteristics. It is stronger than latex and less likely to tear or break. It does not deteriorate with exposure to oil-based products and withstands storage better than latex does.

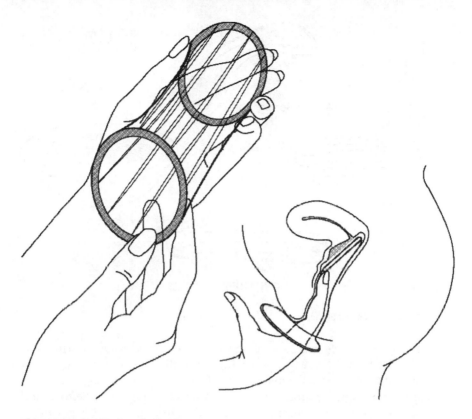

Figure 14–1 Reality Female Condom

Diaphragm. This dome-shaped rubber cup has a flexible rim; it is inserted into the vagina before intercourse so the posterior rim rests in the posterior fornix and the anterior rim fits snugly behind the pubic bone. The dome of the diaphragm covers the cervix; spermicidal cream or jelly applied to the inside of the dome before insertion is held in place near the surface of the cervix. Currently available diaphragms require a prescription, but new products for over-the-counter availability are being tested.

Once in position, the diaphragm may provide effective contraceptive protection for up to 6 hours. If a longer interval has elapsed, insertion of additional, fresh spermicide with an applicator (without removing the diaphragm) is typically recommended, but no evidence supports this practice. After intercourse, the diaphragm must be left in place for at least 6 hours. Wearing it for longer than 24 hours is not recommended because of the possible risk of toxic shock syndrome (TSS).

Diaphragms are available in sizes ranging from 50 mm to 95 mm (diameter) and in several styles (Figure 14–2). The styles differ in the inner construction of the circular rim, and in the case of the *wide-seal* style, the

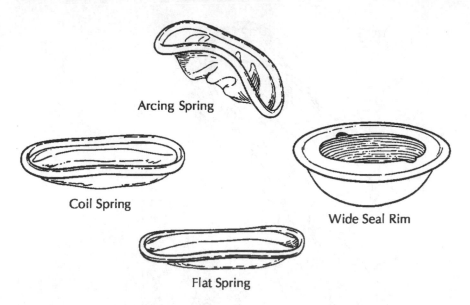

Arcing Spring

Coil Spring

Wide Seal Rim

Flat Spring

Figure 14–2 Types of diaphragms

presence of a flexible flange attached to the inner edge of the rim. The thin, *flat spring* rim has a gentle spring strength that is comfortable for women with firm vaginal muscle tone. The sturdy *coil spring* rim has a firm spring strength suitable for a woman with average muscle tone and an average pubic arch depth. A plastic diaphragm introducer can be used to insert coil or flat spring styles. The sturdy and firm *arcing spring* folds into an arc shape that facilitates correct insertion; it can maintain a correct position despite lax muscle. Wide-seal diaphragms are available with either an arcing spring rim or a coil spring rim.

Contraceptive sponge. This small, pillow-shaped polyurethane sponge contains 1 gram of nonoxynol-9 spermicide. The concave dimple on one side was designed to fit over the cervix and decrease the chance of dislodgement during intercourse (Figure 14–3). The other side of the sponge incorporates a woven polyester loop to facilitate removal. The sponge is a one-size, over-the-counter product. It is moistened with tap water prior to use and inserted deep into the vagina.

The sponge protects for up to 24 hours, no matter how many times intercourse occurs. After intercourse, the sponge must be left in place for at least 6 hours before it is removed and discarded. Wearing the sponge for longer than 24 to 30 hours is not recommended because of the possible risk of TSS.

Lea's Shield. This product is an oval device made of medical-grade silicone rubber, with an anterior loop that assists in removal. It is reusable and is used with spermicide, much like the diaphragm. Like the cap,

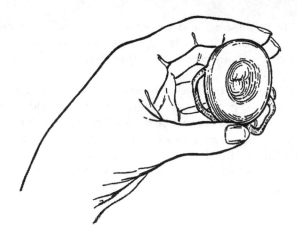

Figure 14–3 Contraceptive sponge

it blocks the cervix, but contains a central valve that allows passage of cervical secretions and air. Lea's Shield has only one size, so fitting is not required. However, in the United States, the device is available by prescription only.

FemCap. This bowl-shaped silicone rubber cap has a brim that flares outward. The concave side of the bowl covers the cervix completely, while the rim fits against the vaginal fornices. The brim is taller on one end than the other. When properly positioned, the larger brim fits into the back of the vagina. Spermicide can be placed on the inside and the outside of the cap. A strap located on the convex side of the bowl could aid in removal. FemCap comes in 3 sizes and is available only by prescription. The FemCap can be worn for up to 48 hours.

Future barrier devices. Other products being developed include devices made of polymers that release spermicide, a custom-molded cap, a diaphragm designed to user preferences, and modifications of the contraceptive sponge.

SPERMICIDES

Gels and creams. Gels, creams, and foam are commonly marketed for use with a diaphragm, but they can also be used alone. One application delivers 52.5 mg to 150 mg of N-9, depending on the product: the spermicide concentration ranges from 8% to 12.5% in foam, and from 2% to 4% in gels and creams.

Suppositories. Spermicide suppositories can be used alone or with a condom. Suppositories have a spermicide concentration of 3% to 5% and provide 100 mg to 125 mg of N-9. Adequate time between insertion and intercourse (10 to 15 minutes depending on the product) is essential for the spermicide to dissolve and disperse. Incomplete dissolution of the suppository may reduce its contraceptive efficacy and may cause an uncomfortable gritty sensation or friction for the woman or the man.

Film. N-9 film can be used alone or with barriers. Each paper-thin sheet of film has a spermicide concentration of 28% and contains 72 mg to 100 mg of N-9. The sheet must be inserted on or near the cervix at least 15 minutes before intercourse to allow time for the sheet to melt and disperse. Placing film on the tip of the penis for insertion is not recommended; the film will not have adequate time to dissolve, and it may not be properly placed so as to cover the cervical os.

EFFECTIVENESS

The contraceptive effectiveness of vaginal barriers and spermicides depends on how correctly and consistently they are used. The pregnancy rates of typical and perfect use for these methods vary because of high levels of inconsistent use (Table 14–1).

Table 14–1 First-year probability of pregnancy* for women using vaginal barrier and spermicide methods

Method	% of Women Experiencing an Unintended Pregnancy Within the First Year of Use		% of Women Continuing Use At One Year
	Typical Use	Perfect Use	
Sponge			
Parous Women	32	20	46
Nulliparous Women	16	9	57
Female Condom	21	5	49
			57
Diaphragm	16	6	
Spermicides	29	18	42
Withdrawal	27	4	43
Latex male condom	15	2	53

* See Table 27–1 for first-year probability of pregnancy for all methods.

VAGINAL BARRIERS

Parity affects the efficacy of some vaginal barriers. From 5% to 9% of nulliparous users and from 5% to 20% of parous users of these methods will become pregnant during the first year of perfect use.[1-4] For parous women, the sponge is substantially less effective than the diaphragm,[2] whereas for nulliparous women, all vaginal barrier devices provide similar contraceptive effectiveness during typical use. For parous women, the sponge and the cap are substantially less effective than the diaphragm or female condom.[2] For nulliparous women, the female condom, diaphragm, cervical cap, and sponge all provide similar contraceptive effectiveness during typical use.

The difference between low failure rates reported in some studies and high rates reported in others is not accounted for entirely by patient diligence or parity. The wide range reflects the profound effect of differences among study populations in fertility characteristics. For example, in one study of the diaphragm,[2] women who used the diaphragm consistently and had intercourse three times weekly or more were almost three times as likely to experience a pregnancy compared with women who had intercourse less than three times weekly.

SPERMICIDES

Reported pregnancy rates among typical spermicide users cover a wide range, from less than 5% to more than 50% in the first year of use.[5] Most published clinical trials of spermicide used alone do not meet modern standards for study design and analysis; thus, we must be cautious when comparing the contraceptive effectiveness of spermicides with that of other contraceptive methods.

A 6-month randomized trial of nonoxynol-9 film and foaming tablets found high unintended pregnancy rates for both products—25% and 28% pregnant in *6 months*, respectively.[6] The population studied was young (58% younger than 25 years) and had frequent coitus (71% more than 10 acts per month). A more recent 6-month randomized trial of five nonoxynol-9 spermicide products conducted in the United States showed somewhat lower pregnancy rates, from 10% to 22% in *6 months*.[7] In this trial, a gel containing 52.5 mg of nonoxynol-9 was less effective at preventing pregnancy than gels containing 100 or 150 mg. However, no difference was found between a gel, a film, and a suppository each containing 100 mg of nonoxynol-9.

The formulation (comfort with using applicator, degree of lubricating effect, or required delay for suppository or film to melt) may influence a woman's ability to use the spermicide effectively. A woman is most likely to succeed with a formulation that is compatible with her sexual routines.

Douching is not a reliable contraceptive, even when a spermicide is in the douching solution, because sperm enter the cervical canal soon after ejaculation. A woman who has used a vaginal spermicide for contraception should not douche until at least 6 hours after sexual intercourse to avoid washing away the spermicide prematurely.

Vaginal Barriers Plus Spermicides

Many vaginal barrier users have wondered whether using spermicide with a diaphragm or cap is really necessary. Although several studies hint that spermicide may be helpful in improving contraceptive effectiveness with some of these devices, the studies have not been large enough to point to clear conclusions.[4] Women using the diaphragm without spermicide had a pregnancy rate of 29 pregnancies per 100 women within 12 months, while those using a diaphragm with spermicide had a rate of 21 per 100 women. In contrast, in a six-month study, women using the new diaphragm-like Lea's Shield device without spermicide experienced almost twice as many pregnancies as those who used spermicide (9.3 vs. 5.6 pregnancies per 100 women over the *6-month* study interval.[8])

ADVANTAGES

Vaginal barrier methods and spermicides have many advantages that make them reasonable for both short-term and long-term contraception. The overall medical safety of these methods, backed up by abortion in case of failure, is comparable to consistent use of male condoms. They do not cause systemic side effects and do not alter a woman's hormone patterns. Vaginal barrier methods and spermicides do not generally require partner involvement in the decision to insert them. For women who need contraception only intermittently, these methods can be available for immediate protection whenever needed, no matter how long the interval between uses. The sponge, female condom, and spermicides can be purchased over-the-counter and do not require the user to seek medical consultation. Finally, these methods offer a simple backup option for a woman who is waiting to start oral contraceptives or have an intrauterine device (IUD) inserted, forgets two or more pills, runs out of pills, suspects her IUD has been expelled, is breastfeeding, or is using a fertility awareness method.

SEXUALLY TRANSMITTED INFECTION (STI) PROTECTION

Potentially, protection against spread of STIs could be the most important noncontraceptive benefit of vaginal barrier use.[9-10] The female condom lines the vagina completely, preventing contact between the penis and vagina. The condom traps semen and is then discarded. The polyurethane in female condoms is strong and impermeable to organisms as small as the HIV virus. Unless the female condom slips out of place or is torn, or the penis gets "misrouted" between the female condom and vaginal wall, the protection against STI exposure should be equivalent to that provided by male condoms. Consistent, correct use of female condoms appears effective in preventing trichomonas reinfection.[11] In addition, supplementing male condoms with female condoms led to slightly lower STI rates in Thailand brothels.[12]

Studies of women who use a diaphragm or sponge differ in their reported reduction of gonorrhea, chlamydia, and trichomoniasis.[13-14] The presence of a mechanical barrier, to reduce exposure of the fragile cervical epithelium to semen and microbes, could theoretically affect infection risk. Nonetheless, in the absence of reliable randomized controlled trials showing that these vaginal barriers effectively protect against infection, be cautious in making recommendations about using vaginal barrier methods for STI protection.

Our currently available spermicides containing nonoxynol-9 are ineffective as microbicides.[15] Thus, do not recommend the use of spermicide alone to prevent HIV or other STIs. Furthermore, frequent use (more than 2 times per day) of spermicides causes more vulvovaginal epithelial disruption,[16] which theoretically could increase susceptibility to HIV.

We have a critical need for female-initiated methods to prevent STIs, including HIV.[17] While male condoms provide protection against most STIs,[18] their use is low among many couples. Methods women can use independently may improve levels of protection. However, the lengthy research required for developing and testing new microbicidal products means these methods are years away.[19-20]

CERVICAL NEOPLASIA PROTECTION

Several weak observational studies show a lower risk of cervical dysplasia and cancer among women using the diaphragm.[21-22] Because cervical infection with certain strains of human papillomavirus virus (HPV) plays an etiologic part in cervical neoplasia, diaphragm use may reduce the risk of HPV similar to the reduced risk observed for other STIs. Alternatively, women who choose to use the diaphragm may be at lower risk for HPV for reasons unrelated to effects of the diaphragm itself.

D ISADVANTAGES

Few serious medical problems are associated with use of vaginal barriers. Most women are medically appropriate candidates for their use. Toxic shock syndrome is potentially life threatening, but rare.

Irritation. Temporary skin irritation involving the vulva, vagina, or penis caused by either local toxicity or allergy is the most common problem associated with spermicide use. When an allergy is suspected, suggest the client try another contraceptive method. Vaginal epithelial disruption has been associated with frequent use (twice a day or more) of spermicides containing N-9.[16] However, epithelial disruption does not always cause noticeable symptoms, and symptoms do not necessarily indicate tissue harm. If any signs of irritation are found, advise the client to use spermicides less frequently or to discontinue their use.

Vaginal and urinary tract infections. Using a diaphragm and spermicide during sexual intercourse is associated with increased vaginal colonization with Escherichia coli.[23]

Toxic shock syndrome (TSS). TSS is a rare but serious disorder caused by toxin(s) released by some strains of Staphylococcus aureus. Most TSS occurs in association with tampon use during menses; nonmenstrual TSS risk is increased for women who use diaphragms.[24] The absolute risk of TSS attributable to vaginal barriers, however, is very low. Nevertheless, patients using vaginal barriers need to be aware of the TSS danger signs and receive instructions consistent with recommended TSS precautions.

Systemic effects and pregnancy exposure. No serious systemic side effects have been reported in association with human use of spermicides in conjunction with vaginal barriers. Safety concerns have centered on the issue of fetal exposure related to their accidental use during early pregnancy. However, composite data show no true association exists between spermicide use and fetal defects.[25]

Removal. Problems with removal of some vaginal barriers are fairly common. Some sponge users have difficulty with vaginal dryness. Foul odor and vaginal discharge are likely to occur if a diaphragm or sponge is inadvertently left in the vagina for more than a few days. Symptoms abate promptly when the device is removed.

Common dislikes. Some women complain about the noise female condoms make during intercourse. The main complaints with spermicides are messiness, having to touch the genitals, and excessive lubrication. Some couples find the taste of spermicide unpleasant when they engage in oral-genital sex. Occasionally, women find the effervescence of foaming vaginal suppositories is unpleasant.

CAUTIONS

The following conditions may make use of one or more of the vaginal barrier methods or spermicides inadvisable:

1. Allergy to spermicide, rubber, latex, polyurethane, the spermicidal agent, or ingredients in the base.

2. Abnormalities in vaginal anatomy that interfere with a satisfactory fit, stable placement, and retention of a vaginal barrier device or spermicide.

3. Inability to learn correct insertion technique.

4. History of TSS (except female condom and spermicide).

5. Repeated UTIs (except female condom).

6. Lack of trained personnel to fit the device or lack of clinical time to provide instruction (for the diaphragm and FemCap).

7. Full-term delivery within the past 6 weeks, recent spontaneous or induced abortion, or vaginal bleeding from any cause, including menstrual flow (for Lea's Shield, FemCap, and sponges).

8. (*For N-9 spermicides*) If STI/HIV exposure is likely, situations that would involve frequent use, defined as 2 times or more a day.

PROVIDING VAGINAL BARRIER METHODS

Help the woman choose which of the available barrier options is most likely to meet her needs (Table 14–2). Women who plan to use female condoms or sponges do not require a pelvic exam. If you perform a routine exam, however, you can make sure the woman does not have an unusual anatomic anomaly such as a septate vagina or duplicate cervices. For a woman who wishes to use a diaphragm, select a device that fits well, or determine that a satisfactory fit is not possible so the patient can choose another contraceptive method.

Be sure each patient has an opportunity to practice inserting and removing her device as part of her visit. After the patient has inserted her device, verify that its position is correct and that the fit is good. New users should try the device initially while still using another method of birth control, such as condoms or oral contraceptives, to be sure it remains in position after intercourse.

Personalizing the barrier method. Vaginal barriers differ in both effectiveness and in rules for their use. These differences may make one option easier or more appealing for a specific woman. For parous women, the diaphragm and female condom provide more effective contraceptive protection than does the sponge. For nulliparous women, the difference in effectiveness is less striking. Because consistent use is so

Table 14–2 Vaginal barrier methods and spermicides—guidelines for use

	Diaphragm	Female Condom	Sponge	Lea's Shield	FemCap Sper	Spermi-cides
Available without prescription	No	Yes	Yes	No	No	Yes
Reusable	Yes	No	No	Yes	Yes	No
May be used with male condoms	Yes	No	Yes	Yes	Yes	Yes
Separate spermicide recommended	Yes	No	No	Yes	Yes	—
Can be used during menses	Yes	Yes	No	No	No	Yes
May be used for multiple sex acts after insertion	Yes[1]	No	Yes	Yes[1]	Yes[1]	No
Recommended waiting times						
Between insertion and sex (minimum minutes)	0	0	0	0	15[2]	0-15
Between insertion and sex (maximum hours)	18[3]	No maximum	24	Not stated	several	1-3
Between sex and removal (minimum hours)	6	—[4]	6	8	6	—
Between insertion and removal (maximum hours)	24	—[4]	30	48	48	—

[1] Insert extra spermicide before each sex act after the first (for diaphragm and FemCap), or before each sex act that occurs more than 40 hours after insertion, if more than 8 hours have elapsed since the previous sex act (for Lea's Shield).

[2] The FemCap should be inserted at least 15 minutes before any sexual arousal.

[3] If more than 6 hours elapse between diaphragm insertion and sex, insert more spermicide into the vagina (without removing the diaphragm) before having sex.

[4] Remove the female condom before standing up after sex to avoid having the semen spill out.

important, a match between the method's characteristics and the woman's personal needs and sexual patterns may improve effectiveness.

Limited evidence. The guidelines for using vaginal barrier methods are based largely on educated opinion rather than scientific evidence. The guidelines balance concerns about convenience of the method, spermicide effectiveness, and possible TSS risk. However, no evidence exists for specifying an unsafe duration of wear to minimize TSS risk. Similarly, the optimal spermicide dose and duration of effectiveness are unknown. Whether an extra application of spermicide for repeated intercourse improves effectiveness for diaphragm users is not known.

CLINICIAN'S ROLE IN BARRIER SUCCESS

You play an important role in helping women make wise decisions about vaginal barrier methods and spermicides and use them successfully:

1. Help the woman assess her own risk of unintended pregnancy. If her risk is low, do not discourage her confidence in vaginal barriers. If her risk is high, however, a vaginal barrier may not be a wise solo method choice. Characteristics that may be associated with higher than average risk of pregnancy include:

   — Frequent intercourse (three times or more weekly)

   — Age less than 30 years

   — Personal style or sexual patterns that make consistent use difficult

   — Previous contraceptive failure with vaginal methods

   — Known abuse of alcohol and/or other drugs

2. Help the woman assess her risk of STI exposure. If the risk is high, encourage her to use male condoms along with her female barrier. (Female condoms should not be used simultaneously with male condoms because the two condoms may stick together.)

3. If unintended pregnancy would be devastating for the woman, or if she is at high risk for vaginal barrier failure, encourage her to consider using either a more effective contraceptive or a combination of barrier methods such as a diaphragm or sponge plus male condoms.

4. Be sure every vaginal barrier user has an accurate understanding of ovulation timing and knows high-risk days for conception begin about 6 to 7 days before ovulation.

5. Be sure every vaginal barrier user is aware of emergency contraception (postcoital treatment) and knows how to obtain it if a contraceptive emergency arises. If possible, provide her with a kit containing an instruction sheet and a supply of pills sufficient for one or more emergency treatment regimens. (See Chapter 6 on Emergency Contraception.)

Practical Caution: Avoid Oil-Based Lubricants and Medications

Lubricants such as mineral oil, baby oil, suntan oil, vegetable oil, and butter; and vaginal medications such as Femstat cream, Monistat cream, estrogen cream, and Vagisil have a rapid, deleterious effect on latex. Their effect on diaphragm integrity has not been studied, but it is reasonable to warn vaginal barrier users to avoid oil products. They will not affect the silicon in Lea's Shield or the FemCap or the polyurethane in the Reality Female Condom. If additional lubrication is needed, a vaginal spermicide or a product intended for use with latex condoms would be reasonable options.

FITTING A DIAPHRAGM

Estimate the diaphragm size that will be needed:

1. Insert your index and middle fingers into the vagina until your middle finger reaches the posterior wall of the vagina.

2. Use the tip of your thumb to mark the point at which your index finger touches the pubic bone.

3. Extract your fingers.

4. Place the diaphragm rim on the tip of your middle finger. The opposite rim should lie just in front of your thumb.

Insert a sample diaphragm of the size you have selected into the patient's vagina. The device should rest snugly in the vagina, but without tension against the vaginal walls. Its rim should be in contact with the lateral walls and posterior fornix, and there should be just enough space to insert one fingertip comfortably between the inside of the pubic arch and the anterior edge of the diaphragm rim.

Choose the largest rim size that is comfortable for the patient. Try more than one rim size before making a final selection. Do not choose a size that is too small; vaginal depth increases during sexual arousal (3 to 5 cm in nulliparous women), and a too-small diaphragm may fail to maintain its position covering the cervix. A diaphragm that is too large, however, may cause vaginal pressure, abdominal pain or cramping, or vaginal ulceration, and may be a factor in recurrent UTI. One practical approach is to have the patient push down while the diaphragm is in place. The largest size that doesn't come out is the right size.

Disinfecting Diaphragms and Rings Used For Fitting

Use universal precautions when fitting diaphragms, as well as when cleaning and disinfecting them after fitting. Use gloves for fittings, and use both eye splash protection and gloves when cleaning diaphragms and rings. Because they come into contact with intact mucous membrane, diaphragms and rings used for fitting are classified as semi-critical devices that require processing with a high-level disinfectant according to OSHA guidelines. After thorough scrubbing with a liquid detergent and water, three disinfection options are recommended.[26]

- Autoclave at 121 degrees Centigrade, 15 pounds per square inch (psi) for 20 minutes unwrapped or 30 minutes wrapped.

- Soak in a solution of one part Clorox to nine parts water (results in a solution of sodium hypochlorite 5,000 ppm) for 30 minutes at room temperature; rinse with tap water; then soak in 70% ethyl or isopropyl alcohol for 15 minutes. Discard all solutions.

- Immerse in Cidex (2% glutaraldehyde) for 20 minutes at room temperature; then rinse and place in boiling water for 30 minutes. Follow manufacturer's instructions concerning preparation and disposal or reuse of Cidex solution.

After disinfection, allow the diaphragms or rings to air dry, then store them in a disinfected container until later use.

FITTING LEA'S SHIELDS

Checking the fit of this device is quite simple since it has only one size. Allow the woman to practice insertion and removal. After she inserts the device, check to see if the cervix is covered, the loop fits behind the symphysis, and the woman is comfortable.

FITTING THE FEMCAP

FemCaps are available in three sizes with internal rim diameters of 22 mm, 26 mm, and 30 mm. Women who have never been pregnant should use the smallest size; women who have miscarried or had a cesarean section should use the middle size; and women who have vaginally delivered a full-term baby should use the largest size. To confirm the fit, insert the Femcap into the vagina by squeezing it and pushing it deep into the vagina with the bowl facing upward and the long rim entering first. When the device is released in place over the cervix, the unfolding dome should create suction between the rim of the cap and the cervix. Check with your finger to make sure that the cervix is completely covered.

To remove the Femcap, rotate the device in any direction that is comfortable for you. Push the tip of your finger against the dome of the device to dimple it. This will break the suction and allow room for your finger to fit between the dome and the removal strap. Hook the strap with your finger and gently pull the device down and out.

PROVIDING SPERMICIDES

Spermicides are currently available over the counter. When providing spermicides in a clinical setting, reinforce instructions for proper use and remind users about common errors that can lead to unintended pregnancy. (See the section on Instructions for Using Spermicides). Counsel users about emergency contraception as a backup. Warn women who have abnormalities of vaginal anatomy (such as a septate vagina or a severe uterine prolapse), which may interfere with proper spermicide placement, that spermicide use may not be effective for them.

MANAGING PROBLEMS AND FOLLOW-UP

Women using vaginal barriers need no special follow-up. Labeling for the diaphragm recommends refitting after a weight gain or loss of 10 pounds or more, after an abortion, or after a full-term pregnancy.[28] However, data suggest that women who have had a change in weight do not commonly require a new diaphragm size, nor do women who have had an abortion. Remind women to avoid wearing vaginal barriers for the last 2 or 3 days before coming for routine exams, if possible, to provide optimal conditions for Pap screening.

When a barrier user returns for a routine exam, ask open-ended questions about how the method is working out. If the woman finds it inconvenient or uncomfortable, offer her an opportunity to consider an alternative method. Refitting her with a different size or rim style may also be helpful.

Problems caused by vaginal barrier methods may require clinical intervention. Recurrent vaginal or introital irritation, with no evidence of vaginal infection, may indicate an allergy or sensitivity to spermicide or to latex. Recurrent urinary tract infection (UTI), recurrent yeast infection, and bacterial vaginosis may be associated with use of contraceptive sponges or a diaphragm.

If a diaphragm user experiences recurring UTIs, consider refitting her with a smaller diaphragm size or an alternative rim style. If her UTI problems persist despite these measures, changing to an alternative method of contraception that does not involve spermicide may be advisable.

A vaginal barrier user who develops signs or symptoms of TSS requires urgent and intensive evaluation and treatment. Treat the patient with antibiotics, and follow her carefully. If her symptoms are severe, she may need hospitalization. Because TSS risk is increased for a woman who has had TSS in the past, the woman should avoid use of vaginal barrier methods in the future.

Spermicide use does not require any special follow-up. Women who experience irritation may seek care. If symptoms persist more than a day or two after the patient discontinues using spermicides, evaluate the underlying factors, such as STI exposure, yeast vaginitis, or bacterial vaginosis. Changing to an alternative product with a different formulation or changing to a less concentrated product may help.

Ask about spermicide use (including condoms lubricated with spermicide) when evaluating a woman with recurrent urinary tract infections. Switching to another contraceptive strategy may help in managing recurrent UTIs.

INSTRUCTIONS FOR USING VAGINAL BARRIERS/SPERMICIDES

1. Use your method every time you have intercourse. Be sure your vaginal barrier method or spermicide is in place before your partner's penis enters your vagina.

2. If you feel unsure about the proper fit or placement of your diaphragm, Lea's Shield, FemCap, or sponge, use male condoms until you see your clinician to be sure your insertion technique is correct.

3. If you are having problems with vaginal or penile irritation, try a different spermicide product. If you have problems with recurring bladder infections or vaginal yeast infections, discuss these with your clinician.

4. You can use male condoms along with your diaphragm, sponge, Lea's Shield, FemCap, or spermicide if you wish. Using this combination, you will have effective protection against both pregnancy and sexually transmitted infection. Do not use a male condom along with a female condom; the two may adhere and increase the chance your female condom will dislodge or male condom will slip off.

5. No conclusive studies show just how long spermicide is fully active or exactly how long the diaphragm or sponge must be left in place after intercourse. The most important thing is consistent and correct use, protecting your cervix.

6. Douching after intercourse is not recommended. If you are using a diaphragm or sponge, and choose to douche, wait at least 6 hours after intercourse to avoid washing away spermicide.

7. If you are using a diaphragm or sponge, learn the danger signs for toxic shock syndrome and watch for them. These signs include sudden high fever, chills, vomiting, diarrhea, muscle aches and sunburn-like rash. If you have a high fever and one or more of the other danger signs, you may have early toxic shock syndrome. Remove the sponge or diaphragm and contact your clinician immediately, or go to a hospital emergency room.

TAKING CARE OF YOUR VAGINAL BARRIER METHOD

1. Store your supplies in a convenient location that is clean, cool, and dark.

2. Wash your spermicide inserter, diaphragm, or cap after each use. Plain soap is best; avoid deodorant soap or perfumed soap. Do not use talcum powder on your diaphragm or cap, or in the case.

3. Contact with oil-based products can deteriorate a diaphragm. Do not use oil-based vaginal medications or lubricants when you are using a diaphragm. Some examples include petroleum jelly (Vaseline), mineral oil, hand lotion, vegetable oil, cold cream, and cocoa butter as well as common vaginal yeast creams and vaginal hormone creams. If you need extra lubrication for intercourse, contraceptive jelly is a good choice, or you can try a water-soluble lubricant specifically intended for use with condoms.

REFERENCES

1. Farr G, Gabelnick H, Sturgen K, Dorflinger L. Contraceptive efficacy and acceptability of the female condom. Am J Public Health 1994;84(12):1960–1964.
2. Trussell J, Strickler J, Vaughan B. Contraceptive efficacy of the diaphragm, the sponge and the cervical cap. Fam Plann Perspect 1993;25(3):100–105, 135.
3. Trussell J, Sturgen K, Strickler J, Dominik R. Comparative contraceptive efficacy of the female condom and other barrier methods. Fam Plann Perspect 1994;26(2):66–72.
4. Cook L, Nanda K, Grimes DA. Diaphragm versus diaphragm with spermicides for contraception (Cochrane review). In The Cochrane Library, Issue Q, 2001. Oxford: Update Software, 2001.
5. Grimes DA, Lopez LM, Raymond EG, Halpern V, Nanda K, Schulz KF. Spermicide used alone for contraception. Cochrane Database of Systematic Reviews 2005, Issue 4.
6. Raymond E, Dominik R, Spermicide Trial Group. Contraceptive effectiveness of two spermicides: a randomized trial. Obstet Gynecol 1999;93(6):896–903.
7. Raymond EG, Chen PL, Luoto J, et al. Contraceptive effectiveness and safety of five nonoxynol-9 spermicides: a randomized trial. Obstet Gynecol 2004;103:430–439.
8. Mauck C, Glover LH, Miller E et al. Lea's Shield: a study of the safety and efficacy of a new vaginal barrier contraceptive used with and without spermicide. Contraception 1996;53(6):329–335.

9. Moench TR, Chipato T, Padian NS. Preventing disease by protecting the cervix: the unexplored promise of internal vaginal barrier devices. AIDS 2001;15(13):1595–1602.

10. Minnis AM, Padian NS. Effectiveness of female controlled barrier methods in preventing sexually transmitted infections and HIV: current evidence and future research directions. Sex Transm Infect 2005;81:193–200.

11. Soper DE, Shoupe D, Shangold GA, Shangold MM, Gutmann J, Mercer L. Prevention of vaginal trichomoniasis by compliant use of the female condom. Sex Transm Dis 1993;20(3):137–139.

12. Fontanet AL, Saba J, Chandelying V et al. Protection against sexually transmitted diseases by granting sex workers in Thailand the choice of using the male or female condom: results from a randomized controlled trial. AIDS 1998;12(14):1851–1859.

13. Cates W Jr, Stone KM. Family planning, sexually transmitted diseases and contraceptive choice: a literature update—Part I [see comments]. Fam Plann Perspect 1992;24(2):75–84.

14. d'Oro LC, Parazzini F, Naldi L, La Vecchia C. Barrier methods of contraception, spermicides, and sexually transmitted diseases: a review. Genitourin Med 1994;70(6):410–417.

15. McCormack S, Hayes R, Lacey CJ, Johnson AM. Microbicides in HIV prevention. BMJ 2001;322(7283):410–413.

16. Roddy RE, Cordero M, Cordero C, Fortney JA. A dosing study of nonoxynol-9 and genital irritation. Int J STD AIDS 1993;4(3):165–170.

17. Stein ZA. More on women and the prevention of HIV infection. Am J Public Health 1995;85(11):1485–1488.

18. Centers for Disease Control and Prevention. Male latex condoms and sexually transmitted diseases. Fact sheet for public health personnel. Update December 12, 2002. www.cdcnpin.org.

19. Stone A. Clinical trials of microbicides. Microbicide Q 2003;1:13–18.

20. Madan RP, Keller MJ, Herold BC. Prioritizing prevention of HIV and sexually transmitted infection: first-generation vaginal microbicides. Current Opinion in Infectious Diseases 2006;19:49–54.

21. Celentano DD, Klassen AC, Weisman CS, Rosenshein NB. The role of contraceptive use in cervical cancer: the Maryland cervical cancer case-control study. Am J Epidemiology 1987;70:410–417.

22. Parazzini F, Negri E, La Vecchia C, Fedele L. Barrier methods of contraception and the risk of cervical neoplasia. Contraception 1989;40(5):519–530.

23. Hooton TM, Roberts PL, Stamm WE. Effects of recent sexual activity and use of a diaphragm on the vaginal microflora. Clinical Infectious Diseases 1994;19:274–278.

24. Schwartz B, Gaventa S, Broome CV et al. Nonmenstrual toxic shock syndrome associated with barrier contraceptives: report of a case-control study. Rev Infect Dis 1989;11 Suppl 1:S43-S48;discussion S48-S49.

25. Food and Drug Administration. Data does not support association between spermicides, birth defects. FDA Drug Bulletin 1986;11–21.

26. Kugel C, Verson H. Relationship between weight change and diaphragm size change. J Obstet Gynecol Neonatal Nurs 1986;15(2):123–129.

Coitus Interruptus (Withdrawal)

15

Deborah Kowal, MA, PA

- Coitus interruptus does not eliminate the risk of sexually transmitted infections (STIs): the pre-ejaculate can contain HIV-infected cells, and lesions or ulcers on the genitals can transmit pathogens.

- It is free, readily available, does not require use of clinical services and providers, does not involve chemicals or other foreign materials.

- Although popularly considered an ineffective method, coitus interruptus provides efficacy similar to that of barrier methods of contraception.

Coitus interruptus is simply the practice of withdrawing the penis from the vagina and away from external genital organs of women before ejaculation, with the intention of avoiding pregnancy. Coitus interruptus, or the withdrawal method, was a natural response to the discovery that ejaculation into the vagina caused pregnancy.[1] The method was probably widely practiced throughout history, playing a predominant role in fertility declines occurring prior to the advent of the pill. Although the 2002 National Survey of Family Growth (NSFG) reports the prevalence of coitus interruptus among women who use a contraceptive is only 4%,[2] this figure belies more widespread practice. When the respondents were asked whether they practiced the withdrawal method during the month of the NSFG interview, 5.4% said 'yes.' When sexually active women were asked if they had *ever* practiced withdrawal, more than half (56%) answered affirmatively, compared with 24.5% in 1992 and 40.6% in 1995. Only pills and condoms were more often reported as methods 'ever used' by the respondents.

In the 1995 NSFG report, 42.3% of young women age 15 to 19 years reported ever having used withdrawal, and in the 2002 report, that percentage increased to 55%.[3] Only 4.7% reported relying on the method during the month of the interview and only 0.8% reported using the method as their current method.[2]

MECHANISM OF ACTION

Coitus interruptus prevents fertilization by preventing the contact between spermatozoa and the ovum. The couple may have penile-vaginal intercourse until ejaculation is impending, at which time the male partner withdraws his penis from the vagina and away from the external genitalia of the female partner. The man must rely on his own sensations to determine when he is about to ejaculate. The pre-ejaculate, which is usually released just prior to full ejaculation, goes unnoticed by both the man and the woman during the course of intercourse and so is not a sign that ejaculation is about to occur.

EFFECTIVENESS

Although coitus interruptus has often been criticized as an ineffective method, it probably confers a level of contraceptive protection similar to that provided by barrier methods. Effectiveness depends largely on the man's ability to withdraw prior to ejaculation. How effective the method would be if used consistently and correctly is highly uncertain. Our best guess is that the probability of pregnancy among perfect users would be about 4% in the initial year of use (Table 15–1). Among typical users, the probability of pregnancy would be about 27% during the first year of use.

As with other methods, withdrawal's efficacy in preventing pregnancy probably depends not only on characteristics of the method, but also on characteristics of the user. Women who are younger and who are married are less likely to experience an accidental pregnancy during the first two years of use.[4] It may be that certain cultural factors influence how successful a couple may be in using withdrawal. A recent study found that Hispanic women were less likely to experience accidental pregnancy than were black or white women.[4] Men who are less experienced with using the method or who have difficulty in foretelling when ejaculation will occur could have a greater risk of failure.

ADVANTAGES AND INDICATIONS

As a method of contraception, withdrawal has several distinct advantages. It costs nothing, requires no devices, involves no chemicals, and is available in any situation. Some couples may select withdrawal as their method because it requires no physical examination or contact with a clinic or pharmacy.[5] Practicing coitus interruptus causes no medical side effects. It also enables men to take a responsible and active role in

Table 15–1 First year probability of pregnancy[a] for couples using condoms, withdrawal, diaphragm, and pill

Method	% of Women Experiencing an Unintended Pregnancy Within the First Year of Use		% of Women Continuing Use at One Year
	Typical Use	Perfect Use	
Withdrawal	27	4	43
Diaphragm	16	6	57
Condom			
Male	15	2	53
Female (Reality)	21	5	49
Pill	8	0.3	68

[a] See Table 27–1 for first-year probability of pregnancy for all methods.

> **Emergency Contraceptive Pills:** Treatment initiated within 120 hours after unprotected intercourse reduces the risk of pregnancy by at least 75%. (See Chapter 6 for more information.)

fertility regulation and may foster a dialogue on contraception and sexuality between the partners.[6,7] Couples who cannot or do not wish to use other contraceptive methods and who can accept the potential for unintended pregnancy may find withdrawal an acceptable alternative. It is also a backup contraceptive that is always available.

DISADVANTAGES AND CAUTIONS

The method is unforgiving of incorrect or inconsistent use, leading to a probability of pregnancy in typical users that is substantially higher than the rates for hormonal methods or intrauterine devices (IUDs). One reason for contraceptive failure may be a lack of the self-control demanded by the method. With impending orgasm, men (and women) experience a mild to extreme clouding of consciousness during which coital movement becomes involuntary.[8] The man may feel the urge to achieve deeper penetration at the time of impending orgasm and may not withdraw in sufficient time to avoid depositing semen in his partner's vagina or on her external genitalia. In addition, some men have difficulty foretelling when they will ejaculate. For some couples, interruption of the excitement or plateau phase of the sexual response cycle may diminish pleasure.

Withdrawal does not completely protect couples from exposure to sexually transmitted infections, because not all pathogens are limited to seminal fluid. Surface lesions, such as those from herpes genitalis or human papilloma virus, may be actively infective.

SPECIAL ISSUES

Studies of stable discordant couples (the man was infected with human immunodeficiency virus [HIV] and the woman was not) demonstrate that coitus interruptus may reduce the risk of infection somewhat better than unprotected intercourse with ejaculation. Coitus interruptus cut the HIV conversion rate of women by half in one study,[9] and by a larger percentage in another study.[10] Because these studies examined only stable heterosexual couples, the findings may not hold true for women with several HIV-infected partners.

Coitus interruptus probably decreases HIV exposure by reducing the amount of semen that enters the woman's vagina. However, the seminal fluid that emerges from the penis prior to ejaculation may contain some HIV.[11–13] Although coitus interruptus may be less likely to transmit HIV than intercourse with ejaculation, women have become infected while their partners consistently practiced withdrawal. Coitus interruptus has not been studied as a way to reduce HIV transmission from woman to man.

Some concern exists that the pre-ejaculate fluid may carry sperm into the vagina. In itself, the pre-ejaculate, a lubricating secretion produced by the Littre or Cowper's glands, contains no sperm. Two studies examining the pre-ejaculate for the presence of spermatozoa found none.[12,13] However, a previous ejaculation may have left some sperm hidden within the folds of the urethral lining. In examinations of the pre-ejaculate in one small study,[14] the pre-ejaculate was free of spermatozoa in all of 11 HIV-seronegative men and 4 of 12 seropositive men. Although the 8 samples containing spermatozoa revealed only small clumps of a few hundred sperm, these could theoretically pose a risk of fertilization. In all likelihood, the spermatozoa left from a previous ejaculation could be washed out with the force of a normal urination; however, this remains unstudied.

USE PATTERNS

Withdrawal can be used in a variety of different patterns. It can be combined with other methods—such as pills, IUDs, or fertility awareness methods—to increase efficacy. Withdrawal can also be used interchangeably with fertility awareness methods or condoms to increase convenience. Some couples may like to share contraceptive responsibility; for example, women may use a modern contraceptive for a while and then men may use withdrawal.[6] Therefore, giving couples information on the fertile period can lower their risk of pregnancy and/or may provide further flexibility and convenience in using the coitus interruptus. Finally, provide the couple with a supply of emergency contraceptive pills and inform them on the use to help decrease failure rates.

INSTRUCTIONS FOR USING COITUS INTERRUPTUS

Most users can learn to use withdrawal on their own and become skillful users.[6] Therefore, the majority of men and women who rely on withdrawal will not be seen in clinical settings for family planning services. Nonetheless, some users or potential users may have questions related to fertile period, emergency contraception, and the risk of any negative health effects, including exposure to sexually transmitted infections.

1. Like all user- and coitus-dependent methods, the efficacy of coitus interruptus depends on its consistent and correct use.

2. When he feels he is about to ejaculate, the man should withdraw his penis from his partner's vagina, making sure that ejaculation occurs away from his partner's genitalia.

3. If more than one intercourse takes place within a relatively short period of time, the man should urinate and wipe off the tip of his penis before intercourse to remove any sperm remaining from a previous ejaculation

4. Withdrawal does not effectively protect against sexually transmitted infections (STIs), including infection with the human immunodeficiency virus (HIV). Abstinence or use of latex or plastic condoms provide better protection.

5. There are no known/documented side effects due to using withdrawal, even among long term users.

6. As a couple, learn what options are available for postcoital protection should any ejaculate come in contact with the vagina. If you think you may have been exposed to a risk of pregnancy, contact your clinician about emergency contraception. (You can also call the toll-free number 1–888-NOT-2-LATE [1–888–668–2528 or go to http://not-2-late.com].

7. Withdrawal is not a good contraceptive method if the man cannot predictably withdraw prior to ejaculation.

REFERENCES

1. Robertson W. An illustrated history of contraception. Park Ridge NJ: Parthenon Publishing Group, 1990.
2. Mosher WD, Martinez GM, Chandra A, Abma JC, Willson SJ. Use of contraception and use of family planning services in the United States: 1982–2002. Advance data from vital health and statistics; no. 350. Hyattsville, MD: National Center for Health Statistics. 2004.
3. Abma JC, Martinez GM, Mosher WD, Dawson, BS. Teenagers in the United States: sexual activity, contraceptive use, and childbearing, 2002. National Center for Health Statistics. Vital Health Stat 2004;23(24). 2004.
4. Ranjit N, Bankole A, Darroch J, Singh, S. Contraceptive failure in the first two years of use: differences across socioeconomic subgroups. Fam Plann Perspect 2001;33: 19–27.
5. Rogow D, Horowitz S. Withdrawal: a review of the literature and an agenda for research. Stud Fam Plann 1995;26:140–153.
6. Ortayli N, Bulut A, Ozugurlu M, Cokar M. Why withdrawal? Why not withdrawal? RHM 2005;13(25):164–173.
7. Schneider J, Schneider P. Sex and responsibility in an age of fertility decline: a Sicilian case study. Social Science and Medicine 1991; 33(8):885–95.
8. Kinsey AC, Pomeroy WB, Martin CE, Gebhard PH. Sexual behavior in the human female. Philadelphia PA: W.B. Saunders Co., 1953.
9. Musicco M, Nicolosi A, Saracco A, Lazzarin A (for the Italian Study Group on HIV Heterosexual Transmission). The role of contraceptive practices in HIV sexual transmission from man to woman. In: Nicolosi A (ed). HIV epidemiology: models and methods. New York: Raven Press, Ltd., 1994:121–135.
10. DiVincenzi I (for the European Study Group). A longitudinal study of human immunodeficiency virus transmission by heterosexual partners. N Engl J Med 1994;331:341–346.
11. Howe JE, Minkoff HL, Duerr AC. Contraceptives and HIV. AIDS 1994;8:861–871.
12. Ilaria G, Jacobs JL, Polsky B, Koll B, Baron P, MacLow C, Armstrong D, Schlegel PN. Detection of HIV-1 DNA sequences in pre-ejaculatory fluid [Letter]. Lancet 1992;340:1469.
13. Zukerman Z, Weiss DB, Orvieto R. Does preejaculatory penile secretion originating from Cowper's gland contain sperm? J Assist Reprod Genet 2003;20:157–159.
14. Pudney J, Oneta M, Mayer K, Seage G, Anderson D. Pre-ejaculatory fluid as potential vector for sexual transmission of HIV-1 [Letter]. Lancet 1992;340:1470.

Fertility Awareness-Based Methods

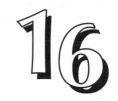

Victoria H. Jennings, PhD
Marcos Arevalo, MD, MPH

- Fertility awareness helps couples understand how to avoid pregnancy or how to become pregnant.
- Regardless of whether they use family planning, or which method they use, most women and men can find value in learning fertility awareness.

Fertility Awareness-Based (FAB) methods of family planning depend on identifying the "fertile window," or the days in each menstrual cycle when intercourse is most likely to result in a pregnancy. Some FAB methods may simply involve keeping track of cycle days to understand on which days of her cycle a woman is most likely to be fertile. Other FAB methods involve observing, recording, and interpreting the body's fertility signs.[1]

To avoid pregnancy, couples either use another method or do not have intercourse during the fertile time. Couples who use a barrier method on fertile days are using a fertility awareness-combined method, while those who abstain are using natural family planning.

MECHANISM OF ACTION

FAB methods of family planning use one or more indicators to identify the beginning and end of the fertile time during the menstrual cycle. These methods are effective when they are used correctly. However, with incorrect use, unprotected intercourse takes place precisely when the woman is potentially fertile.

In most cycles, ovulation occurs on or very near the middle of the cycle.[2] The fertile window of the menstrual cycle lasts for only about 6 days (the 5 days preceding ovulation and the day of ovulation), related to the lifespan of the gametes.[3,4] Even though ovulation does not occur on the same day each cycle, in cycles that range between 26 and 32 days long (approximately 78% of cycles) the fertile window is highly likely to fall within cycle days 8 to 19.[5] In shorter or longer cycles, the fertile window shifts accordingly.

Two FAB methods, the Standard Days Method and the Calendar Rhythm Method, involve counting the days in the menstrual cycle to identify the fertile days. The Standard Days Method requires only that the woman know the day of her menstrual cycle in order to consider herself potentially fertile on days 8 through 19. Prior to starting the Calendar Rhythm Method, the woman must have recorded the length of her previous 6 to 12 menstrual cycles in order to identify the longest and shortest of these cycles. Once these are collected, calculations are performed to identify the probable days of fertility during the current cycle. While survey results show that, in many countries, a significant number of couples state that they are using the "rhythm" or "calendar rhythm" method,[6] most have little understanding of its proper use and simply abstain from intercourse on a few days of the woman's cycle when they believe, often erroneously, that the woman is most likely to become pregnant. It appears that "calendar rhythm" has become a generic term for "occasional abstinence."

Other FAB methods, such as the TwoDay Method, the Billings Ovulation Method and the Symptothermal Method, involve actual observation of fertility signs such as presence or absence of secretions, changes in characteristics of cervical secretions, or changes in basal body temperature. Changes in these signs are caused by fluctuations in circulating hormone levels during the cycle. Women who use these methods identify the start of the fertile time by observing cervical secretions. To identify the end of the fertile time, women can observe their cervical secretions as well as monitor the change in their basal body temperature.

EFFECTIVENESS

Successful use of FAB methods depends on (1) the accuracy of the method in identifying the woman's actual fertile window, (2) a woman's/couple's ability to correctly identify the fertile time, and (3) their ability to follow the instructions of the method they are using—that is, to use a barrier method or avoid intercourse on the days the method identifies as fertile.

There are no recent randomized controlled trials of FAB methods.[7] Efficacy studies of individual FAB methods show that among perfect users (i.e., those who correctly and consistently use a barrier method or avoid intercourse during the fertile time), the percentage of women experiencing an unintended pregnancy during the first year of use ranges from 2% to 5%, depending on the method. In typical use (i.e., correct and consistent use during some cycles, but incorrect or inconsistent use during others), pregnancy rates are higher. (See Chapter 27 on Contraceptive Efficacy.)

Standard Days Method. The first-year probability of pregnancy for women using the Standard Days Method is about 5% if the method is used correctly. When including correct and incorrect use in efficacy trials, as well as data from other field studies, the probability of pregnancy is about 12%.[8] Providers who taught the women participating in the efficacy study how to use the Standard Days Method received 1 to 2 days of training in the method and had no prior experience with it. When the Standard Days Method is offered by experienced providers, efficacy may improve.

Calendar Rhythm Method. Estimates of pregnancy rates for the Calendar Rhythm Method vary widely, partially because the estimates come from flawed studies. One meta-analysis reported a first-year pregnancy rate of 5% with correct use, although the studies included did not identify consistently the parameters of the method.[9] The probability of pregnancy during the first year of typical use of the Calendar Rhythm Method is estimated to be about 13%, based on a meta-analysis of published studies,[10] but no well-designed prospective studies have been conducted.

TwoDay Method. The first-year probability of pregnancy is 3.5% for women who use the method correctly. Adding correct use and incorrect use, the probability of pregnancy, based on the results of clinical trials, is almost 14% in the first year of use. Providers who taught the women participating in the efficacy study how to use the TwoDay Method had no prior experience with any FAB method and received 1 to 2 days of training in the TwoDay Method.[11] Thus, similar to the Standard Days Method, it is possible that failure rates will decrease as provider experience increases.

Billings Ovulation Method. The first-year probability of pregnancy for methods based on using only changes in characteristics of cervical secretions to identify the beginning and end of the fertile time is about 3% among perfect users and 22% among all users in clinical trials.[12,13] Most efficacy studies of the Billings Ovulation Method do not enroll women in the study until they have completed 3 cycles of use, and most use providers with extensive training and experience with the method.

Symptothermal Method. The first-year probability of pregnancy among couples who use two or more fertility indicators (usually cervical secretions and basal body temperature, but others such as cervix position or a calendar calculation may also be used as a "double check" to identify the start and end of the fertile time) is about 2% to 3% among perfect users and as high as 13% to 20% among all users in clinical trials.[14] Several efficacy studies of the Symptothermal Method include women who already had used the method for at least 3 cycles and who had learned the method from experienced providers.

ADVANTAGES AND INDICATIONS

Characteristics of FAB methods that are perceived by some to be advantages may be perceived by others as disadvantages. For example, the importance of the male partner's participation in method use is positive for some couples but difficult to achieve for others. Some women choose FAB methods precisely because of the need for daily awareness of fertility signs while others find this burdensome. For many women, the lack of side effects of FAB methods offsets their higher failure rates. Fertility awareness is important for all women and men, regardless of which family planning method they use or whether they choose to use family planning at all. Fertility awareness increases the users' knowledge of their reproductive potential and enhances self-reliance. Fertility awareness information can be used for a number of purposes:

To avoid pregnancy. For maximum effectiveness, couples should abstain from intercourse or use a barrier method during the entire fertile time.

To become pregnant. Couples have intercourse on days the woman is potentially fertile. Depending on the method used, these may include days 8 to 19 of the cycle, or the days she observes cervical secretions. Women are most likely to become pregnant if they have intercourse within 1 to 2 days of ovulation.[3]

To detect pregnancy. A postovulatory temperature rise (see the section on Basal Body Temperature Charting) sustained for 18 or more days is an excellent early indicator that pregnancy is underway.

To detect impaired fertility. Charting fertility signs costs relatively little and can aid in diagnosing and treating fertility problems due to infrequent or absent ovulation. Women who do not ovulate tend to have a meandering basal body temperature pattern throughout the cycle, rather than the typical pattern (lower in the first part of the cycle and higher in the second). (See Chapter 25, Impaired Fertility.)

To detect a need for medical attention. Changes in cervical secretions, abdominal pain, and other signs or symptoms may indicate the need for medical attention. (See Chapter 21 on Reproductive Tract Infections.)

DISADVANTAGES AND CAUTIONS

FAB methods produce no physical side effects. Like other methods except some barrier methods, however, they offer no protection against sexually transmitted infections, including infection with the human immunodeficiency virus (HIV). Also, lack of the male partner's cooperation will be a distinct obstacle for women who wish to practice abstinence or use an alternative method during the fertile time. Certain conditions may make FAB more difficult to use and require more extensive counseling and follow-up:

- Recent childbirth
- Current breastfeeding
- Recent menarche
- Recent discontinuation of hormonal contraceptive methods
- Approaching menopause

FAB methods are not recommended for women with the following difficulties:

- Inability to abstain or use other methods during the fertile days
- Irregular cycles (Standard Days Method)
- Inability to interpret their fertility signs correctly (Billings Ovulation Method, Symptothermal Method) or to recognize the presence of secretions (TwoDay Method)
- Persistent reproductive tract infections that affect the signs of fertility (Billings Ovulation Method, TwoDay Method, Symptothermal Method)
- Intermenstrual bleeding not distinguishable from menstruation or that impedes noticing secretions

SPECIAL ISSUES

Acceptability

Studies have shown that relatively few family planning providers routinely include information about FAB methods in their discussions with patients. A survey of approximately 500 physicians in the United States found that one-third did not mention FAB methods to their patients at all, while 40% mentioned it to selected women. When asked by a patient for information about a FAB method, most physicians described either calendar rhythm or basal body temperature.[15] In another study, nurse-midwives similarly offered little information on FAB methods, based on their perception that these methods are not effective or are inappropriate for their patients.[16] There appears to be a significant amount of provider bias against FAB methods.

Recent development of FAB methods that are easy to provide and use may increase interest and availability. This could benefit many women, including those who prefer nonmedical methods, those who are dissatisfied with other methods, and the almost 20% of women in the United States between 15 and 44 who ever have used periodic abstinence and the 56% who have used withdrawal.[17] In addition, a discussion of the simpler methods is relatively easy to incorporate in regular clinical services, thus making these simple methods more widely available than those that require extensive counseling.

Some providers and/or program managers consider that using a FAB method will hamper a couple's sexual life, making the method less acceptable and leading to discontinuation of use. Recent statistical analysis of intercourse patterns of users of the Standard Days Method and of the TwoDay Method show that users of these methods have intercourse almost as frequently as users of other modern methods (5.6 vs. 5.5 coital acts per month); however the pattern differs as the couples who use these two FAB methods tend to have sex more frequently during the infertile days before and after the fertile window and avoid sex during their fertile days.[18]

Safety

Because unintended pregnancies among couples who use FAB methods usually result from having intercourse at the beginning or end of the fertile time, concerns have been raised about the risk of birth defects or poor pregnancy outcomes due to aged ovum or sperm. A prospective study showed no significant differences in rates of spontaneous abortion, low birth weight, or preterm birth among women who had an unintended pregnancy while using a FAB method compared with women who had intended pregnancies.[19] Furthermore, fertilization involving aging gametes is not associated with major birth defects and Down syndrome.[20] However, women with a history of spontaneous abortion had a greater chance of having another spontaneous abortion when conception occurred very early or late in the fertile time (23% versus 10% to 15%).[19] Reassure your clients that FAB methods do not pose a threat to the health of mothers and their offspring.

Sex Selection

A study of about 1,000 births showed no association between the timing of conception and the sex ratio at birth.[21] These results do not substantiate claims that couples can select the sex of their child by timing intercourse.

PROVIDING FERTILITY AWARENESS-BASED METHODS

To use FAB methods, couples must adjust their sexual behavior according to their fertility intentions. Users of FAB methods will need to avoid unprotected intercourse for about 10 to 17 days of the woman's menstrual cycle, depending on her cycle length and the method used. Successful use of these methods therefore requires that a couple be able to communicate effectively with each other about sexual matters.

Studies conducted by the Institute for Reproductive Health at Georgetown University have shown that it takes just a few minutes for a woman to learn that she should consider herself fertile on days 8 to 19 of her cycle and to keep track of her cycle days (to use the Standard Days Method) or to learn how to notice the presence of absence of secretions (to use the TwoDay Method).[18] Counseling may be needed to provide the support necessary to help her use the methods correctly. Couples using other FAB methods need an instructor's help to learn how to observe, record, and interpret the woman's fertility signs and patterns. The National Health Service in Great Britain estimates it takes 4 to 6 hours to teach a woman fertility awareness skills, including charting fertility signs (cervical secretions and basal body temperature) and identifying the fertile time.[22] This estimate includes initial classes and follow-up until the woman can use the method without assistance.

A critical component of providing FAB methods is helping women/couples decide how they want to handle their fertile days (i.e. by abstaining or using another method) to avoid pregnancy. Those who choose to use a barrier method (a fertility awareness-combined method) on those days should be instructed on correct method use and counseled accordingly.

INSTRUCTIONS FOR USING FERTILITY AWARENESS-BASED METHODS

STANDARD DAYS METHOD

The Standard Days Method is most appropriate for women who usually have cycles between 26 and 32 days long. Approximately 73% of women can expect to meet this requisite. To use the Standard Days Method, you will need to track the days of your menstrual cycle, starting with the day your menstrual bleeding begins.

1. Count the first day of your menstrual bleeding as day 1.

2. Continue counting every day.

3. On days 1 to 7, you can have unprotected intercourse.

4. On days 8 to 19, you should use a barrier method or avoid inter-course if you do not want to become pregnant.

5. From day 20 through the end of your cycle, you can have unpro-tected intercourse.

6. The Standard Days Method works best for women who usually have cycles between 26 and 32 days long. If you have more than 1 cycle in 1 year that is shorter than 26 days or longer than 32 days, you should contact your provider to discuss the possibility of using another method.

7. **To prevent pregnancy.** Unprotected intercourse is permitted on days 1 to 7 and from day 20 until the end of your cycle. On days 8 to 19, use a barrier method or avoid intercourse.

8. **To become pregnant.** Unprotected intercourse is suggested every other day between day 8 and 19 of your cycle.

Most women who use the Standard Days Method use a specially-de-signed color-coded string of beads called CycleBeads to help them keep track of their cycle days. See Figure 16–1 for an illustration of CycleBeads and instructions for use.

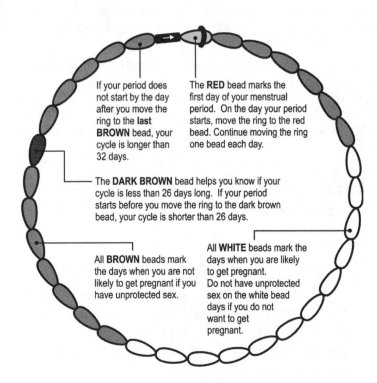

Figure 16–1 CycleBeads for Standard Days method

Table 16–1 How to calculate your fertile period

If Your Shortest Cycle Has Been (# of Days)	Your First Fertile (Unsafe) Day is	If Your Longest Cycle Has Been (# of Days)	Your Last Fertile (Unsafe) Day is
21*	3rd	21*	10th Day
22	4th	22	11th
23	5th	23	12th
24	6th	24	13th
25	7th	25	14th
26	8th	26	15th
27	9th	27	16th
28	10th	28	17th
29	11th	29	18th
30	12th	30	19th
31	13th	31	20th
32	14th	32	21st
33	15th	33	22nd
34	16th	34	23rd
35	17th	35	24th

* Day 1=First day of menstrual bleeding

CALENDAR RHYTHM METHOD

The Calendar Rhythm Method rarely is taught by programs and thus is not described here in detail. To use this method, you will need to follow these steps:

1. Keep a record of your past 6 to 12 menstrual cycle lengths.

2. Find the longest and shortest of your past menstrual cycles.

3. Subtract 18 from the number of days in your shortest cycle to find the first fertile day in your current cycle.

4. Subtract 11 from the number of days in your longest cycle to find the last fertile day in your current cycle.

5. Look on the fertile days chart (see Table 16–1) and apply the "minus 18, minus 11" rule.

6. **To prevent pregnancy.** From the first through the last days identified as fertile, you should use a barrier method or avoid intercourse if you do not want to become pregnant.

7. **To become pregnant.** Intercourse is suggested every other day on the days identified as fertile. (See Chapter 25, Impaired Fertility)

8. Update the calculation every cycle to determine your fertile days.

Example: If the lengths of the past six cycles were 29, 27, 30, 28, 29 and 26 days,

Shortest cycle was 27 days long → 27–18 = 9 (first fertile day)
Longest cycle was 30 days long → 30–11= 19 (last fertile day)

Thus, for the current cycle, probable fertile days are 9 through 19, both inclusive.

Women who have very irregular cycles can use the Calendar-Rhythm method, but would have many days identified as potentially fertile, with many of those being false positives.

TwoDay Method

The TwoDay Method is based on the presence or absence of cervical secretions. If a woman notices cervical secretions of any type TODAY or YESTERDAY, she considers herself fertile TODAY. If she did not notice any secretions TODAY or YESTERDAY she considers herself not fertile TODAY.[23] This algorithm is illustrated in Figure 16–2.

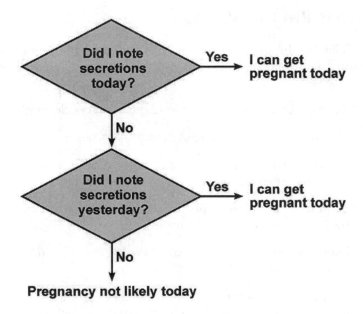

Figure 16–2 TwoDay Method algorithm

1. Check for secretions every day, in the afternoon and in the evening. You can:

   — Look at the secretions in your underwear or in toilet paper, or

   — Touch the secretions in your vulva, or

   — Feel the sensation of wetness at your vulva.

2. Determine whether you are fertile or not TODAY based on the presence or absence of secretions. You can ask yourself these two questions:

   — Did I notice ANY secretions of any type TODAY?

   — Did I notice ANY secretions of any type YESYERDAY?

   — If you noticed any secretions (regardless of their characteristics) TODAY or YESTERDAY, you can become pregnant TODAY. If you did not notice secretions of any type today or yesterday, you are not fertile today.

3. **To prevent pregnancy.** Avoid unprotected intercourse if you noticed any secretions of any type either today or yesterday.

4. **To become pregnant.** Unprotected intercourse is suggested every other day on days with secretions. (See Chapter 25, Impaired Fertility)

5. If you have continuous secretions for more than two weeks, you may have an infection that requires medical attention and should contact your healthcare provider. (See Chapter 21 on Reproductive Tract Infections.)

BILLINGS OVULATION METHOD

Changes in the characteristics of cervical mucus signal the beginning and end of the fertile time, even among those who have irregular cycles. Assistance of a trained instructor is necessary for correct use of the Billings Ovulation Method. Observe your cervical secretions by 'the look, the touch, and the feel':

- *Look* at the secretions on your underwear, fingers, or toilet paper to determine color and consistency.

- *Touch* the secretions to determine their stretch and slipperiness.

- *Feel* how wet the sensation is at your vulva.

When they first appear, the secretions may be scant but sticky and thick with a cloudy or whitish color. Highly fertile secretions are abundant, clear, stretchy, wet, and slippery. Ovulation most likely occurs within 1 day before, during, or 1 day after the last day of abundant, clear, stretchy, slippery cervical secretions (peak day). When you are observing your cervical secretions, do not douche, because it can wash out the secretions, making it very difficult to notice changes. If your secretions do not follow this pattern, you may have an infection that requires medical attention and should contact your healthcare provider. (See Chapter 21 on Reproductive Tract Infections.)

Use your cervical secretions to identify the beginning and end of the fertile time:

1. Observe your cervical secretions every day, beginning the day after your menstrual bleeding has stopped, and record them daily on a special chart (Figure 16–3). To help you avoid confusing cervical secretions with semen and normal sexual lubrication, some counselors advise complete sexual abstinence throughout the first cycle. Alternatively, you can use a condom.

2. Check secretions each time before and after you urinate by wiping (front to back) with tissue paper. Note and record the color and appearance (yellow, white, clear, or cloudy) and consistency (thick, sticky, or stretchy) of the secretions, and feel (dry, wet, or slippery). Record how much they stretch when pulled between your thumb and index finger. Also, note and chart the sensations of dryness, moistness, or wetness at your vulva. Always record the 'most fertile' observations you see during the day.

3. **To prevent pregnancy.** Check for secretions as soon as your menses ends. (Some counselors recommend avoiding intercourse or using a barrier method during menses because it is difficult to detect secretions when they are mixed with menstrual blood.) You can have sexual intercourse on preovulatory days if no secretions are present. (Some counselors recommend abstaining the next day and night following intercourse to allow time for bodily fluids to drain out of your body so you will not confuse semen and arousal fluids with cervical secretions. The following day, check your cervical secretions.) The fertile time begins when cervical secretions are first observed and ends on the 4th day past the peak day.

4. **To become pregnant.** Intercourse is suggested every other day when cervical secretions are present (see Chapter 25, Impaired Fertility). The probability of pregnancy is greatest when the secretions are abundant, clear, stretchy, and slippery.

5. Most women need help in the first few cycles to interpret their cervical secretion patterns and charts to determine the fertile time.

Figure 16–3 Cervical secretion variations during a model menstrual cycle

MENSTRUAL CYCLE DAY	1	2	3	4	5	6	7	8	9	10	11	12	13	14	15	16	17	18	19	20	21	22	23	24
DATES	27	28	29	30	31	1	2	3	4	5	6	7	8	9	10	11	12	13	14	15	16	17	18	19
CERVICAL SECRETIONS (Feel, look & touch) — Wet, slippery, transparent, or stretchy														▓	▓	▓	▓	▓						
Thick, cloudy or sticky										▓	▓	▓	▓						▓					
Dry, no secretions seen or felt						▓	▓	▓	▓											▓	▓	▓	▓	▓
Period	▓	▓	▓	▓	▓																			

Symptothermal Method

Some couples prefer to observe more than 1 indicator of the woman's fertility. Most couples who use a combined or symptothermal approach use cervical secretions and basal body temperature to identify the fertile time. The basal body temperature, the temperature of the body at rest, is lower in the first part of the cycle, rises to a higher level beginning around the time of ovulation, and remains at the higher level for the rest of the cycle. By taking her temperature when she first wakes in the morning and recording her temperature on a chart each day of her menstrual cycle, a woman can retrospectively identify whether she has ovulated and, thus, calculate the end of her fertile time.

To use the Symptothermal Method, follow the steps for the Ovulation Method and, in addition, take and record your basal body temperature as follows to determine the postovulatory infertile time:

1. Take your basal body temperature every morning at the same time before getting out of bed (after at least 3 hours of sleep). A special calibrated thermometer makes temperature reading easier. Take the basal body temperature orally, rectally, or vaginally, but take it at the same site each day so changes in basal body temperature can be detected accurately.

2. Record your basal body temperature readings daily on a chart (Figure 16–4). Connect the dots for each day so a line connects dots from successive days (day 2 to day 3, and so on).

3. Your temperature will probably rise at least 0.4 degrees F° around the time of ovulation and remain elevated until the next menses begins. Your actual temperature and maximum temperature are not important, just the rise over the baseline (preovulatory) temperatures.

4. If you have 3 continuous days of higher temperatures (above the baseline) following 6 days of lower temperatures, you have probably ovulated and your postovulatory infertile time has begun. To see the baseline and rise clearly on the chart, draw a line just above (0.1 degree line) the lower (preovulatory) temperatures. When you record 3 continuous temperatures above this line and the last temperature is 0.4 degrees higher than this line, your postovulatory infertile time has begun.

5. If you cannot detect a sustained rise in basal body temperature, you may not have ovulated in that cycle. A true postovulatory basal body temperature rise usually persists 10 days or longer.

6. Some women notice a temperature drop about 12 to 24 hours before it begins to rise after ovulation, whereas others have no

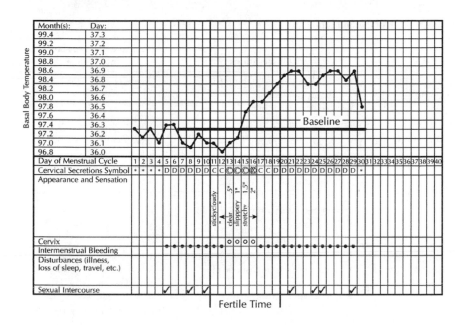

Figure 16–4 Symptothermal variations during a model menstrual cycle

drop in temperature at all. A drop in your basal body temperature probably means ovulation will occur the next day.

7. **To prevent pregnancy.** Rely on your cervical secretions to identify the beginning of your fertile time. Your basal body temperature can help you identify the end of your fertile time. You should use another method or not have intercourse during the fertile time if you do not want to become pregnant.

8. **To become pregnant.** It is often difficult to predict fertile days using basal body temperature. By the time the rise is detected, you are probably in the infertile phase of your menstrual cycle and have missed the opportunity to become pregnant. To become pregnant, you should rely on your cervical secretions.

FAB METHOD COMPARISON

FAB methods differ from each other in terms of the protocol for determining the fertile time and identifying which days to avoid unprotected intercourse. Table 16–2 compares FAB method protocols.

Table 16–2 FAB method protocols

Method	Observations	Days to avoid unprotected intercourse
Standard Days Method	• Track cycle days beginning with first day of menses • Note days 8–19 of cycle	• Days 8–19 of cycle Total: 12 days per cycle
Calendar Method	• Record cycle lengths for 6–12 cycles • Identify shortest and longest cycles • Shortest minus 18: beginning of fertile window • Longest minus 11: end of fertile window	• Days identified as fertile by calculations (repeat calculations every cycle) Total: Depends on cycle-length variability
TwoDay Method	• Note presence or absence of cervical secretions • Record on chart	• All days with secretions • One day following days with secretions Total: Approximately 10–14
Ovulation Method	• Monitor cervical secretions daily • Assess quality and quantity of secretions • Record observations on chart	• Menses • Preovulatory days following days with intercourse • All days with fertile-type secretions • Until 4 days past "peak" day Total: Approximately 14–17 days each cycle
Symptothermal Method	• Monitor cervical secretions daily • Assess quantity and quality of secretions • Take basal temperature daily • Record observations on chart	• Menses • Preovulatory days following days with intercourse • All days with secretions • Until 3 days of higher temperatures following 6 lower temperatures, or 4 days past peak Total: Approximately 12–17 days each cycle

FAB METHODS IN DEVELOPMENT

Home Test Kits for Ovulation Prediction and Detection

There are many products available that can help women identify their fertile days. These include mini microscopes to see ferning of saliva or of cervical mucus (PG53, PC2000, Maybe Baby) as well as handheld computers that measure and correlate day of the cycle with basal body temperature (Babycomp, Ladycomp, Bioself 2000, Cyclotest 2 Plus) or with urinary levels of hormones or their metabolites (Persona, ClearPlan, ClearBlue). Some of them adjust their output as time passes, based on stored information of prior cycles of use. Most of them are now focusing on helping women become pregnant, by recommending intercourse on days identified as fertile. Research done to evaluate potential effectiveness of some of these kits to prevent pregnancy suggests that mini microscope-type devices would have high failure rates.[24] Research to assess the potential contraceptive efficacy of devices with computing capability are mixed.[25-27] Some of them are more user friendly. Others require that the user enter more information or are more difficult to operate. Likewise, the information some of them provide is easier to interpret than others. Cost can be an issue as some of them cost several hundred dollars plus the cost of supplies. Additional research (including efficacy trials) is needed before any of these kits and devices can be confidently recommended for pregnancy prevention.

REFERENCES

1. World Health Organization. Global Handbook for Family Planning Providers (Forthcoming 2007)
2. Lamprecht VM, Grummer-Strawn L. Development of new formulas to identify the fertile time of the menstrual cycle. Contraception 1996; 54:339–343.
3. Wilcox AJ, Weinberg CR, Baird DD. Timing of sexual intercourse in relation to ovulation. N Engl J Med 1995; 333:1517–1521.
4. Wilcox AJ. Dunson D, Baird DB. The timing of the "fertile window" in the menstrual cycle: day specific estimates from a prospective study. BMJ 2000; 321:1259–1262.
5. Arévalo M, Sinai I, Jennings V. A fixed formula to define the fertile window of the menstrual cycle as the basis of a simple method of natural family planning. Contraception 2000; 60:357–360.
6. Chey, Cleland JG, Ali MM. Periodic abstinence in developing countries: an assessment of failure rates and consequences. Contraception 2004; 69(1):15–21.
7. Grimes D, Gallo M, Grigorieva V, Nanda K, Schultz K. Fertility awareness-based methods for contraception: systematic review of randomized controlled trials. Contraception 2005; 72:85–90.
8. Arévalo M, Jennings V, Sinai I. Efficacy of the Standard Days Method of family planning. Contraception 2002; 65:333–338.
9. Dicker D, Wachsman T, Feldbergt D. The vaginal contraception diaphragm and the condom: an evaluation and comparison of two barrier methods with the rhythm method. Contraception 1989; 40:497–503.
10. Kambic RT, Lamprecht V. Calendar rhythm efficacy: a review. Adv Contracept 1996; 12:123–128.
11. Arevalo M, Jennings V, Sinai I. Efficacy of the TwoDay Method. Fertil Steril 2004; 82(4):88–892.
12. Trussell J, Grummer-Strawn L. Contraceptive failure of the ovulation method of periodic abstinence. Fam Plann Perspect 1990; 22:65–75.
13. World Health Organization. A prospective multicentre trial of the ovulation method of natural family planning. II. The effectiveness phase. Fertil Steril 1981; 36:591–598.

14. Frank-Herrmann P, Freundl G, Baur S, Bremme M, Doring GK, Godehardt EAJ, Sottong U. Effectiveness and acceptability of the symptothermal method of natural family planning in Germany. Am J Obstet Gynecol 1991; 165:2052–2054.
15. Stanford JB, Thurman PB, Lemaire JC. Physicians' knowledge and practices regarding natural family planning. Obstet Gynecol 1999; 94(5 Pt 1):672–678.
16. Mikolajczyk RT, Stanford JB, Rauchfuss M. Factors influencing the choice to use modern natural family planning. Contraception 2003; 67(4):253–258.
17. Stanford JB, Lemaire JC, Fox A. Interest in natural family planning among female family practice patients. Fam Pract Res J 1994 Sep; 14(3):237–49.
18. Sinai I, Arevalo M. It's all in the timing: coital frequency and fertility awareness-based methods of family planning. J Biosoc Sci (first published online 2005).
19. Gray RH, Simpson JL, Kambic RT, Queenan JT, Mena P, Perez A, Barbato M. Timing of conception and the risk of spontaneous abortion among pregnancies occurring during use of natural family planning. Am J Obstet Gynecol 1995; 172:1567–1572.
20. Simpson JL, Gray R, Perez A, Mena P, Queenan JT, Barbato M, Pardo F, Kambic R, Jennings V. Fertilization involving aging gametes, major birth defects and Down's syndrome. Lancet 2002; 359:1670–1671.
21. Gray RH, Simpson JL, Bitto AC, Queenan JT, Chuanjun L. Sex Ratio associated in timing of insemination and length of the follicular phase in planned and unplanned pregnancies during use of NFP. Hum Reprod 1998; 13(5):1397–1400.
22. Clubb EM, Pyper CM, Knight J. A pilot study on teaching natural family planning in general practice. Natural family planning: current knowledge and new strategies for the 1990s, Part II 1992:130–132.
23. Sinai I, Arevalo M, Jennings V. The TwoDay algorithm: a new algorithm to identify the fertile time of the menstrual cycle. Contraception 1999; 60(2):65–70.
24. Freundl G, Godehardt E, Kern PA, Frank-Hermann P, Koubenec HJ, Gnoth C. Estimated maximum failure rates of cycle monitors using daily conception probabilities in the menstrual cycle. Human Reproduction 2003; 18(12):2628–2633.
25. Fehring R, Raviele K, Schneider M. A comparison of the fertile phase as determined by the Clearplan Easy Fertility Monitor and self-assessment of cervical mucus. Contraception 2003; 69(1):9–14.
26. Bonnar J, Flynn A, Freundl G, Kirkman R, Royston R, Snowden R. Personal hormone monitoring for contraception. Br J Fam Plann 2000; 26(3):178–9.
27. Guida M, Bramante S, Acunzo G, Pellicano M, Cirillo D, Nappi C. Diagnosis of fertility with a personal hormonal evaluation test. Minerva Ginecol 2003; 55(2):167–73.

Female and Male Sterilization

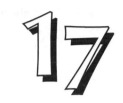

Amy E. Pollack, MD, MPH, FACOG
Lisa J. Thomas, MD, FACOG
Mark A. Barone, DVM, MS

- Permanent contraception requires only a single decision and one simple surgical procedure.

- Sterilization is one of the safest, most effective, and most cost-effective contraceptive methods.

- Reversal of the sterilization procedure is expensive, requires either costly assisted reproductive technology (such as IVF) or highly technical surgery, and results cannot be guaranteed.

- Contraceptive sterilization (female sterilization and vasectomy) is the most widely used method of family planning in the world in both developed and developing countries.

- Patients should be advised that sterilization does not provide any protection against sexually transmitted infections, including HIV infection.

Tubal sterilization and vasectomy are safe and effective permanent methods of contraception. Sterilization continues to be the most commonly used contraceptive method in the United States, with 15 million U.S. women relying on either female or male sterilization.[1] Approximately 700,000 tubal sterilizations[2] and 500,000 vasectomies[3] are performed in the United States annually. Of all women using a contraceptive method (age 15 to 44) in 2002, female sterilization accounted for 27% and male sterilization accounted for 9.2% of method use. This represents minimal change since 1995.[1] Worldwide, 220 million couples use tubal sterilization or vasectomy as their contraceptive method of choice.[4]

Ideally, a couple should consider both vasectomy and female sterilization as options *for permanent contraception*. They are comparable in effectiveness, although vasectomy is simpler, safer, and less expensive.

There is no medical condition that would absolutely restrict a person's eligibility for sterilization. Some conditions and circumstances indicate that certain precautions should be taken. Refer to Chapter 4 on Medical Eligibility Criteria for further information.

FEMALE STERILIZATION

For the past 20 years, the most common methods of female sterilization in the United States have been interval tubal sterilization using a laparoscopic approach under short acting general anesthesia, and postpartum tubal sterilization using a subumbilical minilaparotomy approach. In December 2002, the U.S. Food and Drug Administration approved the Essure microinsert device for interval tubal sterilization. This device is placed transcervically through a hysteroscope, thus avoiding entry into the abdominal cavity. Although current practice in the United States is primarily hospital-based, international practice is office-based using local anesthesia. The number of providers placing the Essure device in the office using local anesthesia is expected to increase given the convenience, safety, and cost benefits. This represents a significant change in the sterilization delivery system. Several other transcervical devices are under development.

EFFECTIVENESS

Following completion of childbearing, women spend approximately twenty years using contraception. Tubal sterilization is far more effective than short-term, user-dependent, reversible contraceptive methods. Contraceptive failure occurs in the first year of use for 80 per 1,000 women using oral contraceptives, 150 per 1,000 women relying on the male condom, and 30 per 1,000 women using injectable methods. See Table 27–1.

Alternatively, failure rates of tubal sterilization are roughly comparable with those of the IUD. The copper T 380A IUD has a 5-year cumulative failure rate of 14 per 1,000 procedures,[5] and levonorgestrel-releasing IUDs range from 5 to 11 failures per 1,000 procedures.[6,7,8]

The U.S. Collaborative Review of Sterilization (CREST), a large, prospective, multicenter observational study of over 10,000 women followed up to 14 years, conducted by the Centers for Disease Control and Prevention in 1996, concluded that although tubal sterilization is highly effective, the risk of sterilization failure is substantially higher than previously reported.[9] Analysis of CREST data found a 5-year cumulative probability of failure of aggregated sterilization methods of 13 per 1,000 procedures.[9] The risk of sterilization failure persists for years after the procedure and varies by several factors including method and age. The younger a woman was at the time of sterilization, the more likely she was to have had a sterilization failure.[9] Postpartum partial salpingectomy had the lowest 5-year and 10-year cumulative pregnancy rates: 6.3 per 1,000 and 7.5 per 1,000 procedures, respectively. It should be noted that the CREST study was done prior to the introduction of the Filshie clip and Essure and that several of the methods studied were evaluated early in their clinical use. Thus, the long-term failure rates with these methods do not necessarily reflect those with current use. Although the Filshie clip was approved in the United States in 1996, experience in the United Kingdom dates back to its introduction there in 1975. The Filshie clip is the predominant occlusion method used today in the United Kingdom and in Canada. The Royal College Working Party on Sterilization in 1999 estimated Filshie clip efficacy to be favorably comparable to other methods with a crude failure rate of 2–3 per 1000 women.[10]

In the two clinical trials on which FDA approval for Essure was primarily based, no pregnancies were reported in the more than 700 patients using the device up to 24 months, and the method was found to be highly acceptable.[11] In an Australian study of 108 women using the device for an average of 17 months, no intrauterine or ectopic pregnancies were reported.[12] Although the method appears to be very highly effective, at the time of this writing there have been rare, anecdotal reports of pregnancies occurring among women who were not part of any clinical trials. Long-term efficacy has not been fully assessed.[13]

Ectopic Pregnancy

Because the risk for pregnancy after sterilization is uncommon, the overall risk of ectopic pregnancy is lower than the general population. However, there is substantial risk that if a pregnancy occurs post-sterilization, it will be ectopic. An analysis of CREST data found that roughly 30% of post-sterilization pregnancies were ectopic.[15] The 10-year cumulative probability of ectopic pregnancy after tubal sterilization by all methods was 7.3 per 1,000 procedures. The risk of ectopic pregnancy did not diminish with the length of time since the tubal sterilization. For all methods except postpartum partial salpingectomy, the probability of ectopic pregnancy was greater for women sterilized before age 30 years than for women sterilized at age 30 years or older. Furthermore, those young women sterilized by bipolar tubal coagulation had a 10-year cumulative probability of ectopic pregnancy of 31.9 per 1000 procedures.[14] As with tubal ligation failures, IUD failures also have an increased risk of ectopic pregnancy—approximately 20% will result in an ectopic pregnancy.[6,9] To date, equivalent long-term efficacy and ectopic pregnancy data with Essure is unavailable.

Intrauterine Pregnancy

When intrauterine pregnancy occurs after tubal sterilization, there is no known added risk to the woman or her fetus. In contrast, when an intrauterine pregnancy is diagnosed in an IUD user and the IUD is not removed, there is substantially greater risk of spontaneous abortion, septic abortion, and preterm birth.[15–17]

MECHANISM OF ACTION

Sterilization for women involves cutting or mechanically blocking the fallopian tubes to prevent the sperm and egg from uniting. (See Figure 17–1.)

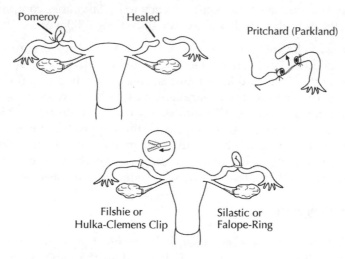

Figure 17–1 Tubal sterilization techniques

ADVANTAGES AND INDICATIONS

Female sterilization is ideal for those women who are certain they wish no further children and need a reliable contraceptive method. Advantages include the following:

- Permanence
- High effectiveness
- High acceptability
- Safety
- Quick recovery

- Lack of significant long-term side effects
- Cost effectiveness
- No need to buy anything
- No need for partner compliance
- No need to interrupt lovemaking
- Privacy of choice

DISADVANTAGES AND CAUTIONS

Female sterilization is not recommended for anyone who is not sure of her desire regarding future fertility. Disadvantages include the following:

- Permanence: Pregnancy after sterilization is difficult though possible; it is expensive, requires either costly assisted reproductive technology (such as IVF) or highly technical major surgery, and results cannot be guaranteed.
- **All surgical procedures carry some risk specific to the nature of the surgery and anesthetic used.**
- Regret for decision is high among some groups of women
- Need for surgeon, procedure room (aseptic conditions), trained assistants, medications, surgical (or hysteroscopic) equipment
- Expense at the time of the procedure
- Higher probability of pregnancy being ectopic if method fails
- Lack of protection against sexually transmitted infections (STIs), including infection with the human immunodeficiency virus (HIV)

Women with medical conditions or other special characteristics may have eligibility criteria for initiation and continuation of contraceptive use that differ from that of healthy women or women without these medical conditions or characteristics. To identify situations in which this is the case, please refer to the table on sterilization in Chapter 4, Medical Eligibility Criteria.

SAFETY

Tubal sterilization is a safe method of contraception. Death from transabdominal tubal sterilization is a rare event, and overall complication rates are low. Mortality rates in the United States have been estimated at 1 to 4 deaths per 100,000 procedures.[18-21] Most deaths in the United States have been associated with anesthetic complications.[22] In the CREST study, no deaths were reported among 9,475 women who underwent interval laparoscopic tubal ligation.[23]

Major complications from transabdominal tubal sterilization are uncommon. Overall complication rates for tubal sterilization are estimated to be 0.9 to 1.6 per 100 procedures.[23] The types of complications vary by the type of surgical procedure and anesthesia. Intraoperative complications include damage to bowel, bladder, or major vessels. If extreme, laparotomy and/or blood transfusion may be required to manage these rare events. Postoperative complications include wound infection and possible prolonged pelvic/abdominal pain. Additional risk factors for complications include previous abdominal or pelvic surgery, obesity, and diabetes.[23]

Based on published literature, major complications from transcervical sterilization using Essure are unreported. Potential complications include hypervolemia from hysteroscopy in less than 1% of cases, and perforation in 1.1% of cases.[24] There are no randomized controlled trials that compare transabdominal and transcervical sterilization safety or post-procedure patient pain.

Anesthetic risk can vary, including idiosyncratic reaction to local anesthesia, or airway control and ventilation complications with the use of general anesthesia. Decreasing the level of anesthesia diminishes the risk of complications.

SPECIAL ISSUES

Cancer Prevention

Case control and cohort studies have consistently shown a reduced risk of ovarian cancer following tubal sterilization.[25,26] The protective effect of tubal sterilization on ovarian cancer persists over many years. A large case-control study showed tubal sterilization was associated with a 39% reduction in the risk of ovarian cancer. The risk remained low up to 25 years after surgery and was irrespective of sterilization technique.[25] Results of a cohort study of more than 65,000 Danish women not only showed an overall decrease in the risk of ovarian cancer, but also a reduced rate of endometrial cancer, although the association was less strong.[26]

The protective effect of tubal sterilization on ovarian cancer risk also extends to carriers of the BRCA1 mutation.[27,28] The risk reduction does not extend to carriers of BRCA2.[28] Combined oral contraceptive (COC) use, especially long term use, confers more protection in BRCA1 carriers; however, the combination of COCs and tubal ligation, conferring, a risk reduction of 72% offered greater protection than either method alone.[28]

The biological mechanism for ovarian cancer reduction in women who have undergone tubal sterilization is unknown. Possible theories include blockage of the ascent of potentially carcinogenic agents such as talc or a nonmeasurable effect on ovarian function or hormone levels.

One prospective cohort study of 619,199 women suggests an inverse association between tubal sterilization and breast cancer mortality.[29] However, it is possible that unmeasured confounding related to differences in screening practices may explain inconsistent study outcomes. Other studies that adjusted for potential confounders reported no protective effect.[26,30]

The impact of the transcervical device, Essure, on these cancers has not been studied.

Menstrual Abnormalities

The long-term health effects of tubal sterilization on menstrual pattern disturbance (post-tubal ligation syndrome) appear to be negligible. Early studies of menstrual disturbances after sterilization failed to account for confounding variables, such as pre-sterilization use of hormonal contraceptives that can mask underlying menstrual dysfunction.[31–33] Most recent studies that account for these factors have found little or no difference in menstrual patterns between women before and after sterilization.[32,34–40]

Ovarian Function, Vascular Changes and Potential Effects

A decrease in the blood supply to the ovaries has been postulated as a possible mechanism by which tubal ligation might protect against ovarian cancer. Several studies have recently evaluated the vascular effects of tubal ligation and subsequent ovarian function as well as possible long-term outcomes such as menopausal symptoms and osteoporosis. A prospective long-term comparison cohort evaluation of ovarian reserve and function in women undergoing laparascopic tubal sterilization using bipolar coagulation showed no functional impact after 5 years.[41] Another prospective study of minilaparotomy and laparoscopic tubal ligation found no difference in uterine or ovarian blood flow or ovarian hormone secretion after 6 months.[42]

Despite relatively strong evidence that ovarian function and vascular resistance do not seem to be affected by tubal ligation,[41–43] there are conflicting reports on the association of tubal sterilization and menopausal symptoms.[44,45] Prospective randomized controlled trials are warranted before definitive conclusions can be made.

Hysterectomy

Although there is no known biologic mechanism to support a causal relationship between tubal sterilization and hysterectomy, the reported association between sterilization and hysterectomy tends to be strong (RR, 1.6–4.4).[38,46–50] Women who undergo tubal sterilization appear to be 4 to 5 times more likely to undergo hysterectomy than those whose partners underwent vasectomy.[46] Increased risk was associated with a pre-sterilization history of menstrual or other benign gynecologic disorders.[46]

Sexuality

A study of female marital sexuality found no detrimental long-term effects from female or male sterilization. Conversely, the study found an increase in coital frequency after 1 year among women who had undergone tubal sterilization as compared with women not planning sterilization.[51]

A CREST study to determine if interval tubal sterilization leads to a change in female sexual interest or pleasure found that interval tubal sterilization is unlikely to result in changed sexual interest or pleasure. Among those women with changes, the majority experienced positive sexual effects.[51,52]

RISK OF REGRET

Most women who choose sterilization as a contraceptive method do not regret their decision; however, women who undergo sterilization before the age of 30 are at greater risk for regret.[53–55] The cumulative probability of regret over 14 years of follow-up in the CREST study was 12.7%.[53] However, the probability was 20.3% for women aged 30 years or younger at the time of sterilization, compared with 5.9% for women older than 30 years at the time of sterilization. The CREST data also shows similar high levels of regret for interval sterilization within 1 year of delivery (22.3%) as for postpartum sterilization after vaginal delivery (23.7%) and cesarean delivery (20.7%) The cumulative probability of regret diminished steadily with the interval between delivery and sterilization.[53] Postabortion sterilization was not associated with increased regret when compared with interval sterilization.[53,56–58]

Analysis of the data from the CREST study showed the 14-year cumulative probability of requesting reversal information was 14.3%, but in women under the age of 24 who underwent sterilization, the request for reversal information was as high as 40.4%.[55] The number of women who requested information about IVF was undocumented.

Risk factors for increased regret include having received less information about the procedure, having had less access to information or support for other contraceptive method use,[59] and having made the decision under pressure from a spouse or because of medical indications.[60,61] Younger women are at greater risk for regret given the longevity of their future fertility and the opportunity for life changes.

Thorough and effective counseling is crucial in reducing regret in women undergoing sterilization. Counseling should be in language the patient can easily understand. Both the patient and her partner (when appropriate) should be counseled, and risk factors for regret should be addressed. The presence of strong risk factors for regret (such as age) should not be used to uniformly restrict sterilization. These risk factors should instead be indicators for more extensive counseling before undergoing sterilization.

Desire for Pregnancy Following Tubal Sterilization

Sterilization should be considered permanent, but even with careful counseling, some women will have a change in personal circumstance and desire more children. In-vitro fertilization or microsurgical tubal reversal can be considered to attempt pregnancy following transabdominal sterilization. Success is not guaranteed with either approach.

The Essure device is, by design, placed in the uterine cornua, and therefore patients are not candidates for microsurgical reversal. In addition, a 6 to 10 mm portion of the coil remains protruding into the uterine cavity after the device is placed, which could be detrimental both to the success of the in-vitro fertilization (IVF) procedure and to the pregnancy, if achieved. Pregnancy outcome data on IVF with the Essure device in place is not currently available. At this time, Essure should be considered an irreversible method of female sterilization.[62]

The choice between IVF and tubal surgery to achieve pregnancy following surgical tubal sterilization is dependent on multiple factors, including the age of the woman at the time of treatment, severity of the tubal damage and remaining tubal length, as well as other fertility factors. With careful case selection and meticulous surgical technique, reasonable pregnancy rates can be achieved following microsurgical reversal of tubal sterilization.[63]

Surgery, especially major abdominal surgery, carries operative risks as well as risks due to anesthesia. Ectopic pregnancy is more common among pregnancies occurring after surgical reversal of female sterilization. Ectopic pregnancy rates range from 1% to 7%—higher rates can be observed in specific anatomical situations.[63] Nonetheless, sterilization reversal may be appealing for younger women, couples who desire more than a single additional pregnancy, or those who are not comfortable with IVF. Both IVF and reversal surgery are costly and are often not covered by health insurance. Finally, those couples utilizing tubal reversal surgery may have the need for future contraception. A large Canadian study showed that 23% of women obtaining tubal reversal following sterilization went on to obtain a subsequent sterilization.[64]

PROVIDING FEMALE STERILIZATION
COUNSELING GUIDELINES FOR FEMALE STERILIZATION

The goal of counseling is to help clients select a contraceptive method that they will use, that will be effective, that is most consistent with their reproductive intentions, and that will not have adverse effects. The permanence of sterilization methods is a significant consideration with respect to counseling.

The factors contributing to an individual's decision about female sterilization vary. Each woman needs to weigh the risks, benefits, effectiveness, and side effects of the various contraceptive options available to her, as well as her personal need to use a barrier method for protection against sexually transmitted infections, especially HIV/AIDS.

1. **Provide choices.** Highly effective, long-acting, temporary methods should be presented as options.

2. **Assess the client's understanding of the procedure.** In the United States, awareness of female sterilization is widespread, and one of the interviewer's tasks is to assure the individual correctly understands the procedure and has no misconceptions.

3. **Facilitate the decision-making process.** Give the client sufficient time to make a thoughtful, informed decision about a permanent method of contraception, especially women having immediate postpartum or postabortion (spontaneous or induced) sterilization. The woman should have decided she wants a permanent method well before delivery or a pregnancy-related event or procedure.

4. Clients should be informed that sterilization is not 100% successful, and that failure occurs, even years after the procedure was performed. Additionally, there is significant risk of ectopic pregnancy if the method fails.

Components of Presterilization Counseling[65]

- Permanent nature of the procedure

- Alternative methods of contraception available (temporary methods as well as vasectomy)
- Reasons for choosing sterilization
- Screening for risk indicators for regret
- Details of the procedure, including risks and benefits of anesthesia
- The possibility of failure and risk of ectopic pregnancy
- The need to use condoms for protection against sexually transmitted diseases, including HIV
- Local regulations regarding interval from time of consent to procedure

Informed Consent

Informed consent is the voluntary decision made by a person who has been fully informed regarding the surgical procedure and its consequences. Provide the information in a language the client can understand. The client must always sign or mark an informed consent form indicating that they understand the type of operation and intended permanence, possibility of failure, and risks and benefits, including the option to decline sterilization without loss of medical or financial benefits. The surgeon or authorized representative must also sign the form.

Policy/Legal Issues. Knowledge of state and local guidelines is important in the counseling and consent process

- Strict adherence to informed choice and consent procedures is mandatory prior to sterilization.[66]
- Partner or spousal consent in the United States is not legally required.[67]
- Clients using federal or state funds for sterilization must be age 21 or older and mentally competent; they must wait 30 days after signing a consent before receiving a sterilization procedure.[68]

Arbitrary decisions by health professionals to restrict access to sterilization have been judged by courts in the United States to violate a woman's basic rights.

The policy and legal status of providing sterilization for mentally challenged individuals remains a problem. Health care providers, policy makers, and the public should be aware of the ethical and legal issues involved in providing voluntary sterilization to those who may not be able to provide informed consent. For further details, see "Sterilization of Women, Including Those with Mental Disabilities" in Ethics in Obstetrics and Gynecology/ the American College of Obstetricians and Gynecologists, 2nd edition: pp 56–59.

TIMING

Tubal sterilization can be performed at the time of cesarean delivery, postpartum, after spontaneous or therapeutic abortion, or as an interval procedure (unrelated in time to a pregnancy). The timing of the procedure influences both the surgical approach and the method of tubal occlusion.

Postpartum Sterilization

Postpartum sterilization is performed after 10% of all hospital deliveries in the United States.[65] Sterilization may be done at the time of cesarean delivery or via minilaparotomy following vaginal delivery and should not extend the patient's hospital stay. Postpartum minilaparotomy should be done prior to the onset of significant uterine involution (within 1 to 2 days following delivery). Local anesthesia with sedation, regional anesthesia, or general anesthesia may be used. A full assessment of maternal and neonatal well-being should be done prior to sterilization; the physician should consider postponing sterilization in the setting of medical or obstetric complications.[65]

Postpartum sterilization requires counseling and informed consent before labor and delivery.[69,70] Consent should be obtained during prenatal care, when the patient can make a considered decision, review the risks and benefits of the procedure, and consider alternative methods of contraception. Federal and state regulations that address the timing of consent should also be considered.[71]

Interval Tubal Sterilization

In the United States, approximately one half of all tubal sterilizations are performed as interval laparoscopic procedures.[2] Although interval tubal sterilization can be done at any time during the menstrual cycle, performing the procedure during the patient's follicular phase reduces the likelihood of concurrent (luteal phase) pregnancy, as does the patient's use of an effective method of contraception before sterilization. Same-day, highly sensitive urine pregnancy tests will detect pregnancies as early as 1 week after conception.[72] The recent introduction of Essure, a transcervical device, offers women a new interval sterilization option.

Postabortion sterilization

Approximately 3.5% of all sterilizations are performed after an elective or spontaneous abortion.[73] Sterilization, either laparoscopically or via minilaparotomy, following uncomplicated abortion, can be provided without added risk over interval sterilization.[74] A single anesthetic for both the abortion and the sterilization may be used to avoid additional risk.

OPTIONS FOR APPROACH

There are 2 basic approaches to female sterilization—transabdominal, provided via minilaparotomy or laparoscopy, and transcervical. The transvaginal approach is rarely used and is associated with an increased rate of postoperative infections and other potential complications. Hysterectomy, whether performed through a vaginal or abdominal approach, carries a much higher risk of morbidity and mortality than other sterilization procedures. Hysterectomy should not be performed for contraceptive purposes alone.

The transabdominal approach is currently the most common approach to tubal sterilization in the United States.[75] *Laparoscopy* is most commonly used for interval sterilization and is usually performed as an outpatient procedure. The advantage of laparoscopy over other surgical approaches includes the opportunity to inspect under direct visualization the abdominal and pelvic organs. Laparoscopy results in barely visible incision scars and a rapid return to full activity for the patient. The disadvantages of laparoscopy include the special training required and the risk of bowel, bladder, or major vessel injuries following insertion of laparoscopic instruments. (See Figures 17-2 and 17-3.)

In the United States, *minilaparotomy* is most commonly used for postpartum procedures prior to involution of the uterus. A small 2 to 3 cm incision is made below the umbilicus, allowing easy access to the fallopian tubes. (See Figure 17-4.) Minilaparotomy requires only basic surgical instruments and training, although there is still a small risk of injury to the bowel, bladder, and other adjacent structures. In developing countries where laparoscopy is not available, suprapubic or minilapartomy can also be used for interval or first trimester postabortion tubal sterilization.

Transcervical approaches to tubal sterilization involve gaining access to the fallopian tubes via the cervix. The Essure device, introduced in 2002, is a soft, flexible, micro-insert hysteroscopically placed in the proximal section of each fallopian tube (Figure 17-5). Special training is needed for insertion of Essure, which can only be done as an interval procedure. In less than 30 minutes, Essure can be provided under local

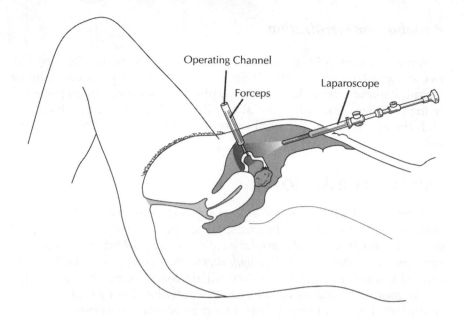

Figure 17–2 Laparoscopy

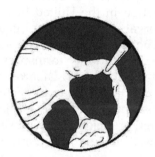

Figure 17–3 A laparoscopy instrument grasps one tube in preparation for electrocoagulation
or application of a ring or clip

anesthesia, with or without sedation, in a physician's office. Successful placement is not guaranteed and the procedure can be abandoned due to abnormal findings at the time of hysteroscopy or with failed attempts to place one or both devices. Data from early prospective multicenter trials reported successful bilateral placement rate of 86% after 1 procedure.[24] A study published in 2004 reported 98% success in single-attempt bilateral placement using a newly designed coil catheter system.[76] Placement may be difficult because of anatomical features or tubal scarring. Effectiveness is dependent on ingrowth and formation of tubal scar tissue. Therefore, an alternate method of reliable contraception must be used for 3 months following placement, until a hysterosalpingogram demonstrates that the device is correctly placed and the tubes are occluded.[77]

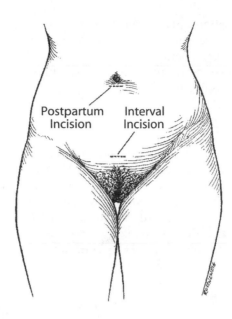

Figure 17–4 Minilaparotomy incision site and size

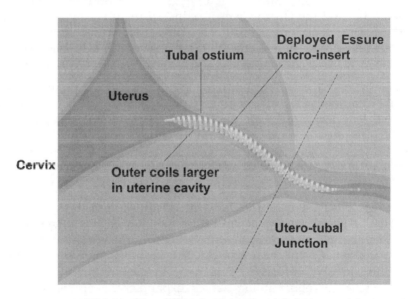

Figure 17–5 Hysteroscopic placement of micro-insert within the tubal lumen

CHOICE OF OCCLUSION METHOD

The choice of occlusion method depends on the provider's training, personal experience, availability of supplies, and ultimately, the approach. The transabdominal minilaparotomy approach allows for ligation and transection of the fallopian tubes, whereas laparoscopic procedures use special instruments to apply clips, bands, or electrocoagulation for complete occlusion. There is currently a single approved device for transcervical tubal occlusion.

Electrocoagulation

Electrocoagulation for tubal occlusion is used exclusively with laparoscopic sterilization. Data from the AAGL 1995 survey suggested that bipolar electrocoagulation was used for interval laparoscopic sterilization by 60% of respondents. Unipolar electrocoagulation is not as commonly used because of a past association with thermal bowel injury. Use of a current meter rather than visualizing tissue blanching during bipolar coagulation more accurately indicates complete coagulation and is associated with improved efficacy rates.[78,79]

Mechanical Methods

Mechanical occlusion devices commonly used with laparoscopic sterilization in the United States include the silastic band (Falope Ring), the Filshie clip, and the Hulka-Clemens clip. All require special applicators and are most commonly used for interval laparoscopic sterilization on normal tubes. None of these methods have an associated risk of electrical burn.[80,81]

The silastic band was first developed in the 1970s in pursuit of a safer nonthermal method. Two centimeters of tube is contained in the constricted loop following application. With this method, it is possible to lacerate the tube and/or surrounding vessels and application may be more difficult when tubal abnormalities are present, such as adhesions or edema. The silastic band is one of the most commonly used tubal sterilization devices worldwide.

In September 1996, the U.S. Food and Drug Administration approved the Filshie clip for use as a new contraceptive device in the United States. The Filshie clip is a good option for patients and clinicians because it is easier to use than other occlusion devices, destroys a minimal amount of the fallopian tube, and has high efficacy.[82] The device is made of titanium with a silicone rubber lining, which expands to keep the tube compressed as it flattens and requires a special applicator for interval laparoscopic sterilization and for postpartum sterilization.[82,83] The Filshie clip compared favorably with other occlusion devices on safety issues. Studies do not support the routine application of multiple clips per tube.

Essure is a mechanical occlusion device and is the only FDA approved transcervical method. The device is placed through a hysteroscope and

Table 17–1 Various Approaches and Occlusion Methods (Advantages and Disadvantages)

Approach	Occlusion Method	Advantages	Disadvantages
Laparoscopy	1. Silastic bands or Falope-rings 2. Filshie or Hulka clips 3. Bipolar electrocoagulation 4. Unipolar electrocoagulation	1. Single incision with either single-punch or double-punch technique 2. Less pain than from minilaparotomy 3. Low complication rate 4. Short recovery time 5. Local or general anesthesia	1. Need for specialist with method-specific training 2. Necessary equipment is often difficult to obtain and maintain. 3. Need a fully equipped operating and recovery room with trained staff.
Transcervical	Essure microinsert device	1. May be performed under local anesthesia 2. No incisions or scars 3. Can be safely performed in an outpatient setting	1. Long-term effectiveness not well known after 3 years 2. Requires initial 3 months of backup contraception and confirmatory HSG
Suprapubic Minilaparatomy	1. Pomeroy and Pritchard (Parkland) techniques 2. Silastic bands or Falope-rings 3. Filshie or Hulka clips	1. Local or general anesthesia. 2. Incision site usually not visible (below pubic hairline)	1. Difficult technique if the woman is obese, the uterus immobile or the tubes have adhesions. 2. Recovery can be more painful than with laparoscopy
Postpartum Sterilization Subumbilical Minilaparotomy	1. Pomeroy or Pritchard (Parkland) technique 2. Filshie clip	1. Convenience 2. Lower costs 3. Ease of surgery 4. Does not necessarily extend hospital stay beyond that for a normal delivery	1. Electrocoagulation not indicated 2. Filshie clip requires special postpartum applicator 3. Counseling must be prior to labor to reduce risk of regret
Cesarean Section	1. Pomeroy or Pritchard (Parkland) technique 2. Filshie clip	1. Convenience 2. Lower costs 3. Anatomy fully visible	1. Cesareans should not be performed solely to occlude the tubes 2. Other disadvantages from subumbilical minilaparotomy apply
Postabortion Sterilization Laparoscopy	1. Silastic bands or Falope-rings 2. Filshie or Hulka clips 3. Bipolar electrocoagulation 4. Unipolar electrocoagulation	1. Convenience 2. Client motivation	1. Need for careful counseling with consideration of risk of regret 2. If using general anesthesia, may increase the amount of blood loss with abortion procedure
Suprapubic Minilaparotomy	Pomeroy and Pritchard (Parkland) techniques	Same as above	Same as above

consists of two concentric metal coils. The outer coil anchors the device in the tubal lumen. The inner coil's synthetic fibers stimulate growth of fibrous tissue, which, over the subsequent few months occludes the tubes. The procedure is irreversible. Since the procedure is not effective immediately, an alternate method of reliable contraception must be used until a hysterosalpingogram demonstrates that the device is correctly placed and the tubes are occluded.

Ligation Methods

Tubal occlusion at the time of Cesarean delivery, minilaparotomy, or laparotomy for other indications is usually performed by ligation and resection of a portion of both fallopian tubes. A variety of techniques have been described, including the Pomeroy[1] and Parkland methods. The Uchida and Irving methods require special training and are rarely used in the United States.[70]

ANESTHESIA AND PAIN MANAGEMENT

Short acting general anesthesia or regional anesthesia is most frequently used for female transabdominal sterilization procedures in the United States. The current trend today is toward out-patient-based surgery. The transcervical device (Essure) may be provided using local anesthesia with oral premedication or minimal intravenous sedation.

Advantages of local anesthesia include lower complication rates, lower cost of the procedure, quicker recovery, better postoperative course with fewer or milder side-effects, and high acceptance by most patients. By not compromising the normal physiological control of vital functions, a high level of safety can be maintained. *All* anesthetic methods, however, need the attention of a trained professional who carefully monitors the patient and the drugs used. Avoid high doses of opioid (narcotic) analgesics and benzodiazepine (tranquilizer) sedatives that can compromise ventilation, sometimes dramatically, and may cause cardiovascular depression.[84] For complete information on anesthetic techniques and regimens go to www.engenderhealth.org (Minilaparotomy for Female Sterilization: An illustrated guide for providers, 2003: pg 27–31.)

MANAGING PROBLEMS AND FOLLOW-UP

Major complications from tubal sterilizations are uncommon and vary by study definition, occurring at levels that range from 1 to 3.5%.[80,81,85] The types of complications vary by the type of surgical proce-

---

[1]The Pomeroy method has undergone a modification whereby plain catgut, which degrades more rapidly, replaces the original chromic suture type. Throughout this text, the term "Pomeroy" means this modification.[84]

dure and anesthesia. The risk of these complications can be reduced by careful screening, use of local anesthesia with light sedation, close monitoring of vital signs, good asepsis, and careful surgical technique. The seriousness of complications can often be minimized by early recognition and aggressive management.

Intraoperative complications recognized during surgery can be avoided or attended to by the experienced surgeon and adherence to protocols. Although complications from laparoscopy are NOT more common than from minilaparotomy some are more severe. Because of the blind entry into the abdomen and the proximity of major blood vessels, bowel and other organs prompt recognition is paramount. No patient should leave the recovery room without both verbal and clear written instructions for followup including 24 hour contact information for concerns or emergencies, immediate self care, and a follow-up visit.

POSTOPERATIVE INSTRUCTIONS: TRANSABDOMINAL FEMALE STERILIZATION

1. **Rest for 24 hours** following surgery. Resume normal activities as you gradually become more comfortable.

2. **Avoid intercourse for 1 week** and when you resume having intercourse, stop if it is uncomfortable.

3. **Avoid strenuous lifting for 1 week** to allow the incisions to heal.

4. Return to the clinic or contact the clinic or provider promptly if you develop:

Condition:	Action:
Temperature: 100+ degrees Fahrenheit	Immediate contact with provider either by phone or for exam.
Fainting: Fainting spells	Contact provider by phone.
Pain: Abdominal pain that is persistent, severe and/or increasing after 12 hours	Immediate contact with provider for exam
Incision sites: Bleeding or spotting from incision sites	1. Put pressure and tape x 12 hours. 2. Keep clean with betadine or peroxide. 3. If condition continues or worsens, contact provider
Pus or discharge from incision sites	1. Clean with betadine or peroxide 2 times/day. 2. If condition continues or worsens, contact provider
Stitch in wound	It will eventually fall out (unless a permanent suture was put in place).

5. Take one or two analgesic tablets at 4- to 6-hour intervals if you need them for pain. Do not use aspirin since it may promote bleeding.

6. You may bathe 48 hours after surgery but avoid putting tension on the incision and do not rub or irritate the incision for 1 week. Dry the incision site after bathing.

7. Stitches will dissolve and do not require removal. (Note to provider: this instruction must be modified if nonabsorbable sutures such as silk are used.)

8. **Return to the clinic** 1 week after the procedure to make sure the healing process is normal.

9. If you think you are pregnant at any time in the future, return to the clinic immediately. Although pregnancy after female sterilization is rare, when it does occur, chances are increased that it will be outside the uterus (an ectopic pregnancy). This is a dangerous life-threatening condition and must be treated immediately.

10. You should know this method of birth control is permanent. Reversal surgery is possible under certain conditions, but it is expensive, requires highly technical and major surgery, and its results cannot be guaranteed.

MALE STERILIZATION

Male sterilization or vasectomy is one of the safest and most effective family planning methods. It is also one of the few contraceptive options available to men. Nearly all vasectomies are performed using local anesthesia. The no-scalpel approach to the vas, developed in China in the mid-1970s, has become common throughout the world. It takes 5 to 10 minutes for preoperative preparation and administration of local anesthesia and then usually 5 to 15 minutes to perform a vasectomy. Recent research results on occlusion techniques and follow-up procedures after vasectomy have led to changes in clinical guidelines and practice in many settings.

EFFECTIVENESS

Vasectomy is highly effective and one of the most reliable contraceptive methods.[86–90] The first-year failure rate in the United States is estimated to be 0.15% (see Table 27–1), with a range of 0% to 0.5% (see Table 27–16). In general, vasectomy failure rates are believed to be similar to those for female sterilization and lower than those for reversible methods.

It is very difficult to interpret the published literature on vasectomy efficacy because follow-up is usually short-term; many studies are retrospective, anecdotal and of low quality; a wide variety of occlusion methods are used; and there is no standard definition of what constitutes failure.[91] In addition, few studies present failure rates based on pregnancies after vasectomy; most report failures as failure to reach azoospermia (i.e., no sperm in the ejaculate). The relationship between sperm counts after vasectomy and the risk of pregnancy is not well understood, nor can it be readily measured. When pregnancy rates are reported, there are two complicating factors. Since vasectomy is not immediately effective, pregnancies may be related to failure to use another contraceptive until sperm are cleared from the reproductive tract. One quarter to one half of pregnancies after vasectomy may occur during this time.[88,89,92] In addition, pregnancies may not always be attributable to the men who underwent the vasectomy. True failure of the technique can result from spontaneous recanalization of the vas, division or occlusion of the wrong structure during surgery, and (rarely) a congenital duplication of the vas that went unnoticed during the procedure. It is clear, nevertheless, that pregnancy can occur long after the vasectomy procedure.

MECHANISM OF ACTION

Sterilization for men involves blocking each vas deferens so that sperm can no longer pass out of the body in the ejaculate.

ADVANTAGES

Vasectomy is simpler, safer, less expensive, and as effective as female sterilization. It is ideal for men and couples who are certain they wish no further children and need a reliable contraceptive method. When both female and male sterilization are acceptable, vasectomy would be the preferred surgical contraceptive method, although individuals and couples need to make their own informed decision. The main advantages of vasectomy are as follows:

- Permanence
- High effectiveness
- High acceptability
- Safety
- Quick recovery
- Lack of significant long-term side effects

- Cost-effectiveness (most cost effective of all contraceptive methods)
- No need to buy anything
- No need for partner compliance
- No need to interrupt lovemaking
- Privacy of choice
- Removal of contraceptive burden from the woman

DISADVANTAGES AND CAUTIONS

Male sterilization is not recommended for anyone who is not sure of his desire to end future fertility. One caution that must be kept in mind is that vasectomy is not effective until all sperm in the reproductive tract are cleared. As a contraceptive method, vasectomy provides indirect protection from pregnancy for women—a woman has to rely on the man being truthful about having had a vasectomy and about knowing that his semen is free of sperm.

The major disadvantages of vasectomy are as follows:

- Permanence: pregnancy after sterilization is difficult, though possible. It is expensive, requires either costly assisted reproductive technology or highly technical major surgery, and its results cannot be guaranteed.
- Risk: although minimal, all surgical procedures carry some risk.
- Regret for decision: regret can be high among some groups of men, for the same reasons that regret is high in some groups of women: being in an unstable marriage at the time of sterilization, being younger than 31, having no children or very young children, or making their decision to be sterilized during a time of financial crisis or for reasons related to a pregnancy.
- Logistical requirements: vasectomy requires a trained physician or other health professional, procedure room with aseptic conditions, trained assistants, medications, and surgical equipment.
- Expense: the procedure carries a cost.
- Lack of protection against STIs, including HIV.

SPECIAL ISSUES

Antisperm Antibodies

Antisperm antibodies appear in 50% to 80% of men following vasectomy,[93] compared to only 8% to 21% of men in the general population.[94]

The theoretical concern that these antibodies may have adverse health consequences has led to numerous studies, results of which have shown no evidence of any immunologic or other diseases related to the formation of antisperm antibodies after vasectomy.[95–97] Antisperm antibodies may play a role in decreased fertility after vasectomy reversal, although conflicting results have been reported. Some studies have shown decreased pregnancy rates due to antisperm antibodies and others have not.[98–100] Current consensus is that fertility following vasectomy reversal is only inhibited by high levels of antisperm antibodies.[101] There is, however, some debate regarding the interpretation and clinical relevancy of different types of antisperm antibody tests.[102,103] In addition, the class of antibody may be more important than the antibody titers themselves, with IgA antibodies leading to greater fertility impairment than IgG antibodies.[103]

Prostate Cancer

The incidence of prostate cancer is rising, and in the United States it is the most commonly diagnosed cancer among men.[104] Little is known about the etiology and pathogenesis of prostate cancer, and few risk factors have been identified.[105] Since the mid-1980s, there have been over a dozen epidemiological studies of the risk of prostate cancer after vasectomy reported in the literature. Results have been difficult to interpret because of conflicting study findings, lack of a convincing biological mechanism for vasectomy causing prostate cancer, and generally weak associations when they have been found (for a review, see Bernal-Delgado, et al. 1998 and Dennis, et al. 2002).[106,107] In addition, the potential for bias in some studies was high and likely led to an overestimation of any effect.[106,107] Based on the results of the published studies to date, there is little evidence for a causal association between vasectomy and prostate cancer.[108] A panel of experts gathered by the U.S. National Institutes of Health in 1993 concluded that no change in the current practice of vasectomy was necessary nor should vasectomy reversal be done as a prostate cancer prevention measure.[109] Studies published after the expert panel report continue to support these conclusions and to find no relation between vasectomy and risk of prostate cancer.[108–111]

Chronic Testicular Pain (also referred to as postvasectomy pain syndrome)

Some men report chronic testicular pain or discomfort after vasectomy. While up to one-third to one-half of men have reported occasional testicular discomfort following vasectomy, only a small percentage of all vasectomized men (no more than 2% to 3%) said the pain had a negative impact on their lives or that they regretted having had the vasectomy because of chronic pain.[112-114] There are limited data on chronic testicular pain in the general population and only one study of postvasectomy pain included a control group. In that study, 47% of vasectomized men reported having occasional testicular discomfort compared to 23% of the controls, with 6% and 2%, respectively, seeking medical advice.[115] None of the men reported they regretted having had a vasectomy because of the pain. The cause of chronic testicular pain after vasectomy is poorly understood but may be related to infection, epididymal or vas congestion, back pressure-induced epididymal tubule rupture, sperm granuloma formation, or nerve entrapment.[116] Conservative therapy such as nonsteroidal anti-inflammatory drugs, sitz baths, antibiotics, or spermatic cord blocks is sufficient treatment in most cases. When this fails, there is some evidence that vasectomy reversal, epididymectomy or denervation of the spermatic cord may be helpful.[116] During counseling it is important to mention that a small percentage of men experience chronic testicular pain following vasectomy.

PROVIDING MALE STERILIZATION

There is no medical reason that would absolutely restrict a man's eligibility for vasectomy. Some conditions and circumstances indicate that certain precautions should be taken or that the procedure should be delayed.[117] These include localized problems that make vasectomy more difficult to perform (such as inguinal hernia, large hydrocele or varicocele, and cryptorchidism) or conditions that may increase the likelihood of complications (such as diabetes, coagulation disorders, or AIDS).

COUNSELING GUIDELINES FOR VASECTOMY

The goal of counseling is to help clients select a contraceptive method that they will use, that will be effective, that is most consistent with their reproductive intentions, and that will not have side effects that are problematic for the client. The permanence of vasectomy is a significant consideration with respect to counseling. Although reversal or assisted reproductive technologies are possible, they are expensive and require technically demanding procedures; results cannot be guaranteed. Vasectomy should be considered permanent. The factors contributing to an individual's decision about male sterilization vary. Each man needs to weigh the risks, benefits, effectiveness, and side effects of the various contraceptive options available to him and his partner, as well as his personal need to use a barrier method for protection against sexually transmitted infections, especially HIV.

Important aspects of counseling men on use of vasectomy include:

1. **Provide choices.** Highly effective, long-acting, temporary methods should be presented as options available to the man's partner.

2. **Assess the client's understanding of the procedure.** In the United States, awareness of vasectomy is fairly widespread, although there are often misconceptions about the procedure. One of the counselor's tasks is to assure that the individual correctly understands the procedure and has no misconceptions. Men should be informed that although rare, chronic testicular pain can occur after vasectomy.

3. **Facilitate the decision-making process.** Give the client sufficient time to make a thoughtful, informed decision about vasectomy, especially when a man's partner has just given birth or had an abortion, or when there are financial, marital, or sexual problems.

4. Clients should be informed that vasectomy, although highly effective, is not 100% successful and that failure occurs, even years after the procedure was performed.

5. The fact that vasectomy will not provide protection against sexually transmitted infections, including HIV for either the client or his partner(s) should be thoroughly explained. Condom use will be necessary if the client is at risk of such infections.

6. Men should be advised that vasectomy is not immediately effective, that success should be confirmed by semen analysis if possible, and that another contraceptive should be used until their provider says they can rely on the vasectomy alone for contraception.

Informed Consent

Informed consent is the voluntary decision made by a person who has been fully informed regarding a procedure and its consequences. Provide the information on vasectomy in a language the client can understand. The client must always sign or mark an informed consent form indicating that they understand the vasectomy procedure, its intended permanence, the possibility of failure, the risks and benefits, and the option to change his mind about having a vasectomy at any time prior to the procedure without loss of medical or financial benefits. The surgeon or authorized representative must also sign the form. Written informed consent should document, but not substitute for, the provider's active involvement in the client's informed decision making process to have a vasectomy, in order to ensure that he has knowingly and freely requested the procedure.

Policy/Legal Issues. See female sterilization section.

Preoperative Screening

Take a preoperative history and evaluate the general health condition of the client with particular attention to assessing the inguinal area, scrotum, and testicles to see if there are factors that might affect the procedure. Laboratory examinations are not routinely performed, but should be available in case the history or physical suggest they might be indicated (e.g., liver function, bleeding and clotting time, etc.). Clip the hair from around the scrotum and penis (if this was not already done at home). Shaving the scrotum is no longer recommended, as this significantly increases the chance of surgical-site infection. Strict adherence to good infection prevention practices and aseptic technique is crucial for the safety of the procedure and essential to prevent both immediate and long-term infectious morbidity and mortality. Both conventional and no-scalpel vasectomies are performed almost exclusively under local anesthesia only, using 1% lidocaine (lignocaine). Pre-medication, sedation or regional or general anesthesia is rarely needed and unnecessarily increases the risk and the costs associated with the procedure.

APPROACHES TO THE VAS

Regardless of the method of scrotal entry, the first step in the vasectomy is to identify and immobilize the vas through the skin of the scrotum, and then to deliver the vas. There are two approaches to delivering the vas: conventional vasectomy and no-scalpel vasectomy.

For conventional vasectomy, the skin and muscle overlying the vas are incised with a scalpel. Generally only the area around the skin entry site is anesthetized. Some surgeons use a single midline incision, and others make two lateral incisions in the scrotal skin, one overlying each vas deferens (Figure 17–6). The incision(s) are typically closed with absorbable suture after the vasectomy is completed.

An alternative approach, no-scalpel vasectomy, is currently being used in many programs around the world, including some in the United States. No-scalpel vasectomy (also known as NSV) was developed in 1974 in China. The anesthetic technique used with NSV includes a deep injection of anesthesia alongside each vas to create a perivasal block, as well as anesthetizing the skin. In addition, two specialized instruments, a ringed clamp and a dissecting forceps, are used in the NSV procedure. Both vasa are reached through the same small midline puncture in the scrotum rather than through a scalpel incision, and sutures are not needed (Figure 17–7). A detailed description can be found in No-Scalpel Vasectomy: An Illustrated Guide For Surgeons.[118]

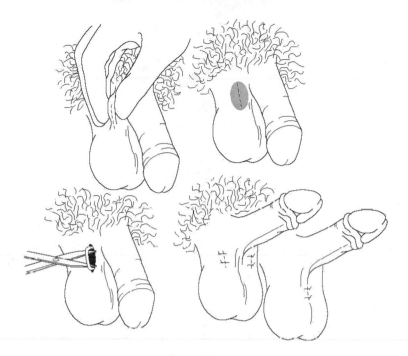

Figure 17–6 Sites of vasectomy incisions

The NSV approach has a number of advantages over the conventional scalpel method: fewer complications, including infection and hematoma, less pain during the procedure and early follow-up period, and earlier resumption of sexual activity after surgery.[6] Several modifications to the NSV approach, successful in the investigator's hands, have been reported in the literature recently.[119–121]

OCCLUSION METHODS

Once the vas has been delivered, it is then occluded. A variety of methods are used, including ligation with sutures, division, cautery, application of clips, excision of a segment of the vas, fascial interposition, or some combination of these. The same techniques are used to occlude the vas whether using conventional or no-scalpel vasectomy.

Ligation and excision of a section of the vas is the most widely used technique worldwide. Another popular occlusion technique is cautery—electrosurgical (electrical coagulation) or thermal. This is done by inserting a needle electrode or a cautery device into the vas lumen and desiccating the luminal mucosa of the vas to create a firm scar that will occlude the vas. Sometimes a segment of the vas is removed as well. Clips can be applied to the vas to compress a narrow segment and block the passage of sperm. With this method, after division of the vas, a clip is ap-

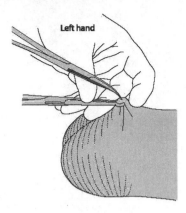

A. Inserting both tips of the dissecting forceps into the puncture site

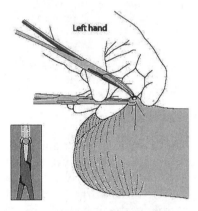

B. Spreading the tissues to make a skin opening twice the diameter of the vas

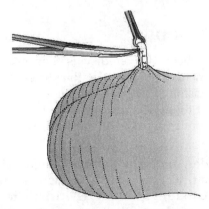

C. Grasping a partial thickness of the elevated vas

Source: Engenderhealth (2002)[86] with permission.

Figure 17–7 No-scalpel vasectomy

plied to both of the cut ends. Sometimes a segment of the vas is removed. A modification performed by some surgeons, which can be used with ligation, cautery, or clips, is to leave the testicular end of the vas open (open-ended vasectomy). Theoretically, success rates for vasectomy reversal may be higher with open-ended vasectomy, but no studies have been reported in the literature. Fascial interposition places a tissue barrier between the cut end of the vas by suturing (or securing with a clip) the thin layer of tissue that surrounds the vas over one of the cut ends. It can be used with any of the occlusion methods described above.

Until recently, there has been little evidence to support the superiority of any one occlusion method over others.[91,122] Results from a number of recent studies, however, suggest that there are some differences in effectiveness among different occlusion techniques. Several studies found higher than expected failure rates for vasectomy by ligation (with suture or clips) and excision of a segment of the vas.[87,88,123,124] Results of a randomized controlled trial demonstrated that use of fascial interposition with ligation and excision significantly improved the effectiveness of vasectomy. Ligation and excision without fascial interposition should no longer be recommended.[125] Cautery has been shown to be highly effective[91,126] and was found to significantly reduce failures compared to ligation and excision with fascial interposition.[127] Data on use of fascial interposition with cautery, differences in the effectiveness of thermal and electrocautery, and the importance of removing a segment of the vas are lacking.

MANAGING PROBLEMS AND FOLLOW-UP

Vasectomy is a minor surgical procedure. Intraoperative complications such as vasovagal reaction, lidocaine toxicity, and excessive bleeding, are unusual and can generally be prevented if appropriate guidelines and procedures are followed. Postoperative complications such as bleeding or infection as well as failure, although infrequent, do occur. Most postoperative complications are minor and subside within one or two weeks. The most frequent complaints after surgery are swelling of the scrotum, bruising, pain, and minor bleeding under the skin. A scrotal support, mild pain medication, and local application of ice are usually sufficient for treatment. More significant complications such as heavy bleeding, hematoma, or infection are quite rare. Careful surgical technique, practicing aseptic technique, early recognition of a problem, and proper postoperative care and follow-up greatly reduce the risks of both minor and major complications after vasectomy.

Vasectomy is a safe method of contraception, and mortality due to vasectomy is extremely rare.[128-130] Although there are few reports on vasectomy-related mortality, the most comprehensive study, based on over 400,000 vasectomies worldwide, found a mortality rate of 0.5 deaths per 100,000 vasectomized men.[130]

LONG-TERM COMPLICATIONS

Vasectomy appears to be largely safe, with risks no greater than those found with any of the contraceptive options for women. For over 25 years, extensive research has been carried out to explore potential physiological effects and long-term sequelae of vasectomy. No significant long-term negative physical or mental health effects have been found. Results of numerous well-designed studies have consistently shown no adverse effects of vasectomy in terms of heart disease, prostate or testicular cancer, immune complex disorders, and a variety of other conditions.[86,131,132] Sexual function remains unaffected and vasectomy does not lead to impotence or other sexual difficulties, nor any reduction in the amount of semen ejaculated. Vasectomy has been reported to have no negative effects on sexuality,[95,133] with some studies demonstrating a positive effect, perhaps because of the reduced worry about unintended pregnancy.[52,134]

Follow-Up After Vasectomy

The standard accepted endpoint of vasectomy has traditionally been achievement of azoospermia, although some have suggested that men with low numbers of nonmotile sperm after vasectomy are at low risk of causing pregnancy and can rely on their vasectomy for contraception.[86] It is generally recommended that men have semen analysis to confirm vasectomy success, although recommendations on when men should return in terms of time and/or number of ejaculations after vasectomy vary widely. In resource-poor settings, semen analysis may not be available or practical. In these settings it had been recommended that men wait 10 to 12 weeks or 15 to 20 ejaculations before beginning to rely on their vasectomy for contraception. Recent research, however, suggests that telling men to use another form of contraception until 12 weeks after vasectomy is more reliable than 20 ejaculations[123,125] and is now recommended to reduce the risk of pregnancy.[135]

RISK OF REGRET

The vast majority of men who have a vasectomy do not regret their decision to do so. Regret among men after vasectomy, most often reported as less than 5%, is lower than the reported regret among women after female sterilization.[136,137] Regret among women whose husbands had a vasectomy has been reported to be slightly higher than men's regret at 6–8%.[54,138] However, reported regret among women whose husbands had a vasectomy (6%) was the same as women who had a tubal ligation (7%).[54] Regret following a vasectomy is more common among men who, at the time of the vasectomy, were less than 30 years old, were in an unstable marriage, had no or very young children, or made the decision to have a vasectomy during a time of financial crisis or for reasons related to a pregnancy.[86,137,139] The need for good counseling prior to vasectomy is underscored by the fact that some men who express regret have had a complication following the procedure or a problem that they perceived to be caused by vasectomy. Men with risk factors for regret should receive more in-depth counseling to make sure that vasectomy is the right contraceptive choice. Men should not be denied the procedure if they decide they want it.

Desire For Pregnancy Following Vasectomy

Vasectomy should be considered permanent, but even with careful counseling, some men will request reversal. The most common reason that men request vasectomy reversal is that they want another child because they have remarried, changed their mind, or lost a child.[86,140] Vasectomy reversal or assisted reproductive technologies can be used; however, success cannot be guaranteed. In addition, these techniques are technically complex, require special skills and are costly.

Both macroscopic and microsurgical techniques have been used for vasectomy reversal. The current consensus is that the microsurgical techniques are more successful.[141] The percentage of men with sperm in the ejaculate ranges from 75% to 100% after microsurgical reversal.[140,142] However, presence of sperm should not be presented to men as the measure of success, since pregnancy is the desired outcome. Reported pregnancy rates are lower, ranging from 38% to 89%.[140,142–144]

The time elapsed between the vasectomy and the reversal is a major factor in the success of reversal; the longer the interval between vasectomy and reversal, the less likely the man is to be fertile after the reversal. Reversal is usually more successful when done within 10 years after vasectomy. Pregnancy rates drop to less than 50% when reversal is performed more than 10 to 15 years after vasectomy.[140,143,144] Other factors that affect the success of vasectomy reversal include the skill of the surgeon, the type of vasectomy procedure originally performed, levels of antisperm antibodies, the age of the female partner, and partial obstruction of the vas after the reversal surgery that prevents movement of sperm through the vas.

Assisted reproduction technologies have been successful in vasectomized men who want children but do not want a vasectomy reversal or have had one or more unsuccessful reversal surgeries. Sperm can be retrieved from the epididymis or the testis and then used for intracytoplasmic sperm injection (ICSI). Pregnancy rates following ICSI with epididymal sperm and testicular sperm are reported to be 25% to 36% and 17% to 36%, respectively.[145] Several studies have found that similar to the case with vasectomy reversal, a negative correlation appears to exist between pregnancy rates and time elapsed from the vasectomy until ICSI.[146-148] However, there are also two reports that found no association between the time since vasectomy and the outcome of ICSI.[149,150]

Vasectomy reversal has been shown to be equally or more successful and less costly than ICSI following epididymal sperm aspiration.[144,147,148] Thus, surgical reversal appears to be a better first choice for vasectomized men who wish to have children.[151,152] This is the case even in men who are undergoing repeat vasectomy reversal surgery due to a previously failed reversal attempt.[153]

USER INSTRUCTIONS FOR VASECTOMY

Preoperative Instructions

1. Be completely sure of your decision to have a vasectomy. You must be certain you understand and desire the permanence of vasectomy. You can change your mind at any time before the operation.

2. Before surgery while you are home, use scissors to cut all hair from around the penis and scrotum to about 1/4-inch in length. Do not shave.

3. Shower or bathe, washing the penis and scrotum thoroughly to remove all loose hairs.

4. If possible, bring someone who can accompany you home after the procedure. Do not ride a bicycle; avoid walking long distances or using other transportation that may rub or put pressure on the scrotum.

5. Plan to remain quiet for about 48 hours following the vasectomy. A 48-hour rest is important to decrease the risk of complications.

Postoperative Instructions

1. Following the surgery, return home and rest for about 2 days. If possible, keep an ice pack on the scrotum for at least 4 hours to reduce the chances of swelling, bleeding, and discomfort. Wear a scrotal support for 2 days (e.g. brief style underwear). You will probably be able to resume your normal activities after 2 or 3 days.

2. Avoid strenuous physical exercise for 1 week. Strenuous exercise means hard physical exertion, lifting or straining that could bring pressure to the groin or scrotum.

3. Do not shower or bathe for the first 24 hours after the vasectomy.

4. The stitches will dissolve and do not have to be removed. (Note to provider: this instruction must be modified if nonabsorbable skin sutures, such as silk, are used or if no skin sutures are used.)

5. You may resume sexual intercourse after 2 or 3 days if you feel it would be comfortable; but remember, you are not sterile immediately. For many men, sperm will not be cleared from the body until after a minimum of 3 months. Until then, use condoms or another contraceptive method to prevent pregnancy. The best way of finding out if you are sterile is to have your semen looked at under a microscope about 3 months after the vasectomy.

6. If you have pain or discomfort, simple analgesics taken at intervals of 4 to 6 hours usually give adequate relief. (Note to provider: name and dose should be specified.)

7. It is important for you to know what is normal and what is abnormal following your surgery. You will probably have some pain and swelling in the scrotal region; the scrotum may be somewhat discolored. These conditions are normal and should not worry you. Occasionally, blood from a tiny blood vessel may escape into the scrotum at the time of surgery, and bleeding may continue. Notify the provider who performed your vasectomy if you have any of the following danger signs or if you notice any other unusual body changes:

Condition:	Action:
Temperature: 100+ degrees Fahrenheit	Contact the provider who performed your vasectomy.
Pain: Unable to sleep or work	If unrelieved by analgesic, contact the provider who performed your vasectomy.
Discharge: Pus or inflammation at incision site	Clean with betadine or peroxide. If redness in skin increases or pus and inflammation persist, contact the provider who performed your vasectomy.
Bleeding: Bleeding from incision site	If after placing pressure on area for 10 minutes the bleeding continues, contact the provider who performed your vasectomy.
Swelling: Greater than twice normal size	Contact the provider who performed your vasectomy.

Condition:	Action:
Nodules: Larger than a nickel, pain and tenderness	Contact the provider who performed your vasectomy.
Stitches: Extreme pulling sensation	Contact the provider who performed your vasectomy.

8. Remember, vasectomy is permanent. Reversal surgery or assisted reproductive technologies are possible under certain conditions, but are expensive and require highly technical procedures. Results cannot be guaranteed.

REFERENCES

1. Mosher W, Martinez G, Chandra A, Abma J, Willson S. Use of contraception and use of family planning services in the United States:1982–2002. Advance data from vital and health statistics;no 350. Hyattsville, Maryland: National Center for Health Statistics. 2004.
2. MacKay AP, Kieke BA Jr, Koonin LM, Beattie K. Tubal sterilization in the United States, 1994–1996. Fam Plann Perspect 2001;33:161–5.
3. Magnani RJ, Haws JM, Morgan GT, Gargiullo PM, Pollack AE, Koonin LM. Vasectomy in the United States, 1991 and 1995. Am J Public Health 1999;89:92–4.
4. EngenderHealth. Contraceptive sterilization: global issues and trends. New York: EngenderHealth, 2002.
5. Fortney JA, Feldblum PJ, Raymond EG. Intrauterine devices. The optimal long-term contraceptive method? J Reprod Med 1999;44:269–74.
6. Andersson K, Odlind V, Rybo G. Levonorgesterel-releasing and copper-releasing (Nova T) IUDs during five years of use: a randomized comparative trial. Contraception 1994;49:56–72.
7. Sivin I, el Mahgoub S, McCarthy T, Mishell DR Jr, Shouope D, Alvarez F, et al. Long-term contraception with the levonorgesterel 20 mcg/day (LNg 20) and the copper T380A intrauterine devices: a five-year randomized study. Contraception 1990; 42:361–78.
8. Luukkainen T, Allonen H, Haukkamaa M, Lahteenmaki P, Nilsson CG, Toivonen J. Five years' experience with levonorgesterel-releasing IUDs. Contraception 1986; 33:139–48.
9. Peterson HB, Xia Z, Hughes JM, Wilcox LS, Tylor LR, Trussell J. The risk of pregnancy after tubal sterilization: findings from the U.S. Collaborative Review of Sterilization. Am J Obstet Gynecol 1996;174:1161–8;discussion 1168–70.
10. Shaw R, Russell I, Settatree R, Templeton A, Filshie GM, Argent VP. Male and female sterilization. Evidence-based guidelines No. 4. London: Royal College of Obstetricians and Gynaecologists;1999.
11. U.S. Food and Drug Administration. FDA approves new female sterilization device. FDA Talk Paper. 2002;T02–41:1–2.
12. Kerin JF, Carignan CS, Cher D. The safety and effectiveness of a new hysteroscopic method for permanent birth control: results of the first Essure™ pbc clinical study. Austral NZ J Obstet Gynaecol 2001;41:364–370.
13. Bril A. First year international commercial experience with Essure hysteroscopic sterilization procedure. J Am Assoc Gynecol Laparosc 2004;11:S30-
14. Peterson HB, Xia Z, Hughes JM, Wilcox LS, Tylor LR, Trussell J. The risk of ectopic pregnancy after tubal sterilization. U.S. Collaborative Review of Sterilization Working Group. N Engl J Med 1997;336:762–7.

15. Chaim W, Mazor M. Pregnancy with an intrauterine device in situ and preterm delivery. Arch Gynecol Obstet 1992;252:21–4.
16. Foreman H, Stadel BV, Schlesselman S. Intrauterine device usage and fetal loss. Obstet Gynecol 1981;58:669–77.
17. Tatum HJ, Schmidt FH, Jain AK. Management and outcome of pregnancies associated with the CopperT intrauterine device. Am J Obstet Gynecol 1976;126:869–79.
18. Escobedo LG, Peterson HB, Grubb GS, Franks AL. Case-fatality rates for tubal sterilization in U.S. hospitals, 1979 to 1980. Am J Obstet Gynecol 1989;160:147–50.
19. Hulka JF, Phillips JM, Peterson HB, Surrey MW. Laparoscopic sterilization: American Association of Gynecologic Laparoscopists' 1993 membership survey. J Am Assoc Gynecol Laparosc 1995;2:137–8.
20. Peterson HB, Ory HW, Greenspan JR, Tyler CW Jr. Deaths associated with laparoscopic sterilization by unipolar electrocoagulation devices, 1978 and 1979. Am J Obstet Gynecol 1981;139:141–3.
21. Peterson HB, Hulka JF, Phillips JM, Surrey MW. Laparoscopic sterilization. American Association of Gynecologic Laparoscopists 1991 membership survey. J Reprod Med 1993;38:574–6.
22. Peterson HB, DeStefano F, Rubin GL, Greenspan JR, Lee NC, Ory HW. Deaths attributable to tubal sterilization in the United States, 1977–81. Am J Obstet Gynecol 1983; 146:131–6.
23. Jamieson DJ, Hillis SD, Duerr A, Marchbanks PA, Costello C, Peterson HB. Complications of interval laparoscopic tubal sterilization: findings from the United States Collaborative Review of Sterilization. Obstet Gynecol 2000;96:997–1002.
24. Essure® Permanent Birth Control System. Instructions for use. 2002 Conceptus, Inc.
25. Green A, Purdie D, Bain C, et al. Tubal sterilization, hysterectomy and decreased risk of ovarian cancer. Int.J. Cancer 1997;71:948–51.
26. Kjaer S, Mellemkjaer L, Brinton L, Johansen C, Gridley G, Olsen J. Tubal sterilization and risk of ovarian, endometrial and cervical cancer. A Danish population-based follow-up study of more than 65 000 sterilized women. Int J Epidemiol 2004; 33:596–602.
27. McGuire V, Felberg A, Millis M, et al. Relation of contraceptive and reproductive history to ovarian cancer risk in carriers and noncarriers of BRCA1 gene mutations. Am J Epidemiol 2004;160:613–18.
28. Narod S, Sun P, Ghadirian P, et al. Tubal ligation and risk of ovarian cancer in carriers of BRCA1 or BRCA2 mutations: a case-control study. Lancet 2001;357:1467–70.
29. Calle E, Rodriguez C, Walker K, Wingo P, Petrelli J, Thun M.. Tubal sterilization and risk of breast cancer mortality in US women. Cancer Causes and Control 2001; 12:127–135.
30. Irwin, KL, Weiss NS, Lee NC, Peterson HB. Tubal sterilization, hysterectomy, and the subsequent occurrence of epithelial ovarian cancer. Am J Epidemiol 1991; 134:362–9.
31. Alder E, Cook A, Gray J, Tyrer G, Warner P, Bancroft J, et al. The effects of sterilization: a comparison of sterilized women with wives of vasectomized men. Contraception 1981;23:45–54.
32. Gentile GP, Kaufman SC, Helbig DW. Is there any evidence for a post-tubal sterilization syndrome? Fertil Steril 1998;69:179–86.
33. Poma PA. Tubal sterilization and later hospitalizations. J Reprod Med 1980;25:272–8.
34. Bhiwandiwala PP, Mumford SD, Feldblum PJ. Menstrual pattern changes following laparoscopic sterilization with different occlusion techniques: a review of 10,004 cases. Am J Obstet Gynecol 1983;145:684–94.
35. DeStefano F, Perlman JA, Peterson HB, Diamond EL. Long-term risk of menstrual disturbances after tubal sterilization. Am J Obstet Gynecol 1985;152:835–41.
36. Foulkes J, Chamberlain G. Effects of sterilization on menstruation. South Med J 1985; 78:544–7.

37. Rivera R, Gaitan JR, Ruiz R, Hurley DP, Arenas M, Flores C, et al. Menstrual patterns and progesterone circulating levels following different procedures of tubal occlusion. Contraception 1989;40:157–69.
38. Rulin MC, Davidson AR, Philliber SG, Graves WL, Cushman LF. Long-term effect of tubal sterilization on menstrual indices and pelvic pain. Obstet Gynecol 1993; 82:118–21.
39. Sahwi S, Toppozada M, Kamel M, Anway MY, Ismail AA. Changes in menstrual blood loss after four methods of female tubal sterilization. Contraception 1989; 40:387–98.
40. Thranov I, Herz JB, Kjer JJ, Andresen A, Micic S, Nielsen J, et al. Hormonal and menstrual changes after laparoscopic sterilization by Falope-rings or Filschie-clips. Fertil Steril 1992;57:751–5.
41. Carmona F, Cristobal P, Casamitjana R, Balasch J. Effect of tubal sterilization on ovarian follicular reserve and function. Am J Obstet Gynecol 2003;189:447–52.
42. Cevrioglu A, Degirmenci G, Acar M, et al. Examination of changes caused by tubal sterilization in ovarian hormone secretion and uterine and ovarian artery blood flow rates. Contraception 2204;70:467–73.
43. Yazici G, Arslan M, Pata O, Utko O, Aban M. Ovarian function and vascular resistance after tubal sterilization. J Reprod Med 2004;49:379–83.
44. Whiteman M, Miller K, Tomic D, Langenberg P, Flaws J. Tubal sterilization and hot flashes. Fertil Steril 2004;82:502–4.
45. Wyshak G. Menopausal symptoms and psychological distress in women with and without tubal sterilization. Psychosomatics 2004;45:403–13.
46. Hillis SD, Marchbands PA, Tylor LR, Peterson HB. Higher hysterectomy risk for sterilized than nonsterilized women: findings from the U.S. Collaborative Review of Sterilization Working Group. Obstet Gynecol 1998;91:241–6.
47. Cohen MM. Long-term risk of hysterectomy after tubal sterilization. Am J Epidemiol 1987;125:410–9.
48. Goldhaber MK, Armstrong MA, Golditch IM, Sheehe PR, Petitti DB, Friedman GD. Long-term risk of hysterectomy among 80,007 sterilized and comparison women at Kaiser Permanente, 1971–1987. Am J Epidemiol 1993;138:508–21.
49. Kendrick JS, Rubin GL, Lee NC, Schulz KF, Peterson HB, Nolan TF. Hysterectomy performed within 1 year after tubal sterilization. Fertil Steril 1985;44:606–10.
50. Stergachis A, Shy KK, Grothaus LC, Wagner EH, Hecht JA, Anderson G, et al. Tubal sterilization and the long-term risk of hysterectomy. JAMA 1990;264:2893–8.
51. Costello C, Hillis SD, Marchbanks PA, Jamieson DJ, Peterson HB. The effect of interval tubal sterilization on sexual interest and pleasure. Obstet Gynecol 2002; 100:511–7.
52. Shain RN, Miller WB, Holden AE, Rosenthal M. Impact of tubal sterilization and vasectomy on female marital sexuality: results of a controlled longitudinal study. Am J Obstet Gynecol 1991;164:763–771.
53. Hillis SD, Marchbanks PA, Tylor LR, Peterson HB. Poststerilization regret: findings from the United States Collaborative Review of Sterilization. Obstet Gynecol 1999; 93:889–95.
54. Jamieson DJ, Kaufman SC, Costello C, Hillis SD, Marchbanks PA, Peterson HB. A comparison of women's regret after vasectomy versus tubal sterilization. Obstet Gynecol 2002;1073–9.
55. Schmidt JE, Hillis SD, Marchbanks PA, Jeng G, Peterson HB. Requesting information about and obtaining reversal after tubal sterilization: findings from the U.S. Collaborative Review of Sterilization. Fertil Steril 2000;74:892–8.
56. Wilcox LS, Chu SY, Eaker ED, Zeger SL, Peterson HB. Risk factors for regret after tubal sterilization: 5 years of follow-up in a prospective study. Fertil Steril 1991; 55:927–33.

57. Cheng MC, Cheong J, Ratnam SS, Belsey MA, Edstrom KE, Pinol A, et al. Psychological sequelae of abortion and sterilization: a controlled study of 200 women randomly allocated to either a concurrent or interval abortion and sterilization. Asia Oceania J Obstet Gynecol 1986;12:193–200.

58. Wilcox LS, Chu SY, Peterson HB. Characteristics of women who considered or obtained a tubal reanastamosis: results from a prospective study of tubal sterilization. Obstet Gynecol 1990;75:661–5.

59. Schmidt JE, Hillis SD, Marchbanks PA, Jeng G, Peterson HB. Requesting information about and obtaining reversal after tubal sterilization: findings from the U.S. Collaborative Review of Sterilization. Fertil Steril 2000;74:892–8.

60. Boring CC, Rochat RW, Becerra J. Sterilization regret among Puerto Rican women. Fertil Steril 1988;49:973–81.

61. Neuhaus W, Bolte A. Prognostic factors for preoperative consultation of women desiring sterilization: findings of a retrospective ananlysis. J Psychosom Obstet Gynecol 1995;16:45–50.

62. Ledger W. Implications of an irreversible procedure. Letter to the editor: Fert Steril 2004.08.005

63. Lee D, Patton P. Tubal surgery and treatment of infertility. GO 04 Vol 5/ Chap 106 Reproductive Endocrinology, Infertility, Genetics.

64. Trussell J, Guilbert E, Hedley A. Sterilization failure, sterilization reversal, and pregnancy after sterilization reversal in Quebec. ObstetGynecol 2003;101:677–84.

65. Pollack AE, Soderstrom RM. Female tubal sterilization. In: Corson SL, Derman RJ, Tyrer LB, editors. Fertility control. 2nd ed. London (ON): Goldin Publishers;1994. p. 293–317.

66. Soderstrom R. Clinical challenges: share warning information, court case teaches. Contra Technol Update 1981;2:8–9.

67. Coe vs. Bolton. United States District Court, Civil Action No. C-76–785-A. September 29, 1976 (N.D. Georgia).

68. Sterilization of persons in federally assisted family planning projects. 42 C.F.R. 50 Subpart B (2004).

69. American College of Obstetricians and Gynecologists. Tubal ligation with cesarean delivery. ACOG Committee Opinion 205. Washington DC: ACOG;1998.

70. Peterson HB, Pollack AE, Warshaw JS. Tubal sterilization. In: Rock JA, Thompson JD, editors. Te Linde's Operative Gynecology. 8th ed. Philadelphia (PA): Lippincott-Raven;1997. p. 529 47.

71. American College of Obstetricians and Gynecologists. Ethics in obstetrics and gynecology. Washington, DC: ACOG;2002.

72. Kasliwal A, Farquharson RG. Pregnancy testing prior to sterilization. BJOG 2000; 107:1407–9.

73. Centers for Disease Control. Surgical sterilization surveillance 1976–1978. Atlanta (GA): CDC;1981.

74. Akhter HH, Flock ML, Rubin GL. Safety of abortion and tubal sterilization performed separately versus concurrently. Am J Obstet Gynecol 1985;152:619–23.

75. MacKay A, Kieke B, Koonin L, et al. Tubal sterilization in the United States, 1994–1996. Family Planning Perspectives 2001;33;161–165).

76. Kerin J, Munday D, Ritossa M, Pesce A, Rosen D. Essure hysteroscopic sterilization: results based on utilizing a new coil catheter delivery system. J Am Assoc Gynecol Laparosc 2004;11(3):388–93.

77. Valle RF, Carignan CS, Wright TC. Tissue response to the STOP microcoil transcervical permanent contraception device: results form a prehysterectomy study. Fertil Steril 2001;76:974–80.

78. Peterson HB, Xia Z, Wilcox LS, Tylor LR, Trussell J. Pregnancy after tubal sterilization with bipolar eclectrocoagulation. U.S. Collaborative Review of Sterilization Working Group. Obstet Gynecol 1999;94:163–7.

79. Soderstrom RM, Levy BS, Engel T. Reducing bipolar sterilization failures. Obstet Gynecol 1989;74:60–3.

80. Sokal D, Gates D, Amatya R, Dominik R.Two randomized control trials comparing the tubal ring and Filshie clip for tubal sterilization. Fertil Steril 2000;74:523–533.

81. Dominik R, Gates D, Sokal D, Cordero M, et al. Two randomized controlled trials comparing the Hulka and Filshie clips for tubal sterilization. Contraception 2000; 62:169–175.

82. Anonymous. Sterilization device to offer ease of use. Contracept Tech Update 1996; 17:53–64.

83. Anonymous. Update on female sterilization. The Contraception Report 1996; 7(3):13–14.

84. Peterson H, Pollack A, Warshaw J. Tubal Sterilization. In: Rock JA , Jones HW III, editors. Te Linde's Operative Gynecology. 9th ed. Philadelphia PA: Lippincott Williams & Wilkins;2003:539, 542.

85. Jameison DJ, Hillis SD, Duerr A, Marchbanks PA, Costello C, Peterson HB. Complications of interval lap tubal sterilization: findings from the US collaborative review of sterilization. Obstet Gynecol 2000;96:997 to 1002.

86. EngenderHealth. Male Sterilization. In Contraceptive Sterilization: Global Issues and Trends. New York NY: EngenderHealth. Chapter 7, pp. 161–177. 2002. Available at www.engenderhealth.org/res/offc/steril/factbook/index.html.

87. Wang D. Contraceptive failure in China. Contraception 2002;66:173–178.

88. Nazerali H, Thapa S, Hays M, Pathak LR, Pandey KR, Sokal DC. Vasectomy effectiveness in Nepal: a retrospective study. Contraception 2003;67:397–401.

89. Jamieson DJ, Costello C, Trussell J, Hillis SD, Marchbanks PA, Peterson HB;US Collaborative Review of Sterilization Working Group. The risk of pregnancy after vasectomy. Obstet Gynecol 2004;103:848–850.

90. Hieu DT, Luong TT, Anh PT, Ngoc DH, Duong LQ. The acceptability, efficacy and safety of quinacrine non-surgical sterilization (QS), tubectomy and vasectomy in 5 provinces in the Red River Delta, Vietnam: a follow-up of 15,190 cases. Int J Gynaecol Obstet 2003;83:S77–85.

91. Labrecque M, Dufresne C, Barone MA, St-Hilaire K. Vasectomy surgical techniques: a systematic review. Biomed Central Medicine 2004;2:21. Available at www.biomedcentral.com/1741-7015/2/21

92. Deneux-Tharaux C, Kahn E, Nazerali H, Sokal DC. Pregnancy rates after vasectomy: a survey of US urologists. Contraception 2004;69:401–406.

93. Ghazeeri GS, Kutteh WH. Autoimmune factors in reproductive failure. Curr Opin Obstet Gynecol 2001;13:287–291.

94. Gubin DA, Dmochowski R, Kutteh WH. Multivariant analysis of men from infertile couples with and without antisperm antibodies. Am J Reprod Immunol 1998; 39:157–160.

95. Petitti DB, Klein R, Kipp H, Kahn W, Siegelaub AB, Friedman GD. A survey of personal habits, symptoms of illness, and histories of disease in men with and without vasectomies. Am J Public Health 1982;72:476–480.

96. Giovannucci E, Tosteson TD, Speizer FE, Vessey MP, Colditz GA. A long-term study of mortality in men who have undergone vasectomy. N Engl J Med 1992; 326:1392–1398.

97. Massey FJ, Bernstein GS, O'Fallon WM, Schuman LM, Coulson AH, Crozier R, Mandel JS, Benjamin RB, Berendes HW, Chang PC. Vasectomy and health: results from a large cohort study. JAMA 1984;252:1023–1029.

98. Huang MK, Wu X, Fu C, Zou P, Gao X, Huang Q. Multiple factors affecting human repregnancy after microsurgical vasovasostomy. Reprod Contracept 1997;8:92–100.

99. Meinertz H, Linnet L, Fogh-Andersen P, Hjort T. Antisperm antibodies and fertility after vasovasostomy: a follow-up study of 216 men. Fert Steril 1990;54:315–321.

100. Newton RA. IgG antisperm antibodies attached to sperm do not correlate with infertility following vasovasostomy. Microsurgery 1998;9:278–280.

101. Lea IA, Adoyo P, O'Rand MG. Autoimmunogenicity of the human sperm protein Sp17 in vasectomized men and identification of linear B cell epitopes. Fertil Steril 1997;67:355–361.
102. Helmerhorst FM, Finken MJ, Erwich JJ. Antisperm antibodies: detection assays for antisperm antibodies: what do they test? Hum Reprod 1999;14:1669–1671.
103. Hjort T. Antisperm antibodies. Antisperm antibodies and infertility: an unsolvable question? Hum Reprod 1999;14:2423–2426.
104. Chan JM, Jou RM, Carroll PR. The relative impact and future burden of prostate cancer in the United States. J Urol 2004;172:S13–6.
105. Bostwick DG, Burke HB, Djakiew D, Euling S, Ho SM, Landolph J, Morrison H, Sonawane B, Shifflett T, Waters DJ, Timms B. Human prostate cancer risk factors. Cancer 2004;101:2371–490.
106. Bernal-Delgado E, Latour-Perez J, Pradas-Arnal F, Gomez-Lopez LI. The association between vasectomy and prostate cancer: a systematic review of the literature. Fertil Steril 1998;70:191–200.
107. Dennis LK, Dawson DV, Resnick MI. Vasectomy and the risk of prostate cancer: a meta-analysis examining vasectomy status, age at vasectomy, and time since vasectomy. Prostate Cancer Prostatic Dis 2002;5:193–203.
108. Peterson HB, Howards SS. Vasectomy and prostate cancer: The evidence to date. Fertil Steril 1998;70:201–203.
109. Healy B. From the National Institutes of Health: does vasectomy cause prostate cancer? JAMA 1993;269:2620.
110. Cox, B. Sneyd MJ, Paul C, Delahunt B, Skegg DC. Vasectomy and risk of prostate cancer. JAMA 2002;287:3110–3115.
111. Lynge E. Prostate cancer is not increased in men with vasectomy in Denmark. J Urol 2002;168:488–90.
112. Choe JM, Kirkemo AK. Questionnaire-based outcomes study of non-oncological post-vasectomy complications. J Urol 1996;155:1284–1286.
113. Ehn, BE, Liljestrand, J. 1995. A long-term follow-up of 108 vasectomized men. Good counselling routines are important. Scandanavian Journal of Urology and Nephrology 29(4):477–481.
114. Manikandan R, Srirangam SJ, Pearson E, Collins GN. Early and late morbidity after vasectomy: a comparison of chronic scrotal pain at 1 and 10 years. BJU Int 2004; 93:571–574.
115. Morris C, Mishra K, Kirkman RJE. A study to assess the prevalence of chronic testicular pain in post vasectomy men compared to non vasectomized men. J Fam Plann Reprod Health Care 2002;28:142–144.
116. Granitsiotis P, Kirk D. Chronic Testicular Pain: an overview. European Urology 2004; 45:430–436.
117. World Health Organization. Improving access to quality care in family planning: medical eligibility criteria for contraceptive use. Third edition. Geneva:World Health Organization, 2004. Available at www.who.int/reproductive-health/publications/mec/srhcare.html
118. EngenderHealth. No-scalpel vasectomy: an illustrated guide for surgeons. Third edition. New York NY: EngenderHealth. 2003. Available at: www.engenderhealth.org/res/offc/steril/nsv/index.html
119. Black T, Francome C. Comparison of Marie Stopes scalpel and electrocautery no-scalpel vasectomy techniques. J Fam Plann Reprod Health Care 2003;29:32–34.
120. Chen KC. A novel instrument-independent no-scalpel vasectomy - a comparative study against the standard instrument-dependent no-scalpel vasectomy. Int J Androl 2004;27:222–227.
121. Jones JS. Percutaneous vasectomy: a simple modification eliminates the steep learning curve of no-scalpel vasectomy. J Urol 2003;169:1434–1436.
122. Cook LA, Vliet H, Pun A, Gallo MF. Vasectomy occlusion techniques for male sterilization. Cochrane Database Syst Rev 2004;3:CD003991.

123. Barone MA, Nazerali H, Cortes M, Chen-Mok M, Pollack AE, Sokal D. A prospective study of time and number of ejaculations to azoospermia after vasectomy by ligation and excision. J Urol 2003;170:892–896.

124. Labrecque M, Nazerali H., Mondor M, Fortin V, Nasution M.: Effectiveness and complications associated with 2 vasectomy occlusion techniques. J Urol 2002; 168:2495–2498.

125. Sokal D, Irsula B, Hays M, Chen-Mok M, Barone MA.. Vasectomy by ligation and excision, with versus without fascial interposition: a randomized controlled trial. Biomed Central Medicine 2004;2:6. Available at www.biomedcentral.com/1741-7015/2/6

126. Barone MA, Irsula B, Chen-Mok M, Sokal D. Effectiveness of vasectomy using cautery. Biomed Central Urology 2004;4:10. Available at www.biomedcentral.com/1471-2490/4/10

127. Sokal D, Irsula B, Chen-Mok M, Labrecque M, Barone MA. A comparison of vas occlusion techniques: cautery more effective than ligation and excision with fascial interposition. Biomed Central Urology 2004;4:12. Available at www.biomedcentral.com/1471-1490/4/12

128. Grimes DA, Satterthwaite AP, Rochat RW, Akhter N. Deaths from contraceptive sterilization in Bangladesh: rates, causes, and prevention. Obstetrics and Gynecology 1982;60:635–640.

129. Grimes DA, Peterson HB, Rosenberg MJ, Fishburne JI Jr, Rochat RW, Khan AR, Islam R. Sterilization-attributable deaths in bangladesh. Int J Gynaecol Obstet 1982; 20:149–54.

130. Khairullah Z, Huber DH, Gonzales B. Declining mortality in international sterilization services. Intl J Gynecol Obstet 1992;39:41–50.

131. Manson JE, Ridker PM, Spelsberg A, Ajani U, Lotufo PA, Hennekens CH. Vasectomy and subsequent cardiovascular disease in US physicians. Contraception 1999; 59:181–186.

132. Coady SA, Sharrett AR, Zheng ZJ, Evans GW, Heiss G. Vasectomy, inflammation, atherosclerosis and long-term followup for cardiovascular diseases: no associations in the atherosclerosis risk in communities study. J Urol 2002;167:204–207.

133. Hofmeyr DG, Greeff AP. The influence of a vasectomy on the marital relationship and sexual satisfaction of the married man. J Sex Marital Ther 2002;28:339–351.

134. Miller WB, Shain RN, Pasta DJ. The pre- and poststerilization predictors of poststerilization regret in husbands and wives. J Nerv Ment Dis 1991;179:602–608.

135. World Health Organization. Selected Practice Recommendations for Contraceptive Use. Second edition. Geneva: World Health Organization, 2005.

136. Shain RN. Psychosocial consequences of vasectomy in developed and developing countries. In: G.I. Zatuchni, et al. (eds). Male contraception: advances and future prospects. Philadelphia: Harper and Row, 1986:34–53.

137. Holman CD, Wisniewski ZS, Semmens JB, Rouse IL, Bass AJ. Population-based outcomes after 28,246 in-hospital vasectomies and 1,902 vasovasostomies in Western Australia. BJU Int 2000;86:1043–1049.

138. Pitaktepsombati P, Janowitz B. Sterilization acceptance and regret in Thailand. Contraception 1991;44:623–637.

139. Potts JM, Pasqualotto FF, Nelson D, Thomas AJ Jr, Agarwal A. Patient characteristics associated with vasectomy reversal. J Urol 1999;161:1835–1839.

140. Belker AM, Thomas AJ Jr, Fuchs EF, Konnak JW, Sharlip ID. Results of 1,469 microsurgical vasectomy reversals by the Vasovasostomy Study Group. J Urol 1991; 145:505–511.

141. Practice Committee of the American Society for Reproductive Medicine. Vasectomy reversal. Fertil Steril 2004;82 Suppl 1:S194–198.

142. Lee HY. Twenty-year experience with vasovasotomy. J Urol 1986;136:413–415.

143. Takihara H. Treatment of obstructive azoospermia in male infertility—past, present, and future. Urology 1998;51:150–155.

144. Boorjian S, Lipkin M, Goldstein M. The impact of obstructive interval and sperm granuloma on outcome of vasectomy reversal. J Urol 2004;171:304–306.
145. Pollack AP, Barone MA. "Reversing vasectomy" In: J. Sciarra (ed). Gynecology and obstetrics. Vol. 6: Fertility regulation, psychosomatic problems, and human sexuality. Lippincott Williams & Wilkins. Philadelphia, 2000, chapter 48.
146. Borges E Jr, Rossi-Ferragut LM, Pasqualotto FF, Rocha CC, Iaconelli A Jr. Different intervals between vasectomy and sperm retrieval interfere in the reproductive capacity from vasectomized men. J Assist Reprod Genet 2003;20:33–37.
147. Kolettis PN, Sabanegh ES, D'amico AM, Box L, Sebesta M, Burns JR. Outcomes for vasectomy reversal performed after obstructive intervals of at least 10 years. Urology 2002;60:885–888.
148. Fuchs EF, Burt RA. Vasectomy reversal performed 15 years or more after vasectomy: correlation of pregnancy outcome with partner age and with pregnancy results of in vitro fertilization with intracytoplasmic sperm injection. Fertil Steril 2002;77:516–519.
149. Sukcharoen N, Sithipravej T, Promviengchai S, Chinpilas V, Boonkasemsanti W. No differences in outcome of surgical sperm retrieval with intracytoplasmic sperm injection at different intervals after vasectomy. Fertil Steril 2000;74:174–175.
150. Nicopoullos JD, Gilling-Smith C, Almeida PA, Ramsay JW. Effect of time since vasectomy and maternal age on intracytoplasmic sperm injection success in men with obstructive azoospermia after vasectomy. Fertil Steril 2004;82:367–373.
151. Kolettis PN, Thomas Jr AJ. Vasoepididymostomy for vasectomy reversal: a critical assessment in the era of intracytoplasmic sperm injection. J Urol 1997;158:467–470.
152. Pasqualotto FF, Lucon AM, Sobreiro BP, Pasqualotto EB, Arap S. The best infertility treatment for vasectomized men: assisted reproduction or vasectomy reversal? Rev Hosp Clin Fac Med Sao Paulo. 2004;59:312–315.
153. Donovan JF Jr, DiBaise M, Sparks AE, Kessler J, Sandlow JI. Comparison of microscopic epididymal sperm aspiration and intracytoplasmic sperm injection/in-vitro fertilization with repeat microscopic reconstruction following vasectomy: is second attempt vas reversal worth the effort? Hum Reprod 1998;13:387–93.

Postpartum Contraception and Lactation

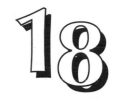

Kathy I. Kennedy, DrPH
James Trussell, PhD

- Breastmilk is the ideal source of nutrition for infants and confers immunological protection against many infections. Family planning clinicians can play an important role in promoting breastfeeding.

- The Lactational Amenorrhea Method (LAM) is a highly effective, *temporary* method of contraception, but must be carefully used. To maintain effective protection against pregnancy, another method of contraception must be used as soon as menstruation resumes, the frequency or duration of breastfeeds is reduced, bottle feeds or regular food supplements are introduced, or the baby reaches 6 months of age.

- Other good contraceptive options for lactating women are (1) barrier methods, such as the male or female condom, which also confer protection against sexually transmitted infections; (2) the Copper T 380A intrauterine device (IUD); (3) *progestin-only methods* such as the minipill, Implanon or Depo-Provera, or the Levonorgestrel intrauterine system (LNG IUS); and (4) the permanent methods, male or female sterilization for women or couples who want no more children.

- The *combined hormonal methods* administered in pills, patches, injectables, or vaginal rings are not good contraceptive options for lactating women because estrogen decreases milk supply.

- HIV can be transmitted through breastmilk. Therefore, in the United States, where safe alternatives to breastmilk are available, HIV-infected mothers are advised to avoid breastfeeding.

After childbirth, a woman soon becomes capable of becoming pregnant again since the postpartum period of infertility may be brief. Although the breastfeeding woman will have a longer period of infertility than will the nonbreastfeeding woman, her fertility usually returns during weaning, as the frequency of breastfeeds decreases. During weaning, the breastfeeding woman should use a contraceptive method so that she may breastfeed for as long as she chooses before becoming pregnant again. Fortunately, most family planning methods are compatible with breastfeeding, and the provider can play an important role in promoting both contraception and breastfeeding. In addition to helping to devise a postpartum plan for contraception, the provider can ensure that the new mother has several essential breastfeeding experiences and lessons while still in the hospital, prior to discharge after delivery (see Figure 18–1[1]). Breastmilk is the ideal source of nutrition for infants and confers immunological protection against many infections. Health experts around the globe have declared that all women should be enabled to breastfeed exclusively for 6 months,[2-7] to continue to breastfeed for 1 year[3,4,7] or 2 years or beyond,[2] and to have access to family planning information and services that allow them to sustain breastfeeding.[8]

POSTPARTUM INFERTILITY

During pregnancy, cyclic ovarian function is suspended. The corpus luteum, which arises from the ovulated follicle, secretes steroids, including estrogen and progesterone, that are essential in maintaining the early weeks of pregnancy. Later, steroids secreted by the placenta emerge to play a more dominant role in hormonal support of the pregnancy. Luteal and placental steroids suppress the mother's circulating levels of follicle stimulating hormone (FSH) and luteinizing hormone (LH) but more importantly disrupt their pulsatile release from her pituitary.[9] When the placenta is delivered, the inhibiting effects of estrogen and progesterone are removed so that levels of FSH and LH gradually rise and the pituitary resumes the pulsatile release of FSH and LH.[10]

Most nonlactating women resume menses within 4 to 6 weeks of delivery, but about one-third of first cycles are anovulatory, and a high proportion of first ovulatory cycles have a deficient corpus luteum that secretes sub-normal amounts of steroids. In the second and third menstrual cycles, 15% are anovulatory and 25% of ovulatory cycles have luteal-phase defects. On average, the first ovulation occurs 45 days postpartum, although few first ovulations are followed by normal luteal phases.[11] The duration of postpartum infertility is variable and unpredictable.

LACTATIONAL INFERTILITY

Lactation, or breastfeeding, further extends the period of infertility and depresses ovarian function.[12] Plasma levels of FSH return to normal follicular phase values by 4 to 8 weeks postpartum in breastfeeding

Clinical Guidelines for the Establishment of Exclusive Breastfeeding

1. Facilitate breastfeeding within the first hour after birth and provide for continuous skin-to-skin contact between mother and infant until after the first feeding

2. Assist the mother and infant in achieving a comfortable position and effective latch (attachment)

3. Keep the mother and infant together during the entire postpartum stay

4. Teach mothers to recognize and respond to early infant feeding cues and confirm that the baby is being fed at least 8 times in each 24 hours

5. Confirm that mothers understand the physiology of milk production, especially the role of milk removal

6. Confirm that mothers know how to wake a sleepy infant

7. Avoid using pacifiers, artificial nipples, and supplements, unless medically indicated

8. Observe and document at least one breastfeeding in each eight-hour period during the immediate postpartum period

9. Assess the mother and infant for signs of effective breastfeeding and intervene if transfer of milk is inadequate

10. Identify maternal and infant risk factors that may impact the mother's or infant's ability to breastfeed effectively and provide appropriate assistance and follow-up

11. Identify any maternal and infant contraindications to breastfeeding

12. If medically indicated, provide additional nutrition using a method of supplementation that is least likely to compromise the transition to exclusive breastfeeding

13. Confirm that the infant has a scheduled appointment with a primary care provider or health worker within five to seven days after birth

14. Provide appropriate breastfeeding education materials

15. Support exclusive breastfeeding during any illness or hospitalization of the mother or infant

16. Comply with the *International Code of Marketing of Breast-milk Substitutes* and subsequent World Health Assembly (WHA) resolutions, and avoid distribution of infant feeding product samples and advertisements for such products

17. Include family members or significant others in breastfeeding education

18. Provide anticipatory guidance for common problems that can interfere with exclusive breastfeeding

19. Confirm that mothers understand normal breastfed infant behaviors and have realistic expectations regarding infant care and breastfeeding

20. Discuss contraceptive options and their possible effect on milk production

Source: International Lactation Consultant Association (2005)[1] Reprinted with permission

Figure 18–1 Clinical Guidelines for the Establishment of Exclusive Breastfeeding

women.[13] In contrast, LH pulsation is disorganized in terms of the frequency or the amplitude of the LH pulse, in the majority of lactating women throughout most of the period of lactational amenorrhea.[14]

Nipple and areola sensitivity increases at birth.[15] Infant suckling stimulates the nerve endings in the nipple and areola. Nerve impulses are passed to the hypothalamus, stimulating the release of various hormones, including prolactin. Prolactin controls the rate of milk production but is not believed to play a major role in suppressing ovarian function.[16] Instead, suckling appears to disrupt the pulsatile release of gonadotropin releasing hormone (GnRH) by the hypothalamus,[13] perhaps by increasing hypothalamic β-endorphin production.[17] The interference with GnRH in turn averts the normal pulsatility of LH, which is required for follicle stimulation in the ovary. Small amounts of secreted estrogen at this time are insufficient to trigger an LH surge necessary to induce ovulation.[13,18]

Ovulation can occur even though the breastfeeding mother has not yet resumed menstruation. Only about 60% of ovulations preceding first menses have an adequate luteal phase.[19] Lactational amenorrhea becomes increasingly unreliable as an indicator of infertility beyond 6 months postpartum. The probability that ovulation will precede the first menses increases over time:[19,20]

- 33% to 45% during the first 3 months postpartum
- 64% to 71% during months 4 through 12
- 87% to 100% after 12 months.

Full or nearly full (unsupplemented) breastfeeding is associated with longer periods of lactational amenorrhea and infertility than is supplemented breastfeeding. Frequent stimulation of the breast by around-the-clock suckling helps maintain the cascade of neuroendocrine events that produces the contraceptive effect.[21] The breastfeeding characteristics that contribute significantly to delay the return of ovulation include a high frequency of breastfeeds, a long duration of each feed, a short interval between breastfeeds, and the presence of night feeds.[20,22] Milk production appears to be reduced far more by supplementary bottle feeds than by supplementary cup and spoon feeds.[20]

CONTRACEPTIVE BENEFITS OF LACTATION

In both traditional societies and developing countries, lactation plays a major role in prolonging birth intervals and thereby reducing fertility.[23] In developed countries, however, breastfeeding has a much smaller contraceptive impact because proportionately fewer infants are breastfed, and those who are breastfed are completely weaned at earlier ages. For example, in Indonesia, 96% of infants are breastfed, and those who are breastfed are not completely weaned until they are 2 years old on average.[24] In contrast, in the United States, only 71% of infants are ever breastfed with only 16% still breastfeeding at one year.[25]

THE LACTATIONAL AMENORRHEA METHOD (LAM) OF CONTRACEPTION

Women who breastfeed can learn to make use of breastfeeding's natural contraceptive effect. If the woman feeds her infant only from her breast (or gives supplemental non-breastmilk feeds only to a minor extent) and has not experienced her first postpartum menses (defined as any bleeding occurring after 56 days postpartum), then breastfeeding provides more than 98% protection from pregnancy in the first 6 months following a birth.[21,26,27] (See Figures 18–2 and 18–3.) The Lactational Amenorrhea Method (LAM) is the proactive application of exclusive breastfeeding during lactational amenorrhea for the first 6 months after delivery. Four prospective clinical studies of the contraceptive effect of this Lactational Amenorrhea Method (LAM) demonstrated cumulative 6-month life-table perfect-use pregnancy rates ranging from 0.5% to 1.5% among women who relied solely on LAM.[28-31] While pregnancy rates during the use of LAM compare favorably with those for many other methods of contraception (see Chapter 27 on Contraceptive Efficacy), even greater efficacy could be achieved by a combination of breastfeeding and use of an additional method of contraception.

LAM requires "full or nearly full" breastfeeding because the infant who obtains nearly all nutritional requirements through breastfeeding is providing maximal suckling stimulation at the breast. As long as additional foods do not decrease this optimal amount of suckling, small amounts of supplementation should have little or no effect on the return of fertility. Thus, if LAM is to be used, supplements should be given only infrequently, in small amounts, and not by bottle. The only real challenge concerning the correct use of LAM is determining the allowable extent of supplementation to the infant's diet, if the mother wishes to supplement. Figure 18–2 defines different infant feeding patterns and can be helpful in determining whether the woman is fully or nearly fully breastfeeding.[26,32] *Milk expression, such as by hand or pump, is not a substitute for breastfeeding in terms of its fertility inhibiting effect.* A study of LAM used by working women reported an elevated pregnancy rate (5.2%) indicating that frequent suckling, despite adequate milk production and full breastfeeding, is necessary to acquire the benefits of LAM.[33]

Experience with LAM in the United States is limited, and it is unknown whether more women would breastfeed if they appreciated the contraceptive effect of lactation (or the other benefits of breastfeeding). Some U.S. women are already highly motivated to breastfeed, and they

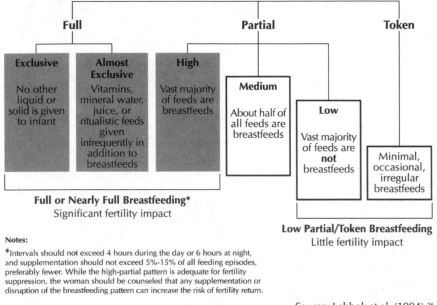

Figure 18–2 Schema for breastfeeding definition

would be good candidates to use LAM as a temporary contraceptive option.[34] Women who choose to use LAM are basically choosing to fully or nearly fully breastfeed for at least some period (up to 6 months), so the choice to use LAM should be associated with the motivation to maintain good breastfeeding practices. In the United States, LAM may be best promoted in the context of breastfeeding support (from the health-care system, friends, employers), which facilitates full/nearly full breast-feeding and maximizes the dura-ation of amenorrhea[35] and the duration for which women can use LAM. The Academy for Breastfeeding Medicine publishes clinical guidelines for the care of breastfeeding mothers and infants at www.bfmed.org/index.asp?menuID=139& firstlevelmenuID=139.

If a woman wishes to avoid becoming pregnant when LAM protection expires, then she must begin to use another contraceptive method at that time.[36,37]

POSTPARTUM SEXUALITY

Most American couples resume sexual intercourse within several weeks of delivery. Among U.S. lactating women, 66% are sexually active in the first month postpartum and 88% are sexually active in the second month postpartum.[38] In small samples of breastfeeding Western women,

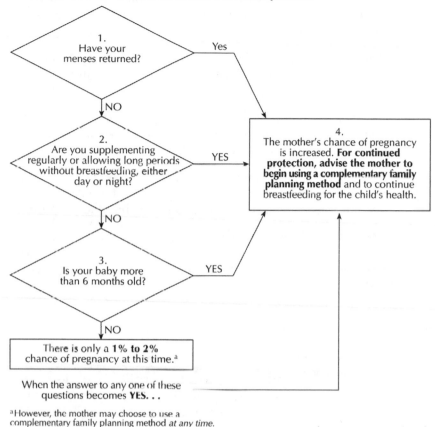

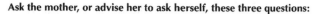

Source: Labbok et al. (1994).[26]

Figure 18–3 LAM: Lactational Amenorrhea Method

monthly coital frequency in the second month postpartum averaged 2.4, increasing to 3.2 to 4.9 in the third postpartum month.[39]

Contraception is only one counseling issue for postpartum women. Women—and men—may experience reduced sexual feelings associated with bodily changes caused by pregnancy and delivery. Discussion of these bodily changes may help to alleviate a couple's anxiety:

- Tenderness in the perineum may make intercourse painful, especially if there has been an episiotomy.

- Reduced postpartum estrogen secretion may result in diminished vaginal lubrication.

- Most women experience a heavy and bloody lochial discharge for a couple of weeks postpartum. This may interfere with a woman's sexual feeling.

- Couples may find that the exhaustion caused by the around-the-clock responsibilities of being a new parent temporarily decreases sexual drive.

- Lactation may diminish the erotic significance of the breasts. Couples need to communicate feelings about whether sucking or touching the breasts is acceptable.

- Bonding between mother and child creates skills and commitment in the mother and trust and security in the infant but may interfere with the mother's emotional availability to her partner.

- Conversely, a birth (especially if planned) can be an exceedingly joyous experience that can enhance sexual intimacy. To some men and women, the shape or fullness of the lactating breast is particularly arousing.

I NITIATING CONTRACEPTIVE USE POSTPARTUM

Counseling for postpartum contraception should begin in the prenatal period because many methods can be provided at the time of delivery or during the hospital stay, such as IUDs, female sterilization and, for nonbreastfeeding women, Implanon or Depo-Provera. For these methods provided immediately upon delivery, it is important to plan in advance, preferably in the prenatal period, so informed choice is valid and method choice and initiation is uncomplicated, convenient, and cost-effective. One large study showed that one-year pregnancy and contraceptive continuation rates were the same whether the women received family planning counseling before or after the delivery; the only exception was that women counseled before delivery in one urban center chose sterilization at a significantly higher rate.[40]

Traditionally, a postpartum follow-up consultation occurred at 6 weeks because the uterus had pretty much involuted and healed by this time. However, a physical exam can reasonably occur at any time between 3 and 8 weeks postpartum. In terms of contraceptive service delivery, routine adherence to the 6-week convention does not seem appropriate. The authors therefore advocate an individual approach to timing postpartum follow-up and contraceptive initiation. Although nearly all contraceptive methods can be used postpartum, the methods vary in terms of when in the postpartum period they can be initiated:[41-43]

- 6 weeks is too late for non-breastfeeding mothers who wish to start using combined oral contraceptives, the patch, the vaginal ring, Lunelle, Implanon or Depo-Provera.[44]

- 3 weeks is too soon for inserting an IUD or fitting a diaphragm.

- 3 weeks if the couple has been unable to select a contraceptive method by the time of hospital discharge.[45]

When the couple's method of choice cannot be initiated during the hospital stay after delivery, they can choose temporary methods such as LAM or the brief use of condoms and plan to initiate a longer-term method later. Schedule the first postpartum visit for the most logical time based on the longer-term method choice. For example, if a breastfeeding woman will be using progestin-only pills, schedule her follow-up visit at 6 weeks postpartum, with the plan for her to use condoms or LAM until that time. To help ensure success, provide a cycle of progestin-only pills (or a prescription) and a package of lubricated condoms at hospital discharge, and instruct her about when to use each. Perhaps most importantly, contact the woman 2 to 4 weeks after delivery to check on her postpartum recovery and to confirm and support her personal contraception plan.

A systematic review of the research concluded that the effectiveness of education about postpartum contraception has not been established.[46] A study of pregnant women revealed that only 30% had discussed family planning options with their provider, and IUD options were inadequately discussed.[47] Apparently, given clinicians' appropriate focus on safe pregnancy and delivery, attention to child spacing is commonly overlooked. The following considerations may prove useful when counseling and providing contraceptives to the postpartum woman, whether or not she is breastfeeding:

- *Withdrawal* may be a good method for couples in the postpartum period. Withdrawal is effective if used correctly and consistently. (See Chapter 27.)

- *Condoms* are attractive options. Postpartum endometritis is a serious complication. The risk of introducing bacteria into the uterus is elevated before cervical closure is complete.

- *Barrier method* use may need to be delayed for methods other than condoms:

  — Episiotomies may still be tender. Fitting a woman for a diaphragm may cause discomfort.

  — Avoid the diaphragm and contraceptive sponge until 6 weeks after delivery. The diaphragm cannot be (re)fitted properly until that time. Moreover, the risk of toxic shock syndrome is increased when blood, including the post-partum lochia, is present.[48] (See Chapter 14.)

— The sponge (though not the diaphragm) has much higher failure rates among women who have delivered a child than among women who have not, *even during perfect use.* (See Chapter 27.) Inform women about this substantial decrease in efficacy for parous women so they can make an informed choice of a contraceptive method.

- *Postpartum abstinence*, if practiced properly, is 100% effective in preventing pregnancy. It can, however, be notoriously difficult to maintain. Counsel women about other contraceptive methods should they desire to resume intercourse.

- *Copper intrauterine devices (IUDs)* (but not the LNG IUS[42]) can be inserted postpartum, either (1) immediately after the expulsion of the placenta (immediate postpartum insertion), or (2) within 48 hours of delivery (delayed postpartum insertion). An IUD can be inserted immediately after a cesarean delivery through the uterine incision.[41,42] Avoid IUD insertion when premature rupture of the membranes, prolonged labor, or fever has occurred, because of the elevated risk of infection.[49,50] Immediate postpartum insertion has not been associated with excessive bleeding or endometritis.[51] Expulsion rates following postpartum insertion are higher than those following interval insertion, but they are lower for immediate than for delayed postpartum insertion.[49] A small study compared the expulsion of Copper T380A IUDs inserted within the first 10 minutes after placental delivery (using a ring forceps inserted through the uterine cervix) with the same type of IUD placed through the hysterotomy site transoperatively in women who delivered by cesarean section. Expulsion was detected by ultrasound and not just clinical examination. In women who delivered vaginally, 50% of the IUDs had been expelled, while none were missing among those who delivered surgically.[52] If insertion is not performed within the first 48 hours postpartum, it should be delayed until 4 to 6 weeks postpartum.[53]

- *Sterilization* presents excellent options for appropriate candidates:

— Vasectomy is an appropriate postpartum choice for couples who want a permanent method. As soon as the health of the mother and infant is determined to be sound, the vasectomy can be performed. If the woman is breastfeeding, a back-up method may not be needed while waiting for confirmation that the vasectomy has taken effect.[14,41] As with tubal ligation, vasectomy requires counseling and reflection under non-stressful circumstances, preferably before delivery.[41,42]

— Tubal ligation performed during the immediate postpartum period can be a more cost-effective and simpler technique than interval sterilization. While tubal ligation is a highly effective method of contraception, a small risk of sterilization failure persists for at least a decade. However, partial salpingectomy performed postpartum carries the lowest known pregnancy risk of any female sterilization procedure.[54] Discuss immediate postpartum sterilization well before the delivery to help ensure that consent is fully informed.[55] Take great care that the woman is confident of this choice[56] since the performance of tubal sterilization during the postpartum period is a risk factor for regret.[57] (See Chapter 17 on Female and Male Sterilization Methods.) After a vaginal delivery, sterilization should be performed by minilaparotomy within 48 hours or else delayed for 4 to 6 weeks. After 48 hours, access to the tubes is reduced and the risk of infection increased.[55] Minilaparotomy can be performed up to 6 days postpartum,[42] but infection precautions must be taken and the procedure will likely be more difficult. Tubal ligation can be performed through the abdominal incision after a cesarean delivery. As with minilaparotomy after vaginal delivery, cesarean sterilization may need to be delayed in the case of complications, such as severe pre-eclampsia, eclampsia, premature rupture of the membranes, sepsis, fever, severe hemorrhage, uterine rupture or perforation.[42,58]

POSTPARTUM CONTRACEPTION FOR THE NONBREASTFEEDING WOMAN

If she wishes to avoid becoming pregnant, the nonbreastfeeding woman should begin using a contraceptive method immediately postpartum or at least by the beginning of the fourth postpartum week.[44] Most nonbreastfeeding mothers have few restrictions placed on which method of contraceptive they can choose. Nonetheless, a few guidelines—in addition to those given above—are warranted:

- Combined oral contraceptives (COCs) and the combined patch, injectable, and vaginal ring may be prescribed immediately postpartum. However, caution women not to use them until 3 weeks after delivery.[41-43] The risk of postpartum thrombophlebitis and thromboembolism is greatest just after delivery.[59] Delaying combined hormonal contraceptive use for at 3 weeks tends to bypass the period of peak risk for postpartum thrombotic complications.[60]

- Caution women that it is difficult to practice fertility awareness before their cycles are reestablished and cyclic signs of fertility return.

- Suggest that lubricated condoms are a good option at least for the short period before the woman becomes better suited to her preferred method.

- Implanon can be inserted and Depo-Provera can be safely injected immediately postpartum. Discuss these options before delivery to ensure that consent is fully informed.

- The LNG IUS should not be inserted during the first 3 weeks after delivery.[42]

POSTPARTUM CONTRACEPTION FOR THE BREASTFEEDING WOMAN

NONHORMONAL METHODS

General comments regarding contraceptive use among postpartum women are given above. In addition, the following considerations are relevant for women who are breastfeeding. Breastfeeding is a condition for which there is no restriction on the use of nonhormonal methods.[42]

Tubal ligation can be performed immediately postpartum, although it can disrupt lactation if it requires general anesthesia or separation of mother and infant. Both problems can be minimized by performing the procedure with only regional or local anesthetic.[61] If tubal ligation does not occur while the mother is on the delivery table, breastfeeding should occur just before, and be delayed immediately after, anesthesia, to reduce the transfer of the anesthetic agent to the infant.[62,63]

Copper T380A IUDs are also good choices for breastfeeding women. The copper on the Copper T does not affect the quantity or quality of breastmilk.[64] (See the following section on Hormonal Methods for information on the IUDs containing a progestin or progesterone.) Some women experience mild uterine cramping when they breastfeed with an IUD in place, but the cramping does not usually interfere with lactation or with the effectiveness of the IUD. IUD insertion is less painful, and pain and bleeding removal rates are lower, for the lactating mother.[65,66] Although case reports and small studies suggested that the risk of uterine perforation is higher among breastfeeding women, larger studies find low rates of perforation in both breastfeeding and nonbreastfeeding women.[50,65–67] Nevertheless, it seems prudent to exercise special care when inserting an IUD postpartum.

Spermicides and barrier methods have no effect on the ability to breastfeed. The lubricated condom is especially useful in the postpartum period because of increased vaginal dryness due to estrogen deficiency. Spermicides also may help offset dryness. In the United States, barrier methods are the most widely used contraceptives among lactating mothers in the first 6 months postpartum.[38] In animal studies, nonoxynol-9 is absorbed through the skin and secreted in breastmilk.[68] The question of whether nonoxynol-9 is secreted in breastmilk has not been completely evaluated in humans. (See Chapter 14 on Vaginal Barriers and Spermicides.)

Lactational Amenorrhea Method (LAM) provides effective protection against pregnancy for up to 6 months postpartum. If continued protection is desired, another method of contraception must be introduced when the LAM criteria indicate a return to the risk of pregnancy. (See the detailed description of LAM earlier in this chapter.)

Fertility awareness methods can be difficult to use during the return of fertility, which can extend for many cycles during lactation.[69] The couple needs to abstain for 2 weeks in order to establish a "basic infertile pattern" of cervical mucus (and other) symptoms. Intercourse can then occur every other night unless/until there is some change in the basic infertile pattern, in which case more abstinence is necessary.[70] The changing fertility symptoms after the first postpartum menses may be especially difficult for new users to identify, and may lead to an increased risk for unplanned pregnancy.[71]

Basal body temperature cannot be ascertained unless a woman has at least 6 hours of uninterrupted sleep. Thus, the woman who gets up in the night to care for her infant is precluded from using the temperature symptom to help determine her fertility status.

The rules for using the symptothermal method during breastfeeding have been found to detect the onset of true fertility extremely well. However, these same rules often necessitate many days of abstinence when there is virtually no risk of pregnancy.[72] However, if they use the proposed new "TwoDay Method," breastfeeding women who want to use a fertility awareness method may need to abstain for fewer days.[73] Recommend LAM to users of fertility awareness methods who are breastfeeding. LAM can eliminate the requirements for abstinence for up to 6 months with no apparent additional risk of unplanned pregnancy.[74] The transition from LAM use to the use of a fertility awareness method begins with the establishment of a basic infertile pattern.[70,72]

HORMONAL METHODS

The use of hormonal contraception by a lactating woman is an area of dispute among experts.[75] Since all steroids pass through the breastmilk to the infant, the World Health Organization (WHO) and the International Planned Parenthood Federation do not consider hormonal methods of contraception to be the category of first choice for breastfeeding women.[41-43,76] Estrogen decreases the volume of milk.

Progestin-only contraceptives such as Implanon, the LNG IUS, Depo-Provera, and minipills do not have adverse effects on lactation, and some studies suggest they may even increase milk volume. They do not have adverse effects on child growth and development.[77-88] In addition, their contraceptive efficacy is high (see Chapter 27), and they are simple to use. Therefore, these methods are good options for lactating women who wish to postpone a subsequent pregnancy.

The WHO recommends that breastfeeding women delay using these methods until 6 weeks after delivery.[42,43] This recommendation is based on the admittedly theoretical concern that early neonatal exposure to exogenous steroids, which have passed from the contraceptive into the milk, should be avoided if possible. The binding capacity of plasma is low, the neonatal liver is not well able to conjugate and oxidize drugs, and the immature kidneys are inefficient in excretion.[14,77] Unable to be cleared from the infant's circulation, exogenous steroids or their metabolites may "compete with natural hormones for receptor sites in sex organs, brain or other tissues."[89] Experts issue their caution because animal literature has indicated long-term effects from inappropriate hormone exposure at critical postpartum periods.[89]

Although progestin-only contraceptives would probably have no adverse effects on lactation or infant health if used soon after delivery, little research has been conducted on their immediate postpartum use, since initiation prior to 6 weeks has been discouraged. A prudent approach would be to share information about the risks and benefits of early use with the client, and, if the client consents, to wait until 6 weeks postpartum before starting progestin-only pills, inserting Implanon capsules, or giving the Depo-Provera injection. However, if a breastfeeding woman requests Implanon insertion before leaving the hospital after delivery (especially if she plans to supplement the infant's diet relatively soon after delivery), and if there is some compelling reason to start the method early (if other more appropriate methods are not available or acceptable), then the real long-term contraceptive benefit of using this method seems likely to exceed the theoretical risks. Because the contraceptive benefit to the lactating woman in obtaining Depo-Provera immediately postpartum is smaller and the theoretical risks might be higher (because the hormonal levels are relatively high in the immediate post-injection days), the case for injecting Depo-Provera before 6 weeks postpartum would be less compelling; a woman unlikely to return for a postpartum visit may be equally unlikely to return for a repeat injection.

COLOR PHOTOS
of Combined and Progestin-Only Oral Contraceptives

The twelve color pages of pills are organized as follows:

Color photos of pills from lowest to highest estrogen dose

- Progestin-only pills with no estrogen: Micronor and NOR-QD

- Lowest estrogen pills with 20 micrograms of the estrogen,
  ethinyl estradiol: Alesse, Levlite, LoEstrin 1/20, and Mircette

- All of the 25-, 30- and 35-microgram pills (all ethinyl estradiol)

- All of the phasic pills

- Highest estrogen pills, with 50 micrograms of estrogen
  (ethinyl estradiol OR mestranol). Mestranol is converted in the body to
  ethinyl estradiol; 50 mcg of mestranol is equivalent to 35 mcg of ethinyl
  estradiol

**Pills which are pharmacologically exactly the same are grouped within
boxes. The color and packaging of pills dispensed in clinics may differ from
pills in pharmacies.*

Pills you can prescribe as emergency contraceptive pills

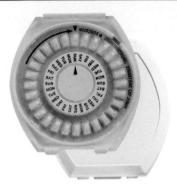

MICRONOR® TABLETS
28-DAY REGIMEN
(0.35 mg norethindrone) (lime green)
Ortho-McNeil

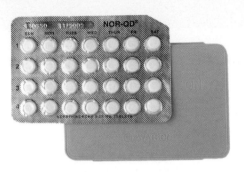

NOR-QD® TABLETS
(0.35 mg norethindrone) (yellow)
Watson

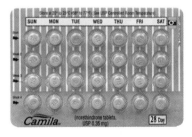

CAMILLA®
(norethindrone tablets, USP 0.35 mg)
(active pills light pink)
Barr Laboratories

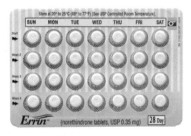

ERRIN®
(norethindrone tablets, USP 0.35 mg)
(active pills yellow)
Barr Laboratories

(B)

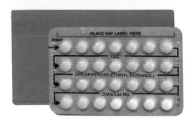

YAZ 28 TABLETS
(3.0 mg drospirenone/
02 mg ethinyl estradiol)
(active pills pink)
Berlex

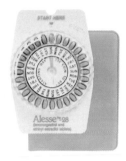

ALESSE - 28 TABLETS
(0.1 mg levonorgestrel/20 mcg ethinyl estradiol)
(active pills pink)
Wyeth

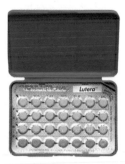

LUTERA
(0.1 mg levonorgestrel/20 mcg ethinyl estradiol)
(active pills white)
Watson

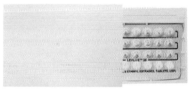

LEVLITE™ - 28 TABLETS
(0.1 mg levonorgestrel/20 mcg ethinyl estradiol)
(active pills pink)
Berlex

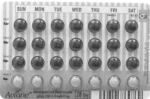

AVIANE®
(levonogestrel/ethinyl estradiol tablets,
USP 0.10 mg/0.02 mg)
(active pills orange)
Barr Laboratories

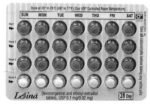

LESSINA®
(levonorgestrel/ethinyl estradiol tablets,
USP 0.1 mg/0.02 mg)
(active pills pink)
Barr Laboratories

(C)

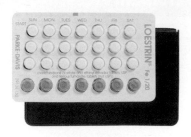

LOESTRIN® FE 1/20
(1 mg norethindrone acetate/20 mcg ethinyl estradiol/
75 mg ferrous fumarate [7d])
(active pills white)
Barr Laboratories

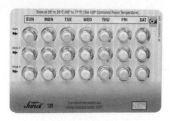

JUNEL ™
(norethindrone acetate and ethinyl estradiol tablets,
USP 1 mg/20 mcg)
(active pills light yellow)
Barr Laboratories

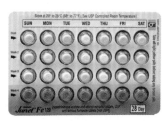

JUNEL ™ Fe
(norethindrone acetate and ethinyl estradiol tablets,
USP and ferrous fumarate tablets 1 mg/20 mcg)
(active pills light yellow)
Barr Laboratories

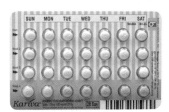

KARIVA®
(desogestrel/estradiol tablets 0.15 mg/0.02
mg and ethinyl estradiol tablets 0.01 mg)
(active pills white and light blue)
Barr Laboratories

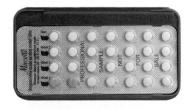

MIRCETTE - 28 TABLETS
(0.15 mg desogestrel/ 20 mcg ethinyl
estradiol X
21 (white)/placebo X 2 (green)/
10 mcg ethinyl estradiol X 5 (yellow)
Barr Laboratories

(D)

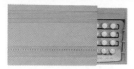

LEVLEN® 28 TABLETS
(0.15 mg levonorgestrel/30 mcg ethinyl estradiol)
(active pills light orange)
Berlex

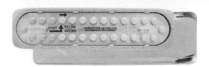

NORDETTE®-28 TABLETS
(0.15 mg levonorgestrel/30 mcg ethinyl estradiol)
(active pills light orange)
Wyeth

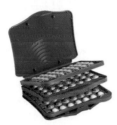

SEASONALE
(0.15 mg levonorgestrel/30 mcg ethinyl estradiol)
84 active pink pills followed by 7 placebo pills
Barr Laboratories

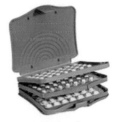

SEASONIQUE
(0.15 mg levonorgestrel/30 mcg ethinyl estradiol)
84 active pink pills followed by 7 pills
with 10 mcg ethinyl estradiol
Barr Laboratories

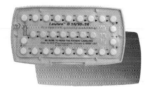

LEVORA TABLETS
(0.15 mg levonorgestrel/30 mcg ethinyl estradiol)
(active pills white)
Watson

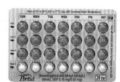

PORTIA®
(levonorgestrel and ethinyl estradiol tablets,
USP 0.15 mg/0.03 mg)
(active pills pink)
Barr Laboratories

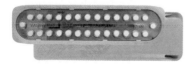

LO/OVRAL®-28 TABLETS
(0.3 mg norgestrel/30 mcg ethinyl estradiol)
(active pills white)
Wyeth

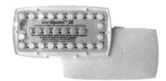

LOW-OGESTREL - 28
(0.3 mg norgestrel/30 mcg ethinyl estradiol)
(active pills white)
Watson

CRYSELLE®
(norgestrel and ethinyl estradiol tablets,
USP 0.3 mg/0.03 mg)
(active pills white)
Barr Laboratories

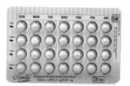

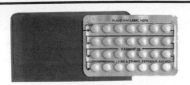

YASMIN 28 TABLETS
(3.0 mg drospirenone/30 mcg ethinyl estradiol)
(active pills yellow)
Berlex

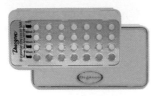

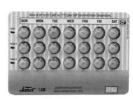

DESOGEN® 28 TABLETS
(0.15 mg desogestrel/30 mcg ethinyl estradiol)
(active pills white)
Organon

**ORTHO-CEPT® TABLETS
28-DAY REGIMEN**
(0.15 mg desogestrel/30 mcg ethinyl estradiol)
(active pills orange)
Ortho-McNeil

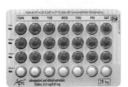

APRI®
(desogestrel/ethinyl estradiol 0.15 mg/0.03 mg tablets)
(active pills rose)
Barr Laboratories

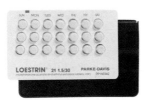

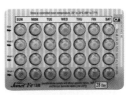

LOESTRIN® 21 1.5/30
(1.5 mg norethindrone acetate/30 mcg ethinyl estradiol)
(active pills green)
Barr Laboratories

JUNEL ™
(norethindrone acetate and ethinyl estradiol
tablets, USP 1.5 mg./30 mcg.)
(active pills pink)
Barr Laboratories

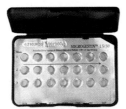

MICROGESTIN 1.5/30 with or without Fe
(1.5 mg norethindrone acetate/
30 mcg ethinyl estradiol)
Watson

JUNEL ™ Fe
(norethindrone acetate and ethinyl estradiol tablets,
USP and ferrous fumarate tablets 1.5 mg/30 mcg)
(active pills pink)
Barr Laboratories

(F)

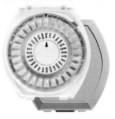

ORTHO-CYCLEN® 28 TABLETS
(0.25 mg norgestimate/35 mcg ethinyl estradiol)
(active pills blue)
Ortho-McNeil

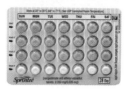

SPRINTEC®
(norgestimate and ethinyl estradiol tablets,
0.250 mg/0.035 mg)
(active pills blue)
Barr Laboratories

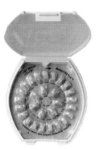

MONONESESSA
(norgestimate and ethinyl estradiol
tablets, 0.250 mg/0.035 mg)
Watson

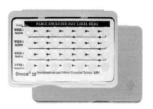

OVCON® 35 28-DAY
(0.4 mg norethindrone/35 mcg ethinyl estradiol)
(active pills peach)
Warner-Chilcott
Now there is a chewable Ovcon-35 pill!

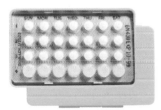

DEMULEN® 1/35-28
(1 mg ethynodiol diacetate/35 mcg ethinyl estradiol)
(active pills white)
Pharmacia - A Division of Pfizer

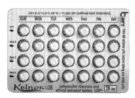

KELNOR™
(ethynodiol diacetate 1 mg. and ethinyl
estradiol 35 mcg, USP)
(active pills light yellow)
Barr Laboratories

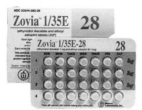

ZOVIA® 1/35E-28
(1 mg ethynodiol diacetate/35 mcg ethinyl estradiol)
(active pills light pink)
Watson

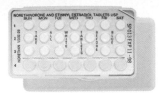

NORETHIN 1/35E–28
(1 mg norethindrone/35 mcg ethinyl estradiol)
(active pills white)
Shire

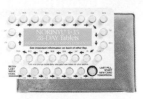

NORINYL® 1+35 28-DAY TABLETS
(1 mg norethindrone/35 mcg ethinyl estradiol)
(active pills yellow-green)
Watson

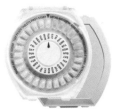

ORTHO-NOVUM® 1/35 28 TABLETS
(1 mg norethindrone/35 mcg ethinyl estradiol)
(active pills peach)
Ortho-McNeil

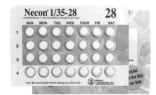

NECON 1/35-28
(1 mg norethindrone/35 mcg ethinyl estradiol)
(active pills dark yellow)
Watson

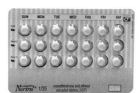

NORTREL®
(norethindrone and ethinyl estradiol tablets,
USP 1/0.035 mg)
(active pills yellow)
Barr Laboratories

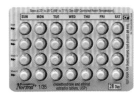

NORTREL®
(norethindrone and ethinyl estradiol tablets,
USP 1.0 mg/0.035 mg 28-day regimen)
(active pills yellow)
Barr Laboratories

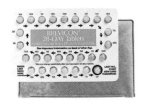

BREVICON®
28-DAY TABLETS
(0.5 mg norethindrone/
35 mcg ethinyl estradiol)
(active pills blue)
Watson

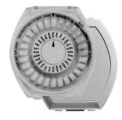

MODICON® TABLETS
28-DAY REGIMEN
(0.5 mg norethindrone/35 mcg ethinyl estradiol)
(active pills white)
Ortho-McNeil

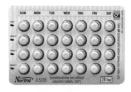

NORTREL®
(norethindrone and ethinyl estradiol
tablets, USP 0.5/0.035 mg)
(active pills light yellow)
Barr Laboratories

(H)

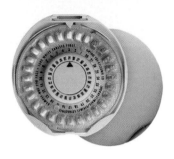

ORTHO TRI-CYCLEN® LO - 28 TABLETS
(norgestimate/ethinyl estradiol)
0.18 mg/25 mcg (7d) (white),
0.215 mg/25 mcg (7d) (light blue),
0.25 mg/25 mcg (7d) (dark blue)
remaining 7 placebo pills are green
Ortho-McNeil

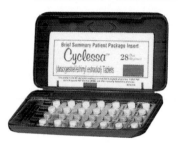

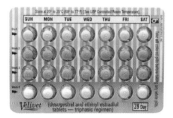

CYCLESSA
(desogestrel/ethinyl estradiol - triphasic regimen)
0.1 mg/25 mcg (7d) (light yellow)
0.125 mg/25 mcg (7d) (orange)
0.150 mg/25 mcg (7d) (red)
Organon

VELIVET®
(desogestrel/ethinyl estradiol tablets - triphasic regimen)
(active pills beige, orange and pink)
Barr Laboratories

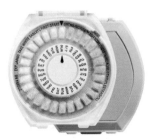

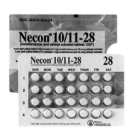

ORTHO-NOVUM® 10/11 - 28 TABLETS
(norethindrone/ethinyl estradiol)
0.5 mg/35 mcg (10d) (white),
1 mg/35 mcg (11d) (peach)
Ortho-McNeil

NECON® 10/11 - 28 TABLETS
(norethindrone/ethinyl estradiol)
0.5 mg/35 mcg (10d) (white),
1 mg/35 mcg (11d) (peach)
Watson

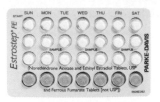

ESTROSTEP® FE - 28 TABLETS
(norethindrone acetate/ethinyl estradiol)
1 mg/20 mcg (5d) (white triangular),
1 mg/30 mcg (7d) (white square),
1 mg/35 mcg (9d), 75 mg ferrous
fumarate (7d) (white round)
Pfizer

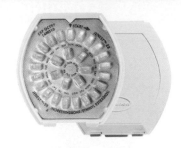

JENEST 28 TABLETS
(norethindrone/ethinyl estradiol)
0.5 mg/35 mcg (7d) (white),
1 mg/35 mcg (14d) (peach)
Organon

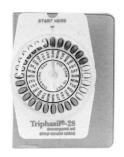

TRIPHASIL®- 28 TABLETS
(levonorgestrel/
ethinyl estradiol—triphasic regimen)
0.050 mg/30 mcg (6d) (brown),
0.075 mg/40 mcg (5d) (white),
0.125 mg/30 mcg (10d) (light yellow)
Wyeth

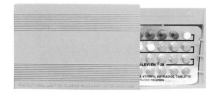

TRI-LEVLEN® 28 TABLETS
(levonorgestrel/
ethinyl estradiol—triphasic regimen)
0.050 mg/30 mcg (6d) (brown),
0.075 mg/40 mcg (5d) (white),
0.125 mg/30 mcg (10d) (light yellow)
Berlex

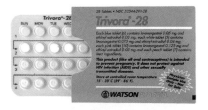

TRIVORA®
(levonorgestrel/ethinyl estradiol—
triphasic regimen)
0.050 mg/30 mcg (6d), 0.075 mg/
40 mcg (5d), 0.125 mg/30 mcg (10d) (pink)
Watson

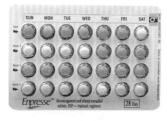

ENPRESSE®
(levonorgestrel and ethinyl estradiol tablets,
USP - triphasic regimen)
(active pills pink, white and orange)
Barr Laboratories

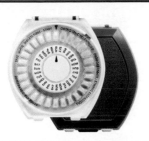

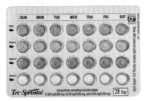

ORTHO TRI-CYCLEN® - 28 TABLETS
(norgestimate/ethinyl estradiol)
0.18 mg/35 mcg (7d) (white),
0.215 mg/35 mcg (7d) (light blue),
0.25 mg/35 mcg (7d) (blue)
Ortho-McNeil

TRI-SPRINTEC®
(norgestimate and ethinyl estradiol tablets -
triphasic regimen)
(active pills gray, light blue and blue)
Barr Laboratories

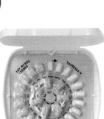

TRINESSA
(norgestimate/ethinyl estradiol)
0.18 mg/35 mcg (7d) (white),
0.215 mg/35 mcg (7d) (light blue),
0.25 mg/35 mcg (7d) (dark blue)
remaining 7 placebo pills are green
Watson

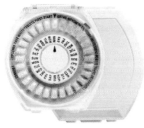

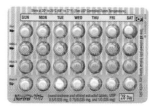

ORTHO-NOVUM® 7/7/7 - 28 TABLETS
(norethindrone/ethinyl estradiol)
0.5 mg/35 mcg (7d) (white),
0.75 mg/35 mcg (7d) (light peach),
1 mg/35 mcg (7d) (peach)
Ortho-McNeil

NORTREL® 7/7/7
(norethindrone and ethinyl estradiol tablets,
USP - triphasic regimen)
(active pills light yellow,
blue and peach)
Barr Laboratories

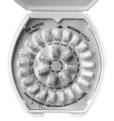

NECON® 7/7/7
0.5 mg/35 mcg (7d) (yellow),
0.75 mg/35 mcg (7d) (blue),
1 mg/35 mcg (7d) (peach)
Watson

(K)

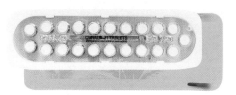

OVRAL - 21 TABLETS
(0.5 mg norgestrel/50 mcg ethinyl estradiol)
(active pills white)
Wyeth

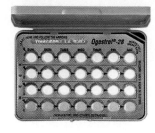

OEGSTREL
(0.5 mg norgestrel/50 mcg ethinyl estradiol)
(active pills white)
Watson

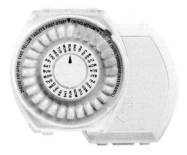

ORTHO-NOVUM® 1/50 - 28 TABLETS
(1 mg norethindrone/50 mcg mestranol)
(active pills yellow)
Ortho-McNeil

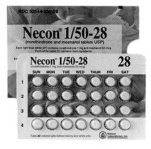

NECON 1/50 - 28 TABLETS
(1 mg norethindrone/50 mcg mestranol)
Watson

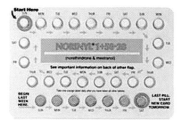

NORINYL® 1/50
(1 mg norethindrone/50 mcg mestranol)
Watson

(L)

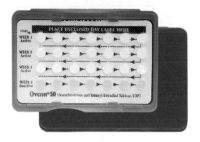

OVCON® 50 28-DAY
(1 mg norethindrone/50 mcg ethinyl estradiol)
(active pills yellow)
Warner-Chilcott

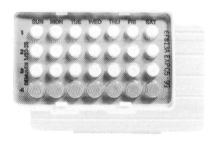

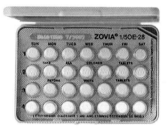

DEMULEN® 1/50-28
(1 mg ethynodiol diacetate/50 mcg ethinyl estradiol)
(active pills white)
Pharmacia - A Division of Pfizer

ZOVIA® 1/50
(1 mg ethynodiol diacetate/50 mcg ethinyl estradiol)
Watson

PILLS AS EMERGENCY CONTRACEPTIVES:
2 Different Approaches: Progestin-Only Pills OR Combined Pills

PROGESTIN-ONLY PILLS

Plan B

1 + 1 pill 12 hours apart OR
2 Plan B Pills *(white)* ASAP after unprotected sex

Plan B available without a prescription in pharmacies to women and men ≥ 18 years old. Plan B is NOT carried in all pharmacies. Check in advance. Ask your pharmacy to carry Plan B.

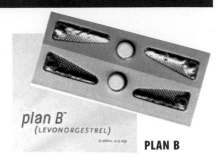

PLAN B

Antinausea meds not necessary

COMBINED ORAL CONTRACEPTIVES

2 + 2 pills 12 hours apart
Ogestrel *(white pills)*
Ovral *(white pills)*

(Ogestrel and Ovral are NOT carried in all pharmacies. Check in advance.)

4 + 4 pills 12 hours apart
Cryselle *(white pills)*
Enpresse *(orange pills)*
Jolessa *(pink pills)*
Low-Ogestrel *(white pills)*
Lo-Ovral *(white pills)*
Levora *(white pills)*
Levlen *(light orange pills)*
Nordette *(light orange pills)*
Portia *(pink pills)*
Quasense *(white pills)*
Seasonale *(pink pills)*
Seasonique *(light blue pills)*
Triphasil *(yellow pills)*
Tri-Levlen *(yellow pills)*
Trivora *(pink pills)*

> **Have your patient take antinausea medication an hour before the first dose if using any of the combined oral contraceptives as emergency contraception. This is not necessary if using Plan B.**

5 + 5 pills 12 hours apart
Alesse *(pink pills)*
Levlite *(pink pills)*
Aviane *(orange pills)*
Lessina *(pink pills)*
Lutera *(white pills)*

Discuss these options before delivery to ensure that consent is fully informed.

Since the precipitous withdrawal of natural progesterone 2 to 3 days postpartum is the physiological trigger for lactogenesis,[90] receipt of a high-dose of exogenous progestin (as with a Depo-Provera injection or in the first week after the insertion of an implant) before the withdrawal may interfere with the stimulus for milk synthesis. This reasoning argues for a delay in commencing progestin-only contraception, especially injectable formulas, until the mature milk has come in.[91] If a woman wants to use Depo-Provera immediately, and no other appropriate methods are available or acceptable, then encourage her to remain in the hospital until her mature milk comes in. Some studies of Depo-Provera and progestin-only pills have found no overall deleterious effect of progestin on milk volume when begun as early as the first week postpartum,[92,93] suggesting that very early exposure to progestin-only contraceptives is not always detrimental to lactogenesis. However, in these studies, progestin might have been initiated after the withdrawal of natural progesterone. Similarly, a study of progestin-only methods saw no effect of progestin method use on breastfeeding duration or child growth, but the average time to administration of the method was more than 2 days postpartum. Also, women were not randomized into the treatment groups, and breastfeeding duration was short for all women.[94] In another non-randomized study, the Implanon implant resulted in the same breastfeeding duration and infant growth as a non-medicated IUD for up to 3 years.[95]

Studies in China and Bolivia showed that breastfeeding women tolerate Depo-Provera's disruption of menstrual cyclicity better than non-breastfeeding women, and their method continuation rates are higher.[96,97] In a phase II clinical trial, a progesterone-releasing vaginal ring was associated with prolonged lactational amenorrhea, which represents a health benefit for the woman.[98] Studies of other progestin-only contraceptives initiated after 6 weeks postpartum show that lactational amenorrhea is prolonged.[99]

As with other progestin-only methods, the LNG IUS is not recommended for use by breastfeeding women until 6 weeks postpartum.[41–43,49,53]

The recommendation to delay the use of progestin-only methods for 6 weeks is not without its detractors. The British Faculty of Family Planning and Reproductive Health Care Clinical Effectiveness Unit believes that it is unnecessary to wait 6 weeks, but these professionals are unable to agree among themselves when it is safe to commence a progestin-only method during lactation.[100] As long as it remains ethically unacceptable to randomize neonates to early exposure to progestins, the risks of this exposure will remain theoretical. This circumstance makes informed choice more important than usual. South African investigators provided women with appropriate information about immediate versus delayed progestin injection, and women were able to make their own decisions about the timing of initiation.[101]

Combined hormonal contraceptives (the combined pill, patch, injectable, and vaginal ring) should not be used by breastfeeding mothers in the first 6 months postpartum unless other more appropriate methods are unavailable or unacceptable.[42,43] A reduction in milk supply, and possibly child growth, has been associated with the estrogen component in combined pills, even those with low-dose preparations.[102,103] A review of the literature has challenged this conclusion, claiming that the studies showing a reduction in milk supply associated with combined pills were flawed.[104,105] Use of combined pills may alter the composition of breastmilk, although results vary among studies; most studies report declines in mineral content.[103]

Just when combined hormonal contraceptives can be provided to lactating women remains a subject of disagreement. It would be ideal to avoid the use of combined hormonal methods entirely during breastfeeding especially since progestin-only methods are available.[106] The International Planned Parenthood Federation states that under normal circumstances combined hormonal contraceptives should not be used by breastfeeding women at all.[41] The World Health Organization (WHO) advises against the use of combined methods until at least 6 months postpartum.[42,43] The use of combined hormonal methods before 6 weeks is judged by WHO experts to represent an unacceptable health risk, and use between 6 weeks and 6 months represents a condition where the theoretical or proven risks usually outweigh the advantages. When a woman's informed choice is to use combined hormonal contraception during breastfeeding, it seems prudent to caution her not to use it until 2 to 3 months after delivery. If she is using the combined pill, she should consume each pill at the beginning of the longest interval between breastfeeds.[107] There are several reasons for this delay in initiation:

- The longer that combined hormonal method use is postponed, the better the ongoing establishment of the milk supply will be facilitated. Nevertheless, milk volume can still be reduced when the combined hormonal contraception is started.[102]

- The risk of postpartum thrombotic complications is highest just after delivery.[59] Women should avoid using any method containing estrogen for 3 weeks as a sensible health precaution.

- The lactating woman is usually at reduced risk of becoming pregnant, especially if she is amenorrheic and fully breastfeeding. Thus, she may opt to use LAM, or she can use condoms or other barrier methods for only a month or two, with efficacy enhanced by lactation itself.

There is no need for breastfeeding women using progestin-only pills to switch to combined pills during lactation. However, if it is the woman's informed choice to make this switch, it is best to do so after 6 months postpartum.[108]

EFFECTS OF HORMONAL CONTRACEPTION ON THE BREASTFED INFANT

Contraceptive steroids taken by the mother can be transferred to the nursing infant through breastmilk. The amounts, however, are small. Nevertheless, it is prudent to avoid exposing the neonate to exogenous steroids, which are not easily bound in plasma, conjugated by the liver, or excreted, and may compete with natural hormones for receptor sites. Also, while concern about the possible effects on the liver, sex organs, and other tissues of the neonate or premature infant is theoretical, exposure should be avoided wherever possible.

- The dose of contraceptive ethinyl estradiol (about 10 nanograms per day) reaching the infant of a mother taking combined pills is comparable to the dose of the naturally occurring estradiol (from 6 to 12 ng per day depending on time of cycle) consumed by nursing infants of ovulatory mothers not taking combined pills.[60]

- The quantity of progestin transferred to mother's milk varies with the type of progestin. The 17-hydroxy compounds (such as medroxyprogesterone acetate) enter the milk at approximately the same level as is found in the mother's blood, whereas the 19-nor compounds (such as norgestrel and norethindrone) enter the milk at only one-tenth the level in the blood.[109]

Combined oral contraceptive use during lactation is not the only possible source of estrogen and progestin exposure for the infant. When a mother becomes pregnant and continues to breastfeed a prior infant, that child is exposed to estrogen and progesterone in the mother's milk. Dairy cattle may also be pregnant at the time that they are milked, so that cow's milk and infant formula made from it may have relatively high levels of estrogen and progesterone.

Although early studies of high-dose oral contraceptives did demonstrate some effect of hormones on nursing babies,[110] most of those reports were anecdotal and have not been corroborated in women using low-dose pills. One study of the male offspring of women who had used depot-medroxyprogesterone acetate (DMPA) found no effect on infant hormone regulation associated with breastfeeding exposure.[111] However, another study found that breastfed infants of mothers using Norplant had higher rates of mild respiratory infections and skin and eye conditions than the infants of breastfed mothers using Copper T IUDs. (Later, the children of the IUD users had more neurological conditions.[85])

EMERGENCY CONTRACEPTION AND THE BREASTFEEDING WOMAN

There is little if any published experience with emergency contraception during breastfeeding. Given what is known in general about both breastfeeding and contraception, the British Faculty of Family Planning and Reproductive Health Care Clinical Effectiveness Unit advises breastfeeding women that a contraceptive failure or unprotected sex before postpartum day 21 does not require the use of an emergency method, and that an IUD can be inserted as emergency contraception beginning in the fourth week[100] (albeit with the elevated risk of expulsion at this time). The World Health Organization indicates that progestin-only pills can be used for emergency contraception without restriction.[42] While this seems reasonable, we also concur with the Royal College, as above, as well as with their view that once a breastfeeding woman starts a hormonal method, she can follow the emergency contraception guidance that corresponds to that method.[100]

BREASTFEEDING: ADVANTAGES TO THE INFANT

Mother's milk has both nutritional and anti-infective advantages for the infant.[112] The particular mixtures of protein, fat, carbohydrate, and trace elements change to meet the infant's evolving needs as breastfeeding proceeds from month to month.[113] Furthermore, breastfeeding may help to cement the psychological bond between mother and infant. This bonding may lead to better psychological and intellectual development, though the evidence is inconclusive.[114] Finally, the infant ingests host-resistant, humoral, and allergy prophylaxis factors. These are particularly concentrated in the colostrum, the high-protein fluid secreted in the first few days postpartum.

Breastfed infants have lower risk of respiratory and gastro-intestinal illness,[113–115] including neonatal necrotizing enterocolitis among preterm infants[116] and sudden infant death syndrome.[117] Breastfed infants are less likely to develop allergies, including eczema, cow's milk allergy, and allergic rhinitis.[113] Whether breastmilk is protective or alternative diets are allergenic cannot be determined from the available evidence.[114] Asthma may be less common and less severe among children who were breastfed.[114] Other benefits include a decreased incidence of otitis media and dental malocclusion and caries.[118] Preterm infants who consume mother's milk in the early weeks of life have higher IQ scores,[119] although the association may not be causal. The benefits of breastfeeding are by no means limited to infants in developing countries. All of the protective effects mentioned here have been demonstrated in children in industrialized nations.[120] Most medications taken by the breastfeeding mother are safe for the infant, and excellent references are available that distinguish those medications which may require an interruption of breastfeeding.[121,122] In the United States there are few contraindications to breastfeeding,[122] and maternal human immunodeficiency virus (HIV) infection is a notable exception.[123]

BREASTFEEDING AND HIV

HIV, which causes acquired immune deficiency syndrome (AIDS), can be transmitted by an infected mother to her infant in utero, during childbirth, and through breastmilk. That HIV-1 can be transmitted by breastfeeding has been conclusively demonstrated by case reports, laboratory data, and epidemiologic studies. Rates of vertical transmission through all three routes combined average 25% to 30%, ranging from 13% to 42% in developing countries and from 14% to 25% in developed settings. The risk of vertical transmission through breastfeeding only is probably 5% to 20%.[124] Thus, the majority of infants who are infected with HIV-1 acquire the infection in utero or during childbirth, and the majority of infants who are breastfed by HIV-positive mothers do not become infected. The risk of perinatal transmission of HIV-2 is much lower than the risk of perinatal transmission of HIV-1.[125]

HIV-1 transmission via breastmilk is greatest when the mother's viral load is high and HIV immune status is poor. The risk of transmission is probably also affected by breast conditions (such as mastitis), the mother's nutritional status, mode of feeding (exclusive breastfeeding is associated with less risk), and possibly HIV-specific anti-infective activities of the milk, (such as inhibiting the binding of HIV-1 glycoproteins to CD4 molecules.[124,126–129] While the duration of breastfeeding is associated with the risk of transmission, studies of mother-to-infant transmission of HIV according to breastfeeding status have produced widely varying results. The differences may be due to methodological limitations and differences among the studies, and to vast differences in the populations studied (such as women in sub-Saharan Africa versus central Europe), and variations in CD4 counts and RNA viral load.[124]

It is clear that breastfeeding can be a route for HIV transmission. It is also clear that breastmilk is normally protective (albeit to an unknown degree) against enveloped viruses such as HIV. However, since the consequence of HIV infection through breastfeeding is virtually always fatal for the infant, it is critical to avoid the risk of infection. According to the World Health Organization, in all countries, "...HIV-positive mothers are recommended to avoid all breastfeeding and use replacement feeding when it is acceptable, feasible, affordable, sustainable and safe to do so. All HIV-infected mothers should receive counseling that includes general information about the risks and benefits of the various infant feeding options and specific guidance in selecting the option most likely to suit their circumstances; they should also have access to follow-up care and support, including family planning and nutritional support..."[124] According to U.S. authorities, HIV-infected mothers *in the United States* should be counseled not to breastfeed or provide their milk to other infants.[122,123,129] Mother to child transmission of HIV during pregnancy and delivery is reduced profoundly through anti-retroviral prophylaxis (and in some places also by cesarean delivery).[130]

BREASTFEEDING: EFFECTS ON THE MOTHER

Breastfeeding has a major protective effect against premenopausal cancers of the ovary, endometrium, and breast.[3,4,131–133] Mother's milk is free and is always available at the right temperature, in contrast to infant formula. Breastfeeding also promotes emotional bonding between mother and infant. Finally, the breastfeeding mother experiences a rapid return of uterine tone. Oxytocin, which induces uterine contraction, is released from the posterior pituitary when the nipple is stimulated by suckling.

During lactation, the body's estrogen levels are very low, and vaginal lubrication may be less than usual and begin later during sexual intercourse. Vaginal lubrication improves when cycling resumes or when the frequency of breastfeeding declines. Nursing mothers have added requirements for calories, protein, calcium, and iron, as well as several vitamins and other micronutrients. The increased needs for specific nutrients can be provided by a well-balanced diet. Supplements are generally unnecessary unless the diet is deficient in one or more of these nutrients.[134,135]

INSTRUCTIONS FOR AND INFORMATION ABOUT BREASTFEEDING

1. Congratulations! Enjoy your baby, rest, and keep in touch with your clinician.

2. Health experts concur that all women should be enabled to breastfeed, and to breastfeed exclusively for 6 months, and to continue supplemented breastfeeding for 12 to 24 months or longer.

3. **If you are not breastfeeding, begin using a contraceptive method before or at your first sexual encounter.** You can

become pregnant before your first menstrual period after childbirth because ovulation can begin before menstruation.

4. **If you are breastfeeding and providing bottle supplements, begin using a contraceptive method as soon as your clinician advises based on the method you have chosen.**

5. **If you are breastfeeding and using the Lactational Amenorrhea Method (LAM) as a temporary method of contraception, breastfeed your baby on demand, avoid any bottle feeds, and provide any minimal supplements by cup or spoon.** Begin using another method of contraception when you resume menstruation (defined as any bleeding after 56 days postpartum), when you reduce the frequency or duration of breastfeeds, when you introduce bottle feeds or regular food supplements, or when your baby turns 6 months old. (See Figures 18–2 and 18–3.)

6. **You can become pregnant while breastfeeding your baby,** although the risk is greatly reduced before your first menstrual period; in the first 6 months of amenorrhea when you feed your baby on demand, avoid any bottle feeds, and provide minimal supplements by cup or spoon, your risk of pregnancy will be about 2%, equivalent to or lower than the risk associated with many other contraceptive methods. Most U.S. women do not follow breastfeeding patterns that confer maximum protection against pregnancy. However, women who choose LAM may adopt breastfeeding behaviors that maximize both milk production and the duration of amenorrhea.

7. **Breastfeeding is a convenient, inexpensive, and nutritious way to feed your baby and it helps to protect the baby against infection, diarrhea, allergy, and sudden infant death syndrome. It also offers you protection against cancer of the breast, ovary, and uterus.**

8. **Neither intercourse nor menstruation affects the quality or quantity of your breastmilk. You do not need to stop breastfeeding because you start having intercourse again or start your period.** You can continue breastfeeding when you start using another contraceptive method.

9. **Lubricants, such as K-Y Jelly, spermicides, or saliva, may make intercourse easier after childbirth** because decreased estrogen production during breastfeeding diminishes vaginal lubrication.

10. **When you are nursing your child, your own nutrition is important.** Women can usually obtain all the calories and nutrients they need to breastfeed through their usual diet. There

is no need to buy any special foods. Just eat a sensible, well-balanced diet, which is always a good idea.

11. **Avoid smoking.** Nursing women who smoke may transfer nicotine to their infant through their breastmilk. Nicotine is a poison that can harm the child. Inhaling smoke is also harmful to the baby. Smoking may also influence your ability to produce milk.

12. **Alcohol that you drink will be passed to your baby through breastmilk.** Your baby will have more difficulty metabolizing alcohol than you do, especially in the first few weeks after delivery. No good studies have been conducted to assess what level of alcohol consumption is safe. Thus it seems prudent to drink only modest amounts of alcohol.

13. **If you are using any medications while breastfeeding, be sure to tell your physician.** You can breastfeed while using virtually all common drugs. However, for some medications you may need advice concerning the best timing for ingestion to decrease infant exposure.

14. **If you are infected with HIV, be sure to get antiretroviral treatment. The virus that causes HIV/AIDS, can be transmitted to your baby through breastmilk.** For this reason, most experts recommend that you not breastfeed your baby.

15. **It is indeed possible to combine work and breastfeeding successfully**, yet any separation of mother from infant for more than a few hours can create challenges to breastfeeding. Working women (or any breastfeeding woman!) should be sure to locate a certified lactation consultant, preferably before delivery, who can help in the event of any difficulty, from engorgement to declining milk supply. Lactation consultants are highly trained to give advice on a broad spectrum of breastfeeding issues, including the storage and transport of expressed milk, and can often help you rent an electric breast pump if you need one. The headquarters of the International Lactation Consultant Association can help you locate a certified lactation consultant near you (Website: www.ilca.org).

RESOURCE MATERIALS

International Lactation Consultant Association (ILCA): Clinical Guidelines for the Establishment of Exclusive Breastfeeding. Raleigh NC: ILCA, June 2005. Can be purchased at www.ilca.org.

REFERENCES

1. International Lactation Consultant Association (ILCA). Clinical guidelines for the establishment of exclusive breastfeeding. Raleigh NC: ILCA, June 2005.
2. World Health Assembly. Infant and young child nutrition. Fifty-fourth World Health Assembly Resolution WHA54.2. Geneva, Switzerland:WHO, 18 May 2001. Available at www.who.int/gb/ebwha/pdf_files/WHA54/ea5515.pdf. Accessed January 14, 2006.
3. American Academy of Pediatrics. Breastfeeding and the use of human milk. Pediatrics 2005;115:496–506. Available at www.pediatrics.org/cgi/content/full/115/2/496. Accessed January 14, 2006.
4. U.S. Department of Health and Human Services, Office of Women's Health. Breastfeeding—HHS blueprint for action on breastfeeding. Washington DC: DHHS, 2000. Available at: . . . . Accessed January 14, 2006.
5. World Health Organization. The optimal duration of exclusive breastfeeding: report of an expert consultation. Geneva, Switzerland, 28–30 March 2001. Geneva, Switzerland: WHO, 2002. WHO/NHD/01.09 WHO/FCH/CAH/01.24. Available at http / whqlibdoc.who.int/hq/2001/WHO_NHD_01.09.pdf. Accessed January 14, 2006.
6. Kramer MS, Kakuma R. The optimal duration of exclusive breastfeeding: a systematic review. WHO, Geneva, Switzerland: WHO, 2002:WHO/FCH/CAH/01.23. Available at www.who.int/child-adolescent-health/publications/NUTRITION/WHO_FCH_CAH_01.23.htm. Accessed January 14, 2006.
7. American Dietetic Association. Position of the American Dietetic Association: promoting and supporting breastfeeding. J Am Diet Assoc 2005;105:810–818.
8. UNICEF. Innocenti declaration on the protection, promotion and support of breastfeeding. New York NY: UNICEF, 1990.
9. Hodgen GD, Itskovitz J. Recognition and maintenance of pregnancy. In: Knobil E, Neill JD, Ewing LL, Greenwald GS, Markert CL, Pfaff DW (eds). The physiology of reproduction. New York NY: Raven Press, 1988:1995–2021.
10. Willson JR. The puerperium. In: Willson JR, Carrington ER, Ledger WJ, Laros RK, Mattox JH (eds). Obstetrics and gynecology. St. Louis MO: CV Mosby Company, 1987:598–607.
11. Gray RH, Campbell OM, Zacur II, Labbok MH, MacRae SL. Postpartum return of ovarian activity in non-breastfeeding women monitored by urinary assays. J Clin Endocrinol Metab 1987;64:645–650.
12. McNeilly AS. Lactational control of reproduction. Reprod Fertil Dev 2001;13:583–590.
13. McNeilly AS. Neuroendocrine changes and fertility in breastfeeding women. Prog Brain Res 2001;133:207–214.
14. Díaz S, Croxatto HB. Contraception in lactating women. Curr Opin Obstet Gynecol 1993;5:815–822.
15. Robinson JE, Short RV. Changes in breast sensitivity at puberty, during the menstrual cycle, and at parturition. Br Med J 1977;1:1188–1191.
16. Díaz S, Seron-Ferre M, Croxatto HB, Veldhuis J. Neuroendocrine mechanisms of lactational infertility in women. Biol Res 1995;28:155–163.
17. Gordon K, Renfree MB, Short RV, Clarke IJ. Hypothalamo-pituitary portal blood concentrations of β-endorphin during suckling in the ewe. J Reprod Fertil 1987; 79:397–408.
18. McNeilly AS, Tay CCK, Glasier A. Physiological mechanisms underlying lactational amenorrhea. In: Human reproductive ecology: interactions of environment, fertility and behavior. New York NY: New York Academy of Sciences, 1994:145–155.
19. Lewis PR, Brown JB, Renfree MB, Short RV. The resumption of ovulation and menstruation in a well-nourished population of women breastfeeding for an extended period of time. Fertil Steril 1991;55:529–536.
20. Campbell OMR, Gray RH. Characteristics and determinants of postpartum ovarian function in women in the United States. Am J Obstet Gynecol 1993;169:55–60.

21. Kennedy KI, Rivera R, McNeilly AS. Consensus statement on the use of breast-feeding as a family planning method. Contraception 1989;39:477–496.
22. Gray RH, Campbell OM, Apelo R, Eslami SS, Zacur H, Ramos RM, Gehret JC, Labbok MH. Risk of ovulation during lactation. Lancet 1990;335:25–29.
23. Becker S, Rutstein S, Labbok MH. Estimation of births averted due to breast-feeding and increases in levels of contraception needed to substitute for breast-feeding. J Bios Sci 2003;35:559–574.
24. Demographic and Health Surveys. Indonesia demographic and health survey 1997. Calverton MD: Macro International Inc., 1998.
25. Li R, Darling N, Maurice E et al. Breastfeeding rates in the United States by characteristics of the child, mother, or family: The 2002 National Immunization Survey. Pediatrics 2005;115;31–37.
26. Labbok M, Cooney K, Coly S. Guidelines: breastfeeding, family planning, and the Lactational Amenorrhea Method—LAM. Washington DC: Institute for Reproductive Health, Georgetown University, 1994.
27. World Health Organization. The WHO multinational study of breastfeeding and lactational amenorrhea: III. Pregnancy during breastfeeding. Fertil Steril 1999; 72:431–440.
28. Kazi A, Kennedy KI, Visness CM, Khan T. Effectiveness of the Lactational Amenorrhea Method in Pakistan. Fertil Steril 1995;64:717–723.
29. Labbok MH, Hight-Laukaran V, Peterson AE, Fletcher V, von Hertzen H, Van Look PFA. Multicenter study of the Lactational Amenorrhea Method (LAM): I. Efficacy, duration, and implications for clinical application. Contraception 1997;55:327–336.
30. Pérez A, Labbok MH, Queenan JT. Clinical study of the Lactational Amenorrhoea Method for family planning. Lancet 1992;339:968–970.
31. Ramos R, Kennedy KI, Visness CM. Effectiveness of lactational amenorrhea in prevention of pregnancy in Manila, the Philippines: non-comparative prospective trial. Br Med J 1996;313:909–912.
32. Labbok M, Krasovec K. Toward consistency in breastfeeding definitions. Stud Fam Plann 1990;21:226–230.
33. Valdés V, Labbok MH, Pugin E, Pérez A. The efficacy of the lactational amernorrhea method (LAM) among working women. Contraception 2000;62:217–219.
34. Hight-Laukaran V, Labbok MH, Peterson AE, Fletcher V, von Hertzen H, Van Look PFA. Multicenter study of the Lactational Amenorrhea Method (LAM): II. Acceptability, utility, and policy implications. Contraception 1997;55:337–346.
35. Valdés V, Pérez A, Labbok M, Pugin E, Zambrano I, Catalan S. The impact of a hospital and clinic-based breastfeeding promotion programme in a middle class urban environment. J Trop Pediatr 1993;39:142–151.
36. Kennedy KI, Labbok MH, Van Look PFA. Consensus statement—Lactational Amenorrhea Method for family planning. Int J Gynaecol Obstet 1996;54:55–57.
37. Van Look PFA. Lactational Amenorrhoea Method for family planning. Br Med J 1996;313:893–894.
38. Ford K, Labbok M. Contraceptive usage during lactation in the United States: an update. Am J Public Health 1987;77:79–81.
39. Visness CM, Kennedy KI: The frequency of coitus during breastfeeding. Birth 1997; 24:253–257.
40. Smith KB, van der Spuy ZM, Cheng L, Elton R, Glasier AF. Is postpartum contraceptive advice given antenatally of value? Contraception 2002;65:237–243.
41. International Planned Parenthood Federation (IPPF). IMAP Statement on breast feeding, fertility and post-partum contraception. IPPF Med Bull 1996;30:1–3.
42. World Health Organization. Medical eligibility criteria for contraceptive use, third edition. Geneva, Switzerland: Reproductive Health and Research Division, World Health Organization 2004. Available at www.who.int/reproductive-health/publications/mec/index.htm. Accessed January 14, 2006.

43. World Health Organization. Selected practice recommendations for contraceptive use, second edition. Geneva, Switzerland: Reproductive Health and Research Division, World Health Organization, 2004. Available at www.who.int/reproductive-health/publications/spr/index.htm. Accessed January 14, 2006.
44. Guillebaud J. Postpartum contraception unnecessary before three weeks. Br Med J 1993;307:1560–1561.
45. Speroff L, Darney PD. A clinical guide for contraception (Second Edition). Baltimore MD: Williams and Wilkins, 1996.
46. Hiller JE, Griffith E, Jenner F. Education for contraceptive use by women after childbirth. Cochrane Database Syst Rev 2005;4.
47. Cwiak C, Gellasch T, Zieman M. Peripartum contraceptive attitudes and practices. Contraception 2004;70:383–386.
48. Faich G, Pearson K, Fleming D, Sobel S, Anello C. Toxic shock syndrome and the vaginal contraceptive sponge. JAMA 1986;255:216–218.
49. O'Hanley K, Huber DH. Postpartum IUDs: keys for success. Contraception 1992; 45:351–361.
50. Treiman K, Liskin L, Kols A, Reinhart W. IUDs—an update. Popul Reports 1995; 22(5). Series B(6).
51. Welkovic S, Costa LOBF, Faúndes A, Ximenes RA, Costa CFF. Postpartum bleeding and infection after post-placental IUD insertion. Contraception 2001;63:155–158.
52. Muller AL, Ramos JGL, Martins-Costa SH et al. Transvaginal ultrasonographic assessment of the expulsion rate of intrauterine devices inserted in the immediate post partum period: a pilot study. Contraception 2005;72:192–195.
53. International Planned Parenthood Federation. IMAP statement on intrauterine devices. IPPF Med Bull 2003;37(2):1–6.
54. Peterson HB, Xia Z, Hughes JM, Wilcox LS, Tylor LR, Trussell J. The risk of pregnancy after tubal sterilization: findings from the U.S. Collaborative Review of Sterilization. Am J Obstet Gynecol 1996;174:1161–1170.
55. Association for Voluntary Surgical Contraception: Safe and voluntary surgical contraception. New York NY: AVSC International, 1995.
56. American College of Obstetricians and Gynecologists. Postpartum tubal sterilization. Int J Gynaecol Obstet 1992;39:244.
57. Wilcox LS, Chu SY, Eaker ED, Zeger SL, Peterson HB. Risk factors for regret after tubal sterilization: 5 years of follow-up in a prospective study. Fertil Steril 1991; 55:927–933.
58. Chi IC, Thapa S. Postpartum tubal sterilization: an international perspective on some programmatic issues. J Biosoc Sci 1993;25:51–61.
59. World Health Organization Task Force on Oral Contraceptives. Contraception during the postpartum period and during lactation: the effects on women's health. Int J Gynaecol Obstet 1987,25(Suppl):13–28.
60. McGregor JA. Lactation and contraception. In: Neville MC, Neifert MR (eds). Lactation. Physiology, nutrition, and breast-feeding. New York NY: Plenum Press, 1983:405–421.
61. Labbok MH. Contraception during lactation: considerations in advising the individual and in formulating programme guidelines. J Biosoc Sci 1985;9(Suppl):55–66.
62. American Academy of Pediatrics Committee on Drugs. The transfer of drugs and other chemicals into human milk. Pediatrics 1994;93:137–150.
63. Burkman RT. Puerperium and breast-feeding. Curr Opin Obstet Gynecol 1993; 5:683–687.
64. Wenof M, Aubert JM, Reyniak JV. Serum prolactin levels in short-term and long-term use of inert plastic and copper intrauterine devices. Contraception 1979; 19:21–27.
65. Chi I, Potts M, Wilkens LR, Champion CB. Performance of the copper T-380A intrauterine device in breastfeeding women. Contraception 1989;39:603–618.

66. Farr G, Rivera R. Interactions between intrauterine contraceptive device use and breast-feeding status at time of intrauterine contraceptive device insertion: analysis of TCu-380A acceptors in developing countries. Am J Obstet Gynecol 1992; 167:144–151.

67. Andersson K, Ryde-Blomquist E, Lindell K, Odlind V, Milson I. Perforations with intrauterine devices: report from a Swedish survey. Contraception 1998;57:251–255.

68. Chvapil M, Eskelson CD, Stiffel V, Owen JA, Droegemueller W. Studies on nonoxynol-9. II. Intravaginal absorption, distribution, metabolism and excretion in rats and rabbits. Contraception 1980;22:325–339.

69. Howie PW. Natural regulation of fertility. Br Med Bull 1993;49:182–199.

70. Parenteau-Carreau S, Cooney KA. Breastfeeding, Lactational Amenorrhea Method, and natural family planning interface: teaching guide. Washington DC: Institute for Reproductive Health, Georgetown University, 1994.

71. Labbok MH, Stallings RY, Shah F, Pérez A, Klaus H, Jacobson M, Muruthi T. Ovulation method use during breastfeeding: is there increased risk of unplanned pregnancy? Am J Obstet Gynecol 1991;165:2031–2036.

72. Kennedy KI, Gross BA, Parenteau-Carreau S, Flynn AM, Brown JB, Visness CM. Breastfeeding and the symptothermal method. Stud Fam Plann 1995;26:107–115.

73. Arevalo M, Jennings V and Sinai I. Application of simple fertility awareness-based methods of family planning to breastfeeding women.Fertil Steril 2003;80:1241–1248.

74. Kennedy KI, Parenteau-Carreau S, Flynn A, Gross B, Brown JB, Visness C. The natural family planning - Lactational Amenorrhea Method interface: observations from a prospective study of breastfeeding users of natural family planning. Am J Obstet Gynecol 1991;165:2020–2026.

75. Johansson E, Odlind V. The passage of exogenous hormones into breast milk—possible effects. Int J Gynaecol Obstet 1987;25(Suppl):111–114.

76. International Planned Parenthood Federation. IMAP statement on hormonal methods of contraception. IPPF Med Bull 2002;36:1–8.

77. Fraser IS. A review of the use of progestogen-only minipills for contraception during lactation. Reprod Fertil Dev 1991;3:245–254.

78. McCann MF, Potter LS. Progestin-only oral contraception—a comprehensive review. Contraception 1994;50:S1-S198.

79. World Health Organization. Progestogen-only contraceptives during lactation: I. Infant growth. Contraception 1994;50:35–53.

80. World Health Organization. Progestogen-only contraceptives during lactation: II. Infant development. Contraception 1994;50:55–68.

81. Sinchai W, Sethavanich S, Asavapiriyanont S, Sittipiyasakul V, Sirikanchanakul R, Udomkiatsakul P, Chantaeyoon P, Roybang K, Trakankamol J, Suti S, Parnraksa W, Dusitsin N. Effects of a progestin-only pill (Exluton) and an intrauterine device (Multiload Cu250) on breastfeeding. Adv Contracep 1995;11:143–155.

82. Coutinho EM, Athayde C, Dantas C, Hirsch C, Barbosa I. Use of a single implant of Elcometrine (ST-1435), a nonorally active progestin, as a long acting contraceptive for postpartum nursing women. Contraception 1999;59:115–122.

83. Reinprayoon D, Taneepanichskul S, Bunyavejchevin S, Thaithumyanon P, Punnahitananda S, Tosukhowong P, Machielsen C, van Beek A. Effects of the etonogestrel-releasing contraceptive implant (Implanon?) on parameters of breastfeeding compared to those of an intrauterine device. Contraception 2000;62:239–246.

84. Massai MR, Díaz S, Quinteros E, Reyes MV, Herreros C, Zepeda A, Croxatto HB, Moo-Young AJ. Contraceptive efficacy and clinical performance of Nestorone implants in postpartum women. Contraception 2001;64:369–376.

85. Schiappacasse V, Díaz S, Zepeda A, Alvarado R, Herreros C. Health and growth of infants breastfed by Norplant contraceptive implants users: a six-year follow-up study. Contraception 2002;66:57–65.

86. Curtis KM, Chrisman CE, Peterson HB. Contraception for women in selected circumstances. Obstet Gynecol 2002;99:1100–1112.

87. Hannon PR, Duggan AK, Serwint JR, Vogelhut JW, Witter F, DeAngelis C. The influence of medroxyprogesterone on the duration of breast-feeding in mothers in an urban community. Arch Pediatr Adolesc Med 1997;151:490–496.

88. Shaamash AH, Sayed GH, Hussien MM et al. A comparative study of the levonorgestrel-releasing intrauterine system Mirena? versus the Copper T380A intrauterine device during lactation: breast-feeding performance, infant growth and infant development. Contraception 2005;72:346–351.

89. Harlap S. Exposure to contraceptive hormones through breast milk—are there long-term health and behavioral consequences? Int J Gynaecol Obstet 1987;25(Suppl): 47–55.

90. Cowie AT, Forsyth IA, Hart IC. Hormonal control of lactation. Berlin, Germany: Springer-Verlag, 1980:164–165.

91. Kennedy KI, Short RV, Tully MR. Premature introduction of progestin-only contraceptive methods during lactation. Contraception 1997;55:347–350.

92. McCann MF, Moggia AV, Higgins JE, Potts M, Becker C. The effects of a progestin-only oral contraceptive (Levonorgestrel 0.03 mg) on breast feeding. Contraception 1989;40:635–648.

93. Moggia AV, Harris GS, Dunson TR, Diaz R, Moggia MS, Ferrer MA, McMullen SL. A comparative study of a progestin-only oral contraceptive versus non-hormonal methods in lactating women in Buenos Aires, Argentina. Contraception 1991; 44:31–43.

94. Halderman LD and Nelson AL. Impact of early postpartum administration of progestin-only hormonal contraceptives compared with nonhormonal contraceptives on short-term breast-feeding patterns. Am J Obstet Gynecol 2002;186:1250–1258.

95. Taneepanichskul S, Reinprayoon D, Thaithumyanon P et al. Effects of the etonogestrel-releasing implant Implanon and a nonmedicated intrauterine device on the growth of breast-fed infants. Contraception 2006;73:368–371.

96. Danli S, Qingxiang S, Guowei S. A multicentered clinical trial of the long-acting injectable contraceptive Depo Provera in Chinese women. Contraception 2000;62:15–18.

97. Hubacher D, Goco N, Gonzalez B, Taylor D. Factors affecting continuation rates of DMPA. Contraception 1999;60:345–351.

98. Massai R, Quinteros E, Reyes MV et al. Extended use of a progesterone-releasing vaginal ring in nursing women: a phase II clinical trial. Contraception 2005; 72:352–357.

99. Díaz S, Zepeda A, Maturana X, et al. Fertility regulation in nursing women. IX. Contraceptive performance, duration of lactation, infant growth, and bleeding patterns during use of progesterone vaginal rings, progestin-only pills, Norplant® implants, and Copper T 380-A intrauterine devices. Contraception 1997;56:223–232.

100. Faculty of Family Planning and Reproductive Health Care Clinical Effectiveness Unit. Contraceptive choices for breastfeeding women. J Fam Plann Reprod Health Care 2004;30:181–189.

101. Hani A, Moss M, Cooper D et al. Informed choice—the timing of postpartum contraceptive initiation. S Afr Med J 2003;93:862–864.

102. Tankeyoon M, Dusitsin N, Chalapati S, Koetsawang S, Saibiang S, Sas M, Gellen JJ, Ayeni O, Gray R, Pinol A, Zegers L. Effects of hormonal contraceptives on milk volume and infant growth. Contraception 1984;30:505–522.

103. Blackburn, R.D., Cunkelman, J.A., and Zlidar, V.M. Oral Contraceptives—An Update. Population Reports, Series A, No. 9. Baltimore, Johns Hopkins University School of Public Health, Population Information Program, Spring 2000. www.infoforhealth.org/pr/a9/a9.pdf Accessed March 13, 2006.

104. Truitt, ST, Fraser, AB, Grimes, DA et al. Combined hormonal versus nonhormonal versus progestin-only contraception in lactation. Cochrane Database Syst Rev 2005;4.

105. Truitt ST, Fraser AB, Grimes DA, et al. Hormonal contraception during lactation: systematic review of randomized controlled trials. Contraception 2003;68:233–238.

106. Guillebaud J. Contraception, your questions answered. New York NY: Churchill, 1993.
107. Erwin PC. To use or not to use combined hormonal oral contraceptives during lactation. Fam Plann Perspect 1994;26:26–30, 33.
108. Visness CM, Rivera R. Progestin-only pill use and pill switching during breastfeeding. Contraception 1995;51:279–281.
109. Toddywalla VS, Mehta S, Virkar KD, Saxena BN. Release of 19-nor-testosterone type of contraceptive steroids through different drug delivery systems into serum and breast milk of lactating women. Contraception 1980;21:217–223.
110. Curtis EM. Oral-contraceptive feminization of a normal male infant. Obstet Gynecol 1964;23:295–296.
111. Virutamasen P, Leepipatpaiboon S, Kriengsinyot R, Vichaidith P, Muia PN, Sekadde-Kigondu CB, Mati JKG, Forest MG, Dikkeschei LD, Wolthers BG, d'Arcangues C. Pharmacodynamic effects of depot-medroxyprogesterone acetate (DMPA) administered to lactating women on their male infants. Contraception 1996;54:153–157.
112. Heinig MJ, Dewey KG. Health Advantages of breastfeeding for infants: a critical review. Nutrition Research Reviews 1996;9:89–110.
113. McCann MF, Liskin LS, Piotrow PT, Rinehart W, Fox G. Breastfeeding, fertility and family planning. Popul Reports 1984;12(2). Series J(24).
114. Kovar MG, Serdula MK, Marks JS, Fraser DW. Review of the epidemiologic evidence for an association between infant feeding and infant health. Pediatrics 1984;74 (4-Suppl):615–638.
115. Howie PW, Forsyth JS, Ogston SA, Clark A, Florey C du V. Protective effect of breast feeding against infection. Br Med J 1990;300:11–16.
116. Lucas A, Cole TJ. Breast milk and neonatal necrotising enterocolitis. Lancet 1990; 336:1519–1523.
117. Woolridge MW, Phil D, Baum JD. Recent advances in breast feeding. Acta Paediatr Jpn 1993;35:1–12.
118. Labbok MH. Consequences of breastfeeding for mother and child. J Biosoc Sci 1985; 9(Suppl):43–54.
119. Lucas A, Morley R, Cole TJ, Lister G, Leeson-Payne C. Breast milk and subsequent intelligence quotient in children born preterm. Lancet 1992;339:261–264.
120. Cunningham AS. Breastfeeding, bottlefeeding and illness: an annotated bibliography, 1986. In: Jelliffe DB, Jelliffe EFP (eds). Programmes to promote breastfeeding. Oxford, England: Oxford University Press, 1988:448–480.
121. American Academy of Pediatrics. The transfer of drugs and other chemicals into human milk. Pediatrics 2001;108:776–789.
122. Lawrence RA. A review of the medical benefits and contraindications to breastfeeding in the United States. Maternal and Child Health Technical Information Bulletin. Arlington VA: National Center for Education in Maternal and Child Health, 1997.
123. American Academy of Pediatrics. Human milk, breastfeeding and the transmission of Human Immunodeficiency Virus in the United States. Pediatrics 1995;96:977–979.
124. World Health Organization. HIV transmission through breastfeeding—a review of the available evidence. Geneva, Switzerland, 2004. Available at www.who.int/child-adolescent-health/New_Publications/NUTRITION/ISBN_92_4_156271_4.pdf. Accessed 15 January 2006.
125. Adjorlolo-Johnson G, De Cock KM, Ekpini E, Vetter KM, Sibailly T, Brattegaard K, Yavo D, Doorly R, Whitaker JP, Kestens L, Ou C-Y, George JR, Gayle HD. Prospective comparison of mother-to-child transmission of HIV-1 and HIV-2 in Abidjan, Ivory Coast. JAMA 1994;272:462–466.
126. Bélec L, Bouquety JC, Georges AJ, Siopathis MR, Martin PMV. Antibodies to human immunodeficiency virus in the breast milk of healthy seropositive women. Pediatrics 1990;85:1022–1026.

127. Newburg DS, Viscidi RP, Ruff A, Yolken RH. A human milk factor inhibits binding of human immunodeficiency virus to the CD4 receptor. Pediatr Res 1992;31:22–28.

128. Van de Perre P, Simonon A, Hitimana DG, Dabis F, Msellati P, Mukamabano B, Butera JB, Van Goethem C, Karita E, Lepage P. Infective and anti-infective properties of breastmilk from HIV-1-infected women. Lancet 1993;341:914–918.

129. Centers for Disease Control (CDC). Recommendations for assisting in the prevention of perinatal transmission of human T-lymphotropic virus type III/lymphadenopathy-associated virus and acquired immunodeficiency syndrome. MMWR 1985; 34:721–726, 731–732.

130. Newell M.Current issues in the prevention of mother-to-child transmission of HIV-1 infection. Transactions of the Royal Society of Tropical Medicine and Hygiene 2006; 100:1–5.

131. Eaton SB, Pike MC, Short RV, Lee NC, Trussell J, Hatcher RA, Wood JW, Worthman CM, Blurton Jones NG, Konner MJ, Hill KR, Bailey R, Hurtado AM. Women's reproductive cancers in evolutionary context. Q Rev Biol 1994;69:353–367.

132. Rosenblatt KA, Thomas DB. Prolonged lactation and endometrial cancer: WHO Collaborative Study of Neoplasia and Steroid Contraceptives. Int J Epidemiol 1995; 24:499–503.

133. Speroff L, Glass RH, Kase NG. Clinical gynecologic endocrinology and infertility (Fifth Edition). Baltimore MD: Williams and Wilkins, 1994.

134. Institute of Medicine (IOM). Nutrition during lactation. Washington DC: National Academy Press, 1991.

135. Worthington-Roberts BS, Williams SR. Nutrition in pregnancy and lactation (Fifth Edition). St. Louis MO: Mosby-Year Book, Inc., 1993:340.

Contraceptive Research and Development

Henry L. Gabelnick, PhD
Jill Schwartz, MD
Jacqueline E. Darroch, PhD

- Developing methods that women can use to protect against both pregnancy and sexually transmitted infections (STIs) including HIV/AIDS, especially methods that can be used with little or no effort required from a male partner, is a high priority for current contraceptive research.

- Research to develop systemic methods for men is ongoing, but the introduction of new options for men is likely to be at least 5 to 10 years away.

- Contraceptive research has the potential to provide improved technologies and also new thinking about regimens and requirements for service delivery. Methods with simpler rules for use and fewer obstacles to regimen initiation could improve a user's ability to use contraceptives more effectively.

- Increased resources are needed for both public and private sectors in the field of contraception. New discoveries in biotechnology, genetics, immunology, and molecular biology have the potential to accelerate innovation; we urgently need methods that provide both pregnancy and STI, HIV/AIDS prevention.

CONTRACEPTIVE RESEARCH OVERVIEW
WHY IS CONTRACEPTIVE RESEARCH NEEDED?

In addition to the intuitive appeal of assuring the latest, best medications and technologies in all medical fields, the need for improvement in the field of contraception is clear from public health statistics. First, data from the National Survey of Family Growth indicate that the percentage of all U.S. women ages 15 to 44 who were at risk for unintended pregnancy (sexually active, able to become pregnant if not using contraception, but wanting not to have a child soon) who were using no method increased from 7.5% in 1995 to 10.7% in 2002.[1] Second, the impact of the HIV epidemic on reproductive-age women has created an urgent need for methods that provide dual protection—against both unintended pregnancy and also sexually transmitted infections (STIs) including HIV/AIDS.[2] Worldwide, this is an imperative problem, but it is also very important for many couples in the United States.

Although couples have a range of family planning methods available now, almost half of all pregnancies in the United States and worldwide are not intended. Many unintended pregnancies occur because the couple was not using a method at the time, but almost half—more than one million annually in the United States—are "failures" that occur despite method use. A small proportion of unintended pregnancies is attributable to technical failure of a method; most failures instead reflect inconsistent or incorrect use of a method, or interruptions in use. Improving the way in which individuals use contraception will require improved education and access to family planning care; improvements in technology can also play an important role.

Contraceptive research in the past focused on finding highly effective methods and on method safety. Newer research priorities include efforts to reduce side effects and develop methods that are easier and more appealing to use. For example, recent research has sought methods that have incidental beneficial effects (non-contraceptive benefits) such as clearer skin or reduced fluid retention. Ideal methods might even have a positive effect on the couple's sexual experience. Methods that are easier to use—simpler, with fewer rules—could potentially improve effectiveness in actual use. Research to reduce obstacles to initiating and continuing a method, and to help providers adopt improved service delivery approaches more quickly, also provides the potential to help reduce unintended pregnancy. New thinking is needed in this field, along with new technologies. The introduction of emergency contraception (EC), for example, has helped prompt a shift in both technology and services. The widening dissemination of EC may turn out to have had an unintended positive effect to the extent that providers and couples begin to understand and respond to contraceptive need as an urgent rather than a "routine" medical issue. Reducing typical delays in initiation of contraception could result in a significant reduction in unintended pregnancy rates.

Medical problems and side effects are not serious obstacles for most couples, but they are important for some. For example, women with serious chronic diseases that make use of hormonal products inadvisable have limited alternative options, as do women who experience unacceptable side effects when using hormonal products. Continued efforts to develop entirely new categories of contraceptives would help both of these groups and might have important advantages for other women as well.

The widening HIV pandemic and the role that STIs play in accelerating HIV spread make it an urgent priority to find methods that can reduce infection. There is some evidence that hormonal contraception alters immune function in the genital tract.[3] Depot-medroxyprogesterone acetate (DMPA) was associated with increased acquisition of cervical chlamydial and gonococcal infections in a prospective cohort study.[4] Concern about a possible association between hormonal contraceptive use and increased risk of HIV infection has triggered research into this question.[5] While no association was found between hormonal contraceptive use and HIV acquisition, among participants who were seronegative for herpes simplex virus-2, hormonal contraceptive users had an increased risk of HIV acquisition.[6] Further research is needed, but if current hormonal methods do turn out to have undesirable effects on infection risk, then new methods based on other mechanisms of action will be desperately needed for women who are at high individual risk for acquiring HIV.

This chapter provides information practitioners can use in supporting or advocating for adequate research funding, and for educational presentations about the future of contraception. It also describes new methods available elsewhere, which are ready for imminent introduction or re-introduction in the United States, and which may become available in the next 5 to 10 years, especially new microbicide and barrier options. The chapter also reviews the status of male methods, although the time horizon for these possibilities may be longer.

A BRIEF HISTORY OF CONTRACEPTIVE RESEARCH

Modern private-sector contraceptive research began in the 1950s and led to the first oral contraceptive pill, (Enovid) approved by the FDA in 1960, and the marketing of IUDs (Lippes Loop and Saf-T-Coil), in the early 1960s (see Table 19–1). At its peak in the late 1970s, significant investments in contraceptive research were being made by at least six large U.S. companies.[7]

Support for basic research prior to 1950, and continuing through the 1980s, was provided principally by three visionary foundations—Rockefeller, Mellon, and Ford—and was critical in establishing the basis for most of the methods available today. Public research funding began when the National Institute of Child Health and Human Development (NICHD) was established at the National Institute of Health (NIH) in 1963. Soon after, U.S. Agency for International Development (USAID) allocated additional research funding.

Table 19–1 Method timeline: date of introduction and/or FDA approval[a]

1839	Condoms mass-produced by Goodyear (vulcanized rubber)
1925	Diaphragms manufactured in United States
1960	Estrogen plus progestin oral contraceptive pill—Enovid
1962	Lippes Loop licensed for use in public programs
1982	Contraceptive sponge (withdrawn in 1994)
1984	Cu T 380A copper-releasing intrauterine device
1988	Prentif cavity-rim cervical cap
1990	Levonorgestrel 6-rod implant device (subsequently withdrawn from sale)—Norplant
1992	3-month progestin injectable—medroxyprogesterone acetate (Depo-Provera)
1994	Female condom—Reality (currently named FC Female Condom)
1996	Levonorgestrel 2-rod implant device (not marketed)—Jadelle
1998	Estrogen plus progestin emergency contraceptive—dedicated product (Preven)
1999	Progestin emergency contraceptive—(Plan B)
2000	Estrogen plus progestin injectable (subsequently withdrawn from sale)—Lunelle
2000	Mifepristone antiprogestin for early abortion
2000	Levonorgestrel-releasing intrauterine system—Mirena
2002	Contraceptive patch—Ortho Evra
2002	Vaginal contraceptive ring—Organon
2002	Lea's Shield
2003	FemCap
2003	Transcervical permanent sterilization device—Essure
2004	Etonogestrel single-rod implant—Implanon
2005	Contraceptive sponge reintroduced—Today
2005	Latex female condom (available for the non-US market)—FC2 Female Condom

[a] Note: This table does not include the many oral contraceptive pill products introduced following the 1960 approval for Enovid, the first "pill." Pill development has provided major improvements, especially with gradual reduction in the hormone dose for both the estrogen and progestin components, and development and introduction of improved progestins and extended use. Intrauterine devices introduced after the Lippes Loop but no longer available also are not listed.

Private-sector involvement after 1970 declined, however, and focused on improvements in hormonal formulations. The level of public and foundation funding for research, after significant growth in the 1960s and early 1970s, also slowed in the 1980s.[8] By 1990, a U.S. Academy of Sciences report concluded that declining and sporadic funding from foundations and public sources and the decreased interest of most pharmaceutical companies threatened to reduce the pool of scientific personnel and resources for the field.[7] The committee noted that resource limitations would be likely to delay the application of new biotechnology, genetic engineering, and molecular biology discoveries that otherwise might provide significant advances in contraception.

During the 1980s and 1990s, the increasing complexity of regulatory review for new drugs and devices along with concerns about product liability and public controversy in the field of contraception also had a detrimental effect on the development of new methods, especially in the United States.[9] Damaging litigation following the Dalkon Shield scandal led to withdrawal of other IUDs from the market in the 1970s, and attacks against Norplant beginning in 1994 were followed by a dramatic decline in its sales.[10] Large companies were logically more reluctant to assume the financial risks involved in development of innovative approaches, and smaller companies lacked sufficient resources to do so. Initial development of new approaches, therefore, became increasingly dependent on public sector resources and research organizations.[8]

Development of a new drug or device is a long and costly process (see Table 19–2). Drug discovery and device invention typically involve many discarded possibilities before an option promising enough to warrant human studies is identified. Human studies require IND (Investigational New Drug) or IDE (Investigational Device Exemption) approval by the Food and Drug Administration (FDA), and applications must include a review of laboratory and toxicology testing in animals. For drugs, human studies are conducted in phases to assess safety (Phase I), effectiveness (Phase II), and extended safety and effectiveness in clinical use (Phase III). Research data from these studies provide the basis for a New Drug Application (NDA) to the FDA. If the product is approved, the data are the basis for product labeling, including dosing, instructions, and indications. When the NDA is approved, the company is entitled to sell and market the drug for the approved indications. FDA processes for reviewing applications for device approval (called PMA—Premarket Approval applications) are similar, although somewhat more complex.[7]

Reviewing available information in 2004, the Institute of Medicine Committee on New Frontiers in Contraceptive Development concluded that development of a new drug takes 10 to 14 years, and involves an investment of $400 million to $800 million.[10] The investment in contraceptive research and development from all sectors is insufficient to develop more than just a handful of new possibilities. Although private sector companies are investing in research on drugs for conditions that primarily affect women, contraception is not a high priority. A 2004 survey of its members reported by PhRMA (the Pharmaceutical Research and Manufacturers of America) identified 371 new drugs in development for diseases that primarily affect women. Only 10 were contraceptives (the single rod implant, 6 new oral contraceptive pill formulations and 3 microbicide candidates). In contrast, this group included 71 new drugs for women's cancers, 55 for arthritis, 45 for autoimmune diseases, 41 for dia-

Table 19–2 The drug development process

Preclinical Development

Concept and synthesis

Production of sufficient drug quantity for research

Formulation to provide suitable dose and administration route

Preclinical Research

Toxicology, safety and effectiveness (animals)	1–3 years

Investigational New Drug Application (IND) Filed

Reviewed by FDA	30 days for FDA staff review but questions can prolong
FDA Acceptance permits research use for human subjects	

Clinical Research (human subjects)

Phase 1 Fewer than 100 subjects to establish safety	6 mo–1 year
Phase 2 100 + human subjects to establish effectiveness	6 mo–2 years
Phase 3 Sufficient subject number (1000 +) to confirm safety, effectiveness and dosage	1–4 years

New Drug Application (NDA) Filed

Reviewed by FDA	2 mo–7 years for FDA review*
FDA Approval for Marketing	

Postmarketing Surveillance

Adverse event reporting

Additional studies as required in FDA Approval Decision

Source: adapted from Mastroianni, 1990.[7]

* Review and decision by FDA staff, with recommendations to FDA from Advisory Committee.

betes, and 31 for psychiatric conditions.[11] Contraceptive research clearly needs continued support for public funding.

The National Institutes of Health (NIH) 2005 appropriation for women's health had the smallest percentage increase in over 19 years and is less than what is needed to keep up with inflation in biomedical research costs.[12] Additional public funding for contraception is also provided through USAID. The public total, however, is modest in relation to the estimated development cost for even a single new product.

The urgent need for methods that women can use to protect against HIV/AIDS and STIs as well as pregnancy has infused the contraceptive development field with new vitality and some new resources. Although the primary sources of funding for this effort have been public sector and foundation grants, private sector organizations have begun to work in this area. The steady increase in contraceptive use in developing countries—a vast potential market for products estimated to include 2.5 billion women by the year 2025—along with the successful introduction of new products, including the hormone-releasing vaginal ring, the patch, the levonorgestrel intrauterine system, and dedicated extended-use oral contraceptives, has helped create renewed interest in contraceptive development at major pharmaceutical companies.

WHAT IS NEEDED?

More public funding. Along with all "women's health" issues, resources for contraceptive development research continue to lag behind research in other areas. Inadequate resources means the opportunity to apply major advances in immunology, genetics, and molecular biology is delayed or lost. These shortcomings are tragic because the human need is great. Contraceptive options that could make a dent in the rate of unintended pregnancy would have a huge health impact—certainly comparable to that of a major heart disease or cancer breakthrough. Not everyone will develop these important diseases, but almost everyone does need effective contraception, and unintended pregnancy involves serious health risks for young people that translate to high losses in years of productive life.

Support for increased participation of private-sector companies. Companies that work in this field should be applauded, and they will be assisted by efforts to increase public awareness of the importance of this research area and to diminish the controversy about family planning and reproductive health in national public policy. Commitment to providing adequate public funding of family planning services and supplies for low income couples in the United States, and as part of international aid, can also fortify the private sector involvement in the field.

Development of innovative approaches. In addition to methods that protect against both infection and pregnancy, investment is needed to pursue entirely new approaches as well as improvements in existing hormonal methods.

CURRENT CONTRACEPTIVE RESEARCH
CONTRACEPTIVE MICROBICIDES

Chemical barriers have been used for contraception in conjunction with cervical caps and diaphragms, and also alone as foams, suppositories, tablets, creams, and gels. Although nonoxynol-9 (N-9)-containing vaginal spermicides have been available over-the-counter for more than 50 years, there has been a paucity of information regarding the effectiveness of these products. A recent multi-center trial evaluating the effectiveness of five N-9 products (52.5 mg gel, 100 mg gel, 150 mg gel, 100 mg suppository, and 100 mg film) found that the 6-month failure rates with typical use (14%-22%) were in the range previously accepted for spermicide and barrier method users (except in the lowest dose, the 52.5 mg gel).[13]

In addition to their spermicidal effect, currently marketed products—N-9 in the United States and similar detergents in other countries—also kill bacteria and viruses when tested in the laboratory. This microbicidal effect led to the initial hope that existing products might also reduce infection risk in actual use. Contrary to the hope, however, research on the effect of N-9 spermicide use by women in a high-risk group found higher HIV incidence with spermicide use than with use of a placebo.[14-16] Vaginal irritation caused by the N-9 may have compromised normal vaginal defenses against infection, leaving women more vulnerable.[17] (See Chapter 14, on Vaginal Barriers and Spermicides.) Other available spermicide detergents also may cause irritation. Because of the potential harm, N-9 use is no longer recommended for women at high risk for HIV/AIDS, and it also should not be used as a lubricant for rectal intercourse. Efforts to find methods to prevent infection have therefore turned to the task of finding entirely new microbicide options.[18]

The challenge in microbicide development is to find an option that is effective in stopping bacterial or viral infection but does not cause irritation. Ideally, a product might even enhance natural infection defenses and protect against irritation. The potential for protecting users against HIV infection or other pathogens is based on the microbicides' ability to kill or inactivate HIV virus or pathogens. Alternatively, a microbicide could act by interfering with essential steps in the infection process, such as cell attachment or entry, or replication of the pathogen. Most of the chemicals and compounds being studied also interfere with sperm fertility or kill sperm. In the future, a product that could safely prevent infection without impairing fertility would also be desirable. Demonstrating safety during conception and through pregnancy, however, would be an even more formidable research challenge than demonstrating infection protection alone.

Research efforts over the last five years have identified several "promising" candidates, and several are already undergoing human safety studies (see the Alliance for Microbicide website [www.microbicide.org] for a current listing of microbicide candidates and clinical trials). Clinical studies to demonstrate effectiveness and extended safety, however, will require several years, so it is unlikely that a new microbicide could be ready for FDA approval before 2008. In the meantime, researchers are also re-assessing lubricants currently marketed for other purposes.[19] Lubrication in itself may be desirable, because its use may decrease irritation and trauma during intercourse, which in turn may reduce infection risk.

It is also possible that the "microbicide" goal could be achieved with a product administered systemically. For example, pre-exposure treatment, or daily treatment, with a drug that could block infection or fortify immune defenses could be considered, as could an agent released continuously from a vaginal ring or barrier device that acted primarily or partially through a systemic effect. Drugs developed for HIV/AIDS treatment and for parasite therapy are being considered for this application.

Research related to microbicide development may also prove to have unanticipated long-term benefits. The microbicide effort has required a major investment in basic research on vaginal physiology and on the pathophysiology of HIV/AIDS and STI transmission. Advances are likely to be helpful in combating common problems such as bacterial vaginosis, and have already produced some important findings. The complex vaginal ecosystem was previously little understood. It is a delicate system that can easily be disrupted by trauma or by chemical alteration. "Mildly" toxic exposures to compounds such as N-9 or a solution that is too acid or too alkaline can disrupt normal vaginal bacteria and impair the normal defenses against infection. Use of "hygiene" products including douching solutions seems to create much more significant problems than previously recognized.

MECHANICAL BARRIER METHODS

Renewed attention has been directed to development of new mechanical barriers in parallel with the emphasis on microbicide development. A mechanical barrier may be helpful for use in conjunction with a new microbicide, and there is also some hope that a barrier may itself provide some protection against transmission of infection. Providing a physical shield for the cervix is a plausible strategy since cervical epithelium is an important infection target: it is the primary site for chlamydial infection and contains a rich supply of immune system cells that are the target for the initial uptake of HIV.[20] A study in Zimbabwe and South Africa is ongoing to evaluate the effectiveness of a diaphragm used with a lubricant in reducing HIV acquisition.

The Today contraceptive sponge, previously marketed for more than a decade in the United States but not available since 1994, returned to the U.S. market in 2005. This product contains N-9 in a small, soft pillow shaped device (see Chapter 14, Vaginal Barrier and Spermicides). At the time of its withdrawal, the manufacturer explained that the investment required to meet FDA-mandated manufacturing equipment upgrades was not feasible. The product was purchased in 1999 by a new company that has struggled persistently to reintroduce the product in the United

States; the product is also marketed in Canada. Other contraceptive sponge options, Protectaid, containing a lower concentration of N-9 along with benzalkonium chloride, and Pharmatex, containing benzalkonium chloride, are available in Canada and in Europe, but are not approved by the FDA.

Research is also ongoing to develop new, improved diaphragm and cap models that are appropriate for use along with a microbicide. Recently approved barrier devices, Lea's Shield and FemCap, are intended for use with a spermicide, but may prove suitable for use with a microbicide in the future. Another device under development, the SILCS diaphragm, is an intravaginal one-size cervical barrier device that has performed well in postcoital testing. The Instead Softcup is being studied as an inexpensive, disposable vaginal barrier that could be marketed with the candidate microbicidal and spermicidal gel Amphora® (also known as ACIDFORM gel). The BufferGel Duet is a disposable, one-size-fits-all, clear diaphragm made of dipped polyurethane that is being studied prefilled with BufferGel, a candidate contraceptive microbicide. Similarly, a small, soft, transparent disposable silicone cervical cap called Oves, available in three sizes, was licensed in accordance with European Union regulations in 1997 and is available in France and in the United Kingdom.[21] There is also research interest in evaluating a method that does not require provider fitting. A method that is available over-the-counter would have the potential to be adopted more widely if the combination of a vaginal barrier and microbicide proves to be effective in helping reduce HIV/AIDS and STI transmission.

New female condom prototypes are under development. The FC2 Female Condom is a second generation female condom with the same design and instructions for use as the FC Female Condom (formerly Reality). It is made of synthetic latex instead of polyurethane, to improve affordability. The Reddy female condom, also known as the VA feminine condom and as V-Amour, is held in place inside the vagina by a soft sponge inside the condom, rather than a ring as used in the FC Female Condom, and has received CE Marking. PATH has a new female condom in development with a dissolving capsule intended to make insertion easier, a polyurethane condom pouch with foam shapes to allow gentle cling to the vaginal walls, and a soft outer ring. In addition, panty condoms such as the Silk Parasol Panty Condom and the Natural Sensation Female Panty Condom have been developed.

New male condom models have been developed with alternative materials other than latex and with design modifications. Synthetic nonlatex materials can be used by people who have latex allergies, can be used with oil-based lubricants, may transmit heat better than latex, and may have longer shelf-lives. Despite male preference for synthetic nonlatex condoms such as Avanti and eZ-on, nonlatex condoms broke or slipped more often than latex condoms; however, most were as effective as latex condoms in preventing pregnancy.[22] Innovative condom designs that are spiral shaped and loose fitting to increase friction and sexual pleasure have been developed and successfully marketed by large companies.

HORMONAL AND SYSTEMIC METHODS FOR WOMEN

Hormonal methods have been the mainstay of reversible contraception because of their safety and effectiveness. New developments have provided methods with a lower hormone dose, improved progestin options, and a drug delivery mechanism that simplifies use. Several options used in other countries, however, are not available in the United States, including implants and injectables that have already received FDA approval and initial marketing here.

The low dose, 6-rod progestin-releasing implant—Norplant—was approved by the FDA in 1990. Sales of the product were stopped in 2000, and the company announced in 2002 that it did not plan to reintroduce the device. The improved, 2-rod version of this method—Jadelle—is currently marketed in Europe by Schering Oy of Finland. Jadelle received FDA approval in 1996 but has not yet been sold in the United States. Another implant option, the single-rod Implanon, has been marketed in Europe and Australia for several years and received FDA approval in July 2006. Implanon should become widely available in the United States in 2007. Implants gained a small but very appreciative user group because of their extremely high efficacy and simplicity of use.

The combination estrogen and progestin injectable, Lunelle, had a history similar to that of Norplant. Although this method is marketed in many other countries, it was available only briefly in the United States, then voluntarily recalled by Pharmacia in 2002. It is not clear when or whether this option will again become available, although it too had a wider-than-expected, enthusiastic user adoption while it was marketed.

Research is being conducted on hormonal methods that have the potential to improve bleeding patterns for women using low-dose, progestin only methods including implants. Implants are a very appealing approach because their efficacy is as good as or better than other long-term methods, including surgical sterilization, and their average continuation rate is higher than that with other reversible methods.[23] New progestins, such as nesterone, have the potential for use in a hormone-releasing vaginal ring and might provide incidental "side benefits" related to the characteristics of the progestin or a method with fewer undesirable side effects. Nesterone rings developed by the Population Council can be made to last at least a year.

The development of approaches to block hormone receptors might also provide new contraceptive options. The anti-progestin mifepristone has been studied for use as an emergency contraceptive after unprotected intercourse, for low-dose, daily use and for use as a once-a-month regimen. Such regimens can provide contraceptive protection, but they have caused menstrual disruption. Further basic research is ongoing to identify and evaluate other members of the anti-progestin family.[24]

In the future, systemic methods may be developed that do not disrupt normal hormone cycles. For example, a narrowly targeted method with effect only on zona pellucida binding of sperm, or factors essential for implantation, might provide effective contraception without the side effects related to hormone disruption. These approaches may lead to the development of methods that could be used monthly. Initial laboratory or animal research has identified two peptides, leukemia inhibitory factor (LIF) and perimplantation factor (PIF), that might be feasible targets for inhibition. The peptide leptin, better known for its role in regulation of hunger, may also play a role in implantation. Development of such options will require more basic research and a better understanding of the molecular biology and biochemistry involved, making it unlikely that these options would be put into clinical use within the next decade.

SYSTEMIC METHODS FOR MEN

Although the percentage of the world's couples that rely on male methods (condoms, withdrawal, and vasectomy) has increased, the development of systemic methods for men has been slow. Part of the reason is that the physiology of male fertility is a difficult challenge: sperm are continuously produced, with maturation and development over an interval of weeks. Part of the challenge is that issues like adverse effects, side effects, acceptability, and affordability are more powerful constraints now than they were in the 1950s when female systemic methods were devised. Three possible approaches include (1) blocking hormonal support for testicular cell function by stopping pituitary LH and FSH, (2) interfering with seminiferous tubule function to stop sperm production, and (3) disrupting maturation, functioning, and/or transport of sperm after they are produced. Targeting the second or third approach would have significant advantages, but except for gossypol, no method has yet been developed sufficiently for clinical studies.[25] Current research has focused on the first option.

Suppression of testicular cells responsible for sperm development has the incidental effect of stopping testosterone production and, along with it, libido and potency. Too much testosterone has unfavorable effects on lipids, acne, weight gain, and possibly mood. Hormonal methods for men, therefore, must provide an ideal amount of testosterone to avoid these effects, but at the same time ensure effective hormonal suppression of sperm production. Regimens most likely to become available first involve androgen (synthetic testosterone) administered along with a progestin sufficient to suppress LH, the normal pituitary stimulus for testicular cell hormone and sperm production. Clinical (human) studies are ongoing to identify an optimal combination. Progestins under consideration include familiar progestins such as levonorgestrel, norethindrone enanthate (NET-EN), etonogestrel, and depot medroxyprogesterone acetate (DMPA). Providing sufficient testosterone had also been a development challenge because available testosterone products would require frequent administration (daily or weekly injections). Longer acting preparations now becoming available such as testosterone undecanoate (TU) or testosterone pellets may provide a more feasible approach.[26] A Phase 2b multi-center clinical effectiveness trial of NET-EN and TU is planned to start in 2007 under the auspices of CONRAD and WHO.

Non-hormonal possibilities have been evaluated as systemic contraceptives for men. Gossypol, derived from cottonseed oil, has been used for clinical research in China. Large studies there have found that it can provide effective sperm suppression without changing testosterone production or libido. Concern about reduced blood potassium levels reported in the initial studies for 10% of subjects, as well as irreversibility of the contraceptive effect in as many as 20% of users, reduced international interest in developing this method further. Subsequent Chinese research, however, found that the low potassium effect was related to the low level of potassium in the diets of study subjects, and a recent review concluded that additional potential for this approach should be explored.[27] Other non-hormonal options being considered for development are anti-cancer drugs such as lonidamine. These agents are known to reduce normal sperm production, and it may be possible to find a compound that has a high effectiveness in reducing sperm but an acceptable toxicity profile in other respects.

INTRAUTERINE DEVICES (IUDs)

Several improvements for existing intrauterine contraceptives are being investigated with the hope of reducing the risk for expulsion, reducing the discomfort and cramping that some women experience, and providing an intrauterine option for women whose uterine depth is too small to accommodate the currently available devices. A smaller sized version of the levonorgestrel-releasing intrauterine system, Mirena, is being tested for use in women at or after menopause. GyneFix carries copper tubes on a string and provides efficacy similar to that provided by the copper T, with (at least) five years duration. It has been approved for marketing in the European Union and is also available in China and Indonesia.[28–30] The Belgian company, Contrel, that markets GyneFix is now developing a second frameless option, the FibroPlant-LNG. Instead of using copper tubes, this model incorporates a levonorgestrel-releasing ethylene vinyl acetate hormone reservoir similar to that of the Mirena T-shaped intrauterine system.[31]

METHODS FOR STERILIZATION

In the United States and worldwide, sterilization surgery is one of the most widely used of all contraceptive options. Research to improve technologies for sterilization therefore has important promise for increasing both safety and effectiveness of sterilization, as well as lowering the cost and simplifying the procedures to avoid the need for surgical facilities and general anesthesia. Minimally invasive transcervical sterilization methods for women are being studied, in addition to the transcervical sterilization device, Essure, approved by the FDA in 2002. One such investigational device is the Adiana transcervical sterilization system, which is a two-step procedure including the creation of a superficial lesion and placement of a small implant through a transcervical catheter using hysteroscopy. Once in place, the implanted device serves as a matrix for growth of tissue that occludes the tube within a few weeks.

Low-tech methods of female transcervical nonsurgical sterilization have been studied since the 1960s by a wide variety of researchers and organizations. The goal is to develop a product that employs a simple method to deliver an active chemical/or device to produce permanent tubal occlusion leading to female infertility.

Of the possible chemical agents evaluated in animal and clinical trials, quinacrine has been the most widely used for female nonsurgical sterilization. The use of quinacrine for nonsurgical sterilization has been halted in several countries due to safety, efficacy, and ethical concerns raised by women's health advocates as well as by WHO. A study of a cancer cluster among women in Chile concluded that the cluster was unrelated to quinacrine, but a single suspicious uterine cancer remained as a provocative finding.[32] Ongoing studies to evaluate the carcinogenic potential of quinacrine should allow researchers to better evaluate the potential carcinogenic risk of quinacrine. So far, a one-year neonatal mouse carcinogenicity study revealed a lack of tumorigenic response to quinacrine in the usual target organs for the neonatal mouse bioassay.[33] However, the carcinogenic risk of quinacrine cannot be fully evaluated with one study alone. A 2-year rat carcinogenicity study with direct intrauterine administration of quinacrine is nearing completion. Also, a case-control study of gynecologic cancers is ongoing in northern Vietnam in the area where quinacrine was most widely used from 1989 to 1993. Meanwhile, a Phase I safety study of quinacrine was conducted in the United States with the FDA concurrence.[34]

In 1999, a reproductive sterilization study in animals identified erythromycin as an alternative agent with the potential to cause sufficient sclerosis to occlude the fallopian tubes.[35] As animal studies continued, another research group conducted a crude Phase I study of crushed erythromycin tablets and concluded that the failure rate of intrauterine insertion of erythromycin was unacceptably high.[36] Some investigators believe additional more carefully designed studies, using an improved erythromycin delivery method and formulation, are warranted.[37]

Both conventional and no-scalpel vasectomies are safe and effective procedures performed almost exclusively under local anesthesia. Investigators have explored alternatives to surgical sterilization for men, including chemical injections and formed in-place plugs, but questions over the safety of these chemicals and material have stalled this research.[38]

IMPROVING USE-EFFECTIVENESS

Since hormonal methods are effective and widely used, recent research has focused on new delivery systems and extended dosing to increase choice and to make methods easier for women to use correctly and consistently. With the knowledge that poor communication between healthcare providers and consumers, including inadequate education regarding emergency contraception, may contribute to the occurrence of unintended pregnancies,[39-40] research into better communication strategies is warranted. Such research suggests that the presentation of pregnancy risk categories rather than standard numeric risk for available methods best conveys pregnancy risks.[41] In addition, active interventions, such as electronic mail reminders, may improve oral contraceptive compliance.[42] Continued research into simple ways of improving regimens, such as the development of novel initiation methods,[43] remove obstacles to use and may improve successful use.

THE 21ST CENTURY

Compared with the extraordinary advances in pharmaceuticals in other fields, progress in development of contraceptives has been modest. Most of the options now in wide use are variations of half-century-old hormonal suppression technology, and realistic possibilities for the next decade are not plentiful. Major innovations are not even apparent on the horizon. It would be a shame to be content with this slow pace when the need is so great, and the public health benefit to be gained so large. Surely this is a time for renewed effort and fortified resources to develop new methods not only for developed countries but also for the billions of couples in less affluent nations whose lives would be so greatly improved.

REFERENCES

1. Mosher WD, Martinez GM, Chandra A, Abma JC, Willson SJ. Use of contraception and use of family planning services in the United States: 1982–2002. Advance Data From Vital and Health Statistics 2004 Dec;(350):1–36.
2. UNAIDS, AIDS Epidemic Update, December 2005.
3. Mostad SB, Overbaugh J, DeVange DM, et al. Hormonal contraception, vitamin A deficiency, and other risk factors for shedding of HIV-1 infected cells from the cervix and vagina. Lancet 1997;350:922–927.
? Prakash M, Patterson S and Kapembwa MS Hormonal upregulation of CCR5 expression on T lymphocytes as a possible mechanism for increased HIV-1 risk J Acquir Immune Defic Syndr 2005 Mar;38 Suppl 1:S14–6.
4. Morrision CS, Bright P, Wong EL, Kwok C, Yacobson I, Gaydos CA, Tucker HT, Blumenthal PD. Hormonal contraceptive use, cervical ectopy, and the acquisition of cervical infections. Sex Transm Dis 2004;31:561–7
5. Morrison CS, Richardson BA, Celentano DD, Chipato T, Mmiro F, Mugerwa R, Padian NS, Rugpao S, Salata RA.Prospective clinical trials designed to assess the use of hormonal contraceptives and risk of HIV acquisition. J Acquir Immune Defic Syndr 2005;38 Suppl 1:S17–8.
6. Morrision CS, Richardson BA, Mmiro F, Chipato T, Celentano DD, Luoto J, Mugerwa R, Padian NS, Rugpao S, Van Der Pol B, Brown JM, Cornelisse, P, Salata RA. Hormonal contraception and the risk of HIV acquisition. ISSTDR, Abstract, July 10–13, 2005
7. Mastroianni LJ, Donaldson PJ, Kane FJ, Jr., editors. Developing new contraceptives: obstacles and opportunities. Washington, D.C.: National Academy Press;1990.
8. Harrison PF, Rosenfield A, editors. Contraceptive research and development: looking to the future. Washington, D.C.: National Academy Press;1996.
9. Harrison PF, Rosenfield A. Research, introduction, and use: advancing from Norplant. Contraception 1998;58:323–334.
10. Nass SJ, Strauss JF III, Editors. New Frontiers in contraceptive research: a blueprint for action. Washington, D.C.: National Academics Press, 2004.
11. 2004 Survey: Medicines in development for women. Washington, D.C.: Pharmaceutical Research and Manufacturers of America;2004 (www.phrma.org).
12. Society for Women's Health Research. Issue: Federal Funding for Women's Health Research. www.womenshealthresearch.org
13. Raymond EG, Chen PL, Luoto J. Contraceptive effectiveness and safety of five nonoxynol-9 spermicides: a randomized trial. Obstet Gynecol 2004;103: 430–439.
14. Roddy RE, Zekeng L, Ryan KA, Tamoufe U, Weir SS, Wong EL. A controlled trial of nonoxynol-9 film to reduce male-to-female transmission of sexually transmitted diseases. N Engl J Med 1998;339:504–510.
15. Roddy RE, Zekeng L, Ryan KA, Tamoufe U, Tweedy KG. Effect of nonoxynol-9 gel on urogenital gonorrhea and chlamydial infection: a randomized controlled trial. JAMA 2002;287:1117–1122.
16. Van Damme L, Ramjee G, Alary M, et al. Effectiveness of COL-1492, a nonoxynol-9 vaginal gel, on HIV-1 transmission in female sex workers: a randomised controlled trial. Lancet 2002;360(9338):971–977.
17. Roddy RE, Cordero M, Cordero C, Fortney JA. A dosing study of nonoxynol-9 and genital irritation. Int J STD AIDS 1993;4:165–170.
18. Richardson BA. Nonoxynol-9 as a vaginal microbicide for prevention of sexually transmitted infections: it's time to move on. JAMA 2002;287:1171–1172.
19. Baron S, Poast J, Nguyen D, Cloyd MW. Practical prevention of vaginal and rectal transmission of HIV by adapting the oral defense: use of commercial lubricants. AIDS Res Hum Retroviruses 2001;17:997–1002.
20. Moench TR, Chipato T, Padian NS. Preventing disease by protecting the cervix: the unexplored promise of internal vaginal barrier devices. AIDS 2001;15:1595–1602.

21. Roizen J, Richardson S, Tripp J, Hardwicke H, Lam TQ. Oves contraceptive cap: short-term acceptability, aspects of use and user satisfaction. J Fam Plann Reprod Health Care 2002;28:188–192.

22. Gallo, MF, Grimes, DA, and Schulz, KF. Non-latex versus latex male condoms for contraception. Cochrane Database of Systematic Reviews 2003;:CD003550. Review

23. Meirik O. Implantable contraceptives for women. Contraception 2002;65:1–2.

24. Van Look PF, von Hertzen H. Clinical uses of antiprogestogens. Hum Reprod Update 1995;1:19–34.

25. Brady BM, Anderson RA. Advances in male contraception. Expert Opin Investig Drugs 2002;11:333–344.

26. Meriggiola MC, Costantino A, Cerpolini S. Recent advances in hormonal male contraception. Contraception 2002;65:269–272.

27. Coutinho EM. Gossypol: a contraceptive for men. Contraception 2002;65: 259–263.

28. Wu S, Hu J, Wildemeersch D. Performance of the frameless GyneFix and the TCu380A IUDs in a 3-year multicenter, randomized, comparative trial in parous women. Contraception 2000;61.91–98.

29. Wildemeersch D, Cao X, Zhang W, et al. Efficacy of a mini version of the frameless GyneFix intrauterine system (IUS) with effective copper surface area of 200 mm². dirk.wildemeersch@contrel.be. Contraception 2002;66:237–241.

30. Wildemeersch D, Batar I, Affandi B, et al. The 'frameless' intrauterine system for long-term, reversible contraception: a review of 15 years of clinical experience. J Obstet Gynaecol Res 2003;29:164–173.

31. Wildemeersch D, Schacht E, Wildemeersch P. Contraception and treatment in the perimenopause with a novel "frameless" intrauterine levonorgestrel-releasing drug delivery system: an extended pilot study. Contraception 2002;66:93–99.

32. Sokal, D. C., A. Dabancens, R. Guzman-Serani, and J. Zipper. 2000. Cancer risk among women sterilized with transcervical quinacrine in Chile: an update through 1996. Fertil Steril 74:169–71.

33. Cancel AM, Smith T, Rehkemper U, Dillberger J, Sokal D and McClain RM. A one-year neonatal mouse carcinogenesis study of quinacrine dihydrochloride. International Journal of Toxicology, in press.

34. Lippes, J., M. Brar, K. Gerbracht, P. Neff, and S. Kokkinakis. An FDA phase I clinical trial of quinacrine sterilization (QS). Int J Gynaecol Obstet 2003;83 Suppl 2:S45–9.

35. Fail PA, Martin P, Sokal D. Comparative effects of quinacrine and erythromycin in adult female rats: a nonsurgical sterilization study. Fertil Steril 2000;73:387–94.

36. Bairagy NR and Mullick BC. 2004. Use of erythromycin for nonsurgical female sterilization in West Bengal, India: a study of 790 cases. Contraception. 2004;69:47–9.

37. Sokal D and Cancel A, Personal communication (01/27/06).

38. Engender Health, Contraceptive Sterilization: Global Issues and Trends, 2002.

39. Jones R, Darroch JE, Henshaw SK. Contraceptive use among U.S. women having abortions in 2000–2001. Perspect Sex Reprod Health 2002;34:294–93.

40. Isaacs JN, Creinin MD. Miscommunication between healthcare providers and patients may result in unplanned pregnancies. Contraception 2003;68:373–76.

41. Steiner MJ, Dalebout S, Condon S, Dominik R, Trusell J. Understanding risk: A randomized controlled trial of communicating contraceptive effectiveness. Obstet Gynecol 2003;102:709–17.

42. Fox MC, Creinin MD, Murthy AS, Harwood B, Reid LM. Feasibility study of the use of a daily electronic mail reminder to improve oral contraceptive compliance. Contraception 2003;68:365–71.

43. Westhoff C, Kerns J, Morroni C, et al. Quick Start: a novel oral contraceptive initiation method. Contraception 2002;66:141–45.

Menstrual Disorders and Related Concerns

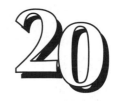

Anita L. Nelson, MD
Susie Baldwin, MD, MPH

- Dysmenorrhea is the most common cause of lost days of school and work for young women.

- PCOS is the most common endocrinopathy among reproductive-age women.

- Dysfunctional uterine bleeding is a diagnosis of exclusion.

- For idiopathic menorrhagia, consider bleeding disorders in your differential.

- Offer therapies that eliminate menses when treating conditions that are worsened by menses.

- Chronic pelvic pain can be caused by a range of gynecologic, gastrointestinal, genitourinary and musculoskeletal causes.

While providing family planning services, reproductive health care providers help women deal with a wide range of gynecologic problems. Many of these problems, including sexually transmitted infections (STIs) and vulvovaginitis, are addressed in other chapters. However, during their reproductive years, women frequently experience disorders in menstrual cycling such as excessive bleeding, infrequent bleeding, or painful menses. In addition, even normal menstrual cycling can be associated with other problems such as premenstrual syndrome (PMS) and menstrual migraine. This chapter focuses on menstrual cycle disorders and related conditions such as endometriosis and chronic pelvic pain. Hormonal contraceptive methods often serve dual purposes of providing birth control and relieving troublesome symptoms.

DYSMENORRHEA

Dysmenorrhea, Greek for painful menstruation, is classified as *primary dysmenorrhea* (intrinsic and usually of early onset) or *secondary dysmenorrhea* (due to some other physical cause and usually of later onset). In a study of young women attending a family planning clinic, 72% of those surveyed reported having experienced dysmenorrhea; for 15%, the symptoms were severe enough to interfere with their normal activities.[1] Among adult menstruating women, dysmenorrhea was reported by 40%; over 10% reported severe limitation of their activities for 1 to 3 days per cycle.[2]

Many women with dysmenorrhea also experience nausea, vomiting, diarrhea, headaches, or lightheadedness. Symptoms often vary in severity from cycle to cycle but generally continue throughout the reproductive years. Dysmenorrhea can incapacitate, causing significant disruption each month. Young women lose days at school, and older women are hampered at home and in the workplace.

PRIMARY DYSMENORRHEA: ETIOLOGY

Primary dysmenorrhea has physiologic, not psychological, causes. While early investigators believed that dysmenorrhea occurred in "maladjusted women who were intensely rejecting their feminine role and suffered from deep hostility,"[3] today we understand that the problem is not in the woman's head but in her uterus. Measurements with intrauterine pressure catheters demonstrate that women with primary dysmenorrhea generate intrauterine pressures similar to those seen during the second stage of labor.[4,5]

Women with primary dysmenorrhea are generally ovulatory and thus produce progesterone in the luteal phase. Progesterone stimulates the production of prostaglandins in the base of the endometrium, which are released when the endometrium sloughs. Women with primary dysmenorrhea produce excessive amounts of prostaglandin F2α,[6] which increases the force of uterine contractions. The uterine contractions reduce uterine blood flow, causing ischemia. This ischemia directly causes pain and sensitizes afferent nerve fibers in the uterus to painful stimuli, which augments the patient's perception of pain. When prostaglandins are injected into the general circulation by uterine contractions, they can induce headache, nausea, vomiting, and diarrhea. Other etiologies of primary dysmenorrhea, such as structural abnormalities of the uterus (blind horns), cervix (stenotic os), or vagina (transverse septa), usually present only with primary amenorrhea or can usually be ruled out by a careful pelvic examination and radiographic studies.

Primary Dysmenorrhea: Therapies

Symptomatic therapies include rest, applying a heating pad, or using teas or over-the-counter medications to treat the discomfort. Vitamin E 200 units given twice a day for 2 days before menses and for 3 days after onset reduces both pain severity and duration.[7] Usually, however, women seeking medical care have already tried many of these measures without success and need therapies targeting the underlying pathophysiology of their complaints. Several complimentary therapeutic interventions are effective for dysmenorrhea, including direct prostaglandin inhibitors, hormonal contraceptives, and gonadotropin suppressants.

Direct Prostaglandin Inhibitors

Prostaglandin synthetase inhibitors such as non-steroidal anti-inflammatory drugs (NSAIDs) and COX-2 inhibitors are more effective than placebo in treating dysmenorrhea; approximately 80% of women with dysmenorrhea feel relief with these agents. The drugs not only improve cramping pain, but also reduce backache, headaches, and gastrointestinal symptoms.[8] Taken at the onset of menses, NSAIDs reduce the release of prostaglandins and significantly reduce menstrual blood loss.[8] In contrast, aspirin is no more effective than placebo for dysmenorrhea and can increase menstrual blood loss. While COX-2 inhibitors do improve dysmenorrhea symptoms, they have been linked to cardiovascular risk and, therefore, are generally not prescribed for this indication.

Hormonal Contraceptives

A significant correlation between the severity of dysmenorrhea and the duration and amount of menstrual blood loss has been reported.[1] Hormonal contraceptives significantly reduce menstrual blood loss and decrease the production of prostaglandins. Within 3 to 4 months of beginning combined oral contraceptive (COC) therapy, 90% of women experience marked decreases in the severity of pain.[9,10]

Women can achieve additional relief from dysmenorrhea by using extended cycle COCs. Extended use of active pills for at least 84 days reduces the number of scheduled bleeding episodes to 4 per year.[11] Ultimately, extended COCs can be used to prevent menses for more prolonged intervals with no known adverse impact. Extended use of other combined hormonal methods, such as the hormonal contraceptive patch or vaginal ring, have not been tested for dysmenorrhea, but these do significantly reduce the days of bleeding and, therefore, would be expected to reduce the pain related to menstruation.

Depo medroxyprogesterone acetate (DMPA) is also helpful in treating dysmenorrhea. After their third injection, nearly half of DMPA users become amenorrheic and avoid dysmenorrhea altogether. The levonor-gestrel-releasing intrauterine system (LNG-IUS) is also an excellent choice for women with dysmenorrhea, because menstrual blood loss and duration of bleeding are significantly reduced. By 12 months of use, 20% of women have amenorrhea; users experience a 70–90% reduction in blood loss overall.

Other Gonadotropin Suppressants

Other medications are also available to achieve amenorrhea, but their use is limited due to side effects and cost. Danazol, an androgen used to treat endometriosis, effectively induces amenorrhea but can be used for only 4 to 6 months due to side effects such as acne, hirsutism, oily skin, clitoral enlargement, and voice deepening. Gonadotropin releasing hormone (GnRH) agonists also induce amenorrhea and, therefore, eliminate dysmenorrhea. However, GnRH use is also limited to 4 to 6 months because it can cause hypoestrogenic side effects such as vasomotor symptoms (hot flashes), vaginal dryness, and loss of bone mineralization. GnRH agonists have been combined with estrogen/progestin "add-back" therapy for long-term treatment of endometriosis, but have not been studied in treatment of primary dysmenorrhea.

In women who fail to respond to these therapies, rule out other causes of pain. Some women who have primary dysmenorrhea early in life may subsequently develop other problems, which complicate their dysmenorrhea later in life (see secondary dysmenorrhea). Women with persistent complaints may benefit from a psychological evaluation and/or treatments for chronic pain, particularly if dysmenorrhea is only one component of their pain syndrome (see below). Some investigators report that a transcutaneous electrical nerve stimulation (TENS) unit reduces dysmenorrhea. Some investigators have suggested that dietary manipulations such as supplementing omega-3 polyunsaturated fatty acids may decrease dysmenorrhea in adolescents.[12] Surgical interventions including presacral nerve ablation, endometrial ablation, and hysterectomy are treatments of last resort; they are reserved for patients who do not respond to medical and other approaches.

SECONDARY DYSMENORRHEA

Women with secondary dysmenorrhea also complain of painful uterine cramping with menses but may have other accompanying complaints, such as dyspareunia or non-menstrual pelvic pain. The pain that women with secondary dysmenorrhea experience is, by definition, due to uterine or pelvic pathology.

The most common causes of chronic secondary dysmenorrhea are adenomyosis, endometriosis, pelvic adhesions, and neoplasia. *Adeno-*

myosis is the presence of endometrial glands and stroma embedded in the myometrium (the deep muscle layer of the uterus). Adenomyosis is commonly found in parous women. Monthly ovarian hormonal swings stimulate this ectopically located endometrial tissue, causing sloughing within the myometrium. Aside from dysmenorrhea, women with symptomatic adenomyosis may also experience heavy menses and perimenstrual pain associated with deep thrusting. On examination, women with adenomyosis have enlarged, somewhat boggy, uteri that can be tender just prior to and during menses.

Implantation of the same endometrial tissue *outside* the uterus is called *endometriosis*. Women with endometriosis experience painful menses due to cyclic shedding of endometriotic implants and the local inflammatory response that shedding incites. Women with endometriosis often report onset of pelvic pain just prior to onset of menses. In cases with established adhesions, dyspareunia from deep thrusting can occur throughout the cycle.

Pelvic adhesions from previous pelvic inflammatory disease (salpingitis or tubo-ovarian abscesses), appendicitis, and pelvic or abdominal surgery can also cause dysmenorrhea. Other pelvic pathology, including uterine fibroids and some types of pelvic masses that may also cause painful menses, can be imaged by ultrasound. Cervical stenosis resulting from LEEP or other processes can increase menstrual pain. Copper intrauterine devices (IUDs) sometimes are associated with heavier or more uncomfortable menses but are an unusual cause of clinically significant secondary dysmenorrhea, unless the device is expelling.

Diagnostic laparoscopy may be needed to evaluate fully the causes of the patient's pain. The treatment of secondary dysmenorrhea should be targeted to the underlying problems and should reflect the patient's desire for fertility. In the absence of problems requiring surgical intervention, the treatments helpful for primary dysmenorrhea (especially those that eliminate menses) often successfully reduce symptoms of secondary dysmenorrhea. If these interventions are not sufficiently effective, or if the patient is seeking fertility, more definitive surgical approaches may be needed. For example, secondary dysmenorrhea caused by pelvic scarring may benefit from surgical lysis of adhesions. For women with dysmenorrhea associated with submucous fibroids not controlled by hormonal therapy, a myomectomy or uterine artery embolization might more effectively reduce menstrual flow and discomfort. Endometrial ablation or hysterectomy is reserved for treatment of incapacitating dysmenorrhea unresponsive to more conservative measures and only in women who do not desire future childbearing.

MENORRHAGIA

Patients may present with complaints of "heavy" periods or "irregular bleeding." Obtaining a more accurate history can clarify the true nature of their problems. Precise use of terminology can help promote effective communication and justify appropriate work-ups and therapies.

Menorrhagia and *hypermenorrhea* refer to menstrual periods that occur at regular intervals but are marked by prolonged bleeding (> 7 days) or excessive blood loss (> 80 cc). *Metrorrhagia* refers to irregular, frequent uterine bleeding of variable amounts. *Menometrorrhagia* is the term used to describe prolonged uterine bleeding occurring irregularly. *Polymenorrhea* is uterine bleeding occurring at short intervals (< 21 days). *Intermenstrual bleeding* is bleeding of variable amounts occurring between regular menses. *Postcoital bleeding* occurs after sexual intercourse.

The "normal" values for the frequency and duration of menses as well as the amount of blood loss each cycle vary widely (see Table 20–1). The "normal values" were derived from population studies without regard to the possible adverse nonmedical impacts they may have.

In obtaining a history from a woman, recognize that her memory of her menses may not be complete. One common pitfall is that women report bleeding-free days rather than total cycle length measured from the first day of bleeding in one cycle to the next. *Menstrual calendars* used prospectively can more accurately document bleeding patterns. Quantifying actual blood loss may be challenging.[13] Estimates derived from numbers of pads or tampons used are complicated by variations in product absorbancy and different degrees of fastidiousness among women. In addition, a large component of the menstrual discharge is not blood, but other fluids.[14] In one study that compared women's perception of their blood loss to measured losses, over one third of women with a 20 to 40cc loss characterized their flows as "heavy" and almost 10% of those with greater than 80cc loss thought their periods were light.[15] By the time excessive menstrual bleeding causes anemia that can be quantified by a physician, the woman has suffered very significant blood loss.

At least as important as the absolute numbers of days or the amount of blood lost is any *change* the patient may perceive from what has been established as normal for her. A woman who has historically bled 3 days

Table 20–1 Range of normal values for menses

	Range	Average
Frequency	21–35 days	28 days
Duration	2–6 days	4 days
Blood Loss	20–80 ml	30–35 ml

per cycle and now notices that she bleeds for 6 to 7 days may still be within an arbitrary range for normal, but she merits an evaluation since she is experiencing a significant change from her baseline pattern. By the same token, even though a woman's total number of days of bleeding or total blood loss may not be excessive, there may be times in her cycle when her flow is so heavy that it interrupts her normal activities. For example, a woman who has 5 days of bleeding with a total blood loss of 75 cc may be completely incapacitated for 4 hours each month when her flow requires that she wear 2 pads at a time and change them every hour. Menstrual bleeding should be considered excessive if the woman considers it excessive. There are other special cases in which menses may be physiologically "normal" but treatment to eliminate them is appropriate. Women with severe developmental disabilities may benefit from induction of amenorrhea for hygiene concerns or to reduce menstrual-related problems.[16]

Causes of excessive uterine bleeding may be classified into several categories to facilitate evaluation. Organic gynecologic disease is the first concern when women present with abnormal bleeding. Pregnancy and pregnancy-related complications (e.g., threatened abortion or ectopic pregnancy) and infection of the cervix, endometrium, or fallopian tubes are primary differential diagnoses for sexually active women. Endometrial and cervical polyps, uterine leiomyoma, and adenomyosis can cause menorrhagia. Endometrial hyperplasia and carcinoma are often associated with heavy and prolonged menses as well as intermenstrual bleeding. Cervical infection or carcinoma more classically present with postcoital bleeding.

Systemic diseases such as thyroid dysfunction, liver cirrhosis, active hepatitis, adrenal hyperplasia, incipient renal failure, and hypersplenism can cause prolonged menses or excessive bleeding by altering estrogen metabolism or hepatic production of coagulation factors. Intrinsic bleeding disorders such as Von Willebrand's disease, idiopathic thrombocytopenia purpura, aplastic anemia, or platelet dysfunction are more frequent causes of menorrhagia than is generally recognized. In a study of 115 women with physician-diagnosed menorrhagia, 47% were found to have hemostatic abnormalities.[17] Platelet dysfunction was the most commonly observed hemostatic defect. Acute problems such as leukemia, severe sepsis, or disseminated intravascular coagulation (DIC) may also induce menorrhagia. Medications such as digitalis, phenytoin, anticoagulants, and plastic and copper IUDs are associated with increased menstrual flow. Heavy menstrual bleeding can result from the presence of a foreign body in the vagina or trauma resulting from sexual abuse.

Dysfunctional uterine bleeding (DUB) is a diagnosis of exclusion. DUB generally results from anovulatory cycling. Anovulation results in unopposed estrogen stimulation, which produces a thick endometrial lining. Without progesterone, there is a dyssynchronous endometrial sloughing and an imbalance in prostaglandins, creating an excess of PGE vasodilation and a relative paucity of PGF2α vasoconstriction. Under these influences, women develop excessive and prolonged bleeding. Anovulatory cycling usually presents during adolescence and perimenopause; today, reproductive age women are more likely to have anovulatory cycling because of the increasing prevalence of obesity.

EVALUATION OF EXCESSIVE UTERINE BLEEDING

Take a complete menstrual history, emphasizing the last several months. The age of the patient and the pattern of her bleeding guide the evaluation. Perform pregnancy tests for reproductive-age women who have abnormal bleeding. If anemia is a concern, determine the patient's hemoglobin or hematocrit level. Rule out vaginal and cervical abnormalities (infection, carcinoma, or polyps) by examination; test as indicated for gonorrhea and chlamydia. Test for cervical cytology only if the patient is late for her routine testing. Biopsy suspicious lesions. Perform a bimanual examination to rule out cervical motion tenderness, to determine the size and shape of the uterus, and to detect ovarian or adnexal masses. Perform thyroid function tests in women with signs or symptoms suggestive of this problem. Evaluate recently menarcheal women with excessive blood loss, as well as women with a life-long heavy or prolonged menses for bleeding disorders.[18] This testing may be most efficiently done in consultation with a hematologist, since the list of needed tests is extensive.[19] To evaluate heavy or intermenstrual bleeding in women with risk factor(s), perform an endometrial biopsy to rule out endometrial hyperplasia or carcinoma. Risk factors include advanced reproductive age (over age 35), obesity, or unopposed estrogen exposure from either exogenous sources (medications) or intrinsic sources (polycystic ovary syndrome [PCOS]). Ultrasound can be used to evaluate the uterus for leiomyoma or other tumors that may affect bleeding. Saline infusion sonography can image the endometrium to identify polyps and fibroids. Hysteroscopy allows visualization as well as directed biopsy, but is more uncomfortable than saline infusion sonography.[20]

TREATMENT OF MENORRHAGIA

Treat any identified problem causing chronic menorrhagia, such as infection, polyps, thyroid dysfunction, or bleeding abnormalities. For women with idiopathic menorrhagia or bleeding due to fibroids or adenomyosis, medical therapy should be the first-line therapy unless significant pelvic pathology requires surgical therapy.

Prostaglandin Synthetase Inhibitors and Iron Supplements

Since a 35 to 40 ml of menstrual blood loss represents the loss of 16 mg of elemental iron, women with excessive blood loss will need routine iron supplementation. Prostaglandin inhibitors are generally first-line therapies for menorrhagia; NSAIDs taken for the first 3 to 5 days of menses each cycle reduces blood loss by 20% to 45%, which was judged by a Cochrane review to be superior to placebo.[21]

No difference in efficacy has been demonstrated among the various NSAIDs. Maximal doses outlined in Table 20–2 are necessary to achieve blood loss reductions; lower doses have no clinical effect. Although gastric or peptic ulcer disease may preclude long-term NSAID therapy, episodic use of high-dose NSAIDs may be well tolerated by women with these problems.

Additional therapy depends on the etiology of the woman's bleeding (whether it is ovulatory or anovulatory bleeding; see Table 20–3), her desire for future childbearing, and her preferences. Surprisingly, given how frequently this problem occurs, only one of the hormonal therapies used to treat menorrhagia in the United States today (cyclic MPA) is FDA-approved. All the other therapies are off-label uses.

Hormonal Therapies

If prostaglandin inhibitors do not adequately control bleeding in women who have heavy monthly menses with *ovulatory* cycling, hormonal interventions often prove effective:

- Progestin-only pills reduce endometrial proliferation.

- COCs taken cyclically reduce blood loss by 30% to 50%.

- Extended cycle COCs and vaginal rings reduce total blood loss in women with menorrhagia.[22,23]

- Both DMPA and the LNG-IUS can reduce menstrual blood loss by 70% to 90%. LNG-IUS improved blood loss significantly better than mefenamic acid did in a randomized clinical trial of women with idiopathic menorrhagia.[24]

Table 20–2 NSAIDs

Ibuprofen 800 mg	3 times daily
Naproxen sodium 550 mg	2 times daily
Mefenamic acid 500 mg	3 times daily
Meclofenamate sodium 100 mg	3 times daily

Table 20–3 Characteristics and treatments of DUB

	Anovulatory DUB	Ovulatory DUB
% of DUB	90%	10%
Timing in life	Early adolescence and perimenopause	Peak reproductive years
Moliminal symptoms	None	Routine
Menses	Unpredictable, irregular	Excessive
Etiologies	Unopposed estrogen stimulation Imbalance of prostaglandins	Imbalance of prostaglandins
Treatment goals	1. Endometrial cycling • Cyclic progestin 2. Endometrial suppression • Combined hormonal contraception • Extended combined hormonal contraception • DMPA, LNG-IUS, progestin-only pills, MPA 5 mg daily • Other: Danazol, GnRH agonist 3. Prostaglandin re-equilibration • NSAIDs	1. Endometrial suppression • Combined hormonal contraception • Extended combined hormonal contraception • DMPA, LNG-IUS, progestin-only pills, MPA 5 mg daily • Other: Danazol, GnRH agonist 2. Prostaglandin re-equilibration • NSAIDs

- Cyclic progestin therapy may *increase* blood loss in ovulatory menorrhagia.[25]

For women with *anovulatory* menorrhagia, prevent a recurrence by pharmacologically inducing cyclic withdrawal bleeding with cyclic combined hormonal contraceptives (pills, patches, or rings) or progestins (medroxyprogesterone 5 mg daily for 10 to 12 days each month) or by suppressing the endometrium with progestin-only COCs, DMPA, combined continuous COCs, or the LNG-IUS.[26]

Surgical Therapies

Women with significant acute bleeding may need a D&C for the immediate control of bleeding as well as for diagnosis. However, the effects of a D&C are only temporary. Initiate medical therapies after surgery to avoid the recurrence of the problem. Other surgical interventions such as endometrial ablation with laser, resectoscope, thermal balloon or roller ball,[27] and hysterectomy are reserved for women who fail to improve with medical therapy and who desire no future fertility. Surgery is also indicated for women who have pelvic pathology.

AMENORRHEA

Amenorrhea, the absence of menses, is also classified as primary or secondary. The workup for *primary amenorrhea* is indicated when there is a lack of any secondary sexual characteristics by age 13, lack of menses by age 15, or no menses within 5 years after initiation of breast development (thelarche) or pubic or axillary hair (pubarche or adrenarche).[28] *Secondary amenorrhea* occurs in women who have previously menstruated. Secondary amenorrhea is defined as the absence of menses for at least 3 months in a woman who previously has had regular monthly menses and for at least 6 to 12 months in a woman who had oligomenorrhea. The absence of menses for a shorter period is referred to as *delayed menses*.

Begin the evaluation of amenorrhea in a sexually active reproductive-age woman with a pregnancy test. History may be helpful in identifying women at risk for pregnancy, but it is not always reliable. Once you have ruled out pregnancy as a cause of the patient's amenorrhea, the evaluation of amenorrhea depends upon its classification. Both primary and secondary amenorrhea have a multitude of causes, so take a systematic approach to find answers in a cost-effective manner.

PRIMARY AMENORRHEA

Usually the evaluation of primary amenorrhea involves consultation with specialists, but a fundamental understanding of the possible etiologies can be helpful in advising the young patient and her often anxious family. A classic efficient evaluation of primary amenorrhea relies on two physical findings: the presence of a uterus and breast development in the absence of any male genitalia suggestive of a hermaphrodite.[29] Figure 20–1 provides testing recommendations based on the four possible combinations of these findings.

SECONDARY AMENORRHEA

The absence of menses in a reproductive-aged woman not using hormonal contraception is an important symptom because it can indicate a systemic medical problem or a problem confined to the reproductive system. Even if a woman does not desire fertility, she must be evaluated because the underlying problem or its consequences require therapy.

Initiate the evaluation of secondary amenorrhea with a thorough history and physical examination. Take a careful menstrual history, asking about ovulatory symptoms (mittelschmerz), moliminal complaints (bloating, cramping, or breast tenderness that typically herald the onset of menses), and any vasomotor symptoms. Question the patient about recent changes in her weight, dietary habits, acne, hair growth, cold or heat intolerance, galactorrhea, recent pregnancy, genital tract procedures, known medical problems, stress, and exercise patterns. On exami-

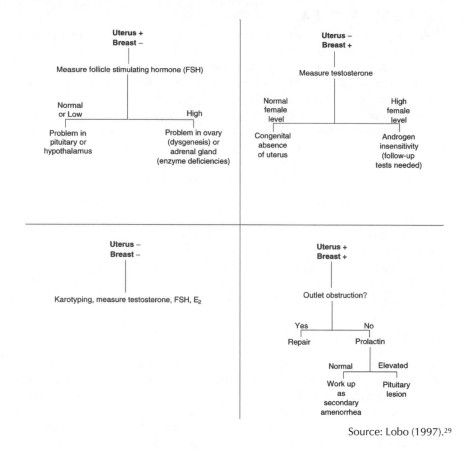

Source: Lobo (1997).[29]

Figure 20–1 Diagnostic evaluation for primary amenorrhea

nation, pay close attention to signs of androgen excess (hirsutism, balding, acne), hypoestrogenism (dry, flattened vaginal mucosa), prolactin excess (galactorrhea), or thyroid dysfunction (skin, pulse, and reflex changes).

Obtain a complete drug history because many classes of medications (prescription, over-the-counter, or street drugs) can induce amenorrhea or oligomenorrhea. Many medications can inhibit hypothalamic dopamine (prolactin inhibiting factor) and raise prolactin levels. Phenothiazine derivatives, phenothiazine-like compounds, reserpine derivative, amphetamines, opiates, diazepams, tricyclic antidepressants, methyldopa, and butyroptrenones all can induce galactorrhea either by depleting dopamine levels or by blocking dopamine receptors. Serum prolactin levels due to medication are usually only mildly elevated (30 to 70 ng/ml). Galactorrhea, which is evident in 30% to 60% of women with medication-induced hyperprolactinemia, should resolve in 3 to 6 months after discontinuation of medicine. Higher serum prolactin levels require imaging studies of the pituitary gland.

If an obvious reason for the woman's amenorrhea emerges from this initial screening, order specifically targeted diagnostic tests to confirm the diagnosis. For example, if the patient has spontaneous galactorrhea, measure her prolactin (PRO) and thyroxine stimulating hormone (TSH) levels. A 20-year-old woman with a recent onset of hirsutism and amenorrhea needs to have her androgen status evaluated to rule out a tumor. On the other hand, a 48-year-old woman who complains of hot flashes and has had no menses for a year needs no specific tests to confirm menopause. Similarly, a woman using DMPA needs no further workup when she develops amenorrhea in the absence of other symptoms.

Frequently, however, no single cause is discovered on the basis of the history and physical examination. Several systematic approaches have been developed by experts in the field, but one particularly cost-effective protocol evaluates the components of the reproductive system in order (see Figure 20–2).[30]

Uterus and Lower Genital Tract

Evaluation begins with the uterus and lower genital tract. Investigate the functional capacity of the uterus and the patency of the lower genital tract with a *progestin challenge test*. Give the patient medroxyprogesterone acetate 5 milligrams (mg) per day for 10 to 12 days. The American Society for Reproductive Medicine guidelines do not call for this step. It is included here because, for women with the most common cause of amenorrhea (chronic anovulation), this step is not only diagnostic, it is also temporarily therapeutic.

- If the patient experiences a withdrawal bleed, then we know that her cervix is patent, that she is producing estrogen, and that her endometrium is functioning. She next needs an evaluation of the higher compartments to determine why she is not ovulating and producing progestin (see the next section).

- If she does not experience a withdrawal bleed, she needs a detailed evaluation of her uterus and cervix. Check for cervical stenosis by passing a uterine sound or a cervical os finder. Assess the responsiveness of the endometrium by priming her uterus with estrogen (such as conjugated equine estrogen 0.625 mg) for 25 days, adding a progestin daily for the last 10 to 12 days.

- If the patient experiences a withdrawal bleed after estrogen/progestin cycling, then it is clear that her endometrium is functioning and that her cervix is patent. Therefore, her higher compartments will need to be tested to determine why she is not making estrogen.

Step 1: *Evaluate Uterus and Lower Genital Tract*

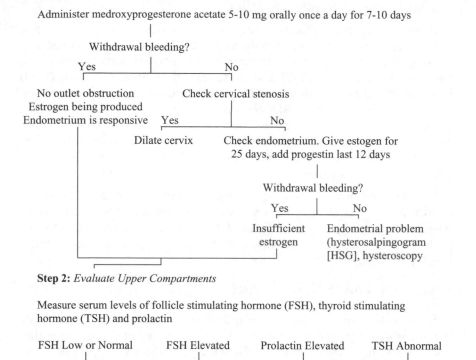

Step 2: *Evaluate Upper Compartments*

Measure serum levels of follicle stimulating hormone (FSH), thyroid stimulating hormone (TSH) and prolactin

Source: Modified from ASRM (2004)[28] and Speroff et. al. (2004).[30]

Figure 20–2 Systematic diagnostic evaluation for secondary amenorrhea

- If she does not have a withdrawal bleed, the endometrium may be scarred (Asherman's syndrome). She will benefit from direct endometrial evaluation by hysteroscopy or hysterosalpingogram (HSG).

Ovaries and Other Endocrinopathy

Evaluate endocrine influences by measuring FSH, prolactin and TSH.

- If the FSH is elevated, she most likely has ovarian failure. In young women, it is generally good practice to reconfirm the findings with measurements of FSH, LH and estradiol.

  — If the diagnosis is confirmed and the woman is younger than 25 years of age, obtain a karyotype to rule out Turner's syndrome or gonadal dysgenesis.

— If she is between 25 and 40 years of age, she will periodically need a more detailed evaluation of other autoimmune endocrinopathies. Recommended tests include calcium, phosphorus, glucose, Free T4, TSH, and antibodies to thyroid, parathyroid and adrenal glands. In any event, treat her as if she were menopausal. Through her 30s and early 40s, offer sex steroid replacement with hormone therapy or combination hormonal contraceptives to reduce the long-term effects of hypoestrogenism, such as osteoporosis.

- If her TSH is abnormal, treat her thyroid dysfunction. Provide progestin to protect her endometrium until therapy has normalized her TSH levels. After treatment, re-evaluate her menstrual status to determine that she has re-established normal cycles.

- If the FSH is low or normal and the TSH is normal, consider hypothalamic amenorrhea or chronic anovulation. If she had withdrawal bleeding with progestin, consider PCOS. See the section on Polycystic Ovary Syndrome.

- Other pathologies such as ovarian insensitivity are rare. Consult with specialists when the patient's endocrine profile does not fit clearly into one of these more common patterns.

- If the prolactin is elevated into the tumor range (usually above 70 to 100), imaging of the pituitary gland is needed. Magnetic resonance imaging (MRI) is preferred, but if it is not available, computerized axial tomography (CT) can be used to determine the presence and size of a prolactinoma. Bromocriptine therapy traditionally has been used to reduce prolactin production and restore ovulatory cycling. The most frequent side effects with bromocriptine are gastrointestinal problems. Newer agents, such as cabergoline, have fewer side effects and less frequent dosing requirements, and can be used in women who do not respond to bromocriptine.

- Other intracranial neoplasms can also cause amenorrhea. Order appropriate imaging studies and consult with neurological experts, especially if the patient has any other symptoms, such as headache, or has abnormal findings on neurologic exam.

- If the FSH is normal or low and she required estrogen stimulation to achieve withdrawal bleeding, it is quite likely that she has hypothalamic amenorrhea. Consider an eating disorder, such as anorexic nervosa or bulimia or excessive exercise. Bulimia can disrupt menstrual cycling, even in a woman of normal weight. One study found that 55% of amenorrheic women had an eating disorder. A woman who has stress due to extreme exercise, eating disorders, or situational factors should have her underlying problems addressed; she also needs hormonal supplementation to maintain adequate estrogen levels to prevent osteoporosis and to protect her endometrium.[31] Young women with hypothalamic amenorrhea have improved bone mineralization when they are given COCs but not when given medroxyprogesterone or placebo.[32] Women with mental disabilities can also have low food intake or swallowing difficulties, resulting in low weight, hypothalamic hypogonadism and oligomenorrhea.[16] Naltrexone, a narcotic antagonist, has been used to treat women with weight-loss-related amenorrhea.[33]

OLIGOMENORRHEA

Oligomenorrhea is appropriately viewed as a being on a continuum between normal ovulatory cycling and secondary amenorrhea. Many of the causes of secondary amenorrhea can, in milder forms, present as oligomenorrhea. When the interval between a woman's menses exceeds 35 days but is not long enough to qualify as being amenorrhea, she has oligomenorrhea. Oligomenorrhea with less than 9 cycles per year requires investigation.[28] It is important to identify the etiology of the oligomenorrhea to reduce other consequences of an underlying endocrinopathy or other medical problems. Most women with oligomenorrhea have anovulatory cycles. Often this menstrual pattern is life-long; many women with PCOS have consistently irregular and infrequent menses (see the next section). Sometimes oligomenorrhea develops because of excessive weight gain or after significant weight loss.

Medical problems such as hypothyroidism, hyperprolactinemia, and liver dysfunction can cause oligomenorrhea, as can certain medications. Women under stress and those who engage in extreme exercise or excessive dieting often develop oligomenorrhea, which can progress to secondary amenorrhea. Cheerleaders and women involved in seasonal sports may have irregular menses during the months in which they participate in those activities. In these women, oligomenorrhea results from *suppressed estrogen production*, which puts these women at risk for estrogen-deficiency problems such as bone loss or vaginal dryness. Adequate sex steroid levels can be maintained with estrogen-containing contraceptives.

On the other hand, women with other causes of oligomenorrhea, such as extreme increases in weight and PCOS usually have *unopposed estrogen*. Unopposed estrogen leads to uninterrupted endometrial stimulation and increases the risk for endometrial hyperplasia and carcinoma. Weight loss and exercise are keys to treatment of such oligomenorrhea. Anovulating women need a source of progesterone to offset the estrogen stimulation. Cyclic administration of progestin or combined hormonal contraceptives (pills, rings, patches), or endometrial suppression with progestin-only pills, DMPA, or the LNG-IUS are reasonable alternatives. Continuous administration of combination COCs protects the endometrium without inducing cyclic bleeding.

POLYCYSTIC OVARY SYNDROME (PCOS)

Previously called Stein-Leventhal syndrome, PCOS is a frequent cause of oligomenorrhea. It is the most common endocrinopathy of reproductive-aged women. In textbook descriptions, women with PCOS are obese, hirsute, oligomenorrheic, and subfertile. In reality, many women with PCOS are not overweight and many do not have hirsutism. Even its name is not defining; many women with polycystic-appearing ovaries (PAOs) do not have PCOS.[31] The common characteristics of PCOS are hyperandrogenism and chronic anovulation. On the other hand, suspect tumors in women who have a rapid onset of hirsutism or dramatic manifestations of hyperandrogenemia, such as clitoromegaly or deepening of voice.

In a routine office practice, the diagnosis of PCOS is generally made clinically by using the 1990 National Institutes of Health (NIH) consensus criteria. These criteria specify that a woman with PCOS has anovulatory cycles (either > 35 day intervals or fewer than 8 periods a year) with either hyperandrogenism (hirsutism, acne, male pattern balding) or hyperandrogenemia (elevated free or total testosterone or elevated DHEAS) in the absence of any other etiology. Therefore, most of the laboratory tests needed to confirm the diagnosis of PCOS are needed to rule out other etiologies, such as thyroid dysfunction, adrenal insufficiency, or androgen-producing tumors. Young women with hirsutism, in particular, should have morning levels of 17-hydroxyprogesterone (17-OHP) measured in the follicular phase to rule out adult-onset (atypical) congenital adrenal hyperplasia (CAH).

The newer 2003 Rotterdam PCOS criteria focus on hirsute women who may have oligomenorrhea and infertility. The diagnosis of PCOS using the Rotterdam criteria is made, once other etiologies have been excluded, if the woman has 2 of the following criteria:

- Oligo-ovulation or anovulation

- Clinical and/or biochemical signs of hyperandrogenism

- Polycystic appearing ovaries, defined as 12 antral follicles in a single ultrasound field.[35]

Recent studies have found that while polycystic-appearing ovaries are not normal, they do not predict a reproductive or metabolic phenotype; performing ultrasound to identify ovarian follicles may not add value in routine practice.[34] Older laboratory tests, such as measuring the LH/FSH ratio, are *not* helpful in establishing the diagnosis of PCOS and should *not* be performed.

PCOS can result from disruptions in the hypothalamic-pituitary axis, the adrenal glands, and/or the ovary. These dysfunctions cause overproduction of androgens (testosterone and DHEAS), which are responsible for the classic PCOS-related problems, such as hirsutism and acne. The excessive androgen levels, paradoxically, also cause relatively high levels of estrogen found in PCOS due to peripheral conversion of androgens to estrone (E1) in adipose, skin, and muscle. Estrone stimulates endometrial proliferation and suppresses pituitary production of FSH. In the absence of FSH stimulation, ovulation and subsequent luteal progesterone production are hampered. Endometrial proliferation continues unchecked, resulting in irregular, uncoordinated endometrial sloughing and an increased risk of endometrial hyperplasia and cancer. With anovulatory cycles, fertility is also compromised. However, *women with PCOS can have ovulatory cycles on an unpredictable, intermittent basis and should not be considered to be protected against unintended pregnancy by their condition.*

Monitor women with PCOS for other associated health risks. Many women with PCOS have insulin resistance with compensatory hyperinsulinemia, which increases their risk of developing overt diabetes.[36] Both obese and lean PCOS women are at risk, but overweight women are at higher risk. Many women with PCOS have unhealthy lipid profiles with high LDL and triglyceride levels; androgenized women with polycystic ovaries have lipid profiles similar to men.[37] Both the lipid and insulin abnormalities are independent risk factors for cardiovascular disease in women. Depression occurs frequently in women with PCOS.

Therapy for PCOS should be designed not only to address the patient's immediate concerns, but also to reduce any long-term adverse health consequences. Encourage weight reduction, exercise, and sensible diet. In obese women with PCOS, a weight loss of at least 5% to 10% can reduce both hyperinsulinemia and hyperandrogenemia.[38] Weight distribution is also important. Women with PCOS with a waist-to-hip ratio greater than 1.2 ("apple shape"), as opposed to a gynecoid distribution with a waist-to-hip ratio less than 0.75 ("pear shape"), are at higher risk for having insulin resistance.[39] Hormonal contraceptives with low androgenicity can be used to treat different aspects of the condition. COCs, patches and vaginal rings with low androgenicity can deal with hirsutism and acne (see below), prevent unopposed endometrial proliferation, and provide contraceptive protection. DMPA or the LNG-IUS can prevent endometrial proliferation and reduce pregnancy risks. Cyclic progestin with 5 mg medroxyprogesterone acetate 12 days each month can reduce the risk of endometrial hyperplasia in an anovulatory woman, but will not provide contraception or ameliorate the cutaneous manifestations of her condition.

Women with acne or hirsutism may be offered estrogenic COCs to suppress ovarian production of androgens and increase sex human binding globulin (SHBG). Increases in SHBG will reduce the serum levels of biologically active, unbound androgens. With lower circulating levels of androgens, further hair growth is reduced and sebum production is reduced, which helps reduce future acne outbreaks. Topical agents and antibiotics can be used as first-line treatment for acne or can be combined with COCs to provide better treatment for mild to moderate cystic acne.[40] See Chapter 11, Combined Oral Contraceptives. Continuous COC administration is superior to cyclic COC use in controlling LH and testosterone levels.[41] To slow the progression of new hair growth, spironolactone can be added to COCs to treat women with androgen sensitivity or hyperandrogenism. If adrenal androgen overproduction is implicated by levels of dehydroepiandrosterone sulfate (DHEAS) greater than 75 mg/ml, corticosteroid therapy may be indicated. Cyproterone acetate-estrogen regimens have been reported to be as effective as spironolactone, although that agent is not available in the United States.[42] Anti-androgens such as flutamide (250 mg daily for the first 10 days of the cycle each month) and finasteride (1 mg daily), which directly inhibit hair growth, represent other approaches to the treatment of hirsutism,[43,44] but hepatic side effects must be monitored; effective contraception must also be provided. Gonadotropin-releasing agonists with estrogen add-back therapies have also been used to block new hair growth, but this approach is still considered experimental. Women with light colored skin benefit from bleaching of their facial hair to reduce its visibility. Removal of existing hair by electrolysis or newer laser treatments is also often advisable after new hair growth stimulation has been slowed. The clinical response to any hormonal therapy is usually slow. Maximal COC impact on acne was seen at 6 months;[40] however, treatment for hirsutism may not achieve its full potential for 1 to 2 years. There is an important PCOS support group for patients at www.pcosupport.org/.

PREMENSTRUAL SYNDROME (PMS) AND PREMENSTRUAL DYSPHORIC DISORDER (PMDD)

Premenstrual syndrome (PMS) is a heterogeneous collection of signs and symptoms that share one common characteristic: a temporal relationship to the menstrual cycle. By definition, PMS is the cyclic appearance of at least one symptom during the luteal phase, followed by an entirely symptom-free interval beginning a few days after the onset of menses. The American College of Obstetrics and Gynecology (ACOG) diagnostic criteria for PMS include the physical symptoms of abdominal

Table 20–4 DSM-IV criteria for premenstrual dysphoric disorder (PMDD)

Need at least five symptoms including:

- At least one of the following:
  — Affective lability

  — Persistent and marked anger or irritability

  — Marked anxiety and tension

  — Markedly depressed mood, feeling of hopelessness

- With one to four of the following:
  — Decreased interest in usual activities

  — Easy fatigability or marked lack of energy

  — Subjective sense or difficulty in concentration

  — Marked change in appetite

  — Sleep disorders

  — Physical symptoms—breast tenderness, headache, edema, joint or muscle pain, weight gain

Source: American Psychiatric Association (2000).[50]

bloating, breast tenderness, headaches, and extremity edema, and the psychological and behavioral symptoms of anxiety, depression, confusion, social withdrawal, angry outbursts, and irritability.[45] Other commonly reported manifestations of PMS include fatigue, thirst, appetite changes, and crying spells. To be considered clinically significant, PMS symptoms must interfere with a woman's work, lifestyle, or interpersonal relationships. PMS can increase relationship strain, sexual dysfunction, social isolation, work absenteeism, and suicide. Studies have demonstrated that PMS results in poorer self-reported mental and physical health, increased use of health services, and higher health care costs for sufferers.[46,47]

While as many as 85% of women of reproductive age experience some premenstrual symptoms, only 20% to 30% of women suffer from moderate or severe symptoms.[48] A smaller number of women (3% to 8%) are debilitated by the condition called premenstrual dysphoric disorder (PMDD).[49] The diagnosis of PMDD, defined by the American Psychiatric Association (APA), requires the manifestation of at least five symptoms present for one to two weeks premenstrually, with relief by the fourth day of menses. See Table 20–4. By definition, at least one symptom must represent a severe change in mood, and the woman must experience functional impairment attributed to the symptoms.[50]

What causes PMS/PMDD? Multiple factors likely play a role in the etiology. Early investigations suggested that PMS was due to a lack of progesterone,[51] but subsequent research failed to find a difference between PMS sufferers and controls in levels of progesterone or any other major hormones including estradiol, FSH, LH, prolactin, SHBG, or testosterone.[52] However, women with PMS may be more biologically vulnerable to normal fluctuations in hormone levels than are women without the syndrome.[53]

Other investigators have theorized that PMS is caused by low beta-endorphin levels,[54,55] low adrenocorticotropin levels,[56] abnormal prostaglandin production, or endogenous hormone allergies, but research has not consistently supported these hypotheses. Nor have studies identified deficiencies of magnesium, zinc, vitamin A, vitamin E, thiamine, or vitamin B6 among PMS sufferers.[57] At least one epidemiologic investigation has revealed an association between post-traumatic stress disorder (PTSD) or trauma and PMS/PMDD.[58]

Scientists now believe that PMS/PMDD likely results from a complex interaction between ovarian hormones, central nervous system neurotransmitters such as serotonin and gamma-aminobutyric acid (GABA), and neurohormonal systems like the renin-angiotensin-aldosterone system.[59,60] Evidence suggests that serotonin dysregulation in particular plays a role in the pathogenesis of many of the psychological elements in PMS, including tension, irritability, and dysphoria.[61] In a large number of clinical trials, drugs that increase serotonin concentrations have significantly improved mood, functional status, and quality of life in women with PMS/PMDD.[62] More information on the use of selective serotonin reuptake inhibitors and other pharmacologic agents in PMS follows in the treatment section below.

DIAGNOSIS OF PMS/PMDD

The differential diagnosis of PMS/PMDD includes dysmenorrhea, other dysthymic and depressive disorders, generalized anxiety disorder, and hypothyroidism. Take a detailed history to begin differentiating between these conditions. For many women, clinical depression and other serious problems worsen premenstrually but never abate completely; women who do not experience a symptom-free interval do not have PMS.[63] Indeed, as many as half the women with self-diagnosed PMS have other problems, which require careful evaluation and therapies different from those for PMS.[64] Some women may have PMS as well as an underlying or concomitant psychiatric problem; in one study, 59% of women with PMDD also had clinical depression or an anxiety disorder.[65]

In general, laboratory tests are not needed to diagnose PMS. In some cases, however, the clinician must rule out hypothyroidism, since a patient with low thyroid hormone levels may present with fatigue, bloating, depression, and irritability. Panels to measure sex steroid hormonal levels are completely unnecessary in the evaluation of PMS.

The key to diagnosing PMS/PMDD is prospective charting of symptoms, by the patient, for at least 2 to 3 menstrual cycles. Research studies have validated a few premenstrual syndrome assessment tools for this purpose, including the Premenstrual Symptoms Screening Tool, the Calendar of Premenstrual Experiences, and the Daily Record of Severity of Problems.[66-68] A woman generally can successfully document her symptoms by taking notes on a regular calendar, writing down the symptoms she experiences each day, along with their severity, and to record the dates of her period. A woman who is overwhelmed by a series of complaints can chart only the 3 to 5 complaints that most profoundly bother her. Ideally, this chart should also include her weight and, if possible, a record of her basal body temperatures or home ovulation test results.

Have the patient return in 2 or 3 months, and at her next visit, carefully study the pattern of her symptoms. Symptoms do not need to recur with equal intensity in each cycle; different symptoms may occur during different cycles. The key to diagnosing PMS/PMDD is the timing of symptoms—they must peak in the luteal phase and disappear with the onset of menses.

TREATMENT OF PMS/PMDD

PMS treatment is strongly influenced by a placebo effect. In a wide range of studies, researchers report that 40% to 94% of patients will improve in the short term regardless of the treatment used. This reinforces the need to rely on placebo-controlled studies rather than case reports and personal testimonials to determine the true efficacy of a particular drug or treatment for PMS. The placebo effect also reminds us to keep an open mind about integrative medicine modalities that improve patients' well-being without doing any harm.

Treatment of PMS/PMDD requires a comprehensive, individualized approach. For women with physiologic menstrual changes, provide reassurance, emotional support, and education. Both the patient and her family may benefit from a discussion of hormonal changes and PMS. Charting the symptoms, along with aiding diagnosis, may help the patient gain more insight into her problem and a greater sense of control. If therapy is initiated, have her continue her charting so that she can identify what interventions improve her symptoms.

For women with mild to moderate PMS, consider directing treatment toward their specific symptoms. Breast tenderness can be eased with a fitted support or sports bra. Abdominal pain and backache respond well to the therapies outlined under the discussion of dysmenorrhea above, including NSAIDS to reduce prostaglandin production and extended cycle hormonal contraceptives.

Increasing evidence underscores the importance of exercise in maintaining physical and mental health.[69] Clinicians should encourage women with PMS, as well as all other patients, to engage in regular physical activity. Vigorous exercise may improve mood as well as reduce stress and physical complaints in PMS.[70,71] Results from one investigation demonstrated that aerobic exercise helped more than body-building exercise in reducing PMS symptoms.[72]

For years, dietary manipulations have been recommended in the treatment of PMS, but for the most part, randomized controlled trials have not validated this approach. Clinicians have traditionally advised patients with PMS to avoid caffeine, chocolate, alcohol, and salt, but no data exist to demonstrate the efficacy of these dietary modifications. The commonly held belief that coffee worsens PMS, for example, stems from two studies in the 1980s that demonstrated an association between caffeinated beverages and PMS.[73] These studies, however, were cross-sectional in design, so it is not possible to conclude that caffeine intake among these women *caused* PMS. An equally plausible explanation of the association observed between PMS and higher caffeine intake is that women with PMS symptoms of fatigue and irritability self-medicated with caffeinated beverages. Carbohydrate-rich food and beverages may reduce food cravings and other symptoms; a small double-blind, randomized controlled trial found that a high-carbohydrate beverage consumed during the late luteal phase reduced not only carbohydrate cravings, but also reduced self-reported symptoms of depression, anger, and confusion among PMS sufferers.[74]

Vitamins and minerals have also been recommended to reduce PMS symptoms. Pyridoxine, vitamin B6, is important in the biosynthesis of neurotransmitters and may help with PMS symptoms, especially breast pain and depression. Most placebo-controlled studies have reported improvement among women with PMS, but an evidence-based review of pyridoxine found "insufficient evidence" to conclusively support its efficacy.[75-77] Since peripheral neuropathy can occur when pyridoxine is taken at daily doses as low as 100 mg to 200 mg, caution patients to use this vitamin with moderation.

Limited but conflicting evidence suggests that supplementation with Vitamin E or magnesium may reduce PMS symptoms, along with dysmenorrhea, perhaps by reducing prostaglandin levels.[78-80] Again, advise patients that more is not always better with supplements, and that their dose of Vitamin E should not exceed 400 IU per day.[81]

Strong evidence does exist for the use of calcium supplementation in PMS. In the Nurses Health Study II, a large longitudinal cohort, women who consumed the most vitamin D and calcium were the least likely to develop PMS during 10 years of follow-up.[82] In addition, randomized controlled trials have demonstrated a reduction of PMS symptoms among women taking 1200 to 1600 mg of calcium carbonate daily.[83,84] Calcium may affect PMS symptomatology through its interaction with estrogen and parathyroid hormone.

Herbal agents have grown in popularity in the United States and are used frequently by women for PMS. Chasteberry tree extract, known in Latin as vitex agnus-castus, is used commonly in Europe for PMS and cyclical breast pain and is approved by the German Commission E for these indications.[85] Small, randomized controlled trials support its use.[86] Evening primrose oil is also popularly used in Europe for PMS and breast tenderness (mastalgia), but randomized controlled studies have not demonstrated the efficacy of this herb in the treatment of PMS.[87]

A variety of other non-pharmacologic approaches to PMS may reduce symptoms. Trials of cognitive therapy, group therapy, and relaxation therapy have shown that these modalities may improve physical and/or psychological symptoms of PMS, although few studies have randomized patients.[88] Biofeedback, acupuncture, reflexology, or light therapy may be helpful for some women.[89–92]

Selective Serotonin Reuptake Inhibitors and Other Psychotropic Medications

Pharmacologic therapy is indicated for women who qualify as having PMDD or other severe manifestations of PMS, as well as for women who do not respond to the treatments and lifestyle modifications described above. The current mainstay of medical treatment for PMS/PMDD is the class of anti-depressant drugs known as selective serotonin reuptake inhibitors (SSRIs). Many randomized, placebo-controlled trials have demonstrated that SSRIs reduce both physical and psychological PMS symptoms.[93–95] While the FDA has specifically approved only three drugs for PMDD (fluoxetine, sertraline, and paroxetine), research has found that other agents in the class are equally effective, including venlafaxine, which selectively inhibits both serotonin and norepinephrine.[96] If one agent is not successful, try another one before abandoning SSRIs as a class, because an individual's response may vary from drug to drug. Recommend that the woman use effective contraception when she is using SSRIs.

Most women tolerate SSRIs without incident, but these medications can cause many side effects, including nausea, decreased libido, and insomnia. Clinicians should counsel patients about these potential side effects and inquire about them at follow-up visits. The risk for side effects is related to dose; the use of low-dose SSRIs (e.g., Prozac 20 mg daily), which often suffice in treatment of PMS/PMDD, may minimize side effects.[97] Reducing the number of days of therapy may reduce side effects; monthly dosing during the luteal phase has also proven effective in PMS/PMDD, with rapid improvement of symptoms noted within a day or 2 of the first dose each cycle.[98]

Anti-depressants without serotonergic activity generally do not improve symptoms of PMS/PMDD. For women who can not tolerate SSRIs but who would benefit from psychotropic medication, anxiolytic medications provide an alternative. Alprazolam has demonstrated efficacy in PMS,[99,100] but the most effective pattern of use has not been defined. Some studies have found therapeutic response with intermittent use of alprazolam (e.g., 4 to 5 days preceding menses) while other studies have found such protocols no better than placebo. The clinician must individualize therapy. To avoid withdrawal symptoms, taper the alprazolam each time it is discontinued. Be careful when prescribing these agents, because they are habit-forming and have potential for abuse; women with histories of alcoholism or other substance abuse are not appropriate candidates. Caution women that the drug may make them feel drowsy; the first dose should be taken at home, before bedtime, to gauge its effect.

Another non-hormonal agent with demonstrated efficacy in PMS is spironolactone, the potassium-sparing diuretic; 25 mg taken 2 to 4 times daily during the luteal phase reduces bloating and improves mood.[101]

Hormonal Therapy

In the past, progesterone supplementation was frequently advocated for treatment of PMS based on anecdotal reports.[51] However, randomized controlled trials failed to confirm the efficacy of this approach. Natural or bio-identical progesterone, in the form of vaginal suppositories or oral micronized progesterone, does not reduce PMS symptoms.[100] Progestin-based contraceptives like DMPA and the LNG-IUS may reduce some menstrual-related PMS symptoms by eliminating or reducing menses.

Ovulation suppressants may also be helpful in the treatment of PMS. COCs sometimes benefit women with mild to moderate symptoms of bloating and breast pain.[102] However, for some COC users, depression, breast tenderness, and bloating increase on the pill, especially during the placebo pill days.[11] Randomized controlled trials of cyclic COC use for treatment of PMS have generated mixed results. Extended-cycle dosing of COCs and other combined hormonal contraceptives and DMPA may aid PMS sufferers not only by suppressing ovulation, but also by reducing the number of withdrawal bleeding episodes (and associated symptoms) they experience each year.

Randomized clinical trials have demonstrated the efficacy of COCs containing drospirenone (a spironolactone derivative) in reducing physical, psychological, and behavioral symptoms of PMS/PMDD when used in a formulation that reduced the numbers of placebo pills per cycle.[103–105]

For women with severe PMS/PMDD for whom other treatments fail, ovulation suppression can be achieved with the use of GnRH agonists (such as leuprolide) or synthetic androgen therapy (such as Danazol). Such treatments function as a medical oophorectomy and may provide relief of symptoms.[106] However, both agents have serious side effects that limit their use to 4 to 6 months. Symptoms often return once these agents are discontinued. Women whose symptoms do not respond to these therapies may need to be re-evaluated because they may have a more serious underlying pathology.

M ENSTRUALLY INDUCED EXACERBATIONS OF OTHER MEDICAL PROBLEMS

MENSTRUAL MIGRAINE

Approximately 1 in 6 women of reproductive age suffers migraine headaches. For many female migraineurs, headache occurs in relation to the menstrual cycle. The 2004 International Classification of Headache Disorders suggested criteria for distinguishing between 2 types of migraine associated with menses. *Pure menstrual migraine* occurs exclusively within 2 days before or 3 days after the onset of menses, while *menstrual-related migraine* occurs within this perimenstrual period as well as at other times during the month. Studies have reported that 7% to 9% of women with migraine experience pure menstrual migraine, while 35% to 51% have menstrual-related migraine.[107–110] Some authors report that menstrual migraine is more severe and more difficult to treat than non-menstrual migraine.[109,111,112]

The precise mechanism of menstrual migraine remains unknown, but declining estrogen levels play a major role. An intriguing set of experiments in the 1970s first demonstrated the link between declining estrogen levels and the onset of menstrual migraine. In the days preceding menses, the investigator administered estradiol to 6 menstrual migraine sufferers, and found that headaches did not occur in these women until estrogen levels fell below 0.2ng/ml, while menses occurred on schedule. In contrast, administration of pre-menstrual progesterone delayed menses but did not affect the onset of headache.[113,114] Estrogen decline may result in migraine through the hormone's effect on pain receptors and blood vessels in the brain.[107] Studies have demonstrated that estrogen interacts with neurotransmitters including noradrenaline, serotonin, and dopamine, and it influences magnesium concentration in vascular smooth muscle cells.[115,116]

An accurate diagnosis of menstrual migraine depends on prospective charting. When menstrual migraine is suspected, ask the patient to keep a headache diary for 3 months. In the diary, the patient should track her menses and the date and duration of each headache she experiences. She should also catalogue other potential migraine triggers such as foods, sleep disruptions, physical activity, medications, illnesses, and other stressors.[107] Review of the calendar at the next visit will differentiate women with true menstrual migraine, menstrual-related migraine, or non-menstrual migraine. Encourage patients to continue keeping headache diaries while they are on therapy to help them identify what works to reduce their suffering.

Acute treatment for menstrual migraine is similar to treatment for non-menstrual migraine. NSAIDs are first-line therapy for migraine and may prove especially useful in women with menstrual migraine, as they also relieve other prostaglandin-mediated menstrual symptoms such as uterine pain and cramping. While acetaminophen alone does not effectively treat migraine, many migraineurs respond to combination aspirin-caffeine-acetaminophen tablets.[117] Other evidence-based therapies for acute migraine include the serotonin agonists known as triptans, which are used orally or subcutaneously, and intranasal dihydroergotamine.[118]

Prophylactic migraine therapy is employed for patients who do not respond to acute therapy, who experience 2 or more attacks resulting in 3 or more days of migraine-related disability per month, or who use abortive therapy more than 2 times per week. Evidence-based prophylactic agents include beta blockers, amitriptyline, and the anti-convulsants divalproex sodium and sodium valproate. One study has demonstrated that women with menstrual migraine can use a home fertility monitor to predict menses in order to more precisely time short-term, prophylactic migraine therapy.[119]

For the most part, only small or open label trials have evaluated hormonal therapy for menstrual migraine. Case reports have shown that severe menstrual migraine responds well to treatment with a GnRH agonist, with or without estrogen/progestin add-back therapy.[120] Others have reported that the anti-estrogen tamoxifen and the androgen danazol provide relief.[121,122] However, all of these therapies may produce unacceptable side effects. Estrogen supplementation alone, through patches or gels, may also prevent menstrual migraine, but the clinician and patient must consider the risks of unopposed estrogen therapy.[117]

Cyclic use of COCs may worsen menstrual migraine, since withdrawal from pharmacologic levels of estrogen during the placebo-pill week is even more dramatic than the physiologic monthly hormone swings. However, continuous use of COCs (or other combined hormonal methods) eliminates estogen withdrawal for long stretches of time.[11,116,123] These extended cycles can be used in women with menstrual migraine without aura. For patients who prefer to have monthly menses, estrogen withdrawal may be minimized by restarting pills, patches, or rings on the first day of bleeding each cycle. In one EE/desogestrel pill formulation, the last 5 pills in the placebo week are replaced with tablets containing 10 mcg EE. Two other formulations have 24 active pills with 4 placebo pills. Another product combines extended cycle active pills (84 pills) with 7 pills containing 10 mcg EE in place of the 7 placebo pills.

Women with migraine headaches are up to 3 times more likely to suffer ischemic stroke, especially if they report migraine with aura.[124] Combined hormonal methods worsen that risk. Women who experience migraine with aura who use estrogen-containing contraceptives have up to a 4-fold risk of stroke. Therefore, WHO rates their use as category 4 in women with migraine with aura. However, for women with menstrual migraine without aura, combined hormonal contraceptives, especially if extended cycle, may be advantageous. DMPA has not been associated with a higher risk of stroke in migraine. Clinicians should also strongly advise migraineurs with aura to refrain from smoking cigarettes, as smoking triples their already increased risk for stroke.[124]

CATAMENIAL SEIZURES

In women with epilepsy, seizures may cluster in relation to the menstrual cycle. Menstrual-related seizure activity, known as catamenial epilepsy, most commonly occurs during the time of menstruation (perimenstrually) but may also occur around the time of ovulation (periovulatory) or during inadequate luteal phase cycles.[125] Doctors first noted the association between seizure activity and menses in the 19th century, but in recent years the relationship has been better characterized.[126] Both estrogen and progesterone significantly affect seizure threshold. While estrogen has an excitatory pro-convulsant effect, progesterone has an inhibitory, anti-convulsant effect on neurons.

Steroid hormones and anticonvulsants are both metabolized by cytochrome p450 hepatic enzymes. Studies have demonstrated that in women with epilepsy, serum levels of anticonvulsant drugs decrease in the luteal phase, likely because of increased metabolism of the drugs by p450 enzymes as estrogen and progesterone peak during that part of the cycle.[125] Many anticonvulsants carry risks for teratogenicity, so women should use effective contraception while on those medications.

Few studies have evaluated hormonal treatments for catamenial epilepsy. Small open trials suggest that progestins and natural progesterone may help with seizure prevention, but no randomized controlled trials confirm this.[127] Many clinicians use DMPA or extended-cycle combined hormonal contraceptives to reduce the hormonal swings and reduce resultant seizure activity associated with ovulation and menses.

OTHER DISEASES

Other diseases that may worsen with menstrual cycling include asthma, diabetes, rheumatoid arthritis, diabetes, and Behçet's disease (oral and genital ulcers as well as ophthalmia).[128]

ENDOMETRIOSIS

Endometriosis is the presence of endometrial implants (glands and stroma) outside the uterus. Endometriosis most frequently involves the peritoneal surfaces of pelvic organs—the cul de sac, ovaries, fallopian tube, uterus, broad ligament, ureters, rectovaginal septum, and utero-sacral ligaments. The bowel, including the appendix, is often involved. Other more unusual sites include surgical scars, the bladder, the vulva, and the lungs.

These lesions often adhere densely to the side wall of the peritoneum. The surrounding fibrosis may involve the fallopian tubes and bowel. Deep infiltrating nodules of endometriosis can also involve the utero-sacral ligaments, vagina, bladder, bowel or ureters. Endometriomas are cystic masses of endometriosis contained within the ovary; these cysts are filled with thick, dark, tar-like brownish fluid, which give the lesions their popular name, "chocolate cysts."

Endometriotic implants are usually transported out of the uterus primarily by retrograde menstruation. Other mechanisms such as hematogenous and lymphatic spread create more distal implants. The initial red endometriotic implants have been thought to respond to monthly sex steroid stimuli the same way the endometrial lining does—by proliferating, hypertrophying, and ultimately sloughing at the end of the cycle. The "local" menstrual blood and the implants themselves incite an inflammatory response, creating adhesions to adjacent structures. Ultimately, the inflammatory reaction leads to fibrosis. The relationship between mild endometriosis and infertility is unclear (see Chapter 25 on Impaired Fertility).

Endometriosis is a common problem: about 3% to 10% of reproductive-age women in the United States have endometriosis. Women undergoing laparotomy for gynecologic diseases have higher rates: ranging from 14% to 21%. Nearly 25% to 35% of infertile women have endometriosis.[129] Rates may be twice as high in Asian women, in women who delay childbearing, and in women with a family history of endometriosis.

CLINICAL PRESENTATION OF ENDOMETRIOSIS

The symptoms associated with endometriosis are variable. Over 50% of affected women complain of severe dysmenorrhea; the pain often precedes the onset of vaginal bleeding. Pain commonly also occurs with deep thrusting; painful defecation and pain with urination are also problems. Lower abdomen pain, back pain, or even loin pain can be due to endometriosis. Some women complain of pain with exercise. In addition to pain, the patient may present with complaints of fatigue, malaise, and sleep difficulties. Endometriosis can cause infertility (see Chapter 25 on Impaired Fertility). The predictive value of these symptoms is low because each of these symptoms can have other causes. Furthermore, there is no consistent relationship between the extent of endometriosis and the degree of a woman's symptoms.

On physical examination, a fixed, retroverted uterus and tender nodular uterosacral ligaments, with or without an adnexal mass, are findings consistent with advanced endometriosis. Ultrasound has no value in diagnosing peritoneal endometriosis, but may be helpful in diagnosing endometriomas and disease involving the bladder and bowel.[130] A definitive diagnosis requires direct visualization, usually via laparoscopy. Biopsies help confirm the visual impression at the time of surgery. A formal classification system has been developed by the American Society for Reproductive Medicine to help stage the extent of disease and guide therapy and counseling.[131]

Treatment of Endometriosis

Therapy can be initiated based on symptoms suggestive of the diseases, and the diagnosis can be supported by response to treatment. Treatment is determined by the nature and severity of the patient's symptoms and disease, as well as her desire for fertility.

Women with endometriosis presenting with dysmenorrhea and pelvic pain can be treated with medical therapy.[130] About 80% to 85% of women improve with any of the medical therapies; selection of treatment often depends upon side effects.[132] NSAIDs may reduce dysmenorrhea, especially if combined with COCs. Continuous use of COCs is particularly helpful in creating a pseudopregnancy state, shrinking the implants and inducing amenorrhea. Progestins have long been a mainstay of therapy. Significant symptomatic relief from endometriosis-related pain can be obtained with DMPA use.[133] The Sub Q 104 DMPA is an FDA-approved treatment for the symptoms of endometriosis.[134] Danazol and GnRH agonists (such as buserelin, goserelin, leuprorelin acetate, nafarelin, and triptorelin) are other FDA-approved medications that are particularly helpful in shrinking and softening the implants to make them more amenable to surgical excision or ablation. They are also useful after surgery to treat residual disease and to prevent re-seeding. Danazol is an androgen that blocks gonadotropins and directly suppresses ovarian hormone production. It can be used for only 6 to 9 months because it causes troublesome side effects, such as acne, hirsutism, and virilization. GnRH agonists block gonadotropin production and reduce circulating estrogen levels to shrink implants.[135] Use of GnRH agonists is limited by hypoestrogenic side effects. Prolonged therapy is possible, if, after initial therapy with GnRH agonists alone for 3 to 6 months, low doses of estrogen and progestin are added to the therapy.

Medical therapy is rarely successful in treating ovarian endometriosis if a disease has caused ovarian enlargement.[136] Surgical removal of larger lesions (> 2–3 cm) is recommended because of the risk of rupture, which can cause a chemical peritonitis. Cystectomy is appropriate for isolated endometriomas. Excision of adhesions and ablation of implants may help women whose symptoms are not relieved by medical therapy.[137] More advanced disease unresponsive to medical therapies may require hysterectomy or bilateral oophorectomy.

CHRONIC PELVIC PAIN

Since women with dysmenorrhea often suffer from underlying chronic pelvic pain, clinicians need to be familiar with the workup, differential diagnosis, and treatments of the major causes of that larger problem. For many years, the condition remained ill-defined, but recently ACOG defined chronic pelvic pain as pain of at least 6 months' duration, unrelated to the menstrual cycle, which localizes to the pelvis, lower back, buttocks, or anterior abdominal wall at or below the umbilicus.[138] While chronic pelvic pain characteristically causes functional disability and prompts the patient to seek medical attention, physical examination, imaging studies, and even exploratory surgery may reveal only normal findings.

Chronic pelvic pain occurs in women of all ages. In the 1990s, population-based and office-based surveys of U.S. women found that 15% to 20% experienced chronic pelvic pain,[139,140] while in the United Kingdom researchers reported a prevalence ranging from 4% to 24%.[141 143] Other authors estimate that the condition accounts for up to 10% of outpatient gynecology visits, and is the primary preoperative condition for 10% to 20% of hysterectomies performed in the United States.[144,145]

Women who suffer from chronic pelvic pain experience interference with work, recreational, physical, and sexual activities and changes in their family dynamics.[141,146] Dyspareunia and dysmenorrhea are more common among patients with chronic pelvic pain, as are mood disturbances, major depression, dysthymic disorder, and substance abuse.[147]

The disability and distress caused by chronic pelvic pain result in significant costs to the health care system and to United States society as a whole. In the mid-1990s, chronic pelvic pain was estimated to cost over $880 million in direct annual expenses for visits to physicians, excluding the costs of surgery and hospitalization. In addition, women with chronic pelvic pain paid an additional $2 billion per year in out-of-pocket expenses. Indirect expenses, due to lost productivity and missed work by affected women, reached over $555 million per year.[141]

Health care costs are high for women with chronic pelvic pain, because patients who suffer from the condition frequently see multiple doctors without ever receiving a diagnosis or satisfactory treatment. Because the pain may be out of proportion to any anatomic or clinical findings, physicians have at times dismissed patients' complaints, telling them the pain is "all in their head" and sending them to a psychiatrist. While mental health care referrals are appropriate and sometimes essentially indicated for chronic pelvic pain, it is also important for the patient's primary care provider or gynecologist to work her up and diligently search for a treatable diagnosis. It is also important to address and treat the patient's pain, irrespective of cause.

DIFFERENTIAL DIAGNOSIS OF CHRONIC PELVIC PAIN

The etiology of chronic pelvic pain may be 1) visceral, arising in the gynecologic, urologic, or gastrointestinal organs; 2) somatic, originating in bones, ligaments, muscles, or fascia; or 3) neurologic, psychiatric, or psychosomatic. Some women have more than one underlying condition contributing to their pelvic pain, complicating the clinical picture.

The most common diagnoses identified in women with chronic pelvic pain are endometriosis, irritable bowel syndrome, interstitial cystitis, pelvic adhesions, physical or sexual abuse, and musculoskeletal disorders. Other causes of pain include pelvic vascular congestion and neurogenic disorders.

Endometriosis. An estimated 15% to 33% of women with chronic pelvic pain have endometriosis. Aside from pelvic pain, endometriosis frequently causes dysmenorrhea and dyspareunia as outlined above.

Irritable bowel syndrome (IBS). IBS affects 10% to 20% of the general population in developed countries, but as many as 33% to 50% of women referred to gynecologists for pelvic pain.[143,148] IBS is functional disorder of the gastrointestinal tract characterized by crampy abdominal pain, gas, bloating, and chronic diarrhea and/or constipation.[149] Typically, symptoms are transiently relieved with defecation. IBS is a functional condition; there are no visible anatomical defects.

Research has demonstrated associations between IBS and dysmenorrhea, dyspareunia, endometriosis, depression, anxiety, and abuse.[143,150] Many of these conditions also occur in women who have chronic pelvic pain without IBS; however, a study of 987 women attending a pelvic pain clinic found that women with IBS were distinct from those without, in that they were significantly more likely to have depression, a history of adult physical abuse, muscular back pain, and pain in 6 to 8 pelvic sites out of 8 palpated on physical exam.[148]

It is important for clinicians to recognize potential cases of IBS among women with pelvic pain, because treatment of IBS may reduce pelvic symptoms.[148] To arrive at a diagnosis of IBS, other diseases of the bowel must first be excluded with blood and stool tests, X-rays, or endoscopy. Referral to a gastroenterologist is often indicated. Pharmacologic treatments for IBS depend on the variant of IBS that a woman has; IBS can induce diarrhea, constipation, or both. Fiber, laxatives, antidiarrheals, anti-spasmodics, antidepressants, and anxiolytic drugs are helpful in different settings. Lifestyle changes such as dietary modification, stress reduction and relaxation, and exercise may also reduce symptoms in women with IBS.[149]

Interstitial cystitis. Another condition commonly identified among women with chronic pelvic pain is interstitial cystitis. Studies have estimated that 38% to 81% of women with chronic pelvic pain have interstitial cystitis, a chronic non-infectious condition of the urinary bladder.[151,152] Along with pelvic pain, patients with interstitial cystitis usually present with urinary frequency and urgency, but urinalysis and cultures reveal no evidence of urinary tract infection. Like other pelvic pain sufferers, people with interstitial cystitis may visit many physicians before receiving a diagnosis. Because clinicians frequently do not recognize interstitial cystitis in its early stages, it is most commonly diagnosed at the advanced stage, when dysuria becomes excruciating and urinary urgency and frequency become debilitating.[153]

Investigators have identified a number of factors that may contribute to the etiology of interstitial cystitis, including dysfunction of the bladder epithelium.[154] Potassium leakage into the bladder wall likely contributes to or causes the pain and injury.[155] The Pelvic Pain and Urgency/Frequency Scale is a very useful diagnostic tool, which enables clinicians to quantify patients' frequency, urgency, and pelvic pain through a questionnaire.[152] High scores on the formalized questionnaire are about 90% accurate in women without infection or tumor. Confirmation of the diagnosis, if needed, can be obtained by performing an intravesical potassium sensitivity test, in which a saline solution and then a potassium solution are infused into the bladder.

Treatments for interstitial cystitis include oral pentosan polysulfate sodium (marketed as Elmiron), intravesical infusion of lidocaine and heparin and oral tricyclic antidepressants.[156–158]

Pelvic adhesions. Investigators have found that as many as 35% of women with pelvic inflammatory disease later develop chronic pelvic pain.[159] Development of chronic pelvic pain after pelvic inflammatory disease does not appear to be related to the severity of initial infection or to whether a woman is treated as an inpatient or outpatient, but women with more than one episode of pelvic inflammatory disease (PID) may be at a higher risk.[160]

It is likely that PID-induced adhesions are responsible for chronic pelvic pain, as adhesion formation from pelvic or abdominal surgery, ruptured appendix, endometriosis, and inflammatory bowel disease can be.[161] Some women with pelvic adhesions, however, report no recognized risk factors.[162] Among women undergoing laparoscopy for chronic pelvic pain, investigators have found adhesions in 27% to 60% although it is not clear that the adhesions are responsible for the pain.[162]

Two randomized controlled trials—one with laparotomy and a more recent one with laparoscopy—have evaluated the therapeutic benefit of adhesiolysis in women with chronic pelvic pain. These studies have not found an improvement in pelvic pain following lysis of adhesions, except among women with dense adhesions involving bowel.[163,164] An NIH study of second-look surgery in endometriosis patients found that surgically removed adhesions re-formed within 2 years 43% of the time, with thick adhesions more likely to re-form than thin ones. New adhesions also formed in most women, often at the site of an endometriosis lesion removed during the previous surgery.[165] A recent Cochrane review of adhesiolysis for chronic pelvic pain concluded that "there is no evidence of benefit, rather than evidence of no benefit" and that more studies are needed.[166]

Musculoskeletal causes. Chronic pelvic pain due to musculoskeletal causes include pregnancy-related pelvic pain, pelvic bone stress, and dysfunction of various pelvic muscles including the levator ani and piriformis.[167] An example of an obstetric cause of chronic pain is peripartum pelvic pain syndrome, which is thought to be due to a strain on ligaments in the pelvis and lower spine. Trauma to other parts of the body, including the neck and back, may contribute to chronic pelvic pain through muscles such as the quadratus lumborum.[168]

Musculoskeletal dysfunction is often associated with the development of trigger points, hyperirritable areas that are tender to palpation and that may cause referred pain. An observational trial showed that trigger point injections of anesthetic agents into the abdominal wall, vagina, and sacrum improved pain in over two thirds of patients.[169] Observational studies also suggest a benefit from pelvic floor muscle exercises and biofeedback, through which patients learn to isolate muscles and relax them.

Sexual and physical abuse. A history of sexual or physical abuse during childhood or adulthood is significantly more common among women with chronic pelvic pain than among other gynecology patients or the general population.[147,170,171] Indeed, as many as 50% to 60% of women with chronic pelvic pain have a history of abuse.[172,173] Not surprisingly, both physical and sexual abuse are associated with increased psychological distress in women with chronic pelvic pain.[174] Studies have also revealed that women with chronic pelvic pain who report a history of abuse are more likely to have somatization and dissociative disorders, along with depression, anxiety, and substance abuse.[173] Past trauma may lower the threshold for pain sensations to be transmitted through the pain gate at the level of the spinal cord. One recent report indicates that compared with healthy controls, women with chronic pelvic pain are more likely to suppress distressing thoughts and negative emotions, a coping style that psychologists consider maladaptive.[175] Referral to a qualified psychiatrist, psychologist, or therapist is especially important for chronic pelvic pain patients with a history of abuse.

Pelvic congestion. The presence of dilated varicose veins in the pelvis, may be another cause of chronic pelvic pain in some women. The dilated vessels often are found in the broad ligament or ovarian plexus, and pain may be associated with activities that increase pelvic or abdominal pressure, such as walking or sexual intercourse. Although not all experts agree that pelvic congestion is a cause of chronic pelvic pain, some have reported treatments with progestin therapy, GnRH agonists, and psychotherapy.[176,177,178]

Neurologic causes. Emerging understanding of chronic pelvic pain shows that it may also have a neurologic or neurogenic component. Unmanaged pain of any etiology can lead to long-term changes in the central nervous system, including biochemical changes that perpetuate pain in the absence of nociceptive stimuli. When neuropathic pain develops, patients report shooting, stinging, or electrical sensations. Evidence-based treatments for neuropathic pain include tricyclic antidepressants, gabapentin, tramadol, and opioid therapy.[179-182]

A recent study investigated patterns of innervation in hysterectomy specimens from patients with chronic pain. Researchers found that uteruses of women with chronic pelvic pain or endometriosis had increased perivascular innervation and significantly more microneuromas than did those of healthy controls.[183] The significance of these findings is not yet clear, but they suggest that biologic processes we do not yet understand may be involved in the etiology of chronic pelvic pain.

EVALUATION OF CHRONIC PELVIC PAIN

The multifactorial nature of chronic pelvic pain demands a thorough, systematic evaluation of the patient, and may require referral to specialists in different disciplines. To facilitate diagnosis and treatment of women with pelvic pain, specialized pelvic pain centers have been established to provide interdisciplinary care. However, individual practitioners can successfully begin a work-up of chronic pelvic pain and take steps to reduce patients' discomfort and frustration. One small study of doctor-patient interactions in chronic pelvic pain visits found that patients who perceived their doctors as direct, sympathetic, and approachable at the initial visit retained a positive impression of that visit 6 months later, regardless of subsequent pain level.[184]

The first step in differentiating between the myriad etiologies of chronic pelvic pain is to take a thorough patient history, eliciting information about bowel function, bladder function, intercourse, sleep and rest, food habits, menstrual history, and obstetric history. One must screen the patient for depression and gently inquire about a history of sexual or physical abuse. Familiarize yourself with domestic violence resources in your community so that you may provide support and appropriate referrals to women who need them. For women who report abuse, ensure that they are not in any immediate danger, and obey local reporting laws. Also, be sensitive to the possibility of drug-seeking behaviors or other situations of possible secondary gain.

Elicit a thorough pain history, as details about the patient's pain may provide clues to its etiology. Ask,

- Where is the pain? Does it move around or radiate?
- When did it begin? How often does it occur? How long does it last?
- What does it feel like? (Sharp, dull, aching, burning, cramping, pinching, shooting?)
- How bad is the pain on a scale of 1–10? (Or on a visual analog scale?)
- Does anything make it feel better or worse?
- What treatments have you tried in the past? What has worked?

On physical exam, observe the patient's posture, affect, and gait. Conduct a careful abdominal exam, looking for scars, hernias, and masses. Assess the abdominal walls and back for muscular tension and trigger points, which are discrete, focal, hyperirritable spots that produce localized or referred pain upon palpation. To differentiate between abdominal wall pain and intraperitoneal pain, have the patient curl forward and tighten her abdominal muscles. If palpation in this position is more painful, her pathology probably rests in her abdominal wall.

On pelvic exam, assess the external genitalia for lesions and point tenderness. The speculum exam may be painful for some women, so approach the patient gently and patiently. Test for sexually transmitted infections as indicated. On bimanual exam, assess uterine size, mobility, and tenderness, and note the presence of adnexal pain or masses. Systematically palpate the vaginal walls to locate trigger points.[169] Palpation of specific pelvic muscles through simple maneuvers can help identify the source of pelvic floor pain.[168] A rectal or rectovaginal exam may reveal posteriorly located lesions or masses.

Laboratory tests that may be indicated in the evaluation of some cases of chronic pelvic pain include complete blood count (CBC), complete metabolic panel, urinalysis and urinary culture, genital cultures, or HIV antibody test. Transvaginal pelvic ultrasound can identify pelvic masses, including endometriomas of the ovary.[185] Ultrasound, computed tomography, magnetic resonance imaging, colonoscopy, and cystoscopy are all available to aid in the work-up of chronic pelvic pain, if indicated.

Women with chronic pelvic pain may require a number of tests and procedures to rule out the pathologies described above. Referral to various specialists—including anesthesiologists, gastroenterologists, and urogynecologists—is often essential for specialized diagnostic studies and treatment. Primary care providers can help patients coordinate these visits and provide ongoing psychosocial support.

TREATMENT OF CHRONIC PELVIC PAIN

Ideally, therapy for chronic pelvic pain relieves suffering, improves quality of life, and prevents future disability. In practice, treatment of chronic pelvic pain often proves challenging, and symptom reduction alone may be a more realistic goal than striving for cure.

Treatment of chronic pelvic pain requires an integrated, comprehensive approach. The clinician should treat the underlying or associated condition, if one has been identified, and/or treat the pain itself. An integrated approach to treatment, addressing somatic, psychological, and environmental factors, is more likely to achieve pain reduction than a standard medical approach.[186] Treatment options include pharmacologic, surgical, and alternative modalities, along with physical therapy and mental health services.

Pharmacologic Treatment Options

Pharmacologic options for chronic pelvic pain include non-steroidal anti-inflammatory drugs, narcotics, progestins, COCs, gonadotropin-releasing agonists, and anti-depressant medications. While randomized controlled trials have not evaluated NSAIDS in chronic pelvic pain, experts consider them a popular first-line treatment.[187] Opioids are an important part of the pharmacologic arsenal for chronic pain, in general, and may be appropriate and helpful for some pelvic pain patients.

Studies have demonstrated that some hormonal agents effectively reduce chronic pelvic pain. Strong evidence supports the use of progesterone in relieving the pain from endometriosis and pelvic congestion syndrome.[188,189] GnRH agonists have proven effective in relieving pain associated with endometriosis, irritable bowel syndrome, interstitial cystitis, and pelvic congestion.[135,190]

While clinical trials have demonstrated the efficacy of SSRIs, tricyclic antidepressants, and gabapentin in other chronic pain disorders, few studies have evaluated the use of these drugs for chronic pelvic pain. One trial of the SSRI sertraline in chronic pelvic pain patients found the drug did not improve pain or emotional functioning compared to placebo.[191] On the other hand, a European study found that over 6 to 24 months treatment of the nerve modulator gabapentin alone or in combination with amitriptyline resulted in greater pain relief than did treatment with amitriptyline alone. However, this study did not include a placebo control.[192]

Surgical Treatment and Physical Therapy Options

Surgical modalities are frequently employed in the treatment of pelvic pain, especially when endometriosis is identified or suspected. In women with intractable pelvic pain, gynecologists may perform hysterectomy. Observational studies suggest that at least 75% of women with chronic pelvic pain improve after hysterectomy.[138] However, as many as 3% to 9% of women develop de novo pain post-hysterectomy, so this therapy must be applied with caution.

Another surgical approach to chronic pelvic pain involves interrupting the nerve plexuses and parasympathetic ganglia in the uterosacral ligaments, which carry pain sensations from the uterus, cervix and other pelvic structures to the spinal cord, through a technique called laparoscopic uterosacral nerve ablation (LUNA). However, while published trials have found that LUNA may improve dysmenorrhea, studies have not demonstrated efficacy in the treatment of non-menstrual, chronic pelvic pain in women with or without endometriosis.[193]

Pre-sacral neurectomy, the surgical removal of the superior hypogastric plexus, also has demonstrated efficacy in the treatment of dysmenorrhea, but it does not appear to alleviate non-menstrual pain.[194]

Physical therapy for the pelvic floor appears to help some women with chronic pelvic pain of musculoskeletal, bladder, or unknown origin.[195,196] Other therapies targeting pelvic floor muscles also hold promise in treating chronic pelvic pain; at least one clinical trial has demonstrated the efficacy of intravaginal electrical stimulation,[197] and another suggests that Botox injections of the pelvic floor muscles may reduce pain with defecation and intercourse and improve quality of life and sexual activity among women with chronic pelvic pain.[198,201] Trigger point injections can provide significant pain relief from musculoskeletal pain and spasm.

Psychological or Psychiatric Treatment Options

Psychological or psychiatric treatment plays an important role in the integrated approach to chronic pelvic pain.[199] The goals of mental health therapy are to improve coping abilities, increase the patient's sense of control, and reduce disability and the impact of pain on the patient's life. Group therapy as well as individual therapy may provide benefit. One randomized clinical trial of psychotherapy among women with pelvic congestion syndrome found that adding psychotherapy to medical treatment improved outcomes.[189]

Complementary or Alternative Medicine Treatment Options

The use of complementary or alternative medicine modalities in chronic pelvic pain remains largely unexplored in the medical literature. One small, randomized controlled trial found that magnetic field therapy applied to trigger points on the abdomen significantly reduced chronic pelvic pain after 4 weeks, but blinding of the study participants was compromised. Randomized controlled trials have demonstrated that acupuncture and acupressure reduce pelvic pain from dysmenorrhea, but their effect on non-cyclical pelvic pain has not yet been evaluated. Massage, yoga, guided imagery, and meditation may all potentially improve health or functioning in women with chronic pelvic pain. However, clinicians can expect that, despite the lack of evidence, many patients will experiment with alternative therapies in their search for symptom relief.

REFERENCES

1. Andersch B, Milsom I. An epidemiologic study of young women with dysmenorrhea. Am J Obstet Gynecol 1982;144:655–60.
2. Avant RF. Dysmenorrhea. Prim Care 1988;15:549–59.
3. Berry C, McGuire FL. Menstrual distress and acceptance of sexual role. Am J Obstet Gynecol 1972;114:83–7.
4. Smith RP. Cyclic pelvic pain and dysmenorrhea. Obstet Gynecol Clin North Am 1993;20:753–64.
5. Wilson L, Kurzrok R. Uterine contractility in functional dysmenorrhea. Endocrinology 1940,27.23–8.
6. Pickles VR, Hall WJ, Best FA, Smith GN. Prostaglandins in endometrium and menstrual fluid from normal and dysmenorrhoic subjects. J Obstet Gynaecol Br Commonw 1965;72:185–92.
7. Ziaei S, Zakeri M, Kazemnejad A. A randomised controlled trial of vitamin E in the treatment of primary dysmenorrhoea. BJOG 2005;112:466–9.
8. Dawood MY. Nonsteroidal anti-inflammatory drugs and reproduction. Am J Obstet Gynecol 1993;169:1255–1265.
9. Milsom I, Sundell G, Andersch B. The influence of different combined oral contraceptives on the prevalence and severity of dysmenorrhea. Contraception 1990; 42:497–506.

10. Robinson JC, Plichta S, Weisman CS, Nathanson CA, Ensminger M. Dysmenorrhea and use of oral contraceptives in adolescent women attending a family planning clinic. Am J Obstet Gynecol 1992;166:578–83.
11. Sulak PJ, Cressman BE, Waldrop E, Holleman S, Kuehl TJ. Extending the duration of active oral contraceptive pills to manage hormone withdrawal symptoms. Obstet Gynecol 1997;89:179–83.
12. Harel Z, Biro FM, Kottenhahn RK, Rosenthal SL. Supplementation with omega-3 polyunsaturated fatty acids in the management of dysmenorrhea in adolescents. Am J Obstet Gynecol 1996;174:1335–8.
13. Chimbira TH, Anderson AB, Turnbull A. Relation between measured menstrual blood loss and patient's subjective assessment of loss, duration of bleeding, number of sanitary towels used, uterine weight and endometrial surface area. Br J Obstet Gynaecol 1980 Jul;87(7):603–9.
14. Fraser IS, McCarron G, Markham R, Resta T. Blood and total fluid content of menstrual discharge. Obstet Gynecol 1985;65:194–8.
15. Hallberg L, Hogdahl AM, Nilsson L, Rybo G. Menstrual blood loss—a population study. Variation at different ages and attempts to define normality. Acta Obstet Gynecol Scand 1966;45:320–51.
16. Quint EH, Schwant A. Menstrual management in adolescents with developmental disabilities. The Female Patient 2005 Nov:13–6
17. Philipp CS, Faiz A, Dowling N, Dilley A, Michaels LA, Ayers C, Miller CH, Bachmann G, Evatt B, Saidi P. Age and the prevalence of bleeding disorders in women with menorrhagia. Obstet Gynecol 2005;105:61–6
18. Claessens EA, Cowell CA. Dysfunctional uterine bleeding in the adolescent. Pediatr Clin North Am 1981;28:369–71.
19. Munro MG, Lukes AS. Abnormal Uterine Bleeding and Underlying Hemostatic Disorders Consensus Group. Abnormal uterine bleeding and underlying hemostatic disorders: report of a consensus process. Fertil Steril 2005;84:1335–7.
20. Kelekci S, Kaya E, Alan M, Alan Y, Bilge U, Mollamahmutoglu L. Comparison of transvaginal sonography, saline infusion sonography, and office hysteroscopy in reproductive-aged women with or without abnormal uterine bleeding. Fertil Steril 2005;84:682–6
21. Lethaby A, Augood C, Duckitt K. Nonsteroidal anti-inflammatory drugs for heavy menstrual bleeding. Cochrane Database Syst Rev. 2002;(1):CD000400.
22. Anderson FD, Hait H. A multicenter, randomized study of an extended cycle oral contraceptive. Contraception 2003;68:89–96. Erratum in: Contraception 2004;69:175.
23. Miller L, Verhoeven CH, Hout J. Extended regimens of the contraceptive vaginal ring: a randomized trial. Obstet Gynecol 2005;106:473–82.
24. Reid PC, Virtanen-Kari S. Randomised comparative trial of the levonorgestrel intrauterine system and mefenamic acid for the treatment of idiopathic menorrhagia: a multiple analysis using total menstrual fluid loss, menstrual blood loss and pictorial blood loss assessment charts. BJOG 2005;112(8):1121–5.
25. Preston JT, Cameron IT, Adams EJ, Smith SK. Comparative study of tranexamic acid and norethisterone in the treatment of ovulatory menorrhagia. Br J Obstet Gynaecol 1995;102(5):401–6.
26. Bayer SR, DeCherney AH. Clinical manifestations and treatment of dysfunctional uterine bleeding. JAMA 1993;269:1823–8.
27. Lethaby AE, Cooke I, Rees M. Progesterone or progestogen-releasing intrauterine systems for heavy menstrual bleeding. Cochrane Database Syst Rev 2005;(4):CD002126.
28. Practice Committee of the American Society for Reproductive Medicine. Current evaluation of amenorrhea. Fertil Steril 2004;82(1):266–72.
29. Lobo RA, Pauson RJ (eds). Mishell's textbook of infertility, contraception and reproductive endocrinology. Boston: Blackwell Science, Ltd, 1997

30. Speroff L, Fritz MA. Clinical gynecologic endocrinology and infertility. 7th ed. Baltimore: Lippincott, Williams & Wilkins, 2004

31. Shangold M, Rebar RW, Wentz AC, Schiff I. Evaluation and management of menstrual dysfunction in athletes. JAMA 1990;263:1665–9.

32. Hergenroeder AC, Smith EO, Shypailo R, Jones LA, Klish WJ, Ellis K. Bone mineral changes in young women with hypothalamic amenorrhea treated with oral contraceptives, changes in young women with hypothalamic amenorrhea treated with oral contraceptives, medroxyprogesterone or placebo over 12 months. Am J Obstet Gynecol 1997;176:1017–25.

33. Genazzani AD, Petraglia F, Gastaldi M, Volpogni C, Gamba O, Genazzani AR. Naltrexone treatment restores menstrual cycles in patients with weight loss-related amenorrhea. Fertil Steril 1995;64:951–6.

34. Legro RS, Chiu P, Kunselman AR, Bentley CM, Dodson WC, Dunaif A. Polycystic ovaries are common in women with hyperandrogenic chronic anovulation but do not predict metabolic or reproductive phenotype. J Clin Endocrinol Metab 2005; 90:2571–9.

35. Rotterdam ESHRE/ASRM-Sponsored PCOS Consensus Workshop Group. Revised 2003 consensus on diagnostic criteria and long-term health risks related to polycystic ovary syndrome. Fertil Steril 2004;81:19–25.

36. Apridonidze T, Essah PA, Iuorno MJ, Nestler JE. Prevalence and characteristics of the metabolic syndrome in women with polycystic ovary syndrome. J Clin Endocrinol Metab 2005;90:1929–35

37. Graf MJ, Richards CJ, Brown V, Meissner L, Dunaif A. The independent effects of hyperandrogenaemia, hyperinsulinaemia, and obesity on lipid and lipoprotein profiles in women. Clin Endocrinol 1990;33:119–31.

38. Pasquali R. Antenucci D, Casimirri F, Venturoli S, Paradisi R, Fabbri R, Balestra V, Melchionda N, Barbara L. Clinical and hormonal characteristics of obese amenorrheic hyperandrogenic women before and after weight loss. J Clin Endocrinol Metab 1989;68:173–9.

39. Lapidus L, Bengtsson C, Larsson B, Pennert K, Rybo E, Sjostrom L. Distribution of adipose tissue and risk of cardiovascular disease and death: a 12 year follow up of participants in the population study of women in Gothenburg, Sweden. Br Med J (Clin Res Ed) 1984;289:1257–61.

40. Redmond GP, Olson WH, Lippman JS, Kafrissen ME, Jones TM, Jorizzo JL. Norgestimate and ethinyl estradiol in the treatment of acne vulgaris: a randomized, placebo-controlled trial. Obstet Gynecol 1997;89:615–22.

41. Ruchhoft EA, Elkind-Hirsch KE, Malinak R. Pituitary function is altered during the same cycle in women with polycystic ovary syndrome treated with continuous or cyclic oral contraceptives on a gonadotropin-releasing hormone agonist. Fertil Steril 1996;66:54–60.

42. Erenus M, Yucelten D, Gurbuz O, et al. Comparison of spironolactone-oral contraceptive versus cyproterone acetate-estrogen regimens in the treatment of hirsutism. Fertil Steril 1996;66:216–9.

43. Marcondes JA, Minnani SL, Luthold WW, Wajchenberg BL, Samojlik E, Kirschner MA. Treatment of hirsutism in women with flutamide. Fertil Steril. 1992 Mar; 57(3):543–7.

44. Tolino A, Petrone A, Sarnacchiaro F, Cirillo D, Ronsini S, Lombardi G, Nappi C. Finasteride in the treatment of hirsutism: new therapeutic perspectives. Fertil Steril 1996;66:61–5.

45. ACOG Committee on Practice Bulletins. Premenstrual syndrome. ACOG Practice Bulletin 15. Washington DC: American College of Obstetricians and Gynecologists, 2000.

46. Borenstein JE, Dean BB, Endicott J, et al. Health and economic impact of the premenstrual syndrome. J Reprod Med 2003;48:515–24.

47. Borenstein J, Chiou CF, Dean B, Wong J, Wade S. Estimating direct and indirect costs of premenstrual syndrome. J Occup Environ Med 2005;47:26–33.
48. Arias RD. Premenstrual syndrome. In: Mishell DR Jr, Goodwin TM, Brener PF (eds). Management of common problems in obstetrics and gynecology, 4th ed. Boston: Blackwell Publishers, 2001.
49. Sternfeld B, Swindle R, Chawla A, Long S, Kennedy S. Severity of premenstrual symptoms in a health maintenance organization population. Obstet Gynecol 2002; 99:1014–24.
50. American Psychiatric Association. Diagnostic and statistical manual of mental disorders, fourth edition text revision (DSM-IV-TR). Washington DC: American Psychiatric Association, 2000:771–774.
51. Dalton K. The premenstrual syndrome and progesterone therapy, 2nd ed. Chicago: Mosby-Year Book Medical Publisher, 1984.
52. Rubinow DR, Hoban MC, Grover GN, Galloway DS, Roy-Byrne P, Andersen R, Merriam GR. Changes in plasma hormones across the menstrual cycle in patients with menstrually related mood disorder and in control subjects. Am J Obstet Gynecol. 1988;158:5–11.
53. Schmidt PJ, Nieman LK, Danaceau MA, Adams LF, Rubinow DR. Differential behavioral effects of gonadal steroids in women with and those without premenstrual syndrome. New Engl J Med 1998;338:209–16.
54. Chuong CJ, Coulam CB, Kao PC, Bergstralh EJ, Go VL. Neuropeptide levels in premenstrual syndrome. Fertil Steril 1985;44:760–5.
55. Straneva PA, Maixner W, Light KC, Pedersen CA, Costello NL, Girdler SS. Menstrual cycle, beta-endorphins, and pain sensitivity in premenstrual dysphoric disorder. Health Psychol 2002;4:358–67.
56. Redei E, Freeman EW. Preliminary evidence for plasma adrenocorticotropin levels as biological correlates of premenstrual symptoms. Acta Endocrinol (Copenh) 1993 Jun; 128(6):536–42.
57. Mira M, Stewart PM, Abraham SF. Vitamin and trace element status in premenstrual syndrome. Am J Clin Nutr 1988;47:636–641.
58. Perkonigg A, Yonkers KA, Pfister H., Lieb R, Wittchen HU. Risk factors for premenstrual dysphoric disorder in a community sample of young women: the role of traumatic events and posttraumatic stress disorder. J Clin Psychiatry 2004;65:1314–22.
59. Mortola JF. Premenstrual syndrome-pathophysiologic considerations. New Engl J Med 1998;338:256–7.
60. Halbreich U, Monacelli E. Some clues to the etiology of premenstrual syndrome/premenstrual dysphoric disorder. Prim Psychiatry 2004;11:33–40.
61. Rapkin AJ. The role of serotonin in premenstrual syndrome. Clin Obstet Gynecol 1992;35:629–36.
62. Eriksson E, Hedberg MA, Andersch B, Sundblad C. The serotonin reuptake inhibitor paroxetin is superior to the noradrenaline reuptake inhibitor maprotiline in the treatment of premenstrual syndrome: a placebo-controlled trial. Neuropsychopharmacology 1995;12:167–76.
63. Rubinow DR, Roy-Bryne P, Hoban MC, et al. Prospective assessment of menstrually related mood disorders. Am J Psychiatry 1984;141:684–6.
64. Harrison WM, Rabkin JG, Endicott J. Psychiatric evaluation of premenstrual changes. Psychosomatics 1985;26:789–92,795,798–9.
65. Fava M, Pedrazzi F, Guaraldi GP, Romano G, Genazzani AR, Facchinetti F. Comorbid anxiety and depression among patients with late luteal phase dysphoric disorder. J Anxiety Disorders 1992;6:325–35.
66. Steiner M, Macdougall M, Brown E. The premenstrual symptoms screening tool (PSST) for clinicians. Arch Women Ment Health 2003;6:203–9.
67. Feuerstein M, Shaw WS. Measurement properties of the calendar of premenstrual experience in patients with premenstrual syndrome. .J Reprod Med 2002;47:279–89.

68. Endicott J, Nee J, Harrison W. Daily record of severity of problems (DRSP): reliability and validity. Arch Women Ment Health 2006;9:41–9.
69. U.S. Department of Health and Human Services. Physical Activity and Health: A Report of the U.S. Surgeon General. Atlanta, GA: U.S. Department of Health and Human Services, Centers for Disease Control and Prevention, National Center for Chronic Disease Prevention and Health Promotion, 1996.
70. Choi PY, Salmon P. Symptom changes across the menstrual cycle in competitive sportswomen, exercisers, and sedentary women. Br J Clin Psychol 1995;34:447–60.
71. Prior JC, Vigna Y, Sciarretta D, Alojado N Schulzer M. Conditioning exercise decreases premenstrual symptoms: a prospective controlled 6 month trial. Fertil Steril 1987;47:402–8.
72. Steege JF, Blumenthal JA. The effects of aerobic exercise on premenstrual symptoms in middle-aged women: a preliminary study. J Psychosom Res 1993;37:127–33.
73. Rossignol AM. Caffeine-containing beverages and premenstrual syndrome in young women. Am J Public Health 1985;75:1335–7.
74. Sayegh R, Schiff I, Wurtman J, et al. The effect of a carbohydrate- beverage on mood, appetite, and cognitive function in women with premenstrual syndrome. Obstet Gynecol 1995;86:520–528.
75. Stevinson C, Ernst E. Complementary and alternative therapies for premenstrual syndrome: a systematic review of randomized controlled trials. Am J Obstet Gynecol 2001;185:227–35.
76. Wyatt KM, Dimmock PW, Jones PW, Shaughn O'Brien PM. Efficacy of vitamin B-6 in the treatment of premenstrual syndrome: systematic review. BMJ 1999;318:1375–81.
77. London RS, Bradley L, Chiamori NY. Effect of a nutritional supplement on premenstrual symptomatology in women with premenstrual syndrome: a double-blind longitudinal study. J Am Coll Nutr 1991;10:494.
78. Facchinetti F, Borella P, Sances G, et al. Oral magnesium successfully relieves premenstrual mood changes. Obstet Gynecol 1991;78:177–81.
79. Girman A, Lee R, Kligler B. An integrative medicine approach to premenstrual syndrome. Am J Obstet Gynecol 2003;188:S56–65.
80. Walker AF, De Souza MC, Vickers MF, Abeyasekera S, Collins ML, Trinca LA. Magnesium supplementation alleviates premenstrual symptoms of fluid retention. J Womens Health 1998;7:1157–65.
81. Miller ER, Pastor-Barriuso R, Dalal D, et al. Meta-analysis: high-dosage vitamin E supplementation may increase all-cause mortality. Ann Intern Med 2005;142:37–46.
82. Bertone-Johnson ER, Hankinson SE, Bendich A, et al. Calcium and vitamin D intake and risk of incident premenstrual syndrome. Arch Intern Med 2005;165:1246–52.
83. Thys-Jacobs S, Ceccarelli S, Bierman A, Weisman H, Cohen M, Alvir J. Calcium supplementation in premenstrual syndrome: a randomized crossover trial. J Gen Intern Med 1989;4:183–9.
84. Thys-Jacobs S, Starkey P, Bernstein D, Tian J. Calcium carbonate and the premenstrual syndrome: effects on premenstrual and menstrual symptoms. Premenstrual Syndrome Study Group. Am J Obstet Gynecol 1998;179:444–52.
85. Blumenthal M. German Federal Institute for Drugs and Medical Devices. Commission E. Herbal Medicine: expanded Commission E monographs. 1st ed. Newton, MA: Integrative Medicine Communications, 2000.
86. Schellenberg R. Treatment for the premenstrual syndrome with agnus castus fruit extract: prospective, randomized, placebo controlled study. BMJ 2001;322:134–7.
87. Budeiri D, Li Wan Po A, Dornan JC. Is evening primrose oil of value in the treatment of premenstrual syndrome? Control Clin Trials 1996;17:60–8.
88. Blake F, Salkovskis P, Gath D, Day A, Garrod A. Cognitive therapy for premenstrual syndrome: a controlled trial. J Psychosom Res 1998;45:307–18.
89. Goodale IL, Domar AD, Benson H. Alleviation of premenstrual syndrome with the relaxation response. Obstet Gynecol 1990;75:649–655.

90. Oleson T, Flocco W. Randomized controlled study of premenstrual symptoms treated with ear, hand and foot reflexology. Obstet Gynecol 1993;82:906–911.
91. Van Zak DB. Biofeedback treatments for premenstrual and premenstrual affective syndromes. Int J Psychosom 1994;41:53–60.
92. Lam RW, Carter D, Misri S, et al. A controlled study of light therapy in women with late luteal phase disorder. Psychiatry Res 1999;86:185–92.
93. Steiner M, Steinberg S, Stewart D, Carter D, Berger C, Reid R, Grover D, Streiner D. Fluoxetine in the treatment of premenstrual dysphoria. N Engl J Med 1995; 332:1529–1534.
94. Yonkers KA, Halbreich U, Freeman E, et al. Symptomatic improvement of premenstrual dysphoric disorder with sertraline treatment. A randomized controlled trial. Sertraline Premenstrual Dysphoric Collaborative Study Group. JAMA 1997; 278:983–8.
95. Steiner M, Hirschberg AL, Bergeron R, et al. Luteal phase dosing with paroxetine controlled release (CR) in the treatment of premenstrual dysphoric disorder. Am J Obstet Gynecol 2005;193:352–60.
96. Freeman EW, Rickels K, Yonkers KA, et al. Venlafaxine in the treatment of premenstrual dysphoric disorder. Obstet Gynecol 2001;98:737–44.
97. Steiner M, Steinberg S, Stewart D, Carter D, Berger C, Reid R, Grover D, Streiner D. Fluoxetine in the treatment of premenstrual dysphoria. N Engl J Med 1995; 332:1529–1534.
98. Halbreich U and Smoller JW. Intermittent luteal phase sertraline treatment of dysphoric premenstrual syndrome. J Clin Psychiatry 1997;58:399–402.
99. Schmidt PJ, Grover GN, Rubinow DR. Alprazolam in the treatment of premenstrual syndrome. A double-blind, placebo-controlled trial. Arch Gen Psychiatry 1993; 50:467–73.
100. Freeman EW, Rickels K, Sondheimer SJ, Polansky M. A double-blind trial of oral progesterone, alprazolam, and placebo in treatment of severe premenstrual syndrome. JAMA 1995;274:51–7.
101. Wang M, Hammarback S, Lindhe BA, Backstrom T. Treatment of premenstrual syndrome by spironolactone: a double-blind, placebo controlled study. Acta Obstet Gynecol Scand 1995;74:803–8.
102. Graham CA and Sherwin BB. A prospective treatment study of premenstrual symptoms using a triphasic oral contraceptive. J Psychosom Res 1992;36:257–66.
103. Freeman EW, Kroll R, Rapkin A, Pearlstein T, Brown C, Parsey K, Zhang P, Patel H, Foegh M. Evaluation of a unique oral contraceptive in the treatment of premenstrual dysphoric disorder. J Womens Health Gend Based Med 2001;10:561–9.
104. Pearlstein TB, Bachmann GA, Zacur HA, Yonkers KA. Treatment of premenstrual dysphoric disorder with a new drospirenone-containing oral contraceptive formulation. Contraception 2005;72:414–21.
105. Yonkers KA, Brown C, Pearlstein TB, Foegh M, Sampson-Landers C, Rapkin A. Efficacy of a new low-dose oral contraceptive with drospirenone in premenstrual dysphoric disorder. Obstet Gynecol 2005;106:492–501.
106. Muse KN, Cetel NS, Futterman LA, Yen SC. The premenstrual syndrome. Effects of "medical ovariectomy". N Engl J Med 1984;311:1345–9.
107. Martin V, Brandes JL. IMED Communications. Strategies for optimizing management of menstrual migraine. J Fam Pract 2005;54(12):S1–7;quiz S8.
108. Cupini LM, Matteis M, Troisi E, et al. Sex-hormone-related events in migrainous females. A clinical comparative study between migraine with aura and migraine without aura. Cephalalgia 1995;15:140–4.
109. Granella F, Sances G, Allais G, et al. Characteristics of menstrual and nonmenstrual attacks in women with menstrually related migraine referred to headache centres. Cephalalgia 2004;24:707–16.
110. Martin VT. Menstrual migraine: a review of prophylactic therapies. Curr Pain Headache Rep 2004;8:229–37.

111. Digre K, Damasio H. Menstrual migraine: differential diagnosis, evaluation and treatment. Clin Obstet Gynecol 1987:30:417–30.
112. Silberstein SD, Merriam GR. Estrogens, progestins, and headache. Neurology 1991; 41:786–93.
113. Somerville BW. The role of estradiol withdrawal in the etiology of menstrual migraine. Neurology 1972;22:355–365.
114. Somerville BW. The role of progesterone in menstrual migraine. Neurology 1971; 21:853–9.
115. Li W, Zheng T, Altura BM, et al. Sex steroid hormones exert biphasic effects on cytosolic magnesium ions in cerebral smooth muscle cells: possible relationships to migraine frequency in premenstrual syndrome and stroke incidence. Brain Res Bull 2001;54:83–89.
116. Allais G, Bussone G, DeLorenzo C, Mana O, Benedetto C. Advanced strategies of short-term prophylaxis in menstrual migraine: state of the art and prospects. Neurol Sci 2005;26 Suppl 2:s125–9.
117. Loder E. Menstrual migraine. Neurol Sci 2005;26 Suppl 2:s121–4.
118. Snow V, Weiss K, Wall EM, et al. Pharmacologic management of acute attacks of migraine and prevention of migraine headache. Ann Intern Med 2002;137:840–9.
119. MacGregor EA, Frith A, Ellis J, Aspinall L. Predicting menstrual migraine with a home-use fertility monitor. Neurology 2005;64:561–3.
120. Murray SC, Muse KN. Effective treatment of severe menstrual migraine headaches with gonadotropin-releasing hormone agonist and add-back therapy. Fertil Steril 1997;67:390–393
121. Powles TJ. Prevention of migrainous headaches by tamoxifen. Lancet 1986;2:1344.
122. Silberstein SD, Merriam GR. Sex hormones and headache. J Pain Symptom Manage 1993;8:98–114.
123. Guillebaud J. The Pill and Other Hormones for Contraception, 5th ed. Oxford: Oxford University Press, 1997.
124. Bousser MG. Estrogens, migraine, and stroke. Stroke 2004;35:2652–6.
125. Herzog AG, Klein P, Ransil BJ. Three patterns of catamenial epilepsy. Epilepsia 1997; 38:1082–8.
126. Foldvary-Schaefer N, Falcone T. Catamenial epilepsy: pathophysiology, diagnosis, and management. Neurology 2003;61:S2–15.
127. Herzog AG. Progesterone therapy in women with epilepsy: a 3 year follow up. Neurology 1999;52:1917–8.
128. Beynon HL, Garbett ND, Barnes PJ. Severe premenstrual exacerbations of asthma: effect of intramuscular progesterone. Lancet 1988;2:370–2.
129. Olive DL, Schwartz LB. Endometriosis. N Engl J Med 1993;328:1759–69.
130. Kennedy S, Bergqvist A, Chapron C, et al. ESHRE guideline for the diagnosis and treatment of endometriosis. Hum Reprod. 2005;20:2698–704.
131. American Society for Reproductive Medicine. Revised American Society for Reproductive Medicine classification of endometriosis: 1996. Fertil Steril 1997;67:817–21.
132. Prentice A. Regular review: Endometriosis BMJ 2001;323:93–5.
133. Vercellini P, De Giorgi O, Oldani S, et al. Depot medroxyprogesterone acetate versus an oral contraceptive combined with very-low-dose danazol for long-term treatment of pelvic pain associated with endometriosis. Am J Obstet Gynecol 1996;175:396–401.
134. Crosignani PG, Luciano A, Ray A, Bergqvist A. Subcutaneous depot medroxyprogesterone acetate versus leuprolide acetate in the treatment of endometriosis-associated pain. Hum Reprod 2006;21:248–56.
135. Prentice A, Deary AJ, Goldbeck-Wood S, et al. Gonadotrophin-releasing hormone analogues for pain associated with endometriosis. Cochrane Database Syst Rev 2000; (2):CD000346.
136. Chapron C, Vercellini P, Barakat H, Vieira M, Dubuisson JB. Management of ovarian endometriomas. Hum Reprod Update 2002;8(6):591–7.

137. Sutton CJ, Ewen Sp, Whitelaw N, Haines P. Prospective, randomized, double blind, controlled trial of laser laparoscopy in the treatment of pelvic pain associated with minimal, mild, and moderate endometriosis. Fertil Steril 1994;62:696–700.

138. ACOG Committee on Practice Bulletins—Gynecology. ACOG Practice Bulletin No. 51. Chronic pelvic pain. Obstet Gynecol 2004;103:589–605.

139. Mathias SD, Kuppermann M, Liberman RF, et al. Chronic pelvic pain: prevalence, health-related quality of life, and economic correlates. Obstet Gynecol 1996;87:321–7.

140. Jamieson DJ, Steege JF. The prevalence of dysmenorrhea, dyspareunia, pelvic pain, and irritable bowel syndrome in primary care practices. Obstet Gynecol 1996;87:55–8.

141. Mathias SD, Kupperman M, Lieberman RF, Lipschutz RC, Steege JF. Chronic pelvic pain: prevalence, health-related quality of life, and economic correlates. Obstet Gynecol 1996;87:321–7.

142. Zondervan KT, Yudkin PL, Vessey MP, et al. Prevalence and incidence of chronic pelvic pain in primary care: evidence from a national general practice database. Br J Obstet Gynaecol 1999;106:1149–55.

143. Zondervan K, Yudkin P, Vessey M, et al. Chronic pelvic pain in the community-symptoms, investigations, and diagnoses. Am J Obstet Gynecol 2001;184:1149–55.

144. Farquhar CM, Steiner CA. Hysterectomy rates in the United States 1990–1997. Obstet Gynecol 2002;99:229–34.

145. Reiter RC. A profile of women with chronic pelvic pain. Clin Obstet Gynecol 1990; 33:130–6.

146. Steege JF, Stout AL, Somkuti SG. Chronic pelvic pain in women: toward an integrative model. Obstetrical and Gynecological Survey 1993;48:95–110.

147. Walker EA, Katon WJ, Hansom J, Harrop-Griffiths J, Holm L, Jones ML, Hickok LR, Russo J. Psychiatric diagnoses and sexual victimization in women with chronic pelvic pain. Psychosomatics 1995;36:531–540.

148. Williams RE, Hartmann KE, Sandler RS, et al. Recognition and treatment of irritable bowel syndrome among women with chronic pelvic pain. Am J Obstet Gynecol 2005; 192:761–7.

149. National Digestive Diseases Information Clearinghouse. Irritable Bowel Syndrome. Bethesda: National Institutes of Health, 2006. Accessed 3/4/06 at: http://digestive. niddk.nih.gov/ddiseases/pubs/ibs.

150. Drossman DA, Camilleri M, Mayer EA, Whitehead WE. AGA technical review on irritable bowel syndrome. Gastroenterology 2002;123:2108–31.

151. Clemons JL, Arya LA, Myers DL. Diagnosing interstitial cystitis in women with chronic pelvic pain. Obstet Gynecol 2002;100:337–41.

152. Parsons CL, Dell J, Stanford EJ, Bullen M, Kahn BS, Willems JJ The prevalence of interstitial cystitis in gynecologic patients with pelvic pain, as detected by intravesical potassium sensitivity. Am J Obstet Gynecol 2002;187:1395–400.

153. Rosenberg M, Parsons CL, Page S. Interstitial cystitis: a primary care perspective. Cleveland Clinic Journal of Medicine 2005;72:698–704.

154. Metts JF. Interstitial cystitis: urgency and frequency syndrome. Am Fam Physician 2001;64:1199–206.

155. Parsons CL, Greenberger M, Gabal L, et al. The role of urinary potassium in the pathogenesis and diagnosis of interstitial cystitis. J Urol 1998;159:1862–7.

156. Nickel JC, Barkin J, Forrest J, et al. Randomized, double blind, dose-ranging study of pentosan polysulfate sodium for interstitial cystitis. Urology 2005;65:654–8.

157. Perez-Marrero R, Emerson LE, Feltis JT. A controlled study of dimethyl sulfoxide in interstitial cystitis. J Urol 1988;140:36–9.

158. Hanno PM. Amitriptyline in the treatment of interstitial cystitis. Urol Clin North Am 1994;21:89–91.

159. Ness RB, Trautmann G, Richter HE, et al. Effectiveness of treatment strategies of some women with pelvic inflammatory disease. Obstet Gynecol 2005;106:573–80.

160. Haggerty CL, Schulz R, Ness R. Lower quality of life among women with chronic pelvic pain after pelvic inflammatory disease. Obstet Gynecol 2003;102:934–9.

161. Brill AI, Nezhat F, Nezhat CH, Nezhat C. The incidence of adhesions after prior laparotomy: a laparoscopic appraisal. Obstet Gynecol 1995;85:269–72.
162. Stovall TG, Elder RF, Ling FW. Predictors of pelvic adhesions. J Reprod Med 1989; 34:345–8.
163. Peters AA, Trimbos-Kemper GCM, Admiraal C, et al. A randomized clinical trial on the benefit of adhesiolysis in patients with intraperitoneal adhesions and chronic pelvic pain. Br J Obstet Gynecol 1992;99:59–62.
164. Swank DJ, Swank-Bordewijk SC, Hop WC, et al. Laparoscopic adhesiolysis in patients with chronic abdominal pain: a double blind randomised controlled multicentre trial. Lancet 2003;361:1247–51.
165. Parker JD, Sinaii N, Segars JH, et al. Adhesion formation after laparoscopic excision of endometriosis and lysis of adhesions. Fertil Steril 2005;84:1457–61.
166. Stones W, Cheong YC, Howard FM. Interventions for treating chronic pelvic pain in women. Cochrane Database Syst Rev 2005;(3):CD000387.
167. Tu FF, As-Sanie S, Steege JF. Musculoskeletal causes of chronic pelvic pain: a systematic review of diagnosis. Obstet Gynecol Survey 2005;60:379–85.
168. Prendergast SA, Weiss JM. Screening for musculoskeletal causes of pelvic pain. Clinical Obstet Gynecol 2003;46:773–82.
169. Slocumb JC. Neurological factors in chronic pelvic pain: trigger points and the abdominal pelvic pain syndrome. Am J Obstet Gynecol 1984;149:536–43.
170. Walling MK, Reiter RC, O'Hara MW, et al. Abuse history and chronic pain in women: prevalences of sexual abuse and physical abuse. Obstet Gynecol 1994; 84:193–9.
171. Jamieson DJ, Steege JF. The association of sexual abuse with pelvic pain complaints in a primary care population. Am J Obstet Gynecol 1997;177:1408–12.
172. Rapkin AJ, Kames LD, Darke LL, et al. History of physical and sexual abuse in women with chronic pelvic pain. Obstet Gynecol 1990;76:92–6.
173. Badura AS, Reiter RC, Altmaier EM, et al. Dissociation, somatization, substance abuse, and coping in women with chronic pelvic pain. Obstet Gynecol 1997;90:405–10
174. Poleshuck EL, Dworkin RH, Howard FM, et al. Contributions of physical and sexual abuse to women's experiences with chronic pelvic pain. J Reprod Med 2005;50: 91–100.
175. Thomas E, Moss-Morris R, Faquhar C. Coping with emotions and abuse history in women with chronic pelvic pain. J Psychosom Res 2006;60:109–12.
176. Cody RF and Ascher SM. Diagnostic value of radiological tests in chronic pelvic pain. Baillieres Best Pract Res Clin Obstet Gynaecol 2000;14:433–66.
177. Farquhar CM, Rogers V, Franks S, et al. A randomized controlled trial of medroxyprogesterone acetate and psychotherapy for the treatment of pelvic congestion. Br J Obstet Gynaecol 1989;96:1153–62.
178. Soysal ME, Soysal S, Vicdan K, Ozer S. A randomized controlled trial of goserelin and medroxyprogesterone acetate in the treatment of pelvic congestion. Human Reprod 2001;16:931–9.
179. McQuay HJ, Tramer M, Nye BA, et al. A systematic review of antidepressants in neuropathic pain. Pain 1996;68:217–27.
180. Serpell MG;Neuropathic pain study group. Gabapentin in neuropathic pain syndromes: a randomized, double blind, placebo controlled trial. Pain 2002;99:557–66.
181. Sindrup SH, Andersen G, Madsen C, et al. Tramadol relieves pain and allodynia in polyneuropathy: a randomized, double-blind, controlled trial. Pain 1999;83:85–90.
182. Eisenberg E, McNicol ED, Carr DB. Efficacy and safety of opiod agonists in the treatment of neuropathic pain of nonmalignant origin. JAMA 2005;293:3043–52
183. Atwal G, du Plessis D, Armstrong G, et al. Uterine innervation after hysterectomy for chronic pelvic pain with, and without, endometriosis. Am J Obstet Gynecol 2005; 193:1650–5.

184. Stones RW, Lawrence WT, Selfe SA. Lasting impressions: influence of the initial hospital consultation for chronic pelvic pain on dimensions of patient satisfaction at follow-up. J Psychosom Res 2006;60:163–7.

185. Okaro E, Condous G. Diagnostic and therapeutic capabilities of ultrasound in the management of pelvic pain. Curr Opin Obstet Gynecol 2005;17:611–7.

186. Peters AA, van Dorst E, Jellis B, et al. A randomized clinical trial to compare two different approaches in women with chronic pelvic pain. Obstet Gynecol 1991;77:740–4.

187. Gambone JC, Mittman BS, Munro MG, et al. Consensus statement for the management of chronic pelvic pain and endometriosis: proceedings of an expert-panel consensus process. Fertil Steril 2002;78:961–72.

188. Harrison RF, Barry-Kinsella C. Efficacy of medroxyprogesterone in infertile women with endometriosis: a prospective, randomized, placebo-controlled study. Fertil Steril 2000;74:24–30.

189. Farquhar CM, Rogers V, Franks S. et al. A randomized controlled trial of medroxyprogesterone acetate and psychotherapy for the treatment of pelvic congestion. Br J Obstet Gynaecol 1989;96:1153–62.

190. Mathias JR, Clench MH, Reeves-Darby VG, et al. Effect of leuprolide acetate in patients with moderate to severe functional bowel disease. Double blind, placebo controlled study. Dig Dis Sci 1994;39:1155–62.

191. Engel CC Jr, Walker EA, Engel AL, et al. A randomized double blind crossover trial of sertraline in women with chronic pelvic pain. J Psychosom Res 1998;44:203–7.

192. Sator-Katzenschlager SM, Scharbert G, Kress HG, et al. Chronic pelvic pain treated with gabapentin and amitriptyline: a randomized controlled pilot study. Wien Klin Wochenschr. 2005;117(21–22):761–8.

193. Johnson NP, Farquhar CM, Crossley S, et al. A double-blind randomized controlled trial of laparoscopic uterine nerve ablation for women with chronic pelvic pain. BJOG 2004;111:950–9.

194. Lee RB, Stone K, Magelssen D, Belts RP, Benson WL. Presacral neurectomy for chronic pelvic pain. Obstet Gynecol 1986;68:517–21.

195. Petros PP, Skilling PM. Pelvic floor rehabilitation in the female according to the integral theory of female urinary incontinence. First Report. Eur J Obstet Gynecol Reprod Biol 2001;94:264–9.

196. Weiss JM. Pelvic floor myofascial trigger points: manual therapy for interstitial cystitis and the urgency-frequency syndrome. J Urol 2001;166:2226–31.

197. de Oliveira Bernardes N, Bahamondes L. Intravaginal electrical stimulation for the treatment of chronic pelvic pain. J Reprod Med 2005;50:267–72.

198. Thomson AJ, Jarvis SK, Lenart M, et al. The use of botulinum toxin type A (Botox) as treatment for intractable chronic pelvic pain associated with spasm of the levator ani muscles. BJOG 2005;112:247–9.

199. Coughlin AM, Badura AS, Fleischer TD, Guck TP. Multidisciplinary treatment of chronic pain patients:its efficacy in changing patient locus of control. Arch Phys Med Rehabil 2000;81:739–40.

LATE REFERENCES

200. Inal MM, Yildirim Y, Taner CE. Comparison of the clinical efficacy of flutamide and spironolactone plus Diane 35 in the treatment of idiopathic hirsutism: a randomized controlled study. Fertil Steril 2005;84(6):1693–1697.

201. Abbott JA, Jarvis SK, Lyons SD, Thomson A, Vancaille TG. Botulinum toxin type A for chronic pain and pelvic floor spasm in women: a randomized controlled trial. Obstet Gynecol 2006;108(4):915–923.

Reproductive Tract Infections, Including HIV and Other Sexually Transmitted Infections

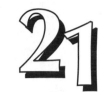

Jeanne M. Marrazzo, MD, MPH
Felicia Guest, MPH, CHES
Willard Cates, Jr., MD, MPH

- Reproductive tract infections (RTI) are frequently encountered by reproductive health professionals. RTI include both sexually transmitted infections and also other common infections of the genital tract, such as bacterial vaginosis and vulvovaginal candidiasis.

- RTIs have four serious health consequences:
  - Tubal occlusion leading to infertility and ectopic pregnancy
  - Pregnancy loss and neonatal morbidity caused by transmission of the infection to the infant during pregnancy and childbirth
  - Genital cancers

    Enhanced transmission of the human immunodeficiency virus (HIV)

- Persistent viral infections, including the human papillomavirus, genital herpes, human immunodeficiency virus (HIV), and hepatitis B virus are common, as are Chlamydia trachomatis and trichomoniasis.

- Every patient should be assessed for risk of RTI, including HIV. Assessing a client's risks for RTI can help the client better select appropriate contraceptive methods and the clinician provide better care. Ask each patient, "What do you do to protect yourself from infection with HIV and other sexually transmitted infections?"

- Preventing RTI and their consequences requires sexually active persons to adopt safer sexual behaviors and clinicians to diagnose and treat existing infections effectively.

- Because reproductive-age women constitute the fastest-growing segment of the HIV epidemic in the United States, reproductive health care settings are a critical conduit to HIV testing. Offer counseling and voluntary HIV testing to each patient.

- Routine HIV testing for all pregnant women is the standard of care for prenatal services. Be certain that HIV-infected pregnant women have access to antiretroviral drug regimens that can improve health status, reduce viral load, and reduce the likelihood of perinatal transmission.

In *Contraceptive Technology*, the generic term RTI covers three types of infections: (1) sexually transmitted infections (STI), (2) vaginal infections including bacterial vaginosis and candidiasis, and (3) iatrogenic infections associated with the insertion of an intrauterine device (IUD) or induced abortion. While prevention of infection through risk reduction and screening/treatment are the most effective ways to reduce the adverse consequences of RTI, recognition and correct management of RTI that do occur can prevent complications in the individual and interrupt transmission in the community. This chapter provides general background about RTI management in the reproductive health care setting.

MAGNITUDE AND RISKS OF RTI

The number of people infected with RTI or affected by their consequences is a major problem for society.[1] The estimated total number of people newly infected each year with curable STI is 15 million in the United States and 340 million worldwide.[2] Approximately 18.9 million new cases of STI occurred in 2000, of which 9.1 million (48%) were among persons aged 15 to 2.[3] In the United States, the annual cost of pelvic inflammatory disease (PID) and its consequences is estimated to be $4.2 billion. Infertility caused by PID accounts for over $1 billion of healthcare costs, as well as significant emotional cost. Although deaths due to some RTI (primarily syphilis and pelvic inflammatory disease (PID)) have declined over the past four decades, bacterial RTI still cause almost one-third of the reproductive mortality in the United States, and HIV-related mortality has become a leading cause of death in reproductive-age persons—particularly women—worldwide.

While the prevalence of RTI by individual pathogen and across different geographic regions varies considerably, some general trends are consistently observed. For example, individuals under 25 years of age account for a majority of RTI cases, with two-thirds of cases of gonorrhea and chlamydia reported in persons less than 25 years of age.[3] Rates of chlamydia, gonorrhea, and PID are highest in adolescents and decline steadily with increasing age. RTI are also concentrated in socio-geographic clusters, so-called "core populations," that generally reflect sexual networks, regional variation in disease prevalence, and, possibly, access to care. In this context, populations vulnerable to higher RTI prevalence include sex workers and illicit drug users (including those who use methamphetamine). Finally, most RTI exhibit a "biological sexism." Compared with men, women suffer more severe long-term consequences, including PID, infertility, ectopic pregnancy, chronic pelvic pain, and cervical cancer. Women may also be less likely to seek health care for assessment of RTI-related symptoms, because a higher proportion of their RTI are asymptomatic or unrecognized as being serious. Finally, due to the transmission dynamics of vaginal intercourse, women are more likely than men to acquire RTI from any single heterosexual encounter. The risk of acquisition increases when trauma occurs to the genital mucosa, as may be the case in sexual assault, but it decreases in the absence of penile-vaginal intercourse, as is the case with sex between women.

TRANSMISSION OF RTI

The probability that unprotected sexual intercourse will lead to RTI or its consequences differs from the probability of unintended pregnancy (Table 21–1). The risk of pregnancy varies according to the menstrual cycle. In contrast, while numerous complex factors probably modulate susceptibility to RTI, the risk of acquisition generally depends on (1) having sex with an infected person, (2) the gender of the infected person, (3) transmissibility of the particular RTI, and (4) use of barrier or other protective measures.[4] For example, the risk of acquiring gonorrhea from a single act of vaginal intercourse (where one partner is infectious) is approximately 25% for men and 50% for women. The probability of suffering consequences from an RTI depends on whether or not proper diagnosis and treatment are effected. In the case of HIV, the quantity of serum (and presumably genital) HIV viral load directly influences risk of transmitting HIV to vulnerable partners. HIV viral load is extremely high in the context of primary infection (the first several months after a person acquires the virus), which is infrequently recognized by both patients and providers alike. Unfortunately, modeling exercises suggest that most sexual transmission of HIV occurs during the period of primary HIV infection,[5] which emphasizes the need for persons at risk to consider protection at all times.

One of the fundamental concepts underlying RTI risk is the "epidemiological synergy" between HIV and other RTI.[6] Organisms that cause genital ulcers (herpes simplex virus (HSV), syphilis, and chancroid) are strongly correlated with the transmission and acquisition of HIV; furthermore, genital herpes increases risk of HIV acquisition even if it is not symptomatic.[7] Moreover, because immune dysfunction caused by HIV

Table 21–1 Comparative risk of adverse consequences from coitus: RTI and unintended pregnancy

Unintended pregnancy/coital act[10]	• 17%–30% midcycle • < 1% during menses
Gonococcal transmission/coital act[11]	• 50% infected male, uninfected female • 25% infected female, uninfected male
PID per woman infected with cervical gonorrhea	• 40% if not treated • 0% if promptly and adequately treated
Tubal infertility per PID episode[12]	• 8% after first episode • 20% after second episode • 40% after third or more episodes

can prolong duration and severity of RTI-related genital ulcers, these infections potentiate each other. RTI that produce vaginal or urethral discharge (such as gonorrhea, chlamydia, and trichomoniasis) have also been associated with higher quantities of HIV both in genital secretions and plasma. Because vaginitis and urethritis are more common than genital ulcers, these syndromes account for a larger proportion of the increased risk of HIV conferred by RTI. For this reason, it is critical to be alert for HIV coinfection in the setting of any RTI.

Research related to preventing sexual transmission of HIV is ongoing. Most recently, studies in Africa indicate that circumcision of male partners can significantly reduce the risk of these men acquiring HIV from their female partners.[8] Suppressive therapy for subclinical genital herpes is also being investigated as a means of reducing sexual transmission of HIV.[9]

RTI RISK ASSESSMENT, PREVENTION AND RISK BEHAVIORS

Different individuals accept different levels of risk. Not everyone will follow every safer sex recommendation but, with the proper knowledge, each person can make his or her own informed choices about reducing risk. Simplistic messages urging absolutist policies are ineffective.[13] While some prevention messages are universal and should be reinforced (for example, barrier methods when appropriate), recent emphasis on client-centered counseling highlights the need to individualize risk assessment and tailor risk reduction plans. The latter may include a discussion on selecting sex partners and building skills for negotiating safer sex.

Preventive measures for avoiding RTI transmission are generally consistent with guidelines for reducing risk of HIV infection. Risk-free options include having a mutually faithful relationship with an uninfected partner or completely abstaining from sexual activities that involve semen, blood, or other body fluids, or that allow for skin-to-skin contact. Examining a partner for lesions, discussing each new partner's previous sexual history, and avoiding partners who have had many previous sex partners can augment other measures to prevent RTI transmission. Educating people about their bodies and teaching them to be active participants in their health care gives them more control over their reproductive health.

Contraceptive Choice

Choice of contraception directly affects the risk of RTI (Table 21–3). Condoms reduce the risks of both bacterial and viral RTIs; the evidence is strongest for condom effectiveness against HIV, trichomoniasis, genital herpes, and gonorrhea.[14] No recent data support spermicides' ability to prevent bacterial or viral infections, including HIV.[15] Diaphragms used with spermicides provide a barrier against cervical infection, but they have been associated with changes in vaginal flora and urinary tract infections. Although oral contraceptives are usually associated with an increase in chlamydia detected in the cervix, they protect against symptomatic PID, but not asymptomatic endometritis.[16] Depot medroxyprogesterone acetate (DMPA) use has been associated with an increased risk of HIV acquisition and of chlamydial RTI infection in some studies.[17,18] IUDs are associated with a transient increased risk of PID in the first month after insertion, but after this, the RTI risk declines to levels seen in women without an IUD. IUDs have a strong record of safety, even for

Table 21–2 Effects of contraceptives on bacterial and viral RTI

Contraceptive Methods	Bacterial RTI	Viral RTI
Condoms	Protective	Protective
Spermicides	No evidence of protection	Not protective
Diaphragms	Protective against cervical infection	Protective against cervical neoplasia
Hormonal Contraceptives	Associated with increased cervical chlamydia Protective against symptomatic PID, but not unrecognized endometritis Effect may depend on estrogen vs. progesterone effects	Not protective
IUD	Associated with PID in first month after insertion	Not protective
Fertility Awareness	Not protective	Not protective

Source: Adapted from Cates and Padian (2000).[20]
See chapters on specific contraceptive methods for details.

HIV-infected women.[19] At present, the data are insufficient to state whether the progesterone-releasing IUD has a differential effect on RTI acquisition or natural history; available data do not suggest that this is likely to be the case.

Microbicides, defined as substances used topically that interrupt the ability of infectious agents to establish infection, hold promise for prevention of both HIV and other STI. (See Chapter 19 on Contraceptive Research and Development.) Currently, no available microbicide offers protection against RTI. In one study, frequent use of nonoxynol-9 gel has been associated with an increased risk of HIV acquisition.[21]

Other Risk Behaviors

In addition to sexual behaviors, other practices have been linked to RTI risk. Routine douching for hygiene has been associated with an increased risk of PID and ectopic pregnancy, and it is a major risk factor for bacterial vaginosis because it eradicates commensal hydrogen peroxide-producing vaginal *Lactobacillus* species.[22] Genital washing or urinating postcoitally have been poorly studied but appear to have little effect, if any, on reducing the risk of acquiring an RTI. In some studies, these practices have been associated with an increased risk of HIV acquisition. Finally, post-exposure prophylaxis (for example, after an unprotected sexual encounter in which RTI is suspected in one partner) has not been well studied for RTI prevention; it is currently recommended only in managing sexual assault.

Drug use influences the transmission of RTI. The risk of blood-borne transmission through needle sharing is especially prominent for hepatitis C, hepatitis B, and HIV. While hepatitis C is not typically considered an RTI, this virus has been identified in genital secretions (particularly in HIV-infected persons[23]), and the risk of sexual transmission, while probably low in the absence of exposure to blood, is not zero. Use of drugs such as methamphetamine and cocaine—whether through intravenous, intranasal, or other routes—has been associated with RTI-related risk behavior. Outbreaks of syphilis, antibiotic-resistant gonorrhea, and chancroid have been linked to drug-related sexual behaviors and to sexual networks in which drug users figure prominently. Crystal methamphetamine currently figures prominently in national outbreaks of syphilis in men who have sex with men, and the drug is especially harmful for its disinhibitory effects on sexual behavior. Abuse of alcohol, particularly binge drinking, has also been associated with risky sexual practices, including not using condoms[24]; alcohol abuse is a notable concern for adolescents.

ASSESSMENT, DIAGNOSIS, AND TREATMENT OF RTI

Professionals in the fields of family planning and RTI have common reproductive health goals:

- Educating all patients about RTI

- Providing diagnostic services that include risk assessment, RTI screening, and voluntary HIV testing

- Ensuring all persons diagnosed with RTI get appropriate treatment, preferably before leaving the facility

- Counseling individuals about the need for simultaneous treatment for their sex partner(s)

- Assisting patients in choosing a contraceptive that will reduce risk of acquiring an RTI

Comprehensive RTI-related care begins with routine risk assessment. Risk assessment should not be discarded due to common assumptions based on prior experience either with the individual patient (for example, a married patient) or with "representative" types of patients (for example, patients who identify as "lesbian"). At a minimum, ask clients about recent numbers of sex partners, anatomic sites exposed during sex (vagina, rectum, oropharynx), and personal protective measures (e.g., condoms). Risk assessment also helps clinicians provide better contraceptive counseling and more cost-efficient RTI management. Balance the variety of demographic, behavioral, and clinical information (other than laboratory test results) to assess the likelihood that clients are infected with an RTI or are at high risk of future infection and to counsel clients in selecting appropriate contraceptive methods. For example, an RTI risk assessment scale can help identify women who may be good candidates for barrier methods or inappropriate candidates for IUDs.[25] With the emergence of HIV infection and acquired immunodeficiency syndrome (AIDS), strongly counsel sexually active clients to use condoms for RTI prevention, even in conjunction with other contraceptive methods for pregnancy prevention.

Laboratory diagnosis of most RTI can be performed in nearly every reproductive health care setting. For example, over the past decade, routine screening for chlamydia has been associated with a decreased prevalence of the infection among clients attending family planning clinics in several regions of the country, and with concomitant declines in PID and ectopic pregnancy.[26] In addition, some family planning clinics have extended their range of services to male clients, including RTI diagnosis, treatment, and counseling. Finally, as family planning staff have become more familiar with the capacity of local STI programs, they are more able to provide appropriate referrals.

Table 21-3 Recommendations for annual screening of women for genital infection with
Chlamydia trachomatis

- All asymptomatic sexually active women < 25 years old
- Women of any age at risk for infection,[a] defined as
  - inconsistent condom use
  - new sex partner in preceding 3 months
  - multiple sex partners in preceding 3 months
- Presence of cervicitis[b]

[a] Other patient characteristics acknowledged by the U.S. Preventive Services Task Force to be associated with a higher prevalence of infection include single marital status, a new male sex partner or ≥ 2 sex partners during the preceding year, African-American race, prior history of STI, and presence of cervical ectopy. The latter four risk factors are endorsed by the American College of Preventive Medicine as formal indicators for routine screening. While individual risk depends on the number of risk markers and local chlamydia prevalence, most experts recommend using the risks listed in the Table as minimum criteria to consider screening in women > 25 years[26]

[b] Although cervicitis represents an indication for _diagnostic_ testing rather than screening, it is generally included in _C. trachomatis_ screening guidelines to emphasize the need for testing for this organism in this context.

Routine screening for RTI. Because most RTI are asymptomatic and do not cause clinical signs, such as cervicitis or PID, routine screening can provide early detection and prompt treatment, thus interrupting the progression to the sequelae of untreated disease. Chlamydial infections are the prototype, since up to 90% of these infections cause neither symptoms nor clinical signs (namely, cervicitis) in women. The U.S. Preventive Services Task Force recommends routine annual screening for target groups of women, as delineated in Table 21-3.[26] Indications for gonorrhea screening are less clear, but take into account the patient's recent history of STI, report of exposures of concern (for example, sex with a partner having chlamydia or gonorrhea, or with a symptomatic partner), and local prevalence.[27] Adults in the United States should be screened for HIV at least once, and more frequently if at ongoing risk of acquisition.[28] Patients should be counseled about the asymptomatic nature of most RTI and that transmission can occur in the absence of symptoms.

COUNSELING PATIENTS ABOUT RTI DIAGNOSIS AND TREATMENT

Counseling patients with RTI requires an approach different than that generally used in family planning settings. For couples trying to prevent unplanned pregnancies, counseling is typically non-directive to allow maximal opportunity for them to make an informed choice of the best contraceptive method. However, for patients who have RTI, _directive_ counseling is important to prevent new infections, increase adherence to treatment and follow-up, and offer guidance on talking to partners about their RTI exposure. Patients must be made aware of both the potential serious consequences of RTI and the behaviors that increase the likelihood of reinfection.

Education about infection and treatment. Make sure patients understand what RTI they have, how it is transmitted, why it must be treated, and exactly when and how to take prescribed medication. Because unpleasant side effects from some medications may discourage patients from continuing treatment, discuss what to expect and ways to minimize side effects. For example, doxycycline taken on an empty stomach may cause nausea that prompts the patient to stop taking the medication. Advise taking the medication with food.

Completion of treatment and abstinence during treatment. Urge patients to finish their entire supply of medication even though symptoms, if present, may diminish or disappear in a few days. Discontinuing antibiotics before the infection is completely cured can lead to recurrent infection and increase the likelihood that hard-to-cure strains of the pathogen may flourish. Advise patients to avoid sex until they complete the full course of therapy.

Partner management. Failure to treat the partners of women with RTI is the major risk factor influencing the high rates of chlamydia and gonorrhea recurrence in the months after initial treatment. An increasing number of family planning professionals are being trained in partner management skills. Confidentiality is crucial, just as it is in all aspects of family planning and RTI care. Sex partner(s) should be notified and treated to prevent both reinfection of the patient and spread of disease through the community. Assist patients in notifying their partners by coaching them in partner notification techniques (patient referral) and using local sexually transmitted disease program staff (provider referral) to help evaluate and treat partners.

Comfort. Provide patients with somatic and emotional comfort to enhance adherence with treatment. Treat nausea, pain, itching, or other physiologic discomforts symptomatically, if possible. Overcoming the psychosocial component of genital discomfort can be exceedingly important in RTI treatment. Patients may be afraid or ashamed to ask a partner to seek treatment, embarrassed to admit their sexual practices, or concerned about confidentiality. Telling patients they have a sexually transmissible *infection* rather than "a disease" may help some people avoid feeling stigmatized.

Concurrent infections. Managing RTI requires that clinicians have a high index of suspicion. A patient may have two or more RTI concurrently. Be alert for symptoms that differ from those normally associated with the primary RTI infection. Treat all presumptive RTI. For example, when a patient has gonorrhea, provide dual therapy for both gonorrhea and chlamydia unless chlamydia has been ruled out by a highly sensitive test (nucleic acid amplification test or NAAT).

STI reporting. All states require that certain STIs, including chlamydia, gonorrhea, syphilis, and chancroid, be reported to public health officials; many states have instituted reporting systems for others, such as genital herpes. Nearly all states require that HIV infection and AIDS be reported. Reporting is not a breach of confidentiality; in fact, statutory protection of patients' names is a crucial part of control strategies. Accurate reporting helps identify trends in disease, gain resources for high-prevalence communities, and evaluate control efforts. Resources to assist with this process can be found online at state STD program websites, which are listed at the National Coalition of STD Directors website at www.ncsddc.org/programsites.htm.

RTI During Pregnancy

Question pregnant women and their sex partners about their risk of RTI; counsel them about the possibility of transmitting an infection to their infant. Because of the severe effects RTI may have on both the pregnancy and the developing fetus, assess whether the pregnant woman should be screened for infections with HIV, syphilis, hepatitis B, chlamydia, gonorrhea, bacterial vaginosis, and trichomoniasis (Tables 21–4 and 21–5). Encourage screening for HIV to detect infected women who could benefit from prophylactic antiretroviral therapy to reduce maternal-to-infant transmission. Routine screening for human papillomavirus (HPV) is not recommended.

The management of specific RTIs is discussed in the Alphabetical Catalog of RTI at the end of this chapter. For more complete information on RTI in pregnant women, refer to Guidelines for Perinatal Care, jointly published by the American College of Obstetricians and Gynecologists and the American Academy of Pediatrics.[29]

RTI and Sexual Assault

In cases of sexual assault and abuse, clinicians must attend not only to physical and psychological trauma, but also to the possibility of pregnancy or RTI. Any of the sexually transmissible infections, including HIV, can be acquired during a sexual assault. Some RTI, such as gonorrhea or syphilis, are almost exclusively sexually transmitted and are therefore useful markers of assault in persons who have not been sexually active. To reduce the risk of pregnancy, offer emergency contraception (see Chapter 6 on Emergency Contraception). To reduce risk of RTI, the Centers for Disease Control and Prevention (CDC) recommends the following approach[30]:

Table 21–4 Risks of sexually transmitted bacteria and related syndromes in pregnancy and childbirth

Organism/Syndrome	Maternal Infection Rate (%)[a]	Infant Effects	Transmission Risk from Infected Mother	Prevention	Treatment of Mother, Neonate
Neisseria gonorrhoeae	1–30	Conjunctivitis, sepsis, meningitis	Approximately 30%	Screening; test mother; apply ocular prophylaxis	Ceftriaxone
Chlamydia trachomatis	2–25	Conjunctivitis, pneumonia, bronchiolitis, otitis media	25%-50% conjunctivitis, 5%-15% pneumonia	Screening in third trimester: test mother, apply ocular prophylaxis	Azithromycin Amoxicillin Erythromycin
Treponema pallidum	0.01–15	Congenital syphilis, neonatal death	50%	Serologic screening in early and late pregnancy	Penicillin
Trichomonas vaginalis	3–35	Low birth-weight, preterm delivery	N/A	Screening	Metronidazole
Bacterial vaginosis	10–35	Low birth-weight, preterm delivery	N/A	Screening	Metronidazole Clindamycin

Source: Adapted from Cates (1995).

[a] Percentage of pregnant women with evidence of infection

Table 21-5 Risks of sexually transmitted viruses and related syndromes in pregnancy and childbirth

Organism/Syndrome	Maternal Infection Rate (%)[a]	Infant Effects	Transmission Risk from Infected Mother	Prevention	Treatment of Mother, Neonate
Hepatitis B Virus	1–10	Hepatitis, cirrhosis	10%–90%	Active HBV immunization	Post-exposure passive HBV immunization
Herpes Simplex Virus	1–30	Disseminated, central nervous system, localized lesions	Recurrent: 3% at delivery; primary: 30% at delivery	Cesarean delivery if lesions present at delivery	Acyclovir
Human Papillomavirus	10–60	Laryngeal papillomatosis	Rare	None	Surgical
Human Immunodeficiency Virus	0.01–40	Pediatric AIDS	27% without ART < 5% with ART	Pregnancy prevention; ART during pregnancy	Antiretrovirals (ART)

Source: Adapted from Cates (1995).

[a] Percentage of pregnant women with evidence of infection

Adult evaluation. If possible, evaluate the victim within 24 hours of the assault and take specimens for culture of N. gonorrhoeae and C. trachomatis. Examine vaginal fluid microscopically for trichomoniasis and bacterial vaginosis (BV). Perform a pregnancy test, and keep a frozen serum sample for possible testing in the future. If treatment is not administered, schedule a repeat evaluation for 2 weeks later. Presumptive treatment may be provided at the victim's request. Advise clients to use condoms until the test results are reported. While no regimen provides coverage against all potential pathogens, the following should be effective against the most frequent RTI:

- Ceftriaxone 125 milligrams (mg) given intramuscularly (IM)
- Metronidazole 2 grams (g) given orally
- Azithromycin 1 g given orally
- Hepatitis B vaccination, first dose
- Post-exposure prophylaxis against HIV, depending on risk assessment

Child evaluation. In general, the presence of an RTI in a child beyond the neonatal period suggests sexual abuse. However, unlike gonorrhea or syphilis, specific infections such as bacterial vaginosis (BV), genital mycoplasmas, and genital warts are not conclusive evidence of sexual abuse. Evaluation is essentially the same as described for adult victims, except culture specimens should be collected from the pharynx and rectum as well as from the vagina or urethra because the child's report of assault may not be complete. Presumptive treatment may be given at the family's request. For more complete information regarding laboratory procedures, diagnosis, and treatment for sexual assault and abuse victims, refer to the CDC 2006 Guidelines for Treatment of Sexually Transmitted Diseases (see www.cdc.gov/std/treatment).[30]

SPECIAL CONSIDERATIONS REGARDING HIV/AIDS IN THE REPRODUCTIVE HEALTH SETTING

Infection with HIV is a global pandemic, with 96% of infected people living in resource-poor countries. Some 40 million people are living with HIV/AIDS (acquired immunodeficiency syndrome), including 17.5 million women.[31] On almost every continent, AIDS is a leading cause of death among young women. In the United States at the end of 2004, approximately 123,405 women were living with HIV/AIDS, 71% of whom contracted the infection through heterosexual contact, and 27% through injection drug use.[32] Most (90%) of children living with HIV/AIDS were exposed perinatally.[32] These women are demographically similar to those who seek reproductive health care in family planning, prenatal, abortion, and STI service sites.

For many young women, reproductive health care clinics may be the only source of health care. Each patient should be asked "What do you do to protect yourself from infection with HIV (the virus that causes AIDS) and other sexually transmitted infections?" Providers may be able to determine readiness for behavior change by assessing this answer. The patient who answers, "I thought I would get some condoms while I'm here today," may be more receptive to behavioral change than the patient who answers, "Who, me?"

With new patients, and with all patients in service areas of ≥ 1% HIV prevalence, consider using a more explicit HIV risk assessment (Table 21–6). Although reproductive health physicians are more likely than other primary care physicians to ask about sex and drug behavior, many are reluctant to risk offending patients. It may be helpful to begin with, "I'm going to ask you some personal questions that I ask everyone, because I think it is so important to your health. Is that all right with you?" If the patient has good literacy skills and is reasonably comfortable with a frank approach to sexual topics (patients at a college campus health service, for example), a risk assessment questionnaire can also be useful. Key considerations are provision of a private setting for these assessments, documentation of only what is critical to good patient care, and rigorous protection of the written record. Some health care providers who use questionnaires choose to return the document to the patient after discussion, with the assurance that only minimal information will be recorded in the chart.

Sex. Have you had an oral, vaginal, or anal sexual experience with another person? If yes, with about how many different people? 1? 2 or 3? 4 to 10? More than 10? Have your partners been men, women, or men sometimes and women sometimes? What about your partner's partners? Have you felt that a sex partner put you at risk for AIDS (injecting drug user, bisexual, lots of partners before you)? Have you had a sexually transmitted infection, such as herpes, gonorrhea, genital warts, or chlamydia? Have you felt forced to have a sexual experience when you

Table 21–6 Assessing HIV risk behaviors

Answer these questions for all the time in your life from 1977 to now.
What are you doing that you think may be putting you at risk for AIDS?
Have you ever had a test for HIV?
What prompted you to have the test?
What was the result?

didn't want to? What do you do to protect yourself from AIDS? Do you use male condoms? Female condoms? Other barriers? Please describe how you use them. Thinking about sex and AIDS, what do you think is the riskiest thing you do?

Drugs. Have you used injecting drugs with shared uncleaned equipment, including street drugs, steroids? Have you had sex with a person who uses injecting drugs and shares uncleaned equipment? How many drinks of beer, wine, and hard liquor have you had in the last 7 days? Have you had sex while stoned, high, or drunk, so that you can't remember details? Have you had sex in exchange for drugs, money, food, or shelter? Do you think alcohol or drugs ever got you into trouble? Thinking about drugs and AIDS, what do you think is the riskiest thing you do?

Blood. Have you shared uncleaned equipment for tattooing or body piercing? Have you had a blood transfusion? Have you had sex with a person who has had a blood transfusion? Do you have hemophilia? Have you had sex with a person with hemophilia? Have you received donor semen, egg, transplanted organ, or tissue? Thinking about blood and AIDS, what do you think is the riskiest thing you do?

Other Key Points. Avoid making assumptions about a patient's sexual and other behaviors based on appearances. In particular, avoid assumptions such as:

- Sexually-experienced people know how to use safer sex techniques.
- People with good jobs and families don't use drugs.
- Single people have lots of partners and risky sex practices.
- Older people have few partners and infrequent sex.
- Married people are heterosexual and don't have sex with same-sex partners.

Remember that terminology can sometimes get in the way of clarity with this type of risk assessment. For example, teens may not know the word "monogamous." Lay people may think "sexually active" means vigorous sex, or many partners. Some people who engage in same-gender sex do not think of themselves as "homosexual."

COUNSELING ABOUT SAFER SEX

Teach safer sex skills, including the correct use of male and female condoms and other latex and plastic barriers, to all at-risk patients (Table 21–7). Be sure to include prevention skills for oral sex, because HIV transmission through unprotected oral sex is possible, especially with activities that expose the mouth to semen.[33] Advise all patients that a crucial time for diligent safer sex practices is the first few months of a new relationship. Delaying intercourse may allow the couple the opportunity to get an HIV test together.

Customize teaching methods for individual patients. Use audiovisual, print, and electronic teaching aids appropriate to the patient's comfort, pleasure, age, language, culture, and learning style. Be sure to make your guidance specific to the patient and related to her particular issues, rather than giving vague, global advice:

- "Starting today, put condoms on the night stand beside the bed," rather than "always use condoms."

- "Maybe you should reconsider whether to date this person, who is also dating other women," rather than "Have fewer, safer partners."

- "Next time you're out with friends and might have sex, avoid getting high on drugs or alcohol," rather than "Have safer sex."

Younger patients may benefit from skill building, such as to how to choose a partner. Consider teaching how to analyze potential partners in categories such as "Don't Even Think About It," "I Deserve Better," and

Table 21–7 Options for sexual intimacy and HIV and STI prevention

Safe	All unprotected sexual activities, when both partners are monogamous and known by testing to be free of HIV and other STIs; also sexual fantasies, massage, hugging, body rubbing, dry kissing, masturbation without contact with partner's semen, vaginal secretions, blood, or broken skin, erotic conversation, books, movies, videos, electronic images, erotic bathing, showering, eroticizing feet, hands, hips, abdomen, ears, other body parts
Low, but Potential Risk	All sexual activities, when both partners are monogamous, but have not been tested; includes wet kissing with no broken skin, cracked lips, or damaged mouth tissue; hand-to-genital touching or mutual masturbation on healthy, intact skin or with a latex or plastic barrier; vaginal or anal intercourse using latex or plastic condom correctly with adequate lubrication; oral sex on a man wearing a latex or plastic condom; oral sex on a woman using a latex or plastic barrier such as a female condom, dental dam, or plastic wrap
Unsafe in the absence of mutual monogamy and HIV testing of both partners	Blood contact of any kind, including menstrual blood; any vaginal or anal intercourse without a latex or plastic condom; oral sex on a woman without a latex or plastic barrier such as a female condom, dental dam, plastic wrap, or modified male condom (especially if she is having her period or has a vaginal infection with discharge); oral sex on a man without a latex or plastic condom, especially if associated with semen in the mouth; oral-anal contact; shared sex toys or douching equipment; Any sex that causes tissue damage or bleeding, such as rough vaginal or anal intercourse, rape, or fisting

"This Could Work." Teach patients to ask about and look for genital tract infections in sex partners.

POSTEXPOSURE PROPHYLAXIS, SEX, AND DRUGS

In cases of isolated high-risk exposures to HIV—unprotected vaginal or anal intercourse, rape, receptive oral sex with ejaculation, or sharing injection equipment when the partner is known or suspected to be infected—consider giving postexposure prophylaxis for HIV (HIV-PEP). Although data on efficacy are limited, an increasing number of health care providers offer treatment to survivors of sexual assault and to other types of patients as well.[34] HIV-PEP should begin as soon as possible, and no later than 72 hours after the exposure. Treatment usually consists of a 1-month course of drugs combined from 2 or 3 antiretroviral drug groups, much like the combination therapy regimens used by persons with HIV. Discuss treatment protocol options with your local rape crisis center, or call the Post-Exposure Prophylaxis Hotline operated by the National HIV/AIDS Clinicians' Consultation Center for guidance on individual cases. The hotline is based at the University of California at San Francisco, and can be reached toll-free 24 hours a day, 7 days a week at 1-888-448-4911. Whether to accept any offered treatment is the patient's decision. Treatment may cost $1,000 to $1,600, and may not be covered by health insurance plans.

FACTORS AFFECTING SEXUAL TRANSMISSION

The likelihood of sexual HIV transmission is variable. The HIV viral load in the infected partner is a major determining factor.[35] Risk of sexual transmission may be increased under certain circumstances:

- During primary HIV infection (the weeks after the infection is acquired), because HIV viral load, and thus infectivity, is very high

- During late HIV infection, when infectiousness often increases as the immune system becomes less effective in controlling the virus, especially in the absence of antiretroviral treatment

- When either partner, but especially the HIV-infected partner, has a concurrent STI including trichomoniasis, gonorrhea, genital herpes, or chlamydia

- When blood or blood secretions are involved, or when tears in the exposed mucous membranes are present

- With anal sex (especially for the receptive partner), relative to vaginal sex

The risk of sexual transmission from an infected partner may be decreased (but not eliminated) under the following circumstances:

- If the HIV-infected partner is on an effective antiretroviral drug regimen and serum HIV viral load is undetectable. This does *not*, however, guarantee that HIV is not present in genital secretions, so transmission is still possible.

- If either the infected or the uninfected male partner is circumcised

Advice for Patients Seeking Contraceptive Services

Until further data are available, it is prudent to advise all patients as follows:

- Use male or female latex or plastic condoms each time you suspect even the slightest risk of HIV but choose to have vaginal or anal intercourse anyway.

- Use latex or plastic condoms for men and latex or plastic vulvar barriers for women any time you suspect any risk of HIV but choose to have oral sex anyway.

- Vaginal spermicides using nonoxynol-9 do not protect against HIV.

- Any tissue damage to the vulva, vagina, anus, or penis could increase susceptibility to HIV. Avoid intercourse until lesions are healed.

SPECIAL CONSIDERATIONS IN RTI/HIV PREVENTION

Romance. It is difficult to hold simultaneously the two thoughts, "I am in love with you," and "You might pose an infection risk to me." Romantic (germ-free) fantasy is a hallmark of midadolescence, and many people never manage to be clear-eyed about romance even when realism pervades other aspects of the adult worldview. Therefore, the reproductive health care provider is frequently in the unenviable position of attempting to foster self-protective health behavior where there is only desire, emotional need, and single-minded devotion to the idealized romantic relationship. Effective RTI/HIV prevention counseling with patients who are in love does not set up the beloved as a bad person, but it stresses that all people can and do harm other people even when they do not intend to and that people who love each other would certainly try to help each other maintain good health.

Power. Sometimes women make a personal commitment to RTI/HIV prevention but have little hope of enlisting the cooperation of the male partner. They say, for example, "You might as well not give me any condoms, because I know he won't use them." In all U.S. cultural groups, women typically lack economic, social, and physical power equal to that of men. Even when couples negotiate and achieve a relationship with equal decision-making power, they are likely to have begun the relationship with a power imbalance. One way to address this issue is to invite women to bring in their partners and to offer prevention skill-building for these men, either together with the female partner or alone. When men cannot or will not come in, offer telephone counseling with a male counselor. When no way exists to speak directly with the patient's partner, give patients audio or print messages to give to men. Remember that community and cultural norms vary substantially in how sexual decisions are made and by whom, so be sure counseling is grounded in the reality of your patient's life. For example, assess her risk of abuse, battering, rape, or abandonment should she try to insist on condom use.

Maintenance of sexual safety. Deciding to protect oneself (and others) from RTI/HIV is not one choice, like flipping a switch, but rather a series of hundreds of choices made day after day in the arenas of sex and drug use. When patients tell their stories, point out to them all their decision points, the places where they made safe and unsafe decisions, and whether they made them actively or passively. An important take-home message for patients is that prevention decisions are made every single day, and one can always learn from past experiences.

HIV TESTING AND COUNSELING

No more important conduit to HIV testing services exists for women than the reproductive health care provider, and such providers are urged to offer testing as a standard component of care.[28,36]

When To Offer Testing

Offer routine HIV testing to *all* women. Moreover, routine, voluntary HIV testing for all pregnant women is the standard of care in the United States.[36] Certain situations outside of the prenatal setting call for the care provider's strong recommendation to seek testing, and extra effort to assure that patients have reasonable access to counseling and testing services:

- Known sexual exposure to an HIV-infected person

- Shared injection equipment with an HIV-infected person

- Possible recent occupational exposure

- Clinical settings with a $\geq 1\%$ HIV seroprevalence

- Settings serving "populations at increased behavioral or clinical HIV risk," such as STI clinics, teen clinics with high rates of RTI, or correctional facilities, regardless of that setting's HIV seroprevalence

- Clinical signs or symptoms suggesting HIV infection (e.g., fever or illness of unknown origin, opportunistic infection without known reason for immune suppression)

- Diagnosis suggesting increased risk for HIV (such as another RTI or bloodborne infection)

- Patient's request

Prenatal testing. Many women learn they have HIV when testing is done as part of routine prenatal care. Some prospective studies have indicated that pregnancy itself may also confer an increased risk of acquiring HIV infection.[37] Acceptance of HIV testing in this setting is fairly high (74% to 95% in one multi-city study).[38] Women in this study were positively influenced to accept the test because they believed that finding and treating HIV would help both them and their offspring, and because their provider strongly endorsed the test. Women who declined testing gave reasons such as not perceiving a risk for HIV, time concerns, and previously having been tested.

Counseling about pregnancy options becomes an important component of post-test counseling if the HIV diagnosis is learned early in pregnancy; the patient may be overwhelmed by the large amount of highly emotional information to absorb. Pregnant women with HIV are faced with the same sorts of reproductive decisions as women without HIV, with similar percentages of terminated pregnancies and live births. For the HIV-infected woman who chooses to continue the pregnancy, consult appropriate guidelines for the use of antiretroviral therapy. Detailed guidelines are available at www.aidsinfo.nih.gov/guidelines.

Test Counseling

The decision to be tested for HIV, as with many other medical procedures, belongs to the patient. The structure of testing and counseling services is up to individual agencies, and must be in accord with local, state, and federal policies that govern the provision of HIV services. Current guidelines stress flexibility in implementing testing services and remind providers to tailor services by considering the characteristics of the patient population, HIV prevalence in the local setting, and available resources.[28,36,39] They describe a number of creative and carefully studied counseling options that are client-centered and allow flexibility for specific situations.

For pre-test services, explain how the test is done, what the routine screening procedure will and will not reveal, implications of anonymous vs. confidential testing, and instructions on how to obtain test results. Some patients tested with routine (rather than rapid) test technologies do not return for test results, so use the pre-test session to teach personalized and explicit risk-reduction skills. A counselor guide (Table 21–8) for the pre-test session and guides for giving negative and positive test results to patients may be helpful. All providers who give positive HIV test results to patients need training to master the skills of breaking bad news. This special encounter must help support the patient first, and then seek to accomplish no more than one or two critical educational goals. Many patients report that they remember little or nothing the care provider said after hearing the word "positive." Test counseling may require training and mastery of new referral sources. Counselors who are experienced at HIV test counseling generally allow 10 to 15 minutes for a pre-test session, 10 to 15 minutes for a negative post-test session, and 30 minutes or longer for a positive post-test session. Be careful to provide sensitive staff training and support both before and after your work setting initiates testing and counseling.

Counseling and Testing Issues

Anonymous and confidential testing. Guidelines stress the importance of having anonymous testing available for patients. Anonymous testing never links a name to the sample presented for evaluation (al-

---

Table 21–8 Components of counseling in the setting of HIV testing

Reason for considering test
- Elicit the patient's reason(s) so a counselor can use a client-centered approach to be as helpful as possible

About the HIV antibody test
- What kind of sample is used for testing: blood, oral mucosal transudate, urine
- What antibodies are
- How soon the test is accurate
- Why this is not a test for AIDS

How people get infected with HIV
- Through unprotected oral, vaginal, or anal intercourse with an infected person
- Through bloodstream to bloodstream contact with an infected person
  - Sharing uncleaned equipment for injectable drugs, steroids, tattoos, skin piercing
  - Transfusion of blood or blood products before March 1985
- From infected woman to child during pregnancy, labor and delivery, or breastfeeding. Risk depends on amount of virus in woman's body. On average, the risk for vertical transmission from untreated U.S. women is 25%, but it can be markedly reduced with antiretroviral therapy

(continued)

Table 21–8 Components of counseling in the setting of HIV testing—*(cont'd)*

Deciding whether to have the test
- Your right to decide whether to be tested
- Voluntary informed consent
- Anonymous vs. confidential testing
- Who will see the results if test is done here, including state laws
- Other sites for testing; home testing options

Benefits of being tested
- Peace of mind; knowing, one way or the other
- If infected:
    - Options for HIV therapy, managing related problems
    - Prevent transmission to others
    - Make informed childbearing decisions
    - Diagnose illness or symptoms
    - Access assistance programs

Difficulties with being tested
- Anxiety, waiting for results
    - If test is positive:
        - Learning you have a very serious illness
        - Telling sex or injecting-drug-equipment-sharing partners (health care agencies can provide help with this task)
        - Possible relationship difficulties with partner, family, friends
        - Possible threat to job
        - Difficulty getting or keeping insurance
        - Few experienced care providers in some locales

What results mean
- If antibody positive:
    - You are infected
    - You can pass the virus on to other people
    - Need to establish care with knowledgeable provider and undergo further assessment for disease staging
- If antibody negative or indeterminate:
    - You are not infected, or
    - You are infected, but antibodies are not yet detectable; infection may have been acquired up to 6 months previously

Reducing risk for HIV
- Develop a personalized risk-reduction plan today with counselor (using Tables 21–1, 21–2, and the CDC's Revised Guidelines for HIV Counseling, Testing, and Referral[9] as starting points)
- Offer condoms and other safer sex supplies
- Referral for drug, alcohol treatment

For more information
- National AIDS Hotline 800–342-AIDS
- HIV InSite: hivinsite.ucsf.edu
- Go Ask Alice: www.goaskalice.columbia.edu

though age, county of residence, sex, and other general demographic characteristics are often recorded). The anonymous patient is given a number code for getting test results. In contrast, confidential testing is name-linked, and information is protected to a degree determined by state law and the formal policies and staff commitment to confidentiality at the testing site. Allow patients to choose the approach they prefer, and be prepared to make a careful referral for anonymous testing if you are unable to provide it on-site. Most laboratories are willing to work out a coding system for anonymous samples, even for private practitioners. Patients not offered anonymous testing and reluctant to have an HIV test on record are likely to go to a test site where they are not known, to use a false name, or both. Another alternative for anonymous testing is home collection of a test sample using an over-the-counter kit, discussed below. Patients should be discouraged from donating blood as a way to learn HIV status; moreover, such donations are not anonymous.

Testing technology. For the past 15 years, HIV testing in the United States typically involved testing serum using an enzyme immunoassay (EIA) screening test and Western blot confirmatory test. Results have generally been available in 1 to 2 weeks. The EIA and Western blot are very sensitive and specific. Neither test is perfect, so an HIV test is reported as positive only after at least two EIAs and one Western blot or other confirmatory test (all using the same test sample) are all positive. As with any screening test, population prevalence is the single biggest factor in determining a test's predictive value; the higher the prevalence, the greater the likelihood that a positive test result means that the person is truly infected. Always regard HIV test results in the context of the total patient history and clinical picture, and re-evaluate when the two are not in accord.

New technologies have added options for testing other body fluids and for providing rapid test results.[40,41] These newer technologies are FDA-approved and provide sensitivity and specificity comparable to traditional tests. Early reports regarding acceptability of these options are reassuring.

- Patients reluctant to visit a care provider can purchase a home collection kit at a pharmacy, collect their own finger-prick blood sample, mail off the sample to a lab, and call for anonymous results and telephone counseling a few days later.

- Rapid HIV screening tests are also available. All provide a definitive negative result and a *preliminary* positive result in a matter of minutes. *Definitive* positive results require a confirmatory test such as a Western Blot. Sensitivity and specificity are comparable to standard EIAs, and costs range from $10 to $14 per test. Check the CDC internet site to track developments in the arena of rapid testing at www.cdc.gov/hiv/rapid_testing/.

Documentation of HIV Test Results. Recording HIV test results is important for ongoing medical care, although problems with confidentiality may result. This dilemma can be addressed by maintaining HIV-related information in a separate chart, by using a code for HIV test results, or by removing HIV-related information before releasing the chart. This latter practice is required by law in some states. State and local professional associations may offer guidance for appropriate, lawful charting that does not compromise the patient, provider, or health care delivery.

CLINICAL CHARACTERISTICS OF HIV INFECTION IN WOMEN

Relative to HIV-infected men, women may manifest immunologic impairment and CD4 cell depletion at HIV viral load levels lower than those in men (by as much as 30% to 50%). This influences the timing at which women seek care for HIV-related symptoms: often, they seek care later in the course of the disease, when CD4 counts have already declined to low levels. Primary HIV infection is typically asymptomatic, but when symptoms occur, they are non-specific and include flu-like symptoms lasting 1 to 4 weeks (fever, generalized lymphadenopathy, skin rash, headache, diarrhea, malaise, and lethargy). Few patients or providers recognize this syndrome as HIV, and this lack of awareness can lead to missed opportunities for early treatment, and also to unsafe behaviors in a time of relatively high infectiousness. After the primary infection period, adults with HIV typically feel well for months or years, then progress (especially in the absence of effective antiretroviral treatment) from minor skin and constitutional symptoms to discrete opportunistic illness, a cascade of illnesses, and then end-stage disease. Specific patterns of immune response to HIV in the first few weeks after infection may predict what pattern of progression the illness will follow. CD4 cell count, viral load, and reproductive health concerns differ according to the stage of HIV infection in women (Table 21–9).

The current standard of care for HIV is highly active antiretroviral therapy (HAART), a combination of oral antiretroviral agents that inhibit different targets of the virus. HAART regimens can be composed of drugs from two, three, or more classes, including nucleoside analog reverse transcriptase inhibitors (NRTIs), non-nucleoside reverse transcriptase inhibitors (NNRTIs), protease inhibitors (PIs) and fusion inhibitors. HAART should be initiated and managed by—or in close consultation with—an experienced HIV clinician in order to prevent the development of resistance to single drugs or to entire classes of drugs. Having an experienced care provider has been shown to be a factor in prolonging life for persons with HIV. HIV mutation and resistance can occur quickly if the regimen is not followed carefully. While single daily dosing regimens and formulations that combine agents from several classes have emerged as the standard of care and have greatly simplified the approach to treatment, side effects still occur, and all regimens are expensive. The decision to initiate therapy is based on assessment of HIV viral load in the plasma, CD4 count, and presence of opportunistic infections. Viral load testing uses DNA or RNA detection assays to measure the actual amount of HIV in plasma, permitting an accurate determination of real-time viral activity and a rapid assessment of antiretroviral drug efficacy. For complete information on recommended regimens, see www.aidsinfo.nih.gov/guidelines/.

Reproductive health care would ideally be managed in the primary care/HIV care setting also, but in some cases these are two providers in two different sites, so careful attention to shared information, shared decision making, and collaboration is essential. Advice on medical management of patients with HIV is available from the National HIV/AIDS Clinicians' Consultation Center based at the University of California at San Francisco. This no-cost "warmline" is staffed Monday through Friday from 6:00 a.m. to 5:00 p.m. Pacific Time, and voicemail is available 24 hours a day, 7 days a week. Call 1–800–933–3413.

A natural role for all care providers is to assist HIV-infected patients with health promotion practices that will engender optimism and contribute to well-being. Provide guidance on nutrition, stress management, exercise, rest, and reduction or elimination of tobacco, alcohol, and drugs.

Gynecologic Management

The keys to successful management of gynecologic infections in women with HIV are a high index of suspicion, prompt diagnosis, aggressive treatment (especially for immunocompromised women), and primary or secondary prophylaxis when appropriate. Table 21-9 outlines general states of HIV infection and related concerns; a discussion of some specific conditions follows.

Table 21–9 Stages of HIV infection and reproductive health concerns

	Primary HIV Infection/ Seroconversion	Symptom-Free	Early Symptoms	Discrete Illness/Cascade of Illness/Endstage
Duration	Average 1–8 weeks	Few months to many years	Few months to several years	Few months to several years
CD4 Cell Count x 106 /L Normal = 500–1600	Normal or slightly low	Typically > 350	Typically < 350	AIDS diagnosis at 200 or less
Viral Load copies/ml Normal = 1600	High	Variable	Rising (without HAART)	High (without HAART)
Characteristics	Self-limited flu-like illness can occur; HIV antibody not detectable 6–12 weeks post-infection,* but serum viral assays positive		Fevers, night sweats, zoster, vulvovaginal candidiasis, oral thrush, hairy leukoplakia, seborrheic dermatitis, weight loss, fatigue, loss of appetite	Mild or severe multiple opportunistic bacterial, viral, fungal, parasitic infections; cancers, including Kaposi's sarcoma, lymphoma, cervical cancer; Neurologic illness including dementia, peripheral neuropathy
Reproductive Health Concerns	Nonspecific presentation if primary infection is symptomatic; sex partner(s) and offspring may be at risk with ongoing risk behavior. Assess contraception, safer sex practices.	Usually asymptomatic, though risk of transmission less than with primary infection. Offer anticipatory guidance on future pregnancy planning. Frequent Paps, aggressive management of abnormal findings. Assess contraception, safer sex practices.	Pregnancy likely to be normal except for transmission risk for offspring. Frequent Paps, aggressive management of abnormal findings. Assess contraception, safer sex practices.	Medications may interfere with hormonal contraception; assess drug interactions. Assist with short-range and long-range child care plans. Pregnancy may result in prematurity, low birthweight, premature rupture of membranes, other complications. Frequent Paps, aggressive management of abnormal findings. Assess contraception, safer sex practices.
Risk of Trans- mission to Offspring	Risk may increase above 25% baseline if primary infection occurs during pregnancy.	25% each pregnancy without treatment. Decreased to about 2% with effective HAART.	25% each pregnancy without treatment. Decreased to about 2% with effective HAART.	25% each pregnancy without treatment. Decreased to about 2% with effective HAART.

Source: Modified from Anderson (ed.) (2001).[43]

* Newer rapid tests may detect antibody to HIV earlier. See www.cdc.gov/hiv/topics/testing/rapid/index.htm for details and updated information.

Vulvovaginal candidiasis (VVC). VVC is common in HIV-infected women and may recur frequently when immune status deteriorates. Non-albicans species may occur and may be relatively less responsive to topical imidazole or oral azole therapy. First-line treatment is a 7-day course of one of the topical imidazole antifungal agents. If topical treatment proves unsatisfactory, consider oral fluconazole (a single dose, 150 mg orally). Boric acid may be useful for women who experience infection with resistant *Candida* species.[42]

Human papillomavirus and cervical disease. Genital warts caused by HPV are common in HIV-infected women and may progress more rapidly in the presence of a declining immune status. These patients have significantly higher rates of Pap smear-detected abnormalities, dysplasia and progression to cervical cancer relative to noninfected women. Consider baseline colposcopy or cervicography, appropriate Pap smear intervals (see below), and prompt colposcopy and excision of any abnormal findings. One-year Pap smear intervals are appropriate for women with a history of normal results. Screen every 6 months for women who have symptomatic HIV, a CD4 < 200, or both. Shorten the interval to 4 to 6 months for ASCUS/LGSIL findings and, following treatment of preinvasive lesions, every 3 to 4 months for a year, then at 6-month intervals.[43]

Pelvic inflammatory disease (PID). In general, immunosuppressed women with PID do not appear to require more aggressive treatment than other women, but the approach should be individualized. Depending on the severity of PID and immune status, providers should consider parenteral therapy and hospitalization, based on factors considered in HIV-negative women.

Genital Herpes. Herpes lesions may be more extensive, more painful, atypical in location or appearance, and slower to heal in the presence of immune dysfunction. Treat in accordance with standard guidelines for HIV-infected persons. Consider daily suppressive therapy for women with frequent recurrences. Some experts recommend daily suppressive therapy in all patients with HIV and genital herpes.

Menstrual problems. Whether HIV or related immunosuppression affects menstrual patterns is not clear. Women may be appropriate candidates for hormonal replacement therapy with the proper indications. Hormonal intervention also may be offered for heavy bleeding and anemia and to ease discomfort. All menstrual irregularities merit a full evaluation; HIV is not always the culprit.

Psychological Care and Support

Women with HIV are likely to be caregivers themselves, accustomed to attending to the needs of children, spouse/partner, parents, and others; they may resist moving into a self-care mode. Women may make sure their children's clinic appointments are kept, for example, but be less diligent about keeping their own appointments. Gently remind the patient that she deserves care as well. Collaborate in establishing family-centered HIV clinics where all family members are cared for at the same time. Often the infected woman is not the only infected person in her household; her spouse or partner and one or more children may also have HIV, so the disruption of daily life may be profound. When infected women discuss their biggest worries and concerns, several fundamental needs are often mentioned:

- Having housing
- Earning an income
- Having a caregiver for children when mother is not feeling well
- Worrying about the health of children
- Feeling dread about disclosing illness to loved ones, especially children
- Fearing loss of the ability to care for oneself
- Worrying about the relationship with a spouse/partner
- Coping with addiction

Any guidance, support, and referral to assist with these fundamental concerns is likely to be welcome and helpful. Remember that for some women—an addicted woman, perhaps, or a woman in poverty—HIV may not be at the top of her list of problems.

Reproductive Health Care

Women with HIV in their reproductive years may make many active or passive decisions about their reproductive lives, including contraceptive practice, desire for pregnancy, outcome of an unintended pregnancy, and prenatal practices to reduce perinatal transmission of HIV. Reproductive decision making is similar to that for uninfected women, and desire for a child is often profound. Counseling for women who are pregnant or contemplating pregnancy includes important medical issues:

- Impact of HIV on pregnancy
- Impact of pregnancy on HIV
- Effect of antiretroviral medication and other drugs on woman and developing fetus
- Risk of perinatal transmission and options for reducing risk
- Risk of breastfeeding for HIV transmission
- Course of HIV in perinatally-infected infants

- Access to HIV-experienced obstetric and pediatric care

- Access to antiretroviral medications

Counseling for pregnancy optimally includes a full understanding of the patient's personal goals, her support network, an understanding of stressors in her life, and her overall physical and emotional status. Once this groundwork is in place, guide the patient through specific questions to help her predict how she would feel, how others would feel, and what might happen:

- Is she able and willing to love and care for a baby, whether or not the baby is infected?

- Does she have the support of a partner, family members, or friends who can help care for a child?

- Who will care for the child—teach the child about his or her culture, remember his or her mother, and raise the child according to her values—if she becomes sick or dies?

- In what ways (good or bad) will having a baby change her life?

- What are the reasons that she wants (or does not want) to have a child?

- Does she feel pressured by others to have (or not have) a child?

- Does she have enough information to make an informed decision?

Clearly, this is difficult counseling work, best carried out by counselors with experience, compassion, and the ability to help with the feelings of grief and loss that these scenarios will likely generate. The goal is to guide each patient to an uncoerced, thoughtful decision.

HIV-infected women who do not wish to become pregnant, like other women, are more likely to succeed with a contraceptive method they have chosen for themselves and feel comfortable using (Table 21-10). The goal is high contraceptive efficacy, low risk of woman-to-partner HIV transmission (if applicable), and low risk of partner-to-woman STI transmission. This goal is met by choices such as oral contraceptives plus male latex or plastic condoms.

Thousands of U.S. women with HIV give birth each year. Generally, HIV-infected women who are immunocompetent have uneventful pregnancies with normal labor and delivery. Just as with any women with serious systemic illness, immunocompromised women may have complicated pregnancies, including prematurity, low birthweight, and premature rupture of membranes. However, the effects of HIV on pregnancy are hard to differentiate from the effects of poverty, poor health care, or addiction. Pregnancy does not appear to speed HIV progression.

Table 21–10 Contraception for the HIV-infected woman

Method	Possible Benefits	Possible Drawbacks
Oral Contraceptives	• Good effectiveness with consistent use • Less blood loss to avoid anemia	• Unclear interaction of steroids and immune function • Possible interaction with certain antibiotics, antiretrovirals, other drugs • Possible increased shedding of virus from genital tract • No RTI protection • No HIV protection for partner
Depo-Provera	Good low-maintenance effectiveness	• Unclear interaction of steroids and immune function • Possible increased shedding of virus from genital tract • Possible increase in cervical inflammation • No RTI protection • No HIV protection for partner
IUD	Good low-maintenance effectiveness	• Risk of infection during insertion interval • No RTI protection • No HIV protection for partner • Increased days of bleeding, possible anemia
Diaphragm	Some RTI protection for the cervix	• Increases vulnerability to UTIs for some users • Requires good technique
Male, Female Condom	Good RTI protection, HIV protection for partner	• Male condom requires partner cooperation; partner cooperation helpful with female condom • Requires good technique
Surgical Sterilization	Good low-maintenance efficacy for women who desire no more children	• No RTI protection • No HIV protection for partner

Sources: Adapted from Anderson (2001)[43] and Cates W Jr. (2001).[14]

Risks of HIV Transmission in the Perinatal Period

Without HAART, each offspring of an infected woman in the U.S. faces approximately a 25% risk of being infected in utero, during birth, or while breastfeeding. With HAART, the risk falls to 2% or less (see below). Regardless of the true infection status of the infant, all infants will test positive for HIV antibody at birth because of the presence of maternal antibodies in infant blood. The HIV antibody screening test becomes accurate for the infant's true status at 15 to 18 months. Repeated measurement of serum HIV viral load is used to reveal the infant's true infection status. This testing is performed at birth, 2 weeks, and 6 weeks of age. If the test is negative at all three points in time, the infant did not acquire HIV. If any of these tests is positive, repeat viral load testing is ordered. If all are positive, the infant has acquired HIV.

Reducing perinatal transmission risk. More than 8,200 U.S. children have developed AIDS because they were born to infected women. Strategies to reduce perinatal HIV transmission continue to evolve rapidly. HAART is recommended for all pregnant women with the goal of suppressing plasma HIV RNA to undetectable levels. This reduces perinatal HIV transmission more effectively than zidovudine alone. Antiretroviral treatment is also recommended for HIV-exposed infants in their first weeks of life. HAART initiation for this purpose may be delayed until the second trimester.

Labor and delivery. In the absence of breastfeeding, an estimated 60% to 75% of perinatal HIV transmissions occur around the time of labor and delivery, and a number of strategies can reduce exposure of the neonate to maternal blood and secretions. In addition to intrapartum HAART, suggested approaches include vaginal disinfection, RTI treatment during pregnancy to lower viral shedding at term, avoidance of intrapartum invasive procedures, and cesarean delivery. Scheduled cesarean delivery before rupture of membranes is recommended for women whose HIV viral load at 36 weeks or later is above 1,000 copies/mL. Avoid delays in delivery once membranes have ruptured. The risk of perinatal HIV transmission can double when fetal membranes rupture more than 4 hours before delivery.

Breastfeeding. Advise infected women in the United States to bottle-feed infants to reduce the risk of postnatal HIV transmission via breast milk. The precise risk of HIV transmission via breast milk is difficult to quantify and may be influenced by the woman's HIV status (with high viral loads during primary infection and late stage disease), her use of HAART, breastfeeding patterns, and other factors. Among infected women who breastfeed, perhaps 10% to 15% of all vertical transmissions are associated with breastfeeding. (See Chapter 18 on Postpartum Contraception and Lactation.) Little is known about the impact of breastfeeding on the HIV-infected woman's nutritional status and overall health, or about the immunoprotective qualities of the breast milk produced by immunocompromised women.

INFECTION CONTROL AND WORKPLACE SAFETY

Workplace safety procedures regarding HIV and other blood-borne pathogens have these essential components:

- Standard precautions or another infection control system for protecting the worker (and patient) from body fluid exposure, including the following—
  - Wash hands or use antiseptic hand cleansers (gels, foams) before and after every patient contact.
  - Dispose of needles and sharps in puncture-resistant containers, and never recap needles.
  - Wear latex or vinyl gloves when likely to touch body fluids, mucous membranes, or broken skin.
  - Wear protective eye wear and mask when eyes and mucous membranes may be splashed.
  - Wear a water-repellent gown when clothing could be soiled with body fluids.
  - Cover any broken skin that could come into contact with body fluids.
- Hepatitis B vaccination for all workers with any risk of exposure to blood or bloody body fluid
- A post-exposure plan for appropriate management of needle sticks and other accidental exposures (see below)
- Appropriate procedures for prompt evaluation and respiratory isolation for known or suspected tuberculosis

Occupationally acquired HIV. Several cases of occupationally acquired HIV are reported annually. Needlesticks and other percutaneous exposures have accounted for 84% of cases. Almost all exposures have been to blood or to concentrated virus in a laboratory setting. No infections have been observed from blood exposure to intact skin, airborne droplets, or environmental surfaces. What proportion of occupationally acquired infections are actually reported is unknown. The rate of occupational HIV infection following a single needlestick or other percutaneous exposure is about 0.3% in 6,498 reported accidental exposures in the United States and other countries. Not all exposures are equally likely to transmit HIV, however. Deep injuries, visibly bloody instruments, instruments previously placed in the source patient's artery or vein, and exposure to source patients who died within 60 days (and presumably had a high viral load) appear to increase risk.

Post-exposure management of persons with potential exposure to HIV. In the event of a workplace exposure to blood or another infectious body fluid from a person known or suspected to have HIV, follow these steps promptly:

- Decontaminate the site thoroughly using a mild bleach solution or topical disinfectant.

- Report the exposure to your facility's staff person designated to handle workplace injury.

- Seek guidance on appropriate chemoprophylaxis from your facility's designated staff person. Other options include calling the National Clinicians' Post-Exposure Prophylaxis Hotline or PEPline at 1–888–448–4911, which is staffed 24 hours a day, 7 days a week. This service is operated by the National HIV/AIDS Clinicians' Consultation Center and based at the University of California at San Francisco. The no-cost resource also assists with occupational exposures to other blood-borne pathogens such as hepatitis B and C. Before the call, identify the source patient if possible. If the source patient is known, learn what you can regarding the patient's HIV status. If the patient is known to have HIV, review antiretroviral medications, recent HIV viral load test results, and any recent HIV drug resistance testing. A post-exposure chemoprophylaxis regimen will be tailored to the specific type of exposure, characteristics of the source patient, and the pregnancy status and wishes of the exposed person. If treatment is recommended, it usually consists of a month long course of two or three antiretroviral agents. Treatment should begin as soon as possible, ideally within an hour of exposure and no less than 72 hours after exposure. Baseline HIV testing should be done immediately as well.

Infected health care providers. Many health care providers have acquired HIV through sex and the other typical transmission routes. Whether HIV infected health care workers place patients at risk is an important question. Retrospective studies using voluntary HIV testing of patients cared for by infected physicians, surgeons, and dentists have found no evidence of transmitted infection in any of the more than 22,000 patients evaluated. Infected dentists, physicians, and other care providers are usually advised to make practice decisions in consultation with their personal physicians, supervisors, and other professional groups as appropriate.

Ultimately, each care provider is responsible for personal safety and must insist on sound workplace policies and procedures, appropriate safety devices, high-quality barriers, and adequate staff training. In emergency situations, take the extra seconds to protect yourself and your coworkers with barriers and careful disposal of sharps. Most important, find a way to maintain compassionate touching, even when a latex barrier must sometimes come between care provider and patient.

ALPHABETICAL CATALOGUE OF REPRODUCTIVE TRACT INFECTIONS

ACUTE URETHRAL SYNDROME (dysuria-pyuria syndrome) is distinct from bacterial cystitis and typically results from a direct urethral infection with the sexually transmitted pathogens C. trachomatis or N. gonorrhoeae. Bacterial cystitis itself is not sexually transmitted per se; however, it can be sexually associated. "Honeymoon" cystitis—that is, cystitis that occurs after frequent vaginal intercourse—is believed to be caused by friction against the urethra during sexual intercourse. In this case, the underlying etiology is mechanical, and coital movements help vaginal organisms ascend into the bladder. Use of the diaphragm with spermicides and spermicidally coated condoms have been associated with a higher risk of acute urethral syndrome.

Prevalence. Urinary tract infections are second in prevalence only to upper respiratory infections. Depending on the population studied, as many as 10% to 25% of reproductive-age women report dysuria during the previous year. Among women with chlamydial infections, approximately 10% are infected at the urethra only.

Symptoms. Painful, urgent, and frequent urination, as well as dyspareunia, characterizes this syndrome. Occasionally, hematuria is the precipitating event for seeking clinical evaluation. Consider pyelonephritis if a patient's temperature exceeds 101° F or if costovertebral angle pain or tenderness are present.

Diagnosis. Women with > 10^5 organisms (coliform bacteria or other uropathogens) per milliliter (ml) of urine have bacterial cystitis; however, a smaller number of organisms may also cause symptoms. Women with dysuria, frequency, pyuria ($\geq$ 10 white blood cells [WBCs] per 400x field on microscopic examination of urinary sediment), and a negative Gram stain of unspun urine have the acute urethral syndrome, and chlamydia should be strongly suspected. A definitive diagnosis of the etiologic organism requires cultures or nucleic acid amplification testing (for gonorrhea and chlamydia) of the urethra or urine. Dysuria may also be caused by vulvovaginitis or genital herpes simplex virus infection.

Treatment. Bacterial cystitis can be treated with a variety of antibiotics that achieve a high concentration in urine. Initial episodes of bacterial cystitis can be treated with appropriate single-dose therapy such as sulfamethoxazole 1.6 g plus trimethoprim 320 mg (Bactrim or Septra). Fluoroquinolones (e.g., ciprofloxacin 250 mg twice a day, OR ofloxacin 200 mg twice a day) can be effective. Three days is the usual course. If bacteriuria is absent in the presence of pyuria, consider presumptive treatment for chlamydial infection.

Potential complications. Left untreated, bacterial infections of the lower genitourinary tract can ascend to the upper tract, leading to pyelonephritis.

Behavioral messages to emphasize. Understand how to take any prescribed oral medications. Drink copious fluids to flush the genitourinary system. If C. trachomatis or N. gonorrhoeae organisms are isolated, refer sex partner(s) for examination. (See the sections on these specific infections.)

BACTERIAL VAGINOSIS (BV) is a clinical syndrome in which several species of vaginal bacteria (including Gardnerella vaginalis, Mycoplasma hominis, and various anaerobes) replace the normal H_2O-producing lactobacillus species and cause vulvovaginitis symptoms. Bacterial vaginosis is a sexually associated condition, but it is not usually considered a specific STI; however, it does occur frequently in lesbians and may represent an STI in this group. Treatment of the male partner has not been found to be effective in preventing the recurrence of BV. Because of the increased risk for postoperative infectious complications associated with BV, screening prior to pelvic surgery is recommended (for example, hysterectomy); some specialists recommend that before performing surgical abortion, providers screen and treat women with BV in addition to providing routine prophylaxis.

Symptoms. Excessive or malodorous discharge is a common finding. Other signs or symptoms include erythema, edema, and pruritis of the external genitalia.

Diagnosis. The presumptive clinical criteria are three of the following four: increased amounts of homogenous discharge; elevated vaginal pH (greater than 4.5); fishy odor on addition of 10% KOH; and identification of clue cells (small coccobacillary organisms associated with epithelial cells) on saline wet mount (> 20% of vaginal epithelial cells). Alternatively, a Gram stain of the vaginal discharge can reveal the relative absence of lactobacilli with replacement of other anaerobic organisms. Cultures for G. vaginalis, M. hominis, or Mobiluncus are not useful and should not be performed.

Treatment. Patients with symptomatic disease should be offered treatment. The three recommended regimens are metronidazole, 500 mg orally twice daily for 7 days; OR metronidazole gel, 0.75%, one full applicator (5 g) vaginally at bed time for 5 days; OR clindamycin cream, 2%, one full applicator (5 g) vaginally at bed time for 7 days. Other alternatives are oral clindamycin 300 mg two times a day for 7 days; clindamycin ovules 100 mg vaginally at bedtime for 3 days; or single-dose sustained-release clindamycin cream, 2%, one full applicator (5 g) vaginally at bed time. During the second and third trimester of pregnancy, 7-day oral regimens of metronidazole 500 mg two times a day or 250 mg three times a day, or clindamycin 300 mg two times a day, are options. Pregnant women who are at low risk for preterm delivery can be treated with metronidazole gel, 0.75%, one full applicator (5 g) vaginally at bedtime for 5 days.

Potential complications. Secondary excoriation may occur. Recurrent infections are common. Bacterial vaginosis is associated with an increased risk of PID, and may also cause cervicitis. Bacterial vaginosis is associated with an increased risk of adverse pregnancy outcomes, including preterm delivery and low birthweight.

Behavioral messages to emphasize. Understand how to take or use any prescribed medications. Return if the problem is not cured or recurs. Avoid drinking alcohol until 24 hours after completing oral metronidazole therapy.

CANDIDIASIS (vulvovaginal candidiasis (VVC)) is caused by Candida species—usually C. albicans—that are dimorphic fungi that grow as oval, budding yeast cells and as chains of cells (hyphae). Candida are normal flora of the skin, mouth, and vagina. VVC is not considered a STI per se; however, sex partners do exchange orogenital strains of Candida. Risk factors for VVC are incompletely understood, but include immuno-suppressed states, glucose intolerance, and (in some women) antibiotic therapy.

Symptoms. Clinical presentation includes whitish vaginal discharge and erythema, edema, and pruritis of the external genitalia. Symptoms or signs alone do not distinguish the microbial etiology. Male sex partners may develop balanitis or cutaneous lesions on the penis.

Diagnosis. The presumptive criteria are typical clinical symptoms of vulvovaginitis and microscopic identification of yeast forms (budding cells) or pseudohyphae in KOH wet-mount preparations of vaginal discharge. VVC is definitively diagnosed when a vaginal culture is positive for C. albicans or other Candida species in a symptomatic woman. Because up to 40% of women are vaginally colonized with Candida species in the absence of VVC, cultures are not recommended unless chronic suppressive therapy is under consideration, in which case they are recommended to confirm both the etiology and ideally susceptibility to antifungal agents.

Treatment. Single-dose oral fluconazole, 150 mg, is a convenient therapy. In addition, many topical formulations provide effective candidiasis treatment. Examples include miconazole vaginal suppositories, 200 mg intravaginally at bedtime for 3 days; OR miconazole, 2%, vaginal cream, one full applicator (5 g) intravaginally at bedtime for 3 days (and applied externally for vulvitis); OR clotrimazole vaginal tablets, 100 mg intravaginally, daily for 3 days; OR butoconazole cream, 2%, 5 g intravaginally for 3 days. A variety of other effective treatment regimens exist. In general, more severe infections may need treatment of longer duration. Over-the-counter preparations for intravaginal administration of miconazole, clotrimazole, and butaconazole are available. Women with resistant VVC may benefit from treatment with boric acid, provided as 600 mg in a gelatin capsule administered vaginally once daily for 2 weeks (avoid in pregnancy).

Potential complications. Secondary excoriation may occur. Recurrent infections are common, particularly with antibiotic use, immunosuppression, or diabetes.

Behavioral messages to emphasize. Understand how to take or use any prescribed medications. Return if the problem is not cured or recurs. Wear a sanitary pad to protect clothing. Change pads frequently. To reduce moisture in the area, avoid panty hose, tight fitting clothing, and non-cotton panties. Store suppositories in a refrigerator. Continue taking medicine even during menses.

CERVICITIS is a term used to refer to the syndrome of cervical inflammation that can accompany infection with some STI, notably Chlamydia trachomatis and Neisseria gonorrhoeae and occasionally trichomoniasis and genital herpes. It is defined as the presence of endocervical mucopurulent discharge, easily induced bleeding, and/or edematous ectopy. Cervicitis can have non-infectious causes, including chemical trauma, and may also be promoted by progesterone-based hormonal therapy or bacterial vaginosis.

Prevalence. Based on extrapolation from local studies, cervicitis probably occurs more frequently than male urethritis. Up to 3 million cases per year may occur annually.

Symptoms. Cervical mucopurulent discharge may be exuded from the cervix and may be perceived as abnormal vaginal discharge, and cervical bleeding may manifest as intermenstrual bleeding.

Diagnosis. Diagnosis is made by visualizing either mucopus on a swab of endocervical secretions or friability (bleeding) on gentle passage of a cotton-tipped swab. In most cases, a microbial organism cannot be identified. A definitive etiologic diagnosis is made when either chlamydia or gonorrhea (or less commonly, another STI) is isolated.

Treatment. Presumptive treatment should be provided based on the individual patient's risk for chlamydial and/or gonococcal infections, and it should be directed at these organisms (particularly chlamydia). In women at low risk for these STI, the results of sensitive diagnostic tests for C. trachomatis or N. gonorrhoeae should determine the need for treatment. Chlamydia is treated with azithromycin 1 g orally in a single dose OR doxycycline 100 mg orally twice a day for 7 days. The section on

Gonorrhea contains the range of recommended treatment regimens for this infection.

Potential complications.   PID (with subsequent infertility) may complicate infection. In addition, neonatal chlamydial infections, such as ophthalmia or pneumonia, may be acquired during delivery if the mother has an infected cervix. If a pregnant woman is infected, she may be at risk for postpartum endometritis.

Behavioral messages to emphasize.   If infection involves C. trachomatis or N. gonorrhoeae, refer your sex partner(s) for examination and treatment. Avoid sex until you and your partner(s) have completed the prescribed course of medication and/or for one week after treatment was started. Understand how to take prescribed oral medications. Return early if symptoms persist or recur. Use condoms to prevent future infections.

CHANCROID is a type of genital ulcer disease caused by Hemophilus ducreyi, a gram-negative bacillus. Chancroid is implicated as potentiating HIV transmission.

Prevalence.   Chancroid occurs more frequently in the developing than in the developed world. However, chancroid is endemic in selected areas of the United States, and outbreaks have occurred in settings where sex is exchanged for drugs or money.

Symptoms.   Women are frequently asymptomatic, but ulcers may occur internally and go unnoticed. Usually a single painful ulcer, surrounded by erythematous edges, appears in men. Ulcers may be necrotic or severely erosive with a ragged serpiginous border. Painful inguinal lymphadenopathy (bubo) presents in about half of the cases and may rupture in 25% to 60% of cases. Ulcers usually occur on the coronal sulcus, glans, or shaft of the penis.

Diagnosis.   A painful ulcer, particularly if accompanied by a unilateral bubo, could suggest chancroid, but keep in mind that the overwhelming majority of genital ulcer disease in the United States is caused by herpes simplex virus. Because syphilis also causes genital ulcers (known as chancres), all new ulcers not known to be genital herpes should be examined with darkfield microscopy when adequate facilities exist. If chancroid is identified, perform serologic tests for syphilis and HIV. The diagnosis is definitive when H. ducreyi is recovered by culture or appropriate selective media.

Treatment.   Azithromycin 1 g orally in a single dose OR ceftriaxone 250 mg IM in a single dose OR ciprofloxacin 500 mg orally twice a day for 3 days OR erythromycin base 500 mg orally four times a day for 7 days. Persons infected with HIV have higher rates of treatment failure with single-dose therapy. The susceptibility of H. ducreyi to this combination of antimicrobial agents varies throughout the world. Evaluate the results of therapy after a maximum of 7 days, and continue therapy until ulcers or lymph nodes have healed. Fluctuant lymph nodes should be aspirated through healthy, adjacent, normal skin. Incision and drainage or excision of nodes will delay healing and are contraindicated. Apply compresses to ulcers to remove necrotic material. All sex partners should be simultaneously treated.

Potential complications. Systemic spread is not known to occur. Lesions may become secondarily infected and necrotic. Buboes may rupture and suppurate, resulting in fistulae. Ulcers on the prepuce may cause paraphimosis or phimosis.

Behavioral messages to emphasize. Because genital ulcers can be a risk for HIV infection, get an HIV test at baseline treatment and again in 3 months. Refer sex partner(s) for examination as soon as possible. Return for evaluation 3 to 5 days after therapy begins and thereafter return weekly for evaluation until the infection is entirely healed. The prepuce should remain retracted during therapy, except in the presence of preputial edema.

CHLAMYDIA is the common name for infections caused by Chlamydia trachomatis. Genital chlamydial infection is the leading cause of preventable infertility and ectopic pregnancy. Chlamydia is now the most commonly reported infectious disease in the United States. An estimated 3 million new cases occur annually. Like viruses, chlamydiae are obligate intracellular parasites and can be isolated in the laboratory only by cell culture. Unlike viruses, C. trachomatis is susceptible to antibiotics. Because many chlamydial infections are asymptomatic and probably chronic, widespread screening is necessary to control this infection and its sequelae. CDC recommends that all sexually-active women age 25 years or younger be screened annually for C. trachomatis (Table 21–3). For further information about the syndromes caused by C. trachomatis, see the sections on Cervicitis, Acute Dysuria Syndrome, Nongonococcal Urethritis, and Pelvic Inflammatory Disease (PID) in this chapter. The recommended regimens for all sites of uncomplicated chlamydial infection are azithromycin 1 g orally in a single dose OR doxycycline 100 mg orally twice a day for 7 days. Alternatives are ofloxacin 300 mg orally two times a day for 7 days OR levofloxacin 500 mg orally for 7 days OR erythromycin base 500 mg orally four times a day for 7 days OR erythromycin ethylsuccinate 800 mg orally four times a day for 7 days. During pregnancy, the recommended regimens are Azithromycin 1 g orally in a single dose OR amoxicillin 500 mg orally three times daily for 7 days. Alternatives are erythromycin base 500 mg orally four times daily for 7 days OR erythromycin base 250 mg orally four times daily for 14 days OR erythromycin ethylsuccinate 800 mg orally four times a day for 7 days OR erythromycin ethylsuccinate 400 mg orally four times a day for

14 days. In general, erythromycin-based regimens are inferior to the other drugs listed and should be viewed as second-line therapy. If these regimens are used, a test-of-use at 1 month after treatment is required.

GENITAL HERPES is caused by herpes simplex virus (HSV) types 1 and 2 DNA viruses that cannot be distinguished clinically; however, initial infection with HSV-1 is typically less severe and causes less frequent (and sometimes no) recurrences related to HSV-2. HSV type 2 (HSV-2) is more common in genital disease and is responsible for nearly all recurrent genital herpes.

Prevalence. Symptomatic primary (or initial) HSV infections affect an estimated 200,000 persons each year. Recurrent HSV infections are much more common. An estimated 45 million Americans are infected with genital HSV, though most infections are asymptomatic.[44] Persons without symptoms transmit most HSV infection.

Symptoms. Single or multiple vesicles, which are usually pruritic, can appear anywhere on the genitalia. Vesicles spontaneously rupture to form shallow ulcers that may be very painful. Lesions resolve spontaneously with minimal scarring. The first clinical occurrence is termed first episode infection (mean duration 12 days). Subsequent, usually milder, occurrences are termed recurrent infections (mean duration 4.5 days). The interval between clinical episodes is termed latency. Viral shedding from the cervix, vulva or penile skin occurs intermittently without clinical symptoms during latency. HSV-2 genital infections are more likely to recur than is HSV type 1 (HSV-1), thus identification of the type of infecting strain at initial infection has prognostic value.

Diagnosis. When typical genital lesions are present or a pattern of recurrence has developed, suspect herpes infection. An HSV tissue culture demonstrates the characteristic cytopathic effect following inoculation of a specimen from the cervix, the urethra, or the base of a genital lesion. Several type-specific HSV serologic assays may help in the diagnosis of unrecognized infection, in management of sex partners of those with HSV, or, in pregnant women, to diagnose HSV susceptibility or recent infection.[45]

Treatment. No cure for HSV exists; however, antiviral drugs are helpful in reducing or suppressing symptoms. Oral administration is more effective than topical, both in treating clinically symptomatic episodes and in suppressing or reducing recurrent outbreaks. Initial episodes can be treated with any of the following oral regimens, each given for 7–10 days:

- Acyclovir
  - 400 mg three times a day OR
  - 200 mg capsules five times a day

- Famciclovir
  - 250 mg five times a day
- Valacyclovir
  - 1.0 g two times a day

Recurrent infections can be treated with any of the following oral regimens:

- Acyclovir
  - 400 mg three times a day for 5 days OR
  - 800 mg twice a day for 5 days OR
  - 800 mg three times a day for 2 days
- Famciclovir
  - 125 mg twice a day for 5 days
  - 1000 mg twice a day for 1 day
- Valacyclovir
  - 500 mg twice a day for 3 days OR
  - 500 mg twice a day for 5 days OR
  - 1.0 g once a day for 5 days.

Daily prophylaxis with valacyclovir by HSV-infected persons reduces the risk of transmission to uninfected partners.[46] Regimens given orally to prevent recurrences include the following:

- Acyclovir 400 mg twice a day OR
- Famciclovir 250 mg twice a day OR
- Valacyclovir
  - 500 mg once a day OR
  - 1.0 gram once a day.

Intravenous regimens are used to treat uncommon disseminated forms of herpes infection requiring hospitalization. Famciclovir and valacyclovir offer more convenient dosing but are not more effective clinically than acyclovir. For persons infected with HIV, increased dosages and/or extended duration of therapy is recommended.[30]

Potential complications. *Men and women*: HSV infection can cause neuralgia, meningitis, ascending myelitis, urinary retention, urethral strictures, and lymphatic suppuration. These outcomes are generally more common in women. *Women*: Pregnancy loss and preterm delivery have been associated with HSV infections, usually in primary infection occurring in the third trimester. *Neonates*: During vaginal delivery, virus from an active genital infection can cause neonatal herpes. This condition ranges in severity from clinically inapparent infections to local infections of the eyes, skin, or mucous membranes or to severely disseminated infection that may involve the central nervous system. Full-blown neonatal herpes has a high fatality rate, and survivors often have ocular or neurologic sequelae.

Behavioral messages to emphasize. Because both initial and recurrent lesions shed high concentrations of the virus, abstain from sexual activity while ulcers are present. The risk of HSV transmission also exists during asymptomatic intervals. Condoms offer some protection from HSV acquisition.[30] Prophylactic valacyclovir reduces HSV transmission risks. The risk of transmission to the neonate from an infected mother is highest among women with primary herpes infection (the first time they have been infected with either HSV-1 or HSV-2) during the third trimester, lower among women with nonprimary first episodes of the disease and least among women with recurrent herpes. At the onset of labor, describe any symptoms and get examined for lesions. If you have no symptoms or signs, your infant may be delivered vaginally. Infants delivered through an infected birth canal should be cultured and followed carefully. Genital herpes (and other diseases causing genital ulcers) have been associated with an increased risk of acquiring HIV infections. Clinically evaluating asymptomatic partners has little value for preventing transmission of HSV; however, some recommend considering serologic screening of pregnant women to identify those at risk for HSV acquisition during pregnancy.[47]

GONORRHEA is caused by Neisseria gonorrhoeae, a gram-negative bacterium seen as a diplococcus on Gram stain. About 650,000 new cases of gonorrhea occur each year, making it the second most commonly reported infectious disease in the United States.

Symptoms. Women are most commonly asymptomatic, but may have abnormal vaginal discharge, abnormal menses, or dysuria. Symptomatic men usually have dysuria, increased frequency of urination, and purulent urethral discharge. An estimated one-fourth of infected men can be asymptomatic. Pharyngeal gonorrhea can occasionally produce symptoms of pharyngitis, but most infections are asymptomatic.

Diagnosis. In men, presumptive diagnosis relies on microscopically identifying typical gram-negative intracellular diplococci on smear of urethral exudates. In women, Gram stain of endocervical secretions of infected women is positive only half the time and is not commonly performed. Definitive diagnosis, especially in women, requires recovery of bacteria either by culture or molecular testing (NAAT). Ideally, all gonorrhea cases should be diagnosed by culture to facilitate antimicrobial susceptibility testing. However, increasing use of non-culture tests has increased the number of women tested. A definitive diagnosis by culture is required if the specimen is extragenital or from a child or if is important for medico-legal reasons.

Treatment. In many areas of the United States, about one-fourth of men and two-fifths of women with gonococcal infections also have a coexisting chlamydial infection. For this reason, use both a single-dose anti-gonococcal drug AND an anti-chlamydial regimen, unless sensitive diagnostic tests (nucleic acid amplification tests) for chlamydia are negative. The recommended therapies for gonorrhea include cefixime 400 mg orally once; OR ceftriaxone 125 mg IM once; OR ciprofloxacin 500 mg orally once; OR ofloxacin 400 mg orally once; OR levofloxacin 250 mg orally once. However, the latter three drugs (quinolones) should be avoided in persons who may have acquired their infection outside the United States or in California or Hawaii, where rates of quinolone resistance are considerable, or in bisexual men (who have high rates of quinolone-resistant gonorrhea). See the CDC's website on this topic for frequent updates (www.cdc.gov/std/treatment). See the Chlamydia section for discussion of treatment regimens. Pharyngeal gonorrhea may be more difficult to treat and appropriate regimens should be used.[30]

Potential complications. Up to 40% of untreated women with cervical gonorrhea develop PID and are at risk for its sequelae (see the section on PID), including involuntary sterility and pelvic abscesses. Men are at risk for epididymitis, urethral stricture, and sterility. Newborns are at risk for ophthalmia neonatorum, scalp abscess at the site of fetal monitors, rhinitis, or anorectal infection. All infected untreated persons are at risk for disseminated gonococcal infection.

Behavioral messages to emphasize. Understand how to take any prescribed oral medications. Refer sex partner(s) for examination and treatment. Avoid sex until patient and partner(s) have been treated.

GRANULOMA INGUINALE (Donovanosis) is caused by Calymmatobacterium granulomatis (formerly known as Donovania granulomatis), a bipolar, gram-negative bacterium (Donovan body) that in a crush preparation, appears in vacuolar compartments within histiocytes, white blood cells, or plasma cells.

Prevalence. Granuloma inguinale is rare in the United States. However, it is endemic in certain less developed countries including India, Papua New Guinea, Central Australia, and Southern Africa.

Symptoms. Initially, single or multiple subcutaneous nodules appear at the site of inoculation. Nodules erode to form granulomatous, heaped ulcers that are painless, bleed on contact, and enlarge slowly. Spread by autoinoculation is common.

Diagnosis. The typical clinical presentation is sufficient to suggest the diagnosis. Resolution of the lesions following specific antibiotic therapy supports the diagnosis. The patient's or partner's history of travel to endemic areas helps substantiate the clinical impression. A microscopic examination of biopsy specimens from the ulcer margin reveals the pathognomonic Donovan bodies. Tissue culture of C. granulomatis is not feasible.

Treatment. Recommended initial regimens are doxycycline 100 mg orally twice a day OR trimethoprim-sulfamethoxazole, 1 double-strength tablet twice a day until all lesions have completely healed (usually a minimum of 3 weeks). Alternatives are ciprofloxacin 750 mg orally twice a day OR erythromycin 500 mg orally four times a day OR azithromycin 1 mg orally once a week—all for at least 3 weeks.

Potential complications. Lesions may become secondarily infected. Fibrous, keloid-like formations may deform the genitalia. Pseudo-elephantoid enlargement of the labia, penis, or scrotum occurs. Necrosis and destruction of the genitalia may result.

Behavioral messages to emphasize. Understand how to take prescribed oral medications. Return for evaluation 3 to 5 days after therapy begins. Assure examination of sex partner(s) as soon as possible. Return weekly or biweekly for evaluation until the infection is entirely healed.

HEPATITIS A is caused by hepatitis A virus (HAV), an RNA virus that is typically transmitted by the fecal-oral route. For this reason, HAV can be transmitted through oral-anal sex.

Symptoms. The majority of infections are symptomatic, causing fatigue, anorexia, nausea, vomiting, headache, fever, dark urine, jaundice, and moderate liver enlargement with tenderness.

Diagnosis. HAV infection is clinically indistinguishable from other forms of hepatitis. Routine viral hepatitis serology should be performed in such patients. Serum IgM anti-HAV is almost always detectable at the onset of symptoms, and IgG anti-HAV levels rise soon thereafter. Measurement of serum IgM anti-HAV is the diagnostic test of choice.

Treatment/Prevention. No specific therapy exists; therapy is supportive. Vaccines made from recombinant genetic material are available. Specific vaccination and post-exposure prophylaxis strategies are of proven efficacy in preventing hepatitis A infection. Vaccinating all men who have sex with men, persons who use illicit drugs, and travelers to endemic areas against hepatitis A is currently recommended.

Potential complications. Long-term sequelae are rare. Rarely, acute fulminant hepatitis can occur, resulting in hepatic failure and death.

Behavioral messages to emphasize. HAV vaccination is strongly encouraged for target groups. Consult public health authorities regarding recommendations for post-exposure prophylaxis of household contacts and sex partners.

HEPATITIS B is caused by hepatitis B virus (HBV), a DNA virus with multiple antigenic components. In the United States, about 5% of the general population show evidence of past HBV infections. An estimated 120,000 new cases of HBV infection are transmitted sexually each year. Heterosexual intercourse is now the predominant mode of HBV transmission.

Symptoms. Most HBV infections are not clinically apparent. When present, symptoms include a serum sickness-like prodrome (skin eruptions, urticaria, arthralgias, arthritis), lassitude, anorexia, nausea, vomiting, headache, fever, dark urine, jaundice, and moderate liver enlargement with tenderness.

Diagnosis. HBV infection is clinically indistinguishable from other forms of hepatitis. A patient with the typical clinical symptoms and exposure to a patient with definitive or presumed HBV infection may be presumed to have HBV infection. Serodiagnosis of HBV infection is the best method for clinicians to reach a definitive diagnosis. Positive results of the following tests are reliable:

- Hepatitis B surface antigen (HBsAg): Acute HBV infection or, with no acute disease exposure, the chronic active state (infectious)

- HBe antigen: More infectious than if just HBsAg-positive, because the virus is actively replicating

- Anti-HBs (surface antibody): Past infection or immunization with present immunity

- Anti-HBc (core antibody): Past or current infection; see reference 30 for discussion

Treatment. No specific therapy exists. Provide supportive and symptomatic care. Vaccines made from recombinant genetic material are available. Specific vaccination and post-exposure prophylaxis strategies are of proven efficacy in preventing hepatitis B. Vaccinating all newborn infants and adolescents against hepatitis B is currently recommended. In addition, the Advisory Committee on Immunization Practices recommends HBV vaccination for all persons with recent STI and those who have a history of sexual activity with more than one partner in the previous 6 months. Subsidized HBV vaccine programs are available in many states.

Potential complications. Long-term sequelae include chronic, persistent, active hepatitis, cirrhosis, hepatocellular carcinoma, hepatic failure, and death. Rarely, the course may be fulminant with hepatic failure.

Behavioral messages to emphasize. HBV vaccination is strongly encouraged for all young, sexually active clients. The full vaccination regimen is necessary for maximum protection. Patients with hepatitis B should be followed to document seroconversion to immunity or persistence of chronic carrier state.

HEPATITIS C is caused by hepatitis C virus (HCV), an RNA virus that is typically transmitted by the parenteral route (needle sharing or transfusion to contaminated blood). HCV has been detected in genital secretions, but is probably infrequently sexually transmitted unless exchange of blood or bloody secretions occurs.

Symptoms. The majority of infections are asymptomatic, but occasionally can present with fatigue, anorexia, nausea, vomiting, headache, fever, dark urine, jaundice, and moderate liver enlargement with tenderness.

Diagnosis. HCV infection is clinically indistinguishable from other forms of hepatitis. Routine viral hepatitis serology should be performed in such patients. Serum IgM anti-HCV is almost always detectable at the onset of symptoms, and IgG anti-HCV levels rise soon thereafter. Measurement of serum IgM anti-HCV is the diagnostic test of choice in the setting of acute hepatitis.

Treatment/Prevention. No specific therapy exists; therapy is supportive. No vaccine is available. Patients should be educated about ways to avoid transmission through contaminated needles or by sharing such items as razors with household or sexual contacts who are infected.

Potential complications. Long-term sequelae include chronic, persistent, active hepatitis, cirrhosis, hepatocellular carcinoma, hepatic failure, and death. Rarely, the course may be fulminant with hepatic failure.

Behavioral messages to emphasize. Sex partners already in an established relationship do not need to change their sexual practices if one partner is found to be HCV-infected; the partner of unknown status should be screened. Persons with HCV who are embarking on new sexual relationship are advised to use safer sex precautions as applicable for routine STI protection (e.g., condoms).

HUMAN IMMUNODEFICIENCY VIRUS (HIV) See "Special Considerations Regarding HIV/AIDS in the Reproductive Health Setting," above.

HUMAN PAPILLOMAVIRUS (HPV) are common viruses that include over 100 types specific to the human genital tract. Two major clinical syndromes arise from these infections: genital warts and epithelial (notably, cervical) neoplasia. Genital warts are discussed below; cervical neoplasia is discussed in Chapter 22.

GENITAL WARTS (Condyloma acuminata) are caused by several of the many types of human papillomavirus (HPV), a small, slowly growing DNA virus belonging to the papovavirus group. Types 6 and 11 usually cause visible genital warts. Other HPV types in the genital region (16, 18, 31, 33, 35) are associated with vaginal, anal, and cervical dysplasia.

Prevalence. Genital warts account for more than 1 million physician office visits annually, making condyloma the most common symptomatic viral RTI in the United States. The most sensitive measures of HPV indicate up to 80% of all sexually active young women are infected with this virus. Cases of condyloma have been correlated with earlier onset of sexual activity, multiple sex partners, and a higher frequency of casual relationships than in controls.

Symptoms. Single or multiple soft, fleshy, papillary or sessile, painless keratinized growths appear around the vulvovaginal area, penis, anus, urethra, or perineum. Women infected with condyloma may exhibit typical growths on the walls of the vagina or cervix and may be unaware of their existence. Regular genital self-examinations may be helpful in detecting such growths on the external genitalia of both women and men. From 60% to 90% of male partners of women with condyloma have HPV infection on the penis, although infection may not be visible to the naked eye.

Diagnosis. No evidence supports the use of HPV DNA tests in the routine diagnosis or management of visible genital warts.[30] A diagnosis is made from the typical clinical signs on the external genitalia. Colposcopy is valuable for diagnosing flat warts, which are difficult to see. Exclude the possible diagnosis of condylomata lata by obtaining a serologic test for syphilis. A biopsy is usually unnecessary but would be required to make a definitive diagnosis. When neoplasia is a possibility, take a biopsy of any atypical lesions or persistent warts before initiating therapy.

Treatment. Several different treatment regimens can be used, depending on client preference, available resources, and the experience of the health care provider. None of the currently available treatments is superior to others or are ideal for all patients. The currently available treatments for visible genital warts consist of two types: (1) patient-applied therapies and (2) provider-administered therapies.

Patient-applied therapies:

- *Podofilox* 0.5% solution or gel. Patients apply podofilox solution with a cotton swab, or a podofilox gel with a finger, to visible genital warts twice daily for 3 days, followed by 4 days of no therapy. This process may be repeated up to a total of four times. Podofilox should not be used during pregnancy.

- *Imiquimod* 5% cream. Patients should apply imiquimod cream with a finger, at bed time, 3 times a week, for up to 16 weeks. They should wash with mild soap and water after 6 to 10 hours. Imiquimod should not be used during pregnancy.

Provider-administered therapies:

- *Cryotherapy* with liquid nitrogen or cryoprobe. Repeat applications every 1 to 2 weeks.

- *Trichloroacetic acid (TCA) or bichloroacetic acid (BCA)* 80% to 90%. Apply a small amount to only the warts and allow to dry, at which time a white "frosting" develops. Repeat weekly as needed.

- *Podophyllin resin* 10% to 25% in tincture of benzoin. A small amount of podophyllin should be applied to each wart and allowed to air dry. Avoid normal tissue. Wash off thoroughly in 1 to 4 hours to reduce local irritation. Podophyllin should not be used during pregnancy and is not recommended for vaginal use.

- *Surgical removal.* Scissor or shaving excision, curette, or electrosurgery are possible.

HPV infection is an infectious condition even when asymptomatic. However, for most persons, it has a benign natural history, and some individuals may not be infectious for long periods of time. No therapy completely eradicates the virus, although the burden of HPV appears to decline in the years following initial infection. HPV has been demonstrated in adjacent tissue even after attempts to eliminate subclinical HPV by extensive laser vaporization of the anogenital area. The effect of genital wart treatment on HPV transmission and the natural history of HPV is unknown. Therefore, the goal of treatment is the temporary removal of visible genital warts and the amelioration of symptoms and signs, *not* the eradication of HPV.

Potential complications. Lesions may enlarge and destroy tissue. Giant condyloma, while histologically benign, may simulate carcinoma. In pregnancy, warts enlarge, are extremely vascular, and may obstruct the birth canal to necessitate a cesarean delivery. Neither routine HPV screening tests nor cesarean delivery for prevention of the transmission of HPV to the newborn is indicated. The perinatal transmission rate is unknown, although probably low. Persons with HIV disease can have rapidly growing genital warts. Women infected with HIV have an increased risk of progressive HPV-cervical disease.

Prevention. A vaccine to prevent up to four types of genital HPV (6, 11, 16, 18) is now available. Large multicenter studies in young women indicate that the vaccine is nearly 100% effective in preventing infection with these HPV types and importantly, in preventing associated cervical neoplasia. Recommendations for targeted immunization of young women target pre-adolescent girls age 10 to 12 years, prior to the onset of sexual activity; however, the vaccine is approved and recommended for women up to 25 years in the event that HPV acquisition has not yet occurred (www.cdc.gov/nip/acip).

Behavioral messages to emphasize. Return for regular treatment until lesions have resolved. Once warts have responded to therapy, no special follow-up is necessary. If you have anogenital warts, you are contagious to uninfected sex partners. Because most partners are probably already infected, examination of sex partners is not necessary. To reduce risks of sequelae from cervical cancer, regular Pap smears are crucial for all women with documented HPV infection. HPV testing may be useful in triaging women with Pap smears showing ASCUS. Smoking cessation will reduce the risk of HPV and neoplasia.

LYMPHOGRANULOMA VENEREUM (LGV) is caused by serovars L1, L2, or L3 of Chlamydia trachomatis. LGV infections are endemic in Asia and Africa and were thought to be relatively rare in the United States. However, beginning in 2003, outbreaks of rectal LGV (proctitis) were documented in several U.S. cities among men who reported unprotected receptive anal sex (most of whom were also HIV-infected).

Symptoms. The primary lesion of LGV is a 2 to 3 mm painless vesicle or nonindurated ulcer at the site of inoculation. Patients commonly fail to notice this primary lesion. Regional adenopathy follows a week to a month later and is the most common clinical symptom. A sensation of stiffness and aching in the groin, followed by swelling of the inguinal region, may be the first indications of infections for most patients. Adenopathy may subside spontaneously or proceed to the formation of abscesses that rupture to produce draining sinuses or fistulae. In patients who acquire the infection from receptive anal intercourse, proctitis can result and may be severe.

Diagnosis. LGV is often diagnosed clinically and may be confused with chancroid because of the painful adenopathy. LGV-specific serology has been validated for the classical form of the disease, in which the complement fixation test is sensitive, and 80% of patients have a titer of 1:16 or higher. Levels of 1:64 are considered diagnostic. However, these tests have not been well validated for the diagnosis of LGV proctitis. Because the sequelae of LGV are serious and preventable, do not withhold treatment pending laboratory confirmation. A definitive diagnosis requires isolating C. trachomatis from an appropriate specimen and confirming the isolate as an LGV immunotype. However, these laboratory diagnostic capabilities are not widely available.

Treatment.   Give doxycycline 100 mg orally two times a day for 21 days OR erythromycin 500 mg orally four times a day for 21 days. Aspirate fluctuant lymph nodes as needed. Incision and drainage or excision of nodes will delay healing and are contraindicated.

Potential complications.   Dissemination may occur with nephropathy, hepatomegaly, or phlebitis. Large polypoid swelling of the vulva (esthiomene), anal margin, or rectal mucosa may occur. The most common severe morbidity results from rectal involvement: perianal abscess and rectovaginal or other fistulae are early consequences, and rectal stricture may develop 1 to 10 years after infection.

Behavioral messages to emphasize.   Understand how to take prescribed oral medications. Return for evaluation 3 to 5 days after therapy begins. Assure examination of sex partner(s) as soon as possible. For all patients with LGV proctitis, knowledge of HIV status is essential given the epidemiology of the current outbreak.

MOLLUSCUM CONTAGIOSUM is caused by molluscum contagiosum virus, the largest DNA virus of the poxvirus group.

Prevalence.   As an STI, molluscum contagiosum occurs infrequently, about 1 case for every 100 cases of gonorrhea. Outbreaks have been reported among groups at high risk for other RTIs.

Symptoms.   Lesions are 1 to 5 mm, smooth, rounded, firm, shiny flesh-colored to pearly-white papules with characteristically umbilicated centers. They are most commonly seen on the trunk and anogenital region and are generally asymptomatic. Exceptions to this occur in immunosuppressed patients (particularly HIV with low CD4 counts), in whom the lesions can be diffuse or become bulky.

Diagnosis.   Infection is usually diagnosed on the basis of the typical clinical presentation. Microscopic examination of lesions or lesion material reveals the pathognomonic molluscum inclusion bodies.

Treatment.   Lesions may resolve spontaneously without scarring. However, they may be removed by curettage after cryoanesthesia. Treatment with caustic chemicals (podophyllin, trichloroacetic acid, silver nitrate) and cryotherapy (liquid nitrogen) have been successful. If every lesion is not extirpated, the condition may recur.

Potential complications. Secondary infection, usually with staphylococcus, may occur. Lesions rarely attain a size greater than 10 mm in diameter.

Behavioral messages to emphasize. Return for reexamination 1 month after treatment so any new lesions can be removed. Sex partner(s) should be examined.

MYCOPLASMA GENITALIUM is a bacterium that has recently been associated with urethritis in men and cervicitis and PID in women. No specific diagnostic test is currently available. Studies are underway to determine the prevalence in representative populations and the best approach to treatment.

PELVIC INFLAMMATORY DISEASE (PID) can be caused by varying combinations of N. gonorrhoeae, C. trachomatis, anaerobic bacteria, facultative gram-negative rods (such as E. coli), Mycoplasma hominis, and a variety of other microbial agents. Clinical PID is usually of polymicrobial etiology. N. gonorrhoeae and C. trachomatis may cause antecedent inflammation, which makes the tubes susceptible to invasion by anaerobic organisms.

Prevalence. PID accounts for nearly 180,000 hospitalizations every year in the United States. More than 1 million episodes occur annually. Among American women of reproductive age, 1 in 7 reports having received treatment for PID.

Symptoms. Based on retrospective reports, many women with PID have atypical or no symptoms. Women may have pain and tenderness involving the lower abdomen, cervix, uterus, or adnexae, occasionally with fever, chills, and elevated white blood cell (WBC) count and erythrocyte sedimentation rate (ESR). The condition is more likely if the patient has multiple sex partners or a history of PID or is in the first 5 to 10 days of her menstrual cycle. More specific criteria, such as endometrial biopsy, magnetic resonance imaging, or diagnostic laparoscopy, are warranted only in selected instances.

Diagnosis. Women who have the typical clinical symptoms are presumed to have PID if other serious conditions, such as acute appendicitis or ectopic pregnancy, can be excluded. The diagnosis of PID is often based on imprecise clinical findings.[30] Maintain a low threshold for diagnosing PID, because even mild or moderate PID has the potential for reproductive sequelae. Use objective criteria to monitor response to antibiotics, especially if ambulatory treatment is given. Direct visualization of inflamed (edema, hyperemia, or tubal exudate) fallopian tube(s) during laparoscopy or laparotomy confirms the diagnosis of PID. Cultures of tubal exudate may help establish the microbiologic etiology.

Treatment. Because the causative organism is usually unknown at the time of the initial therapy, use treatment regimens that are active against the broadest possible range of pathogens. Antimicrobial coverage should include N. gonorrhoeae, C. trachomatis, anaerobes, Gram-negative facultative bacteria, and streptococci.

Hospitalization and inpatient care: Since hospitalization is no longer synonymous with parenteral therapy, the decision to hospitalize is based on the clinician's discretion. Consider hospitalizing patients with acute PID when (1) surgical emergencies, such as appendicitis and ectopic pregnancy, are not definitely excluded; (2) severe illness precludes outpatient management; (3) the woman is pregnant; (4) the woman is unable to follow or tolerate an outpatient regimen; or (5) the woman has failed to respond to outpatient therapy. Special consideration may be given to adolescents both to preserve their fertility and to improve their adherence.

Combined drug therapy is recommended in all cases since the full bacterial etiology of PID is not clear and is generally polymicrobial.

Parenteral treatment: Two parenteral regimens are recommended for both inpatient and outpatient care:

- *Regimen A:* Either cefotetan 2.0 g IV every 12 hours, OR cefoxitin 2.0 g IV every 6 hours for at least 24 hours after the patient clinically improves PLUS doxycycline 100 mg orally or IV every 12 hours. Continue doxycycline 100 mg orally twice daily after discharge to complete at least 14 days of therapy.

- *Regimen B:* Clindamycin 900 mg, IV three times a day, PLUS gentamicin 2 mg per kilogram (kg) IV loading dose and maintenance 1.5 mg/kg IV every 8 hours. Continue oral therapy as above.

Oral treatment: Either of two oral regimens is recommended:

- *Regimen A:* Ofloxacin 400 mg twice daily OR levofloxacin 500 mg once daily; add metronidazole 500 mg two times a day for 14 days if bacterial vaginosis is present.

- *Regimen B:* Ceftriaxone 250 mg IM; OR Cefoxitin 2.0 g IM along with probenecid 1.0 g orally PLUS doxycycline 100 mg taken orally twice daily for 14 days.

Potential complications. Potentially life-threatening complications include ectopic pregnancy and pelvic abscess. Other sequelae are involuntary infertility, recurrent or chronic PID, chronic abdominal pain, pelvic adhesions, premature hysterectomy, and depression.

Behavioral messages to emphasize. For outpatient therapy, return for evaluation 2 to 3 days after initiation of therapy. Return for further evaluation 4 days after completing therapy. Refer sex partner(s) for evaluation and treatment (even if they are asymptomatic). Avoid sexual activity throughout the course of treatment. Understand how to take prescribed oral medications.

SYPHILIS is caused by Treponema pallidum, a spirochete with 6 to 14 regular spirals and characteristic motility.

Prevalence. Because of recent syphilis elimination efforts, primary and secondary syphilis currently are declining in the United States among women. Congenital syphilis is also on the wane. However, syphilis rates are increasing among men who have sex with men, and it remains an important STI, with serious sequelae if not treated. In heterosexual populations, southeastern states have the highest rates of both syphilis and congenital syphilis, although recent outbreaks have occurred in the Southwest.

Symptoms. *Primary:* The classical chancre is a painless, indurated ulcer, located at the site of exposure. The differential diagnosis for all genital lesions should include syphilis.

Secondary: Patients may have a highly variable skin rash, mucous patches, condylomata lata (fleshy, moist tissue growths), lymphadenopathy, alopecia, or other signs. *Latent:* Patients are without clinical signs of infection.

Diagnosis. The 2006 CDC STD Treatment Guidelines discuss the types of serologic testing that are available.[30] *Primary:* Patients have typical lesion(s) and either a positive darkfield exam; a fluorescent antibody technique in material from a chancre, regional lymph node, or other lesion; or they have been exposed to syphilis within 90 days of lesion onset.

Secondary: Patients have a typical clinical presentation and a strongly reactive serologic test; condyloma lata will be darkfield positive. *Latent:* Patients have serologic evidence of untreated syphilis without clinical signs.

Primary and secondary syphilis are definitively diagnosed by demonstrating T. pallidum with darkfield microscopy or fluorescent antibody technique, but can be presumptively diagnosed in the setting of a compatible clinical presentation and reactive serology. A definitive diagnosis of latent syphilis cannot be made under usual circumstances.

Treatment. *Primary, secondary, or early syphilis of less than 1 year duration:* benzathine penicillin G 2.4 million units IM in a single dose. Alternative regimens include ceftriaxone 1 gram IV or IM daily for 8–10 days. The regimen of doxycycline 100 mg orally twice daily for 14 days is inferior, and not recommended unless no other alternatives are available. *Syphilis of indeterminate length or of more than 1 year duration:* benzathine penicillin G 7.2 million units total; 2.4 million units IM, weekly, for 3 successive weeks. *Patients allergic to penicillin:* Doxycycline 100 mg orally two times a day. [Note: Duration of therapy depends on the estimated duration of infection. If duration has been less than 1 year, treat the infection for 14 days; otherwise, treat for 28 days.] *Penicillin-allergic pregnant women or for doxycycline-intolerant patients only:* Consult the 2006 Guidelines for Treatment of Sexually Transmitted Diseases.[30] *Congenital syphilis or if the patient is simultaneously infected with syphilis and HIV:* Refer to the 2006 Guidelines for Treatment of Sexually Transmitted Diseases.[30]

Potential complications. Late syphilis and congenital syphilis, both complications of early syphilis, are preventable with prompt diagnosis and treatment. Sequelae of late syphilis include neurosyphilis (general paresis, tabes dorsalis, and focal neurologic signs), cardiovascular syphilis (thoracic aortic aneurism, aortic insufficiency), and localized gumma formation.

Behavioral messages to emphasize. Because genital ulcers may be associated with HIV infection, get an HIV test. Return for follow-up syphilis serologies at 3 and 6 months for early syphilis, and at 6 and 12 months for late latent disease. HIV-positive patients should return 1, 2, 3, 6, 9, and 12 months after therapy; pregnant partners should be followed monthly. Understand how to take any prescribed oral medications. Refer sex partner(s) for evaluation and treatment. Avoid sexual activity until treatment is completed. Use condoms to prevent future infections.

TRICHOMONIASIS is caused by Trichomonas vaginalis, a motile protozoan with an undulating membrane and four flagella.

Prevalence. Trichomoniasis is the most common curable STI in the United States and worldwide. Each year an estimated 3 million U.S. women become infected.

Symptoms. Excessive, frothy, diffuse, yellow-green vaginal discharge is common, although clinical presentation varies from no signs or symptoms to erythema, edema, and pruritis of the external genitalia. Dysuria and dyspareunia are also frequent. The type of symptoms or signs alone does not distinguish the microbial etiology. Male sex partners may develop urethritis, balanitis, or cutaneous lesions on the penis; however, the majority of males infected with T. vaginalis are asymptomatic.

Diagnosis. Trichomoniasis is diagnosed when a vaginal culture or antigen test is positive for T. vaginalis OR typical motile trichomonads are identified in a saline wet mount of vaginal discharge. Examine vaginal secretions to verify the finding of trichomonads on a Pap smear, as this test is relatively non-specific for the diagnosis.

Treatment. Metronidazole 2.0 g orally at one time. Alternative regimens are metronidazole 500 mg orally twice daily for 7 days or tinidazole 2 g orally at one time. Most treatment failures are due to failure to treat the index patient's sex partners; initial management should include retreatment of the patient and partners with single-dose metronidazole (2.0 g). Metronidazole-resistant T. vaginalis, although uncommon, can occur. Most treatment failures respond to higher doses of metronidazole therapy or to a single dose of tinidazole (2 g). Sex partners should be simultaneously treated with the same regimen as the index client.

Potential complications. Secondary excoriation may occur. Recurrent infections are common. Trichomoniasis has been associated with an increased risk of salpingitis, low birthweight, prematurity, and acquisition of HIV.

Behavioral messages to emphasize. Understand how to take or use prescribed medications. Return if the problem is not cured or recurs. Make sure sex partner(s) are treated. Use condoms to prevent future infections. Avoid drinking alcohol until 24 hours after completing metronidazole therapy.

URETHRITIS, INCLUDING NONGONOCOCCAL URETHRITIS (NGU) is caused by Chlamydia trachomatis about 30% of the time. Other sexually transmissible agents, which cause 10% to 45% of NGU, include Trichomonas vaginalis, Mycoplasma genitalium, and herpes simplex virus; Ureaplasma urealyticum may also contribute. The etiology of the remaining cases is unknown.

Prevalence. NGU appears more frequently than gonorrhea in both public STI clinics and private practices. More than 1 million cases annually are estimated to occur in men.

Symptoms. Men usually have dysuria, urinary frequency, and mucoid to purulent urethral discharge. Many men have asymptomatic infections.

Diagnosis. Men with typical clinical symptoms are presumed to have NGU when their gonorrhea tests are negative and they have either white blood cells (WBCs) on Gram stain of urethral discharge or sexual exposure to an agent known to cause NGU. Asymptomatic men with negative gonorrhea tests are also presumed to have NGU if > 5 WBCs per oil immersion field appear on an intraurethral smear. Chlamydia testing is strongly recommended for a specific diagnosis. Gonococcal and nongonococcal urethritis may coexist in the same patient.

Treatment. When the etiology is C. trachomatis, or unknown, the following treatment is recommended: azithromycin 1 g orally in a single dose OR doxycycline 100 mg orally twice daily for 7 days. For patients who fail their first trial of antibiotics and whose partners have been treated, the persistent urethritis should be documented (either by visual examination of discharge or microscopy to quantify WBC). In this case, the patient should be treated with metronidazole 2.0 g orally as a single dose, and if not previously treated with azithromycin, treated with azithromycin 1.0 g orally as a single dose. For herpes simplex infections, see the sections of this chapter that deal specifically with these agents.

Potential complications. Urethral strictures or epididymitis may occur. If C. trachomatis is transmitted to female sex partners, the condition may result in mucopurulent cervicitis and PID. If C. trachomatis is transmitted to a pregnant woman, complications may include neonatal infections such as conjunctivitis or pneumonia.

Behavioral messages to emphasize. Understand how to take any prescribed oral medications. If chlamydial infection or other STI is diagnosed, refer sex partner(s) for examination and treatment. Avoid sex until treatment is completed. Use condoms to prevent future infections.

VAGINITIS is a general term that refers to the syndrome of abnormal vaginal discharge and related patient complaints, which may include abnormal odor and vulvovaginal pruritis or nonspecific discomfort. Specific causes of vaginitis discussed in this catalogue include bacterial vaginosis (BV) and vulvovaginal candidiasis (VVC). Other causes of vaginitis that reproductive health clinicians might encounter include:

Desquamative inflammatory vaginitis (DIV) is a relatively uncommon, but probably underdiagnosed, form of vaginitis in which women complain of copious, purulent vaginal discharge, typically accompanied by vaginal pain or burning and dyspareunia. DIV may be more common in older (peri- or postmenopausal) women, though the epidemiology is poorly defined. Occasionally frank vestibulitis or excoriations will occur. On examination of vaginal fluid, the characteristic findings are elevated vaginal pH (usually 5.5 to 7.4), few lactobacilli, and numerous Gram-positive cocci. Group B streptococcus may be involved in the pathogenesis of this condition. Treatment includes a relatively prolonged course of clindamycin 2% cream administered vaginally at bedtime, usually given for at least 14 days OR 10% hydrocortisone cream 5 g administered nightly at bedtime for at least 14 days. Longer courses of therapy are often required.

Irritant/chemical vaginitis occurs commonly, though few population-based data are available. Any substance that can elicit a mucosal inflammatory response, including douches, some spermicides, soaps or other cleansing agents, or other "feminine hygiene" products, can be responsible if administered vaginally. This condition may result in vaginal discharge characterized by numerous WBC. When evaluating women for vulvovaginal complaints take a careful history of use of any vaginal products or of products applied directly to the vulva.

References

1. Eng TR, Butler WT, Committee on Prevention and Control of Sexually Transmitted Diseases IoMUS, Division of Health Promotion and Disease Prevention. The hidden epidemic confronting sexually transmitted diseases. Washington, DC: National Academies Press, 1996.

2. Cates W, Jr. Estimates of the incidence and prevalence of sexually transmitted diseases in the United States. American Social Health Association Panel. Sex Transm Dis 1999;26:S2–7.

3. Weinstock H, Berman S, Cates W, Jr. Sexually transmitted diseases among American youth: incidence and prevalence estimates, 2000. Perspect Sex Reprod Health 2004;36:6–10.

4. Rothenberg R. STD transmission dynamics: some current complexities. 2002 Thomas Parran Award Lecture. Sex Transm Dis 2003;30:478–82.

5. Pilcher CD, Tien HC, Eron JJ, Jr., et al. Brief but efficient: acute HIV infection and the sexual transmission of HIV. J Infect Dis 2004;189:1785–92.

6. Fleming DT, Wasserheit JN. From epidemiological synergy to public health policy and practice: the contribution of other sexually transmitted diseases to sexual transmission of HIV infection. Sex Transm Infect 1999;75:3–17.

7. Serwadda D, Gray RH, Sewankambo NK, et al. Human immunodeficiency virus acquisition associated with genital ulcer disease and herpes simplex virus type 2 infection: a nested case-control study in Rakai, Uganda. J Infect Dis 2003;188:1492–7.

8. Auvert B, Taljaard D, Lagarde E, Sobngwi-Tambekou J, Sitta R, Puren A. Randomized, controlled intervention trial of male circumcision for reduction of HIV infection risk: the ANRS 1265 Trial. PLoS Med 2005;2:e298.

9. Celum C, Levine R, Weaver M and Wald A. Genital herpes and human immunodeficiency virus: double trouble. Bull World Health Organ 2004;82:447–53.

10. Trussell J, Kost K. Contraceptive failure in the United States: a critical review of the literature. Stud Fam Plann 1987;18:237–83.

11. Anderson RM. Transmission dynamics of sexually transmitted infections. In: Holmes KK, et al., ed. Sexually Transmitted Diseases. 3rd ed. New York: McGraw Hill, 1999:25–37.

12. Westrom L, Joesoef R, Reynolds G, Hagdu A and Thompson SE. Pelvic inflammatory disease and fertility. A cohort study of 1,844 women with laparoscopically verified disease and 657 control women with normal laparoscopic results. Sex Transm Dis 1992;19:185–92.

13. Cates W, Jr., Hinman AR. AIDS and absolutism—the demand for perfection in prevention. N Engl J Med 1992;327:492–4.

14. Cates W, Jr. The NIH condom report: the glass is 90% full. Fam Plann Perspect 2001;33:231–3.

15. Cates W, Jr. Review of non-hormonal contraception (condoms, intrauterine devices, nonoxynol-9 and combos) on HIV acquisition. J Acquir Immune Defic Syndr 2005;38 Suppl 1:S8–10.

16. Ness RB, Keder LM, Soper DE, et al. Oral contraception and the recognition of endometritis. Am J Obstet Gynecol 1997;176:580–5.

17. Martin HL, Jr., Nyange PM, Richardson BA, et al. Hormonal contraception, sexually transmitted diseases, and risk of heterosexual transmission of human immunodeficiency virus type 1. J Infect Dis 1998;178:1053–9.

18. Morrison CS, Bright P, Wong EL, et al. Hormonal contraceptive use, cervical ectopy, and the acquisition of cervical infections. Sex Transm Dis 2004;31:561–7.

19. Grimes DA. Intrauterine device and upper-genital-tract infection. Lancet 2000;356:1013–9.

20. Cates WJ, Padian NS. The interrelationship of reproductive health and sexually transmitted diseases. In: Goldman M, Hatch M, ed. Women and Health. San Diego, California: Academic Press, 2000:381–9.

21. Van Damme L, Ramjee G, Alary M, et al. Effectiveness of COL-1492, a nonoxynol-9 vaginal gel, on HIV-1 transmission in female sex workers: a randomised controlled trial. Lancet 2002;360:971–7.
22. Martino JL, Vermund SH. Vaginal douching: evidence for risks or benefits to women's health. Epidemiol Rev 2002;24:109–24.
23. Nowicki MJ, Laskus T, Nikolopoulou G, et al. Presence of hepatitis C virus (HCV) RNA in the genital tracts of HCV/HIV-1-coinfected women. J Infect Dis 2005;192:1557–65.
24. Leigh BC. Alcohol and condom use: a meta-analysis of event-level studies. Sex Transm Dis 2002;29:476–82.
25. Cates W, Jr. A risk-assessment tool for integrated reproductive health services. Fam Plann Perspect 1997;29:41–3.
26. Screening for chlamydial infection: recommendations and rationale. Am J Prev Med 2001;20:90–4.
27. Screening for gonorrhea: recommendation statement. Ann Fam Med 2005;3:263–7
28. Chou R, Huffman LH, Fu R, Smits AK, Korthuis PT. Screening for HIV: a review of the evidence for the U.S. Preventive Services Task Force. Ann Intern Med 2005;143:55–73.
29. American College of Obstetrics and Gynecology and American Academy of Pediatrics. Guidelines for Perinatal Care. 5th ed. Washington, D.C.: American College of Obstetrics and Gynecology and American College of Pediatrics, 2002.
30. Centers for Disease Control and Prevention. Sexually transmitted disease treatment guidelines. MMWR 2006:55 (RR-11).
31. Joint United Nations Programme on HIV/AIDS. AIDS epidemic update: 2004, 2005: Available at www.unaids.org.
32. Centers for Disease Control and Prevention. *HIV/AIDS Surveillance Report, 2004.* Atlanta: US Department of Health and Human Services, Centers for Disease Control and Prevention, 2005:Available at: www.cdc.gov/hiv/stats/hasrlink.htm.
33. Royce RA, Sena A, Cates W, Jr. and Cohen MS. Sexual transmission of HIV. N Engl J Med 1997;336:1072–8.
34. Centers for Disease Control and Prevention. Antiretroviral postexposure prophylaxis after sexual, injection-drug use, or other nonoccupational exposure to HIV in the United States: recommendations from the U.S. Department of Health and Human Services. MMWR 2005;54.
35. Gray RH, Wawer MJ, Brookmeyer R, et al. Probability of HIV-1 transmission per coital act in monogamous, heterosexual, HIV-1-discordant couples in Rakai, Uganda. Lancet 2001;357:1149–53.
36. CDC. Revised recommendations for HIV testing for adults, adolescents, and pregnant women in healthcare settings. MMWR 2006;55 (RR-14).
37. Gray RH, Li X, Kigozi G, et al. Increased risk of incident HIV during pregnancy in Rakai, Uganda: a prospective study. Lancet 2005;366:1182–8.
38. Fernandez MI, Wilson TE, Ethier KA, Walter EB, Gay CL and Moore J. Acceptance of HIV testing during prenatal care. Perinatal Guidelines Evaluation Project. Public Health Rep 2000;115:460–8.
39. Centers for Disease Control and Prevention. Revised guidelines for HIV counseling, testing, and referral and revised recommendations for HIV screening of pregnant women. Mor Mortal Wkly Rep 2001;50.
40. Spielberg F, Branson BM, Goldbaum GM, et al. Choosing HIV Counseling and Testing Strategies for Outreach Settings: A Randomized Trial. J Acquir Immune Defic Syndr 2005;38:348–55.
41. Spielberg F, Levine RO, Weaver M. Self-testing for HIV: a new option for HIV prevention? Lancet Infect Dis 2004;4:640–6.
42. Sobel JD, Chaim W, Nagappan V, Leaman D. Treatment of vaginitis caused by Candida glabrata: use of topical boric acid and flucytosine. Am J Obstet Gynecol 2003;189:1297–300.

43. Anderson JR (ed.) .A guide to the clinical care of women with HIV. 1st ed. Rockville, MD: HIV/AIDS Bureau, Health Resources and Services Administration, 2001. Available at http:/hab.hrsa.gov/womencare.htm.

44. Xu F, Sternberg MR, Kottiri BJ, et al. Trends in herpes simplex type 1 and type 2 seroprevalence in the United States. JAMA 2006; 296;964–973.

45. Wald A, Ashley-Morrow R. Serological testing for herpes simplex virus (HSV)-1 and HSV-2 infection. Clin Infect Dis 2002;35:S173–82.

46. Corey L, Wald A, Patel R, et al. Once-daily valacyclovir to reduce the risk of transmission of genital herpes. N Engl J Med 2004;350:11–20.

47. Baker DA. Risk factors for herpes simplex virus transmission to pregnant women: a couples study. Am J Obstet Gynecol 2005;193:1887–8.

Female Genital Tract Cancer Screening

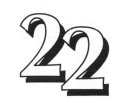

Michael S. Policar, MD, MPH

- The goal of Pap smear screening is to detect and treat CIN 2 and 3 cervical lesions, adenocarcinoma precursors, and cervical cancers. CIN 1 is a benign lesion with a high regression rate, especially in adolescents.

- Pap smear screening should begin 3 years after the onset of sexual activity (or by age 21) and should be discontinued after total hyster-ectomy for benign disease or in women older than 65 to 70 years old who have a history of 3 or more normal Pap smears in the prior 10 years.

- Women age 30 and older who have had 3 consecutive negative tests should receive Pap smears every 2 to 3 years, while women under 30 should have conventional Pap smears annually or liquid-based Pap smears every 1 to 2 years.

- Oral contraceptive use for 10 years or longer reduces the risk of ovarian cancer by as much as 80%.

- Most guidelines recommend breast cancer screening by mammog-raphy every 1 to 2 years for women age 50 and older. Newer guide-lines recommend that women between 40 to 49 years old who choose to have mammograms do so yearly.

A reproductive health care visit represents an ideal opportunity to offer periodic health screening services, including screening for genital tract cancers. As early as the 1920s, the prevalent philosophy of the American medical community was that individuals of all ages should re-ceive an annual physical examination and a battery of routine screening tests to detect early, asymptomatic disease.[1] Over the past decade, how-ever, the wisdom of this practice has been challenged, and research studies and health policy discussions have focused upon the optimal content of periodic health screening: which tests should or should not be performed, how often each screening test should be done, and whether each test should be performed routinely or limited to persons with certain risk factors. While many approaches to periodic health screening have been proposed, the recommendations of the United States Preventive Services Task Force (USPSTF) are considered the blueprint for the screening guidelines developed by most state Departments of Health, professional specialty societies, and health plans.[2] Using an evidence-based methodology, the USPSTF guidelines gauged both the strength of each recommendation and the quality of the research studies used to develop each guideline. The guidelines emphasize that the most important clinical contribution to maximizing a person's health status is by avoiding the development of disease through primary prevention based on focused risk assessment and counseling interventions, rather than on periodic physical examination or laboratory testing.

In the past, the concept of an "annual well woman exam" was coupled with the recommendation that Pap smears be performed yearly in women who had initiated sexual activity or who had reached 18 years of age. However, owing in part to the changes in cancer screening recommendations listed below, many women will no longer require yearly visits for the purpose of receiving screening tests, irrespective of their choice of contraceptive method. In addition, most medical specialty societies, with the notable exception of the American College of Obstetricians and Gynecologists[3], no longer recommend annual "check up" visits, instead promoting the concept of "opportunistic prevention" at the time of problem-oriented visits. As it relates to contraceptive practice, it is reasonable to recommend that women seek a "check-up" visit once every one to three years, depending upon her underlying health status, the risk level of her sexual behaviors, the recommended intervals of the screening tests that she requires, and her own personal preferences.

Another issue that may arise at a health screening visit is whether to provide comprehensive preventive health services or only those related to reproductive health. Increasingly, patients will have an established relationship with a primary care provider from whom they will receive some or all necessary preventive health services. If so, it is important for the reproductive health care provider to avoid duplication of tests already provided, and ideally, with the permission of the patient, to transmit the record of the reproductive health care visits to the primary care provider. In other cases, the only opportunity available to a woman to receive preventive health care services is during her reproductive health care visit. Consequently, if you are equipped to do so in your practice, it is appropriate to offer her the full range of recommended preventive interventions. Two helpful sources of age-specific disease prevention guidelines are the USPSTF (www.ahcpr.gov/clinic/uspstfix.htm) and "Preventing Cancer, Cardiovascular Disease, and Diabetes: A Common

Agenda of the American Cancer Society, the American Diabetes Association, and the American Heart Association".[4]

Over the years, annual periodic health screening also has been linked with the provision of prescription hormonal contraceptives. In many cases, a woman could get a prescription for combined oral contraceptives (COCs) only when she underwent an annual "well woman" exam, which necessarily included a breast exam and a Papanicolaou (Pap) smear. In this way, women have been compelled to receive desirable screening tests as a by-product of their need for contraception. However, many reproductive health programs no longer require genital tract cancer screening for the provision of prescription contraceptives, based on the position that beneficial screening tests must be supported on their own merits, and any unnecessary barriers to contraceptive services should be removed.[5-7] In addition, for every hormonal contraceptive method, the 2004 WHO Selected Practice Recommendations for Contraceptive Use[8] do not recommend breast or genital tract examination, cervical cancer screening, STI assessment or lab test screening, hemoglobin determination, or routine lab tests as "contributing substantially to safe and effective use of the contraceptive method." However, the guidelines specify that, if available, it is desirable to have a blood pressure measurement taken before initiation of combined oral contraceptives, combined injectable contraceptives, progestin-only pills, progestin-only injections, and implants. Furthermore, hormonal methods need not be restricted or withheld from a woman solely because she has an abnormal Pap smear. There is no reason to believe that the use of any contraceptive method will hasten the progression of an existing cervical lesion. All too often, the unfortunate result of withholding contraceptive methods from a woman with cervical dysplasia is unintended pregnancy, which makes diagnosis more difficult and often delays treatment.

SCREENING FOR CERVICAL CANCER

The Pap smear, more than any other screening test, has proven its cost-effectiveness over the years.[9] Based upon current screening patterns in the United States, early detection and treatment of pre-invasive lesions prevents at least 70% of potential cervical cancers. Of the 10,370 American women[10] who will develop new cases of cervical cancer each in 2005[11,12]—

- One-half had not had a Pap smear in the past 3 to 5 years.

- One-half had received a Pap smear within 3 to 5 years, but there was either a falsely negative result, the patient was not managed correctly, or there was inadequate follow-up of the patient.

False negative results occur in 20% or more of Pap smears and can occur because the lesion exfoliated too few cells be detected, there was a sampling error by the clinician, or an interpretive error in the cytopathology lab. In 1996 the U.S. Food and Drug Administration (FDA) approved a number of new technologies aimed at improving the quality of Pap smears and to facilitate computerized readings. One approach, liquid based cytology (LBC) with thin layer preparation technique (Thin Prep Pap Test, AutoCyte Prep, SurePath), may improve accuracy by increasing the number of cells sampled and by removing blood, mucus, and debris from the background of the smear. Another approach is to evaluate the Pap smear by routine microscopy and then re-screen the negative smears with computer-based evaluation techniques (AutoPap QC System) to detect abnormal smears that should be re-evaluated microscopically.

Some studies suggest that these newer approaches improve Pap smear accuracy over current practices;[13,14] however, a 2003 statement of the USPSTF concludes that "the evidence is insufficient to recommend for or against the routine use of these technologies to screen for cervical cancer."[33] Controversy persists whether the additional cost associated with these tests justifies their use or, in contrast, if the increased cost of screening actually may lead to fewer Pap smears being performed.[15,16]

PATHOPHYSIOLOGY

The cervix consists of two types of epithelium:

- Squamous epithelium, which covers the vagina and the portio vaginalis of the cervix

- Columnar epithelium, which covers the endocervical canal, and in younger women, the area around the external cervical os

At menarche, the vaginal pH drops into an acidic range and causes the fragile columnar epithelial cells around the cervical os to be replaced by squamous epithelium, a process referred to as squamous metaplasia. As this process proceeds over decades, the advancing edge of the squamous epithelium (referred to as the squamocolumnar junction) migrates centrally toward the cervical os and ultimately into the endocervical canal.

Because squamous cell cancers and their precursors virtually always develop within the field of metaplasia (also called the transformation zone), both cytological and colposcopic evaluation focus upon this area. There is now widespread agreement that the cause of cervical dysplasia is an accumulation of DNA mutations in immature metaplastic cells as a consequence of human papilloma virus (HPV) infection in concert with other carcinogenic co-factors. Although more than 100 DNA-types of HPV have been identified, only a limited number are associated with premalignant and malignant epithelial lesions of the lower genital tract:

HPV types 16 and 18 account for about 70 percent of CIN 3 lesions and cervical cancers while the remaining 30 percent are due to HPV types 31, 33, 35, 39, 45, 51, 52, 56 and 58.[17] The high-risk HPV types exert their cancer-causing effects through a series of events leading to the degradation of the p53 tumor suppressor protein in infected cells, reducing the host's ability to reject cells with random DNA mutations. However, HPV infection alone is insufficient to initiate this process. A facilitating agent, or co-factor, appears to be necessary to act in concert with HPV to initiate these premalignant changes. For example, cigarette smoking has been identified as a powerful co-factor, doubling a smoker's risk of cervical cancer.[18,19] Infections due to HPV types 6 and 11, the cause of genital warts and most low-grade cervical lesions, are felt to exhibit very low or no malignant potential.

HPV infections are widespread among sexually active adults, costly to characterize virologically through HPV DNA testing, and cannot be eradicated with anti-viral drugs. The duration of HPV infection remains controversial; while older studies inferred that HPV infection is lifelong, newer studies suggest that HPV infections are transient in a majority of infected individuals.[20,21] In addition, the role of evaluating and treating the male sexual partner in preventing recurrences of cervical dysplasia in treated women and in preventing spread of the virus to uninfected women is uncertain.[22] From a public health viewpoint, it makes more sense to prevent cervical cancer and its precursors through HPV vaccination and to detect and treat high grade pre-invasive lesions, before life-threatening invasive cervical cancers have a chance to develop, rather than to rely on a behavioral strategy that focuses on the transmissibility of HPV.

RISK FACTORS FOR CERVICAL CANCER

Epidemiological observations are consistent with the biological mechanism of cervical cancer. The following are primary epidemiological risk factors for the development of cervical cancer:

- Early onset of intercourse (defined as a sexual debut before 20 years old). Metaplasia is most active during adolescence, making a young woman more vulnerable to cell changes.

- Three or more sexual partners in one's lifetime. The greater the number of sexual partners, the greater the risk of acquiring a high-risk type of HPV.

- Male sexual partner who has had other partners, especially if a previous partner had cervical cancer.

- Clinical history of condyloma acuminata. Infection with a low-risk type of HPV is a risk marker for co-infection with a high-risk type.[22]

- Infection with the human immunodeficiency virus (HIV) and other medical conditions associated with immunodeficiency. These illnesses decrease the ability of the immune system to recognize and reject abnormal cells.

Behavioral protective factors include virginity, long-term celibacy, life-long mutual monogamy, and long-term use of condoms. Factors that appear to have no effect on cervical cancer risk include history of herpes simplex virus infection, circumcision status of the male partner, or religious background. The effect of race and socioeconomic status are controversial. Studies show higher rates of cervical cancer among African American women and women of lower socio-economic status;[23] however, it is unclear whether the higher rates are related to poor access to medical care and, consequently, Pap smear services, or other undetermined factors.

HPV VACCINATION

Vaccination against high risk HPV holds great promise for primary prevention of cervical cancer. The FDA approved a quadrivalent HPV vaccine (Gardasil), which includes antigens for HPV types 6, 11, 16, and 18, in June 2006, and other products may soon follow. The vaccine consists of three injected doses of "virus like particles" (VLPs), rather than the virus itself, to stimulate the production of anti-HPV antibodies. Research has shown[72] that the vaccine is extremely effective in preventing high grade CIN lesions due to HPV 16 and 18 when provided to virus naïve women who are between 9–26 years old. In addition, the vaccine also provides a high degree of protection against vulvar and vaginal intraepithelial lesions, which could lead to squamous cell cancers of the vulva and vagina, respectively, and genital warts. The vaccine provides protection for at least 4 years (the length of the trial follow-up) and appears to cause no serious side effects. However, because one-third of high grade CIN lesions contain high risk HPV types not included in the vaccine, women who have been vaccinated are advised to continue to receive routine Pap smears at currently recommended intervals. The CDC's Advisory Committee on Immunization Practices (ACIP) is expected to issue guidelines regarding the use of HPV vaccine in the near future.

HIV Infection and Cervical Cancer Risk

Studies have demonstrated that the natural history of genital tract HPV infection, as well as that of pre-invasive and invasive cervical lesions, is different in HIV-seropositive women when compared to untreated HIV seronegative women.[24] While the prevalence of dysplasia in reproductive-age women is below 3%, its prevalence is 36% among HIV-positive women and 64% among women with acquired immune deficiency syndrome (AIDS). Although an early uncontrolled study suggested that HIV-positive women had substantially higher rates of falsely negative Pap smears, more recent studies show that the accuracy of Pap smears is the same in HIV-positive as in HIV-negative women.[25,26] When cervical dysplasia occurs in an HIV-infected woman, the lesion may progress more rapidly, especially if she is immunocompromised. It also has been observed that HIV-positive women treated for cervical dysplasia have loop electrosurgical excision (LEEP) failure rates of 40% to 60% (even higher if the woman is immunocompromised) compared with failure rates of 10% for HIV-negative women.[27] In 1992, the Centers for Disease Control and Prevention changed its surveillance definition of AIDS to include cervical cancer in an HIV-positive woman as an indicator of AIDS.[28] Women with HIV also are more likely to develop multifocal vulvar intraepithelial neoplasia (VIN), as well as pre-invasive and invasive squamous cell cancers of the anus.[25] Three clinical recommendations can be made:

1. Because of more rapid progression rates of CIN in HIV-seropositive women, immunocompetent women should receive Pap smears twice in the first year after diagnosis, then annually, while those who are immunocompromised or who have been treated for dysplasia since the time of HIV diagnosis should receive Pap smears more frequently. No major organization recommends that baseline colposcopy should be performed routinely for all HIV-seropositive women.

2. There is no role for expectant management when an HIV-positive woman has an abnormal Pap smear result. Perform a colposcopy after a single reading of atypical squamous cell of undetermined significance (ASC-US) or squamous intraepithelial lesion (SIL). During this examination, check the vagina, vulva, and anus for neoplastic changes.

3. Do not assume that treatment is futile for the woman who has both HIV and premalignant or malignant cervical disease. Aggressive treatment of cervical disease will prolong her life in most cases.

TECHNICAL ASPECTS OF CYTOLOGICAL SCREENING

High accuracy in cytological screening depends on a good quality cervical sample, appropriately performed slide preparation, and competent cytopathologic interpretation.

- **Timing.** A Pap smear may be performed whenever heavy menstrual bleeding is not present. However, the optimal timing is at midcycle in a woman who has not had intercourse for 24 hours and has not placed any substances in her vagina for at least 48 hours.

- **Sampling.** Moisten the speculum with warm water or a small amount of lubricating gel, neither of which will negatively impact the accuracy of the Pap smear.[29] Using a large cotton-tipped applicator in a gentle wiping motion, remove excess cervical mucus. The order in which cervical specimens are obtained is critical, in that samples most easily contaminated by blood should be taken early in the sampling sequence. DNA probe and amplification tests (LCR, PCR) for chlamydia and gonorrhea should be performed before the Pap smear. If non-DNA tests are used, take the Pap sample first, collect the sample for gonorrhea culture next, and sample for chlamydia testing last.

- **Slide preparation.** First sample the exocervix by rotating a wooden or plastic spatula 360 degrees around the exocervix, then sample the endocervical canal using a brush sampling device, or if one is not available, a saline-moistened cotton-tipped applicator. Place the spatula sample on a glass slide, creating a thin layer that covers most of the slide's surface. Then gently roll the brush or swab on top of the first sample. Apply fixative immediately in order to avoid air drying. Unless specifically requested by the cytopathology laboratory, separate slides are not needed for each sample, nor is segmenting the slide into a section for the exocervical sample and another for the endocervical sample. Sampling of the vaginal pool is not helpful and actually may decrease the quality of the sample by adding degenerating cells and other debris.

CYTOLOGICAL SCREENING INTERVALS

The issue of Pap smear screening intervals has been a contentious one, often resulting in inconsistent practices among providers in various specialty groups. Until recently, most providers followed the 1987 Pap Smear Consensus Statement:

> All women who are or who have been sexually active or who have reached 18 years old (should) have an annual Pap test and pelvic exam. After a woman has had three or more consecutive, satisfactory, normal annual exams, the Pap test may be performed less frequently at the discretion of the physician and the patient.

Consequently, most national women's health care organizations, including ACOG and the U.S. Title X Family Planning Program,[30] recommended Pap smear intervals based upon a woman's risk factors for cervical cancer; that is, high-risk women were screened annually while low-risk women were screened less frequently. However, compelling evidence from mathematical modeling shows that the time interval of disease progression and screening error rates are the most important factors in computing screening intervals, and that risk factors for cervical cancer should not be considered, as long as the woman is not immunocompromised.[31] This is biologically plausible, as the presence or absence of behavioral or clinical risk factors does not affect the rate at which cervical disease progresses in immunocompetent women.

Since 2002, three major national organizations have issued recommendations regarding Pap smear periodicity (Table 22–1). While there is a great deal of overlap between the guidelines, minor differences exist among them, which prevents the existence of a single "national standard" regarding Pap smear periodicity. Clinicians (or entire practices) should adopt one of the guidelines, or develop a composite "practice-specific" policy, which then is followed consistently for all women, regardless of the number or degree of an individual's risk factors. The guidelines also specify that these recommendations apply to asymptomatic women who are being screened for cervical cancer, while those who are "under surveillance" for prior abnormal Paps or who are in the first year after treatment of a pre-invasive cervical lesion should be followed under other protocols.[32]

A major contribution of the new guidelines is the explicit categorization of when screening should start, when it can be discontinued, and how often it should be performed in between these points. From the viewpoint of contraceptive services, the most significant new recommendation is that Pap screening need not be initiated until 3 years after the first episode of vaginal intercourse or 21 years of age, whichever comes first. This recommendation is based on the following observations.[32,35]

- HSIL and cervical cancer are rarely seen in this young age group
- Many cytologic abnormalities and some CIN 2 and 3 lesions will resolve spontaneously and will never be clinically relevant
- Cervical excisional treatments, which may be the outcome of positive screening, have been associated with adverse obstetrical outcomes

To summarize the recommendations of the American Cancer Society, "Screening before the 3-year period may result in an over diagnosis of cervical lesions that will regress spontaneously leading to inappropriate interventions that may do more harm than good."

Table 22–1 Pap smear screening intervals

	American Cancer Society[32]	U.S. Preventive Services Task Force[33]	American College of Obstetricians and Gynecologists[34]	Rationale
When to start	• 3 years after the onset of vaginal intercourse • Start no later than 21 years old, unless reliable history of virginity	Within 3 years of onset of sexual activity or age 21 whichever comes first	Approximately 3 years after the onset of sexual intercourse, but no later than age 21	• HSIL and cervical cancer are extremely rare within 3 years of sexual debut • Upper age limit (21) needed for providers who do not take a sexual history or for adolescents unwilling to disclose sexual history
	Virginal women should be counseled regarding the benefits and risks of screening			HSIL and cervical cancer are extremely rare in the absence of vaginal intercourse
When to stop	Women ≥ 70 years old with intact cervix and 3 consecutive negative tests and no abnormal tests in prior 10 years	Women > 65 years with negative tests, who are not otherwise at high risk for cervical cancer	Inconclusive evidence to establish upper age limit; determine on an individual basis	• Cervical cancer in older women is almost entirely confined to the un- and underscreened. • If sexually active, very low risk of new lesion since little active metaplasia.
Post total hysterectomy	Discontinue if for benign reasons and no prior history of high grade CIN	Discontinue if for benign reasons	Discontinue if for benign reasons and no prior history of high grade CIN	• Squamous cell cancer of the vagina is extremely rare. • Abnormal vaginal smears are uncommon and rarely important.

(continued)

Table 22–1 Pap smear screening intervals—(cont'd)

	American Cancer Society[32]	U.S. Preventive Services Task Force[33]	American College of Obstetricians and Gynecologists[34]	Rationale
Interval				
Until age 30				
Conventional smears	Annually	At least every 3 years	Annually	Progression to HSIL may be more rapid in younger women
Liquid-based smears	Every 2 years	Insufficient evidence	No separate recommendation	LBC has poorer specificity; excess false positives if done annually
30 years old and older	If three consecutively normal smears, screen every 2–3 years	No separate recommendation	Every 2–3 years with 3 negative cytology tests	Progression to HSIL may be slower in women over 30 years old
HPV+ Pap co-screening	Every 3 years if HPV negative and Pap negative	Insufficient evidence	Every 3 years if HPV negative, cytology negative	Risk of a new lesion is negligible and likelihood a false positive HPV test is significant
Special Circumstances				
• Immuno-compromise (organ transplant, chemotherapy, chronic steroid use • HIV seropositive	Twice in the first year after diagnosis, then annually	No separate recommendation	"More frequent cervical screening"	Immunocompromise can hasten progression rate from SIL to invasive cancer
DES exposure in utero	As for women under 30 years old	No separate recommendation	"More frequent cervical screening"	Reduced sensitivity for glandular cancers (DES)
Hysterectomy for high grade dysplasia	Screen until 3 consecutive normal tests and no abnormals within the prior 10 years	No separate recommendation	Screen annually until three consecutive, negative vaginal Paps; then discontinue routine screening.	To evaluate for residual or recurrent CIN at the vaginal cuff

Another significant modification in the guidelines is the recommendation that well screened women over 30 years of age should have Pap smears performed every 2 to 3 years. Many industrialized countries, including the United Kingdom, Canada, and Japan, have recommended 3-year Pap screening intervals for decades. However, this represents an important departure from the longstanding U.S. public health recommendation that women receive annual Pap smear screening, and both clinician-initiated discussions and public educational campaigns will be necessary to re-educate consumers regarding the reason for this change.[36] A number of studies have shown that most women believe that they need to have annual Pap smears and many are suspicious that the recommendations for longer Pap screening intervals are economically, rather than clinically, motivated.[37,38] When a well-screened woman over 30 years old requests an annual Pap smear, it seems expedient for a clinician to acquiesce to her request and provide one. However, studies show that performing Pap smears more often than necessary can do more harm than good, since the hazards of a false positive test will exceed the negligible benefit of the shorter screening interval. For example, in a study by Sawaya, in order to prevent a single case of cervical cancer in a cohort of 100,000 well-screened women between 45 to 59 years old by screening annually instead of every 3 years, an additional 209,324 Pap smears and 11,502 colposcopies would be required.[39]

HPV Testing as an Adjunct to Pap Smear

A newer approach to cervical cancer screening is the performance of a simultaneous Pap smear and a HPV DNA test. This combination approach significantly improves the sensitivity of screening for high-grade squamous intraepithelial lesions (HSIL)/cancer to at least 92% when compared to a sensitivity of 80% for a Pap smear alone.[40] Of equal importance is the negative predictive value of this approach, since women who are both Pap negative and HPV negative have an extremely low risk of developing HSIL within the next 10 years. Either LBC or a conventional Pap smear can be used, but the later requires "co-collection" of an HPV DNA sample. The HPV DNA test utilized should test for high-risk HPV types only, as the presence of low-risk HPV types is not relevant to management. Additionally, the combined approach is not recommended for women who are under 30 years old, who are immunocompromised, or who have had a hysterectomy for benign disease and no longer have a cervix. Most importantly, women who are HPV-DNA negative and who have a benign Pap smear result should not be re-screened before 3 years, since the risk of a new lesion is negligible and likelihood a false positive test is significant. The combination of a negative Pap smear and a positive HPV test is followed with a repeat of both tests in 6 to 12 months, during which time the woman may experience considerable anxiety, knowing that she carries high-risk HPV. Women who have a reading of ASC-undetermined significance (ASC-US) and a positive HPV test need colposcopy, as well as women with ASC-cannot exclude HSIL (ASC-H), low-grade squamous intraepithelial lesions (LSIL), HSIL and atypical glandular cells (AGC) results, irrespective of HPV result. If you intend to perform combination cervical cancer screening, it is critical to inform the patient in advance of sampling that she is being screened for HPV and that she need not be re-screened earlier than 3 years if both tests are negative.

MANAGEMENT OF ABNORMAL PAP SMEAR RESULTS

The classification system recommended by the third Bethesda workshop (the 2001 Bethesda System)[41] contained a number of modifications to include new screening technologies, as well as to remedy points of confusion between pathologists and clinicians. Cervical cytology reports conforming to the 2001 Bethesda System format include comments in each of the following categories, as applicable:

- Specimen type (conventional smear vs. liquid-based vs. other)

- Specimen adequacy (satisfactory or unsatisfactory for evaluation)

- General categorization (Negative, Epithelial cell abnormality, Other)

- Interpretation/Result (see Table 22–2)

- Automated review and ancillary testing (including HPV reflex results, if done)

- Educational notes and suggestions (optional)

Negative, with Comments Regarding Specimen Adequacy

While the 2001 Bethesda System has eliminated the category of "satisfactory, but limited by..." (SBLB), comments regarding suboptimal specimen quality still may be made. The finding that most often limits interpretation is a paucity of endocervical cells. Their presence confirms that in the process of sampling the transformation zone, the active squamocolumnar junction was included. Even with the best of sampling efforts, however, endocervical cells are absent in up to 10% of Pap smears obtained from premenopausal women and as many as 50% from postmenopausal women.[42] In addition, fewer endocervical cells may be present in smears from women who use oral contraceptives or are pregnant. If a negative result is reported, take the next Pap smear at a routine interval. A result that describes inadequate or absent endocervical cells

Table 22–2 2001 Bethesda System interpretation/result categories

	Negative For Intraepithelial Lesion Or Malignancy
Organisms	• Trichomonas vaginalis • Fungal organisms morphologically consistent with Candida sp. • Shift in flora suggestive of BV • Bacteria morphologically consistent with Actinomyces sp. • Cellular changes consistent with herpes simplex virus
Other non-neoplastic finding	• Reactive cellular changes associated with inflammation, radiation, or intrauterine contraceptive device • Glandular cells status post hysterectomy • Atrophy
Other Endometrial cells	Endometrial cells, cytologically benign, in a woman ≥ 40 years of age

Epithelial Cell Abnormalities	
Squamous cell	• Atypical squamous cells (ASC) — of undetermined significance (ASC-US) — cannot exclude HSIL (ASC-H) • Low-grade SIL (LSIL) • High-grade SIL (HSIL) • Squamous cell carcinoma
Glandular cell	• Atypical glandular cells (AGC) — specify endocervical, endometrial, or glandular cells NOS (not otherwise specified) • Atypical glandular cells, favor neoplastic — specify endocervical or NOS • Endocervical adenocarcinoma in situ (AIS) • Adenocarcinoma — specify: endocervical, endometrial, extrauterine, or NOS

but provides no other general categorization or result must be managed as an unsatisfactory smear (see the next subsection).

The proportion of Pap smears with this reading provides an important opportunity to monitor Pap smear technique. If the percentage of Pap smears with no endocervical cells present exceeds 10%, remedial action is necessary. If clinician education regarding Pap smear technique and a switch to brush sampling devices does not result in improvement, the laboratory's cytopathologist should be consulted in order to determine whether the problem lies with the laboratory or the provider and to define further steps necessary to rectify the problem.

Unsatisfactory for evaluation. Inadequate sampling, air drying, excessive red or white blood cells, or other factors make interpretation impossible. Because unsatisfactory smears have a greater likelihood of being abnormal,[43] repeat the smear, preferably when the woman is at midcycle and has not had intercourse or used vaginal products for at least 24 hours. Do not repeat the Pap smear earlier than 6 weeks from the previous smear; repetitive sampling over short periods of time may increase the risk of falsely negative smears due to decreased exfoliation of abnormal cells and a greater likelihood of reparative changes. Postmenopausal women with one or more unsatisfactory Pap smears due to vaginal atrophy should apply topical vaginal estrogen cream daily for 4 to 6 weeks, and then receive a repeat Pap smear no earlier than 1 week after completing the medication. Unless a woman has a history of endometrial hyperplasia, progestin withdrawal is not necessary after this short course of estrogen exposure. If the proportion of unsatisfactory smears within a practice is greater than 5%, remedial action in consultation with the cytopathologist is recommended.

Negative for Intraepithelial Lesion or Malignancy: Organisms

Trichomonas vaginalis. While the Pap smear is a relatively insensitive test for the detection of Trichomonas (it detects trichomonads in only about one-half of infected women), its specificity is as high as 98%.[44] Since the prevalence of trichomonas vaginal colonization in reproductive aged women is about 5%, the positive predictive value of a Pap smear reporting trichomonas is about 72%. When the Pap report indicates presence of Trichomonas, review the woman's medical record to determine whether the infection was recently treated. If it has been, no further action is required. If it has not been treated, offer treatment to avoid horizontal transmission to a new sexual partner and to prevent conversion of asymptomatic Trichomonas colonization into an uncomfortable case of symptomatic vaginal trichomoniasis. The practice of requiring microscopic saline suspension to confirm vaginal trichomonads is illogical because the sensitivity of this test is only 60%. Instead, if the saline suspension is negative and confirmation is desired, use a test with high sensitivity and specificity, such as a DNA test or Diamond's media culture. Repeat the Pap smear after the next routine screening interval, unless the narrative report mentions obscuring inflammation and indicates the need to repeat the Pap smear after treatment.

Fungus morphologically consistent with **Candida spp.** In most cases, Candida detected on Pap smear is due to normal vaginal colonization with low levels of Candida, rather than frank vaginal candidiasis. Candida colonization is not dangerous to the affected woman or her sexual partner. Repeat the Pap only if the inflammation due to the candidiasis is of sufficient severity that the cytopathologist recommends that the Pap smear be repeated after treatment is complete.

Shift in flora suggestive of bacterial vaginosis. This reading refers to changes detected in the bacterial flora of the vagina in which the normal Lactobacillus are not abundant but coccobacilli are seen in numbers greater than normal. While this description was devised to suggest the possibility of bacterial vaginosis (BV), it is both an insensitive and non-specific indicator of BV. The clinical diagnosis of BV is made solely on clinical findings (see Chapter 21 on Reproductive Tract Infections), and neither vaginal culture nor Pap smear findings have any role in the diagnosis of this condition. Management is controversial. Many clinicians feel that no further evaluation is necessary and that the next Pap smear should be performed at the routine interval, while others feel that the woman should be informed that BV is inferred from findings on the smear and be offered clinical evaluation for BV.

Bacteria morphologically consistent with **Actinomyces** *spp.* *Actinomyces israelii* is an anaerobic bacteria capable of causing a rare, but severe, pelvic infection called pelvic actinomycosis, especially in long-term IUC users over 35 years of age. The vast majority of intrauterine contraceptive (IUC) users with "Actinomyces-like organisms (ALO)" on their Pap smears have an asymptomatic cervical colonization (not infection) that does not require either antibiotic therapy or removal of the IUC. However, IUC users with Actinomyces on their Pap smear should have a bimanual pelvic examination to determine whether they have evidence of pelvic infection. If symptoms or physical findings suggest pelvic actinomycosis, remove the IUC and initiate intensive antibiotic therapy. Advise the woman to use another method of contraception. (See Chapter 7 on Intrauterine Devices.)

Cellular changes consistent with herpes simplex virus (HSV). Although an insensitive indicator of cervical herpes simplex shedding, the Pap smear is a specific indicator. If the patient requests confirmation, a positive HSV-2 type-specific serology will confirm prior infection, but an HSV culture should be avoided, since viral shedding is intermittent and unpredictable. Advise the infected woman to tell her obstetrical care provider so that precautions may be taken to minimize the risk of vertical transmission to a newborn. Unless inflammation interferes with the interpretation of the Pap smear, the next Pap smear should be performed at the routine interval.

Negative for Intraepithelial Lesion or Malignancy: Other Non-Neoplastic Findings

Reactive cellular changes associated with inflammation. Nonspecific reactive inflammatory changes may be associated with benign metaplasia, mechanical or chemical irritation, post-traumatic repair, chlamydial or gonococcal endocervicitis, trichomoniasis, viral infection, invasive cervical cancer, or other unknown factors. Of these possibilities, the only infectious conditions amenable to antibiotic therapy are gonococcal and chlamydial endocervicitis and vaginal trichomoniasis. Women who recently have been evaluated for these organisms and found to be uninfected do not require further evaluation or antibiotic therapy. Evaluate women who have not been screened recently by performing gonorrhea and chlamydia tests and treating women who test positive. Empirically treating women with inflammatory Pap smears with topical antibiotic sulfa creams is of no value in either the treatment of cervical infection or the resolution of abnormal Pap smears and is to be avoided.[45]

Rarely, the only Pap smear finding in a woman with an invasive cervical carcinoma is the persistent finding of inflammation. Although not evidence-based, some experts recommend that women who have had consecutive Pap smears with unexplained inflammation be evaluated by colposcopy; others contend that this practice is unnecessary because of the extremely low likelihood of detecting a cervical cancer in this circumstance.

Cytological changes associated with the use of an IUD detected on Pap smear are of a benign nature and do not require further investigation.

Atrophy. Atrophy is most common in postmenopausal women or those with estrogen-deficiency states. Treatment of the vaginal atrophy is indicated only if the woman has symptomatic atrophic vaginitis; it is not necessary for the asymptomatic woman. Pap smear screening intervals do not need to be modified, and the woman does not need to be notified.

Endometrial cells, cytologically benign, in a woman ≥ 40 years of age. Endometrial cells found on Pap smear are an insignificant finding in premenopausal women with normal ovulatory cycling. However, because the endometrium normally is atrophic in postmenopausal women, the finding of endometrial cells may be the result of exfoliation from a focus of endometrial hyperplasia or adenocarcinoma. For this reason, consider the finding of endometrial cells in a postmenopausal woman as a danger sign and sample the endometrium. Because a premenopausal woman with chronic anovulation also is at risk for endometrial hyperplasia, manage the finding of endometrial cells in the same way.

Epithelial Cell Abnormalities: Squamous Cell

The atypical squamous cell (ASC) category refers to the finding of cells with nuclear atypia that are not normal, yet not diagnostic of SIL. The majority of ASC-US smears are due to benign HPV infections, although 2.5% of women over 40 years old and 11% under 40 years old with this reading have CIN 2 or worse, and very rarely, invasive cancer.[46] Because of confusion regarding the meaning of the ASC reading, the 2001 Bethesda System encourages the cytopathologist to further qualify the reading as either ASC-US and ASC-H. ASC-US refers to findings that suggest LSIL, but not meeting criteria, and ASC-H is suggestive of HSIL, but which lack criteria for definitive interpretation.

The ASCCP 2001 Consensus Guidelines[47] describe three acceptable options for the management of women with ASC-US results: perform colposcopy, follow with a shorter Pap screening interval, or use HPV typing to differentiate women who are at high risk for having, or progressing to, HSIL (also called intermediary triage).

While clinicians should advise women of the advantages and disadvantages of each approach, the option of reflex HPV testing is most appropriate for women 30 years of age and older, since HPV positivity rates are substantially lower in this age group and the sensitivity remains high.[35] Adolescents with an ASC-US result may be better served with a repeat cytology strategy, since time is afforded for the resolution of a transient HPV infection. If this approach is adopted, "reflex HPV test for ASC-US" need not be ordered when submitting the Pap smear request to the cytopathology laboratory. Furthermore, the ACOG Practice Bulletin[48] states that as an alternative to colposcopy, adolescents with ASC-US and positive HPV may be monitored with cytology at 6 and 12 months or a single HPV test at 12 months.

Management recommendations for other abnormal Pap smear results from the American Society for Colposcopy and Cervical Pathology (ASCCP)[47] are contained in Table 22–3.

Epithelial Cell Abnormalities: Glandular Cell

Atypical glandular cells (AGC). AGC may result from HPV infection of glandular cells, adenocarcinoma-in-situ (AIS), adenocarcinoma, or in some cases, an SIL lesion. Because adenocarcinomas of the cervix are associated with a rate of false-negative Pap smears as high as 40%,[49] women with AGC require aggressive evaluation in order to exclude a cancer diagnosis. There is no role for observation (repeat Pap smear) in this situation.

Table 22–3 ASCCP Consensus Guidelines for Management of Women With Cervical Cytological Abnormalities[47]

	Initial Intervention	Management of Initial Findings	Subsequent Follow up
ASC-US	**Either:** Repeat cytology at 6 months ***Preferred for adolescents***	• Negative: repeat cytology at 6 mos • ≥ ASC-US: colposcopy	→• Negative: routine cytology • ≥ ASC-US: colposcopy
	Or: HPV DNA testing (reflex test)	• Negative: repeat cytology at 12 mos • Positive: colposcopy (in adolescent, may manage as LSIL/adolescent, below)	→• Negative: routine cytology • ≥ ASC-US: colposcopy
	Or: Colposcopy	• No CIN, HPV pos: cytology at 6 and 12 mos **or** HPV testing at 12 mos • No CIN, HPV neg: cytology at 12 mos • CIN: per ASCCP CIN guideline[51]	→• Negative: routine cytology →• ≥ ASC-US or HPV (+): repeat colposcopy
ASC-US postmenopause	**Either:** Colposcopy or HPV DNA testing	• Per management of ASC-US	
	Or: Intravaginal estrogen for 4–6 weeks, then repeat cytology	• Negative: repeat cytology at 4–6 mos • ≥ ASC: colposcopy	→• Negative: routine cytology • ≥ ASC-US: colposcopy
ASC-H	Colposcopy (with ECS)	• No CIN: cytology at 6 and 12 mos **or** HPV testing at 12 mos • CIN/cancer: per ASCCP CIN guideline[2]	→• Negative: routine cytology • ≥ ASC-US or HPV (+): colposcopy
LSIL	Colposcopy	• No CIN: cytology at 6 and 12 mos **or** HPV testing at 12 mo • CIN/cancer: per ASCCP CIN guideline[2]	→• Negative: routine cytology • ≥ ASC-US or HPV (+): colposcopy

(continued)

Table 22–3 ASCCP Consensus Guidelines for Management of Women With Cervical Cytological Abnormalities[47]—(cont'd)

	Initial Intervention	Management of Initial Findings	Subsequent Follow up
LSIL postmenopause	**Either:** HPV DNA at 12 mos	• Negative: repeat cytology at 12 mos • Positive: colposcopy	→ • Negative: routine cytology • ≥ ASC-US: colposcopy
	Or: Repeat cytology at 4–6 mos	• Negative: repeat cytology at 4–6 mos • ≥ ASC-US: colposcopy	→ • Negative: routine cytology • ≥ ASC-US: colposcopy
	Or: Vaginal estrogen for 4–6 weeks, then repeat Pap	• Negative: repeat cytology at 4–6 mos • ≥ ASC-US: colposcopy	→ • Negative: routine cytology • ≥ ASC-US: colposcopy
LSIL adolescent	**Either:** Cytology at 6 mos *Preferred*	• Negative: repeat cytology at 6 mos • ≥ ASC-US: colposcopy	→ • Negative: routine cytology • ≥ ASC-US: colposcopy
	Or: HPV DNA at 12 mo	• Negative: repeat cytology at 12 mos • Positive: colposcopy	→ • Negative: routine cytology • ≥ ASC-US: colposcopy
	Or: Colposcopy	• Per management of LSIL	

HSIL	Colposcopy (with ECS)	• See and treat LEEP (if CIN 2 or 3 likely)
		• Unsatisfactory colposcopy:
		  • CIN biopsy: per ASCCP CIN guideline[51]
		  • No lesion*: DEP
		• Satisfactory colposcopy:
		  • CIN 2/3 biopsy: per ASCCP CIN guideline[51]
		  • No CIN or CIN 1* biopsy: DEP
			NOTE: if HSIL cytology and no cervical lesion seen at colposcopy, perform endocervical sampling and evaluate vagina with Lugol's solution for vaginal intraepithelial neoplasia (VaIN)

AGC: Atypical endometrial cells	Endometrial sampling	• Negative endometrial sampling: colposcopy + ECS	

(continued)

CONTRACEPTIVE TECHNOLOGY

Table 22–3 ASCCP Consensus Guidelines for Management of Women With Cervical Cytological Abnormalities[47]—(cont'd)

	Initial Intervention	Management of Initial Findings	Subsequent Follow up
AGC **All other** **sub-categories**	Colposcopy + ECS **And:** Endometrial sampling (if ≥ 35 years old or abnormal bleeding)	• Invasive cancer: refer to specialist • Pap= AGC-favor neoplasia or AIS: DEP • Pap= AGC –not specified (NOS): 　• Bx= CIN/AIS: per ASCCP guideline[51] 　• No CIN/AIS: cytology at 4–6 month intervals **four times**	• All 4 negative: routine cytology • ASC or LSIL: repeat colposcopy →• HSIL or AGC: DEP

* After pathologist review of material, including referral cytology, colposcopic findings, and all biopsies

ECS = endocervical sampling with endocervical curettage or cervical brush

DEP = diagnostic excisional procedure, e.g., LEEP cone, (cold-knife) cone biopsy, or laser cone biopsy

Table 22–4 Indications for colposcopy

- Papanicolaou (Pap) smear showing ASC-H, HSIL, or suspicion of cancer
- Pap showing LSIL, unless adolescent or post-menopausal and using alternate management pathway
- Pap smear showing atypical glandular cells (AGC), other than AGC-atypical endometrial cells
- Pap smear showing ASC-US
  - Women who are HIV-positive or immunocompromised
  - Women who are unlikely or unwilling to return for frequent follow-up
  - Women not entering HPV testing or repeat cytology management pathways
  - Finding of another ASC or worse on Pap smear performed during observation period
  - High-risk HPV DNA present at initial or subsequent testing (except in adolescents, as noted above)
- Cervical leukoplakia (white lesion visible to the naked eye without the application of acetic acid) or other unexplained cervical lesion, regardless of Pap smear result
- Unexplained or persistent cervical bleeding, regardless of Pap smear result

TREATMENT OF SQUAMOUS INTRAEPITHELIAL LESIONS

Since the early 1990s, management protocols have become much more conservative, due to the recognition that most LSIL lesions will regress without treatment, rather than progress to higher-grade lesions or cancer. Once a diagnosis of CIN I (LSIL) is made in a patient with a fully visible cervical lesion, she should be followed until there is evidence of HSIL or persistence of LSIL over the period of 1 year. The preferred approach to follow-up is either cytology alone at 6 and 12 months or HPV DNA testing at 12 months, although an acceptable alternative is colposcopy plus cytology at 12 months. If any of these alternatives is chosen, both the provider and the patient must be diligent with follow-up. Alternatively, if the patient is uncomfortable with being observed and requests treatment, or if she is a poor follow-up risk, immediate treatment is an acceptable choice.

Typical papillary condyloma accuminata of the cervix, once histologically proven by cervical biopsy, should be treated rather than observed. This aggressive approach decreases the amount of friable cervical tissue, which will reduce receptivity to HIV infection and may decrease the risk of viral transmission to a partner. Cryotherapy is the least invasive and most inexpensive treatment modality in most cases, although some situations may require the use of LEEP or laser. The use of trichloroacetic acid, topical 5-fluorouracil (FU), or imiquimod for the treatment of cervical condyloma and SIL is considered investigational and is not recommended.

There is universal agreement that high-grade SIL must be treated, because the risk of progression to cervical cancer is both more likely and more immediate. Consensus guidelines for the management of CIN lesions have been published by the American Society for Colposcopy and Cervical Pathology.[50,51]

OVARIAN CANCER SCREENING

In the United States in 2005, about 22,200 women were diagnosed with ovarian cancer,[10] making this cancer the fifth most common among American women. However, because of the low 5-year survival rates with this disease, especially in the later stages when it is more commonly diagnosed, it is the leading cause (53%) of gynecologic cancer deaths, accounting for 16,200 deaths in the United States. The average age at diagnosis is 60 years. A woman's lifetime risk of ovarian cancer is about 1 in 70.

Although some risk factors for ovarian cancer are well known, a majority of women diagnosed with this condition have none.[52] Geographic differences are marked; rates in Sweden and the United States are 13 to 15 cases per 100,000 women per year, while the rate in Japan is 3 cases per 100,000 women per year. This difference in part may be related to dietary fat intake, which is higher in the United States and Scandinavia and lower in Japan. A long interval of ovulatory cycles also is associated with ovarian cancer, and low parity, delayed childbearing, and infertility are weak risk factors. Familial predisposition accounts for 5% to 10% of cases, and the risk of ovarian cancer is 5% if one first-degree relative had ovarian cancer and 7% if two or more first-degree relatives had the condition. A site-specific familial ovarian cancer syndrome also has been described, which is mediated through a highly penetrant autosomal dominant gene; in these cases, the risk to a first-degree relative is up to 50%. In addition, women with BRCA-1 and BRCA-2 mutations are at greater risk of both ovarian and breast cancer. Because there is no accurate method to detect early ovarian cancer in these high-risk women, some experts recommend prophylactic oophorectomy for women who have two or more first degree relatives with ovarian cancer and who have completed childbearing.[53]

Conversely, oral contraceptive use reduces the risk of ovarian cancer by as much as 80% in women age 40 to 59 years. Not only does longer duration of use provide more protection, but the effect lasts for as long as 15 years after oral contraceptives are discontinued.[54] There is a decreased risk of ovarian cancer in women who are chronic anovulators (i.e., polycystic ovary syndrome); protection also is seen with increasing parity and greater duration of lactation. Contraceptive sterilization is associated with a 40% to 50% reduction in the risk of ovarian cancer, and hysterectomy (without oophorectomy) with a 35% reduction.

Ovarian Cancer Screening Techniques

Ovarian cancer typically is diagnosed during an evaluation of a symptomatic woman, but it may be detected as a mass found incidentally during pelvic examination or ultrasound. While early ovarian cancer has been long considered a "silent cancer," a recent study showed that 70% of women recalled having symptoms for 3 months or longer before their diagnosis.[55] Ovarian cancer can be associated with pelvic pain, abdominal discomfort and distention, bloating after meals, indigestion, constipation, nausea, urinary frequency, and irregular vaginal bleeding. In advanced stages, ovarian cancer is often accompanied by fatigue, nonspecific gastrointestinal symptoms, poor appetite and weight loss, increased abdominal girth, or shortness of breath due to pleural effusion. Currently, it appears that the best way to promptly diagnose ovarian cancer is for both the patient and her clinician to have a high index of suspicion when characteristic symptoms occur.

A number of techniques have been suggested to screen for the early stages of asymptomatic ovarian cancer: periodic bimanual pelvic examination, serum CA-125 measurement, and transvaginal ultrasound examination. Conducting a bimanual pelvic examination as part of periodic health examination is inexpensive and safe and may provide valuable information, but it is insensitive, has poor specificity, and has not been found to be cost-effective when the visit and examination are done for the sole purpose of ovarian cancer screening. Screening with the serum tumor marker CA-125 will detect up to 80% of women with advanced non-mucinous ovarian cancers, but the test is only 50% to 70% sensitive for early-stage cancers and has poor specificity (many false positives), which may lead to unnecessary invasive and costly workups. Screening with this test is not cost-effective because of the low prevalence of ovarian cancer and the test's moderate sensitivity, poor specificity, and high cost. Vaginal-probe pelvic ultrasound also has been suggested as a screening test because of its high sensitivity (98%), but it has poor specificity and the highest cost of any of the screening modalities. While there is general agreement that asymptomatic low-risk women should not be screened routinely with any of these interventions, either alone or in combination, many experts believe that they should be offered annually to women who have familial risk factors for ovarian cancer, starting at 25 to 30 years old. The current USPSTF guidelines make the following recommendations regarding ovarian cancer screening:[56]

- Screening asymptomatic women for ovarian cancer with ultrasound, tumor markers, or physical exam is not recommended. [D recommendation]

- There is insufficient evidence to recommend for or against testing in asymptomatic women at increased risk of ovarian cancer. [I recommendation]

BREAST CANCER SCREENING

In 2005, breast cancer was the second leading cause of cancer deaths in women in the United States, accounting for one-third of all cancer cases and 15% of cancer deaths in women (40,400 deaths per year).[10] Incidence rates of breast cancer have increased 1% per year since 1973, although mortality rates have started to fall as a result of earlier diagnosis and improved treatments.[57] A woman's lifetime risk of breast cancer, assuming she lives to old age, is about 1 in 9. Risk factors are helpful indicators of risk, but do not predict the development of breast cancer in the majority of cases. Of women with breast cancer, 21% of women age 30 to 54 years have risk factor(s), as do 29% of women between 55 and 84 years old (Table 22–5).[56] Given the multiplicity of breast cancer risk factors, and their relative contribution to breast cancer risk, it is challenging for a clinician to forecast an individual patient's likelihood of acquiring breast cancer. Two free internet-based programs are available to quickly calculate a patient's breast cancer risk:

The Breast Cancer Risk Assessment Tool, sponsored by the National Cancer Institute, projects a woman's individualized of risk for invasive breast cancer over a 5 year period and her lifetime. It can be found at http://bcra.nci.nih.gov/brc/ or use www.cancer.gov/bcrisktool.

The Detailed Breast Cancer Risk Calculator produces estimates using each of the Gail Model 1 and NSABP model-2. It is located at www.halls.md/breast/risk.htm

BREAST CANCER SCREENING TECHNIQUES

Breast self-examination (BSE). The longstanding recommendation that all adult women practice monthly BSE is now being questioned.[60] Although BSE may provide women with a sense of empowerment and occasionally may result in earlier detection of a breast mass than might occur by coincidence, two very large randomized clinical trials have shown that breast cancer survival is no greater in women who practice BSE than in those who do not. The larger study, involving 266,000 women in Shanghai, China, concluded that BSE actually may cause more hazard than benefit, owing to the many false positives that result from BSE.[61] From a public health standpoint, these studies suggest that financial and educational resources should not be used to implement population-based BSE programs. For individual women, the message in these studies is that a formal, timed regimen of BSE is no more effective in preventing death from breast cancer than the incidental discovery of unusual breast changes. Nonetheless, women still should be counseled to take note of changes in their breasts, and when they occur, and bring the finding to the attention of their clinician.

Table 22–5 Risk characteristics of breast cancer

Factor	High-Risk Group	Low-Risk Group
Relative risk > 4.0		
Age	Old	Young
Country of birth	North America, Northern Europe	Asia, Africa
Two first-degree relatives with breast cancer diagnosed at an early age	Yes	No
History of cancer in one breast	Yes	No
Relative risk = 2.1–4.0		
Nodular densities on mammogram (postmenopausal)	Densities occupy > 75% of breast volume	Parenchyma composed entirely of fat
One first-degree relative with breast cancer	Yes	No
Biopsy-confirmed atypical hyperplasia	Yes	No
High-dose radiation to chest	Yes	No
Oophorectomy before age 35	No	Yes
Relative risk = 1.1–2.0		
Socioeconomic status	High	Low
Place of residence	Urban	Rural
Race/ethnicity: —Breast cancer at ≥ 40 years —Breast cancer at < 40 years	Caucasian Black	Asian Asian
Religion	Jewish	Adventist, Mormon
Age at first full-term pregnancy	≥ 30 years	< 20 years
Age at menarche	< 12 years	> 14 years
Age at menopause	> 55 years	< 45 years
Obesity (postmenopausal)	Obese	Slender
Breastfeeding	None	Several years
Hormonal contraceptives	Yes	No

Source: Hulka BS, et al. (1995)[59]

For women who continue to practice BSE, the optimal time for performing BSE is 1 to 7 days after the end of the menses. Performing the exam after a shower, while the skin still is wet, may improve accuracy. After inspecting her breasts while she is sitting or standing in front of a mirror, the woman should palpate each breast in turn, with her hand on the side of the breast being examined placed behind her head. The objective of BSE is to detect a significant change in the breasts from one month to the next, not necessarily the finding of a dominant nodule.

Clinical Breast Examination (CBE). While most consensus guidelines include CBE as a component of the periodic health examination in adult women, there is disagreement regarding age of initiation and frequency of screening. The USPSTF states that evidence is insufficient to recommend CBE alone (without mammography), while the American Cancer Society recommends that CBE should be performed at least every 3 years from 20 to 39 years old and annually thereafter.[62] CBE is not a highly accurate screening test, having a sensitivity of only 54% and a false positive rate of 6%. However, one benefit of CBE is that about 5% to 15% of breast cancers missed on mammography are found on CBE, the combination thereby improving detection rates. Consequently, CBE should be considered as an adjunct to mammography and offered to all women starting no later than when they are 40 years old.

When performing CBE,[63] examine the breasts while the woman is sitting with her hands on her hips or behind her head. Repeat the exam while the woman is lying down. Examine each breast in vertical strips. Palpate with flat portion of your fingers rather than your fingertips. If a woman has very pendulous breasts, place your hand between her breast and chest wall, then palpate tissue between your hands. Be sure to include the axillary tail of the breast in the examination. Lymph node examination of the supraclavicular and axillary nodes is an integral component of the examination. Draw a diagram in the medical record indicating the position and size of abnormalities, noting that dominant nodules have measurable dimensions, while fibrocystic change does not.

MAMMOGRAPHY

When used as a screening test, the purpose of mammography is to detect pre-clinical breast cancer before a mass can be palpated clinically. Large-scale studies show that in women who receive at least biennial mammograms over a 10-year period, breast cancer mortality is reduced by an average of 24% , with an even greater reduction in women over 50 to 69 years old. The accuracy of mammography as a screening test has improved over the last two decades, resulting in a false-negative rate of 5% to 15% and a false-positive rate of 3% to 6% .

The USPSTF recommends screening mammography every 1 to 2 years for women aged 40 and older,[64] while the American Cancer Society recommends annual mammography beginning at age 40.[62] Both guidelines are in agreement that women 40 to 49 years of age who choose to have screening mammograms should do so annually, given that breast cancer grows more rapidly among younger women and mammograms are more likely to be falsely negative in this age group. However, the benefit of mammography in younger women must be balanced against a lower prevalence of breast cancer among women in their 40s, as well as a higher rate of false positive mammograms because of a greater breast density and a higher likelihood of benign breast conditions.[65-67] When compared to film mammography, digital mammography does have a greater sensitivity for women who are under 50 years old, premenopausal, and those with dense breasts.[68]

For women 50 and older, USPSTF guidelines state there is no advantage of annual over biennial (every other year) screening, because in older women breast cancers grow more slowly than in younger women.[64,69] Additionally, mammography has a lower false negative rate in post-menopausal women, since tumors more are surrounded by fatty tissue and therefore are more detectable. ACS guidelines recommend that women under 40 years of age who have increased risk for breast cancer might benefit from additional screening strategies, including initiation of mammographic screening at 30 years old, shorter screening intervals, and the addition of ultrasound or MRI screening.[65]

A new reporting system for mammogram results, developed by the American College of Radiologists and adopted internationally, is entitled BI-RADS (Breast Imaging Reporting and Data System).[70] The six categories of assessment and management of each are contained in Table 22–6. Women with assessments of BI-RADS 4 or 5 should be referred immediately for breast biopsy. Pay special attention to women with category "zero" results, as they will need to receive additional imaging studies, and those with category 3 results, since they will need further follow-up imaging studies at an interval specified by the radiologist. Women with a BI-RADS a category 3 result who are at increased risk of breast cancer should be referred to a breast specialist.[71]

When used as a diagnostic test in a woman with a breast abnormality, mammography can suggest malignancy at the location of the finding and exclude malignancy elsewhere in the same or opposite breast. In the presence of a dominant breast nodule, a negative diagnostic mammo-

Table 22–6 BI-RADS mammogram reporting system

Category	Assessment	Recommendation
0	Incomplete	Further diagnostic imaging studies needed until a final category can be assigned
1	Negative	Routine screening interval
2	Benign finding	Routine screening interval
3	Probably benign	Follow-up 4–6 months for 2 years (or longer) until stability can be demonstrated
4	Suspicious	Biopsy
5	Highly suspicious	Biopsy

gram does not exclude the diagnosis of breast cancer. In this case, tissue sampling, either by fine-needle aspiration cytology or open biopsy, is the only definitive procedure to exclude cancer.

Useful algorithms describing the management of women with abnormal mammograms and other breast complaints or clinical findings have been developed by the California Department of Health Services and can be found at http://qap.sdsu.edu/screening/breastcancer/bda.[71]

REFERENCES

1. American Medical Association. Periodic health examination: a manual for physicians. Chicago: American Medical Association, 1940.
2. U.S. Preventive Services Task Force. Guide to clinical preventive services: report of the United States Preventive Services Task Force (2nd edition) Baltimore MD: Williams & Wilkins, 1996.
3. ACOG Committee Opinion. Primary and preventive care: periodic assessments. Obstet Gynecol. 2003 Nov;102 (5 Pt 1):1117–24.
4. Eyre H, Kahn R, et.al. Preventing cancer, cardiovascular disease, and diabetes: a common agenda for the American Cancer Society, the American Diabetes Association, and the American Heart Association. CA Cancer J Clin. 2004 Jul-Aug;54(4):190–207.
5. Stewart FH, Harper CC, Ellertson CE, Grimes DA, Sawaya GF, Trussell J. Clinical breast and pelvic examination requirements for hormonal contraception: Current practice vs. evidence. JAMA 2001;285(17):2232–9.
6. Grimes DA. Over-the-counter oral contraceptives—an immodest proposal? [editorial]. Am J Public Health 1993;83:1092–1094.
7. Trussell J, Stewart F, Potts M, Guest F, Ellertson C. Should oral contraceptives be available without prescription? Am J Public Health 1993;83:1094–1099.
8. World Health Organization, Selected practice recommendations for contraceptive use, 2nd edition 2004. Accessed at http://whqlibdoc.who.int/publications/2004/9241562846.pdf
9. Koss LG. The Papanicolaou test for cervical cancer detection. A triumph and a tragedy. JAMA 1989;261:737–743.
10. F. Jemal A, Murray T, et.al. Cancer Statistics 2005 CA A Cancer Journal for Clinicians 2005;55:10–30
11. Harlan LC, Bernstein AB, Kessler LG. Cervical cancer screening: who is not screened and why? Am J Public Health 1991;81:885–891.
12. Kristensen GB, Skyggebjerg KD, Holund B, et. al. Analysis of cervical smears obtained within 3 years of the diagnosis of invasive cervical cancer. Acta Cytol 1991;35: 47–50.
13. Hessling JJ, et al. Effectiveness of thin-layer preparations vs. conventional Pap smears in a blinded split-sample study. Extended cytologic evaluation. J Repro Med 2001;46:880–886.
14. Wertlake P. Results of AutoPap system-assisted and manual cytologic screen comparison. J Reprod Med 1999;44:11–17.
15. Hutchinson ML. Assessing the costs and benefits of alternative rescreening strategies [editorial]. Acta Cytol 1996;40–48.
16. Sawaya GF, Grimes DA. New technologies in cervical cytology screening: A word of caution. Obstet Gynecol 1999; 94:304–307.
17. Munoz N, Bosch FX, de Sanjose S, Herrero R, et al. Epidemiologic classification of human papillomavirus types associated with cervical cancer. N Eng J Med 2003; 348:518–527.

18. Brinton LA, Schairer C, Haenszel W, Stolley P, Lehman HF, Levine R, Savitz DA. Cigarette smoking and invasive cervical cancer. JAMA 1986;225(23):3265–3269.
19. Winkelstein W, Jr. Smoking and cervical cancer—current status: a review. Am J Epidemiol 1990;131:945–957.
20. Ho, GY et. al. Natural history of cervicovaginal HPV in young women. NEJM 1998;338:423.
21. Moscicki, et. al. The Natural History of HPV Infection as Measured by Repeated DNA Testing in Adolescent and Young Women. J Pediatrics 1998;132:277.
22. Centers for Disease Control and Prevention. Sexually transmitted diseases treatment guidelines 2002. Centers for Disease Control and Prevention. MMWR Recomm Rep. 2002 May 10;51(RR-6):1–78.
23. Centers for Disease Control. Black-white differences in cervical cancer mortality— United States, 1980–1987. MMWR 1990;39:245–248.
24. Korn AP, Landers DV. Gynecologic disease in women infected with human immunodeficiency virus type 1. J Acq Immune Defic Syndr Hum Retrovirol 1995;9:361–370.
25. Korn AP, Autry M, DeRemer PA, Tan W. Sensitivity of the Papanicolaou smear in HIV-infected women. Obstet Gynecol 1994;83:401–404.
26. Adachi A, Fleming I, Burk RD, Ho GY, Klein RS. Women with human immunodeficiency virus infection and abnormal Papanicolaou smears, a prospective study of colposcopy and clinical outcome. Obstet Gynecol 1993;81:372–377.
27. Wright TC, Koulos J, Schnoll F, Swanbeck J, Ellerbrock T, Chaisson M, Richart RM. Cervical intraepithelial neoplasia in women infected with the human immunodeficiency virus: outcome after loop electrosurgical excision. Gynecol Oncol 1994;55:253–258.
28. Centers for Disease Control. 1993 revised classification system for HIV infection and expanded surveillance case definition for AIDS among adolescents and adults. MMWR 1992;41(RR-17):1–19.
29. Amies AM, Miller L, Lee SK, Koutsky L. The effect of vaginal speculum lubrication on the rate of unsatisfactory cervical cytology diagnosis. Obstet Gynecol. 2002 Nov;100(5 Pt 1):889–92.
30. Department of Health and Human Services. Improving the quality of clinician Pap smear technique and management, client Pap smear education, and the evaluation of Pap smear laboratory testing: a resource guide for Title X family planning projects. Washington DC: U.S. Department of Health and Human Services, Public Health Service, Office of Population Affairs, Office of Family Planning, 1989:3–4, 59.
31. Frame PS, Frame JS. Determinants of cancer screening frequency: the example of screening for cervical cancer. J Am Board Fam Pract 1998 Mar-Apr;11(2):87–95.
32. Saslow D, Roncowicz CD, et al. American Cancer Society Guideline for the Detection of Cervical Neoplasia and Cancer. CA Cancer J Clin 2002;52:342–362.
33. U.S. Preventive Services Task Force, Screening for Cervical Cancer. 2003. Accessed at www.ahcpr.gov/clinic/uspstf/uspscerv.htm.
34. ACOG Committee on Practice Bulletins. ACOG Practice Bulletin: clinical management guidelines for obstetrician-gynecologists. Number 45, August 2003. Cervical cytology screening. Obstet Gynecol 2003 Aug;102(2):417–27
35. Sawaya GF. A 21-year-old woman with atypical squamous cells of undetermined significance. JAMA 2005;294:2210–2218
36. Rolnick SJ, LaFerla JJ, Jackson J, Akkerman D, Compo R. Impact of a new cervical Pap smear screening guideline on member perceptions and comfort levels. Prev Med 1999 May;28(5):530–534.
37. Schwartz LM, Woloshin S, Fowler FJ Jr, Welch HG. Enthusiasm for cancer screening in the United States. JAMA 2004 Jan 7;291(1):71–8.
38. Sirovich BE, Woloshin S, Schwartz LM. Screening for cervical cancer: will women accept less? Am J Med 2005 Feb;118(2):151–8.

39. Sawaya GF, McConnell KJ, Kulasingam SL, Lawson HW, et al. Risk of cervical cancer associated with extending the interval between cervical-cancer screenings. N Engl J Med 2003 Oct 16;349(16):1501–9.

40. Wright TC Jr, Schiffman M, Solomon D, Cox JT, Garcia F, Goldie S, Hatch K, Noller KL, Roach N, Runowicz C, Saslow D. Interim guidance for the use of human papillomavirus DNA testing as an adjunct to cervical cytology for screening. Obstet Gynecol 2004 Feb;103(2):304–9.

41. Solomon D, Davey D, et al. The 2001 Bethesda System: terminology for reporting results of cervical cytology. JAMA 2002;287:2114–2119.

42. Kivlahan C, Ingram E. Papanicolaou smears without endocervical cells. Are they inadequate? Acta Cytol 1986;30:258–260.

43. Ransdell JS, Davey DD, Zalesky S. Clinicopathologic correlation of the unsatisfactory Papanicolaou smear. Cancer 1997;81:139–143.

44. Krieger JN, Tam MR, Stevens CE, et al. Diagnosis of trichomoniasis: comparison of conventional wet mount examination with cytologic studies, cultures, and monoclonal antibody staining of direct specimens. JAMA 1988;259:1223–1227.

45. Reiter RC. Management of initial atypical cervical cytology: a randomized, prospective study. Obstet Gynecol 1986;68:237–240.

46. Kinney WK, Manos MM, Hurley LB, et al. Where's the high grade cervical neoplasia? the importance of minimally abnormal Papanicolaou diagnoses. Obstet Gynecol 1998;91:973–976.

47. Wright TC, Cox JT, et al. 2001 Consensus guidelines for the management of women with cervical cytological abnormalities. JAMA 2002;287:2120–2129. May be accessed at www.asccp.org/consensus/cytological.shtml.

48. American College of Obstetricians and Gynecologists, ACOG Practice Bulletin: Management of abnormal cervical cytology and histology. Obstet Gynecol 2005;106:645–664

49. Hurt WG, Silverberg SG, Frable WJ, Belgrad R, Crooks LD. Adenocarcinoma of the cervix: histopathologic and clinical features. Am J Obstet Gynecol 1977;129:304–315.

50. Wright TC, Cox JT, et al. 2001 consensus guidelines for the management of women with cervical intraepithelial neoplasia. Am J Obstet Gynecol 2003;189:295–304.

51. American Society for Colposcopy and Cervical Pathology. Algorithms from the consensus guidelines for the management of women with histological abnormalities, 2003. Accessed at: www.asccp.org/consensus/histological.shtml.

52. Whittemore AS, Harris R, Itnyre J. Characteristics relating to ovarian cancer risk. Collaborative analysis of 12 US case-control studies. II. Invasive epithelial ovarian cancers in white women. Am J Epidemiol 1992;136:1184–1203.

53. National Institute of Health Consensus Development Panel on Ovarian Cancer, NIH consensus conference. Ovarian cancer. Screening, treatment, and follow up. JAMA 1995;273:491–497.

54. Rosenberg L, Palmer JR, Zauber AG. A case control study of oral contraceptive use and invasive epithelial ovarian cancer. Am J Epidemiol 1994;139:654–661.

55. American College of Obstetricians and Gynecologists Committee on Gynecologic Practice. The role of the generalist obstetrician-gynecologist in the early detection of ovarian cancer. ACOG Committee Opinion number 280. Obstet Gynecol 2002;100:1413–1415.

56. U.S. Preventive Services Task Force, Screening for Ovarian Cancer, May 2004. Accessed at www.ahcpr.gov/clinic/uspstf/uspsovar.htm.

57. Berry DA, Cronin KA, Plevritis SK, Fryback DG, et al. and Cancer Intervention and Surveillance Modeling Network (CISNET) Collaborators. Effect of screening and adjuvant therapy on mortality from breast cancer. N Engl J Med. 2005 Oct 27;353(17):1784–92.

58. Hoskins KF, Stopfer JE, Calzone KA, et. al. Assessment and counseling for women with a family history of breast cancer: a guide for clinicians. JAMA 1995;273:577–585.

59. Hulka, BS, Stark AT. Breast cancer: cause and prevention. Lancet 1995;346:883–887.

60. Ellman R, Moss SM, Coleman D, et al. Breast self-examination programmes in the trial of early detection of breast cancer: ten year findings. Br J Cancer 1993;65:208.

61. Thomas DB, Gao DL, Self SG, et al. Randomized trial of breast self-examination in Shanghai. Final Results. J Natl Cancer Inst 2002;94:1445–1457.

62. Smith RA, Cokkinides V. Eyre HJ. American Cancer Society guidelines for early detection of cancer 2006. CA Cancer J Clin 2006;56:11–25

63. Barton MB, Harris R, Fletcher S. Does this patient have breast cancer? The screening clinical breast exam: should it be done? How? JAMA 1999;282:1270.

64. U.S. Preventive Services Taskforce. Screening for Breast Cancer; 2002 Release. Accessed at www.ahcpr.gov/clinic/uspstf/uspsbrca.htm.

65. Smith RA, Saslow D, et al. American Cancer Society guidelines for breast cancer screening: Update 2003. CA Cancer J Clin 2003;54:141–169.

66. Esserman L, Kerlikowski K. Should we recommend screening mammography to women aged 40–49? Oncology 1996; 10:357–364.

67. Kerlikowski K, Grady D, Barclay J, Sickles E, Ernster V. Effect of age, breast density, and family history on the sensitivity of first screening mammography. JAMA 1996;276:33–38.

68. Pisano ED, Gatsonis C, Hendrick E, Yaffe M, et al. and Digital Mammographic Imaging Screening Trial (DMIST) Investigators Group. Diagnostic performance of digital versus film mammography for breast-cancer screening. N Engl J Med. 2005 Oct 27;353(17):1773–83

69. Wai ES, D'yachkova Y, Olivotto IA, Tyldesley S, et al. Comparison of 1- and 2-year screening intervals for women undergoing screening mammography. Br J Cancer. 2005 Mar 14;92(5):961–6.

70. Liberman, A.F. Abramson, F.B. Squires et al. The Breast Imaging Reporting and Data System: positive predictive value of mammographic features and final assessment categories. AJR 171 (1998), 35–40.

71. Cancer Clinical Services Quality Assurance Project. Breast diagnostic algorithms for primary care clinicians, 2005. Accessed at http://qap.sdsu.edu/screening/breastcancer/bda/index.html.

LATE REFERENCE

72. Villa LL, Costa RL, Petta CA, et al. Prophylactic quadrivalent human papillomavirus (types 6, 11, 16, and 18) L1 virus-like particle vaccine in young women: a randomised double-blind placebo-controlled multicentre phase II efficacy trial. Lancet Oncol. 2005 May;6(5):271–8.

Pregnancy Testing and Management of Early Pregnancy

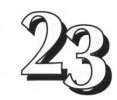

Mary Fjerstad, NP
Felicia Stewart, MD

- Providing immediate scheduling for a pregnancy confirmation exam, as soon as the woman suspects she may be pregnant, is an essential family planning service.

- With early pregnancy diagnosis, a woman planning to continue her pregnancy can begin prenatal precautions and medical care during the early, most vulnerable stages of fetal development.

- A woman considering abortion will have time for adequate counseling and decision making. Abortion can be performed when it is safest—early in pregnancy. A woman considering medication abortion will be able to arrange for care within the first 9 weeks following her last normal menstrual period, when this option is possible. In the context of this chapter, medication abortion refers to abortion in the first 9 weeks of pregnancy dated from the last menstrual period (LMP), provided with mifepristone and misoprostol.

- Early pregnancy diagnosis helps ensure that ectopic pregnancy can be detected early. Early detection reduces the risk of life-threatening ectopic pregnancy complications. Early diagnosis and treatment are more likely to preserve the affected fallopian tube.

Optimal pregnancy outcomes for both mother and fetus depend on advance planning to provide the best environment for conception and pregnancy. All women and men need to know about pre-pregnancy health measures long before a pregnancy occurs. These measures include steps to protect future fertility and maintain good general health as well as steps needed when a woman contemplates pregnancy in the near future. Pregnancy affords an important opportunity to encourage women to adopt healthier behaviors. For example the 22% of women who smoke and 20% who drink alcohol can improve their chances for a healthy baby by stopping (or reducing) these exposures.

Prevention of reproductive tract infections before and during pregnancy is an important priority. Infections can cause infertility or ectopic pregnancy, and if present during pregnancy, pose multiple risks to mother, fetus, and neonate. For some women, pregnancy is an important time to use condoms. Correct and consistent use is vital. Every effort should be made to avoid primary Herpes Type 1 or 2 infection during pregnancy as well as the acquisition of HIV, syphilis, gonorrhea, hepatitis, or chlamydia.

Offer clinical assessment and pregnancy testing as soon as the patient seeks these services. Promptly evaluate and refer if the woman wishes to consider abortion, especially medication abortion (see Chapter 2 on Abortion), which is provided only during the very first weeks of pregnancy—the first 63 days following the woman's last normal menstrual period. Pregnancy is not likely to be suspected or confirmed before day 28, when the woman's next period is due. That means the interval for pregnancy confirmation, referral, and provision of medication abortion is short, only 35 days. A delay in scheduling a visit is obviously not wise.

ESSENTIAL PRE-PREGNANCY INFORMATION FOR EVERYONE

A pregnancy test visit as well as every family planning visit or routine periodic exam is an opportunity to provide preconception education and care. Ask each patient about plans for pregnancy in the future. Counsel about effective contraceptive use; how an optimal pregnancy outcome is correlated with its intendedness and the woman's ability to prepare in advance. Assess lifestyle and personal health risk factors. If appropriate, provide screening and offer preventive services (Table 23–1). Check for diabetes in any woman with risk factors such as family history of diabetes, obesity, or abnormal sugar levels during a prior pregnancy. Diabetes is common and often unsuspected. Poor control of blood sugar during the very early weeks of pregnancy is associated with a marked increase in risk for fetal abnormality.[2]

Some situations pose unique opportune "teachable moments," when education about optimal pregnancy is likely to be directly relevant to the patient:

- A negative pregnancy test result
- Diagnosis and management of a reproductive tract infection
- Identification of possible risk of infection with the human immunodeficiency virus (HIV)

Table 23–1 Pre-pregnancy health precautions

Avoidance of toxic exposure	Tobacco, alcohol, and illicit drugs are potentially toxic to fetal development. Minimize caffeine intake. Avoid exposure to abdominal x-ray and to potentially toxic chemicals.
Folic acid (prenatal vitamin) intake	Reduce the risk for neural tube defects such as spina bifida, beginning several months before pregnancy, by taking a vitamin that contains at least 400 micrograms (mcg) of folic acid (folate) every day. Cereals, breads and vitamins are usually fortified with folic acid.
A healthy diet is a top priority	Dieting for weight-loss is not recommended during pregnancy. A well-balanced diet includes fresh fruits and vegetables. Ensure a total intake of 1500 mg calcium; drink 3 glasses of milk daily or take calcium supplements. Do not eat fish that may contain high levels of methyl mercury such as shark, swordfish, king mackerel, tilefish, and fish from non-commercial sources. Eat no more than 6 ounces of canned tuna per week, and no more than one serving of farm-raised salmon per month.
All medications should be reviewed with a clinician	All prescription and non-prescription drugs such as pain remedies (ibuprofen) and medications for seizures as well as herbal or other remedies should be reviewed with the clinician providing prenatal care. Avoid megadoses of anything, including vitamins.
Review immunization status	Immunizations should be up to date, especially rubella, rubeola, varicella, Hepatitis B, and polio; ideally, these immunizations will be provided at least three months before conception.
Medical and family history review of the pregnant woman and the baby's father	If either the pregnant woman or the baby's father has a family history of genetic abnormalities (e.g., cystic fibrosis or sickle cell anemia), counseling or testing may be helpful. Discuss serious medical problems before the pregnancy. Diabetic patients need careful management before and during early pregnancy to reduce the risks of birth defects.
Elevated body temperature or fever	Avoid exposure to contagious illnesses like flu, or activities such as sauna or hot tubs that might elevate core body temperature, which can increase the risk of abnormal fetal development.
Review menstrual cycle dates	Review the record of the first day of each menstrual period to help determine the pregnancy due date accurately. This is especially important if tests are needed during pregnancy or if labor induction or a C-section will be indicated.
Sexually transmitted infection (STI)	Prior to conception and during pregnancy, the pregnant woman should avoid intercourse or use condoms carefully if there is any chance at all of STI exposure; infection such as herpes, syphilis, gonorrhea, chlamydia, or HIV/AIDS acquired during pregnancy is a very serious risk for the fetus. Get testing and treatment promptly for any symptoms that suggest an STI.

(continued)

Table 23–1 Pre-pregnancy health precautions—*(cont'd)*

Toxoplasmosis, Listeriosis and other uncommon infectious organisms	Acquiring toxoplasmosis infection during pregnancy is a serious risk for the fetus; avoid handling kitty litter (someone else should empty it every day), wear gloves for handling soil outdoors and wash your hands with soap and water after gardening. Also avoid eating raw meat or fish, or drinking unpasteurized milk or cheese. Avoid certain soft cheeses such as feta, brie, Camembert, Roquefort, queso blanco, queso fresco or Panela unless the label states they are made with pasteurized milk.
Confirm pregnancy early	When you think you may be pregnant, if you can't get an appointment to be tested and examined within two weeks of missing a period, do a home pregnancy test. Follow the instructions carefully. If the home pregnancy test is positive, or you have any pregnancy symptoms (even if the home pregnancy test was negative), make an appointment to be tested and examined in the health center as soon as possible.

- Diagnosis of a reproductive tract abnormality
- Identification of a substance abuse problem
- Diagnosis of a significant medical problem

In each of these situations, provide information about the possible consequences and discuss planning for an optimal future pregnancy.

If pregnancy occurs accidentally, the opportunity to prepare is lost; this is one of the important health reasons for avoiding unintended pregnancy. Integration of preconception care into routine gynecological services is recommended to assure systematic review of a medical history, completion of recommended screening tests and immunizations, and planning for pregnancy care, including initiation of folic acid.[1]

Negative pregnancy test visits are a common and under-exploited opportunity for intervention. As many as one-quarter of all adolescent girls who conceive have previously had one or more visits to learn that their pregnancy test was negative.[3] Clearly, this is a group at high risk for unintended pregnancy.

PRECONCEPTION CARE SERVICES

A preconception care visit offers services and education to help a woman improve her lifestyle and health habits. Risk assessment identifies the woman at risk for a poor pregnancy outcome or for whom pregnancy will endanger her health. Screening tests reveal a mother's underlying medical and genetic conditions that may require medical intervention or may require her to make a decision about how to manage a pregnancy or whether to even attempt carrying a pregnancy. Identify health problems that indicate caution in undertaking aerobic exercise

Table 23–2 The preconception care visit

Action	Risk Reduction
Review contraceptive use	Prevent unintended pregnancy
Supplement with folic acid	Decrease risk of neural tube defects
Improve nutrition and fitness	Decrease risk of pregnancy loss Improve maternal health and well-being Decrease risk of low-birthweight infant and congenital anomalies
Advise smoking cessation (or at least a decrease in # of cigarettes smoked)	Decrease risk of pregnancy loss Increase birth weight
Advise abstinence from alcohol	Prevent fetal alcohol syndrome
Screen for HIV infection	Decrease perinatal transmission by giving antiretroviral medication treatment Avoid transmission via breast milk
Screen for hepatitis B	Protect the neonate from infection by administering vaccine and by using condoms
Screen for other sexually transmissible infections	Protect maternal fertility Prevent fetal and neonatal infection
Immunize	Prevent vaccine-preventable infections
Control diabetes	Decrease risk of congenital anomalies
Counsel about domestic violence	Prevent injuries
Screen for genetic diseases	Provide choices about pregnancy outcome
Review psychosocial status	Improve emotional support and well-being

during pregnancy. Encourage exercise in pregnancy as long as there is no trauma to the uterus and the level of exertion is moderate. Test women for rubella at the first prenatal visit. Women without immunity to rubella should be immunized and should wait three months after immunization to become pregnant.

Early pregnancy diagnosis is an essential part of every family planning program. Screening very early in pregnancy can avert serious complications and provide the pregnant woman with an opportunity to learn about precautions needed during pregnancy and prenatal care resources, or about options for abortion care. Early evaluation also provides an opportunity to screen for infection with the human immunodeficiency virus (HIV). Nonjudgmental, supportive counseling and information are also important, including accurate and specific referral options for abortion, adoption services, and prenatal care.

Inexpensive pregnancy test kits, sensitive enough to provide accurate results for most women by 28 days since the last menstrual period

(LMP), are widely available and simple to use. Thus, there is no reason to impose an arbitrary delay in pregnancy evaluation based on the date of the woman's last menstrual period. Clinical assessment and pregnancy testing should be offered as soon as the patient seeks these services. When there is concern about a possible pregnancy, retesting a week later even after a negative pregnancy test is essential. Promptly evaluate and refer women who wish to consider medication abortion (see Chapter 24 on Abortion), which is provided only during the first 9 weeks of pregnancy.

In addition to a preconception care visit, some couples need referral for more detailed evaluation and counseling by a genetics specialist or perinatologist. Arrange a referral well in advance to allow time for testing or planning for prenatal testing during the first trimester for persons with the following conditions:[2,4]

- The woman is age 35 or older.

- Either partner has had a child with a birth defect or cystic fibrosis.

- Either partner has a birth defect, genetic disorder, cystic fibrosis, chromosome abnormality, or has a family history of birth defects or genetic disorders.

- Either partner's ethnicity indicates risk for genetic diseases such as Tay Sachs disease (Ashkenazic Jewish, French Canadian), sickle cell anemia (African-American), or thalassemia (Mediterranean ancestry) if carrier status is not already known.

- Either partner has previously experienced three or more pregnancies ending in spontaneous abortion.

- The woman has a serious medical condition.

PREGNANCY EVALUATION

The clinical evaluation for a woman who may be pregnant should include a review of pertinent history and symptoms, and an exam and/or lab tests to confirm pregnancy and provide accurate pregnancy dates. In most though not all cases, the last menstrual period date provides an accurate estimate of gestational age. A pelvic exam can confirm pregnancy test results and correlate uterine enlargement with menstrual dates. The pelvic exam is essential in identifying the possibility of abnormal pregnancy or uterine abnormalities (i.e., fibroids, etc.). Pregnancy diagnosis has several goals:

1. Determine whether or not the woman is pregnant.

2. Identify possible problems that require further evaluation (such as threatened abortion) or urgent intervention, such as ectopic gestation.

3. Assess gestational age accurately (in days or weeks).

4. Help the patient make and implement her own plans for prenatal care or abortion.

5. Screen for Chlamydia. Screening for gonorrhea is also indicated if the woman is at high risk because of high community prevalence or exposure to multiple partners. Screen for HIV and syphilis if indicated. Screen even if the patient is considering abortion, because these infections are statistically associated with an increased risk of post-abortal infection.

Definitions used for dating the pregnancy and timing early pregnancy events.   Menstrual age dates the pregnancy beginning from the first day of the LMP. Menstrual age is stated in days LMP or weeks LMP. The normal pregnancy duration is 40 menstrual weeks. The term gestational age is often used interchangeably with menstrual age. When the actual date of conception is known (e.g., as in assisted fertility), the pregnancy can be dated according to conceptual age. Assuming that a woman ovulates mid-cycle, the conceptual age of a full-term pregnancy is 38 weeks. This chapter will refer to pregnancy dating with the terms 'LMP' or 'menstrual age.'

Figure 23–1 provides a visual format for landmarks in very early pregnancy.

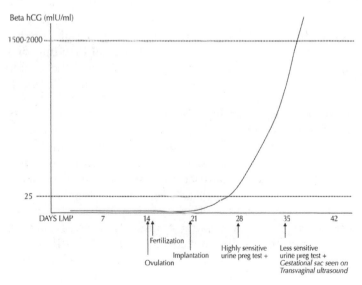

Figure 23–1 Very early pregnancy timeline (based on 28-day cycle)

Fertilization of the ovum (egg) by sperm occurs within the fimbria of the fallopian tube (distal end). The embryo (fertilized egg) moves through the tube to the uterus over the next 5 days to become a blastocyst. By the end of the 3rd week (21 days LMP), the blastocyst begins to implant into the thickened endometrium. The tissue of the blastocyst is divided into two important layers. The trophoblast, the outer cell layer, eventually forms the chorionic membranes and the placenta. As trophoblastic cells form placental tissue, the placental tissue produces human chorionic gonadotropin hormone (hCG). The inner cell layer of the blastocyst develops into the embryo, amnion, umbilical cord, and primary and secondary yolk sacs.

History and symptoms. The most common sign that prompts a woman to seek pregnancy evaluation is an overdue menstrual period. Often the woman herself suspects pregnancy or has reason to believe that she could be pregnant. A particularly useful question to ask is simply: Do you think you are pregnant now? An unusually light or mistimed period may mean fertilization actually occurred before the LMP, and for this reason, the date of the previous menstrual period (PMP) should be determined. The date when pregnancy symptoms began can help corroborate the fertilization date. Breast tenderness and nipple sensitivity typically begin around 3 to 4 weeks LMP; fatigue, nausea, and urinary frequency at 4 weeks LMP.

Bleeding, spotting, or lower abdominal pain may signal ectopic gestation or threatened spontaneous abortion. An abnormally light menses may also indicate an ectopic pregnancy. Note that women who have had a previous ectopic pregnancy may seek evaluation slightly earlier in pregnancy than do women experiencing a first ectopic pregnancy, so they are less likely to have experienced abnormal bleeding or spotting that could indicate a possible ectopic location with the current pregnancy.[5]

However, an episode of light bleeding can also occur in the early weeks of a normal, continuing pregnancy. The early pregnancy (blastocyst) becomes fully imbedded in the uterine myometrium during the 4th week LMP. As trophoblastic tissue invades the endometrium, vaginal bleeding may occur and be confused clinically with menstrual bleeding.[6]

Physical examination. Cervical softening and uterine softening are early signs of pregnancy, appearing around the time of the first missed menses. If the uterine size does not correspond to the estimated length of gestation based on last menstrual period, consider the possible reasons for the discrepancy (Table 23–3). Ultrasound evaluation often is helpful in this situation.

Table 23–3 Possible reasons for discrepancy between uterine size and menstrual dates

Uterus Smaller Than Expected	Uterus Larger Than Expected
Fertilization later than dates suggest	Fertilization earlier than dates suggest
Ectopic pregnancy	Uterine leiomyomata (fibroids)
Incomplete or missed, spontaneous abortion	Twin gestation
Error in pregnancy test	Hydatidiform mole*
Uterine anomaly (i.e., unicollate uterus)	

* In 28% of molar pregnancies, uterine size is larger than expected; in 14%, the uterus is smaller than expected, and in the rest, the uterus is normal size for dates.[7]

BETA HCG LEVELS IN PREGNANCY

Pregnancy tests detect the beta subunit of hCG in a pregnant woman's urine or serum. Elevated beta hCG can be detected in the woman's serum at low levels as early as 21 days LMP, very soon after implantation occurs. Serum level of hCG reaches 50 to 250 mIU/ml by the time of the first missed menstrual period; hCG reaches a peak approximately at approximately 10 to 12 weeks LMP and then declines to a plateau that is maintained until delivery (Figure 23–2).

The original data regarding doubling time of beta hCG levels was derived from a population of women receiving fertility treatment when timing of ovulation was known. A linear pattern of beta hCG rise was identified for the first 30 days of gestation (30 days from ovulation) with

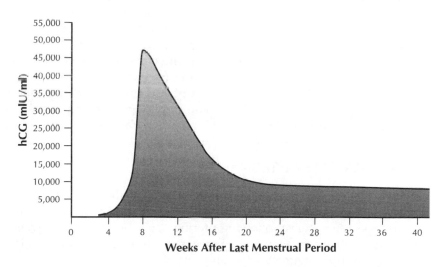

Source Braunstein (1976)[8] with permission.

Figure 23–2 hCG levels during normal pregnancy

a doubling time of 2.2 days.[9] However, for most women, the precise timing of ovulation is not known.

The mean increase of hCG levels for an early viable intrauterine pregnancy is 124% in 2 days. Levels of hCG can rise as rapidly as 81% in 1 day, 228% in 2 days and nearly a 10-fold increase in 4 days. The lower limit of normal is a 53% rise in 2 days.[10] A rise slower than this indicates that the gestation is experiencing abnormal growth, but it does not determine the location of the pregnancy; slower-than-normal beta hCG rise may be seen both in an ectopic or a failing intrauterine pregnancy.

In abnormal pregnancies, hCG levels often increase abnormally, plateau, or decrease. Elevated levels are normal with a multiple gestation, reflecting the increased placental mass. Extremely high hCG production, with hCG levels as high as one million mIU/ml, can occur with a molar pregnancy (hydatidiform mole or gestational trophoblastic disease). Abnormally low hCG levels often occur before a spontaneous abortion or with an ectopic pregnancy. The rate of rise of beta hCG in ectopic pregnancy generally is lower than for intrauterine pregnancies, but the curves overlap. Beta hCG patterns in ectopic pregnancy will be discussed in more detail later in the chapter in the section, Managing Problems in Early Pregnancy. Until the location and status of the pregnancy are confirmed, follow the hCG levels until the curve is outside of that expected, a definite diagnosis is made by ultrasound, the patient becomes symptomatic, or the hCG values fall to non-pregnant levels.

Low levels of beta hCG may simply indicate that a normal pregnancy is earlier in gestation than menstrual dates suggest. A single beta hCG result alone is usually not meaningful; assess the *pattern* of rise, fall, or plateau in combination with the clinical picture, sonogram (if performed), and risk factors for ectopic pregnancy. (See Table 23–6, Risk Factors for Ectopic Pregnancy.) Following the clinical course of a stable patient when the location and status of the pregnancy are unknown is both art and science because interruption of a desired pregnancy that is viable and intrauterine should be avoided, yet it is also imperative to avoid evolution of ectopic pregnancy to the point of rupture.

hCG LEVELS AFTER PREGNANCY

After a pregnancy is terminated by delivery or abortion, blood and urine hCG levels gradually decrease. Figure 23–3 below represents the hCG disappearance curve following uterine aspiration at 7 to 13 weeks (upper curve), miscarriage at 6 to 15 weeks (middle curve), and surgical treatment of ectopic pregnancy (bottom curve).

The initial decrease in beta hCG (β hCG) after full-term delivery is quite rapid, so that an hCG level following the delivery will have

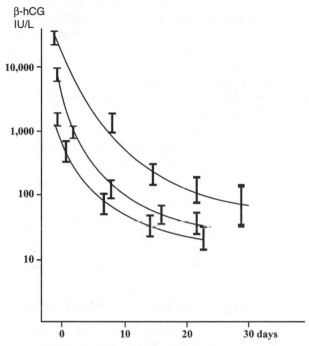

Disappearance curves of serum β hCG in three groups of women. Semilogarithmic scale. Upper curve represents women (n=36) who had elective vacuum aspiration abortion at 7–13 weeks LMP. Middle curve represents women (n=35) with spontaneous abortion at 6–15 weeks LMP treated with uterine aspiration. Lower curve represents women (n=35) with ectopic pregnancies diagnosed 2.5–11.0 weeks after LMP and removed surgically.

Source: Steier et al. (1984)[11] with permission.

Figure 23–3 Disappearance curve of hCG after abortion, miscarriage and surgical treatment of ectopic pregnancy

dropped to less than 50 mIU within 2 weeks, and hCG will be undetectable after 3 to 4 weeks.[12] In the case of first-trimester abortion, if hCG is clearing normally from the bloodstream as expected, the hCG level should decline steadily, halving at least every 48 hours. However, initial hCG levels are at the peak at 8 to 10 weeks LMP, as high as 150,000 mIU; therefore even 2 weeks after first trimester abortion, the hCG levels may still be 1,500 mIU, high enough that all pregnancy tests will still be positive. hCG is likely to be detectable by sensitive tests, including commonly-bused office urine test kits, for as long as 60 days after first-trimester abortion.[13]

When patients have medication abortion, beta hCG continues to increase following mifepristone but then declines precipitously after administration of misoprostol.[14] By the first follow-up visit 5–17 days after taking mifepristone, beta hCG levels drop to 20% of the initial value (measured on the day of mifepristone) in 98.5% of successful medication abortions.[15] In contrast to the usual pattern of sharp drop in hCG after medication abortion, it is possible for hCG levels to have a lengthy plateau even though the patient has a clinically normal course without need for surgical intervention. Patients who require surgical intervention less than 15 days after medical abortion due to prolonged bleeding or pain generally have higher absolute and relative beta hCG values than women with normal courses whose beta hCG values drop sharply. However, there is an overlap in absolute and relative beta hCG values between patients with lengthy plateau who in the end have successful medication abortion and those who will require uterine aspiration.[14] Beta hCG measurement is merely a supplement to the general clinical evaluation in determining whether intervention is indicated.

If intrauterine pregnancy continues to evolve after medication or surgical abortion, an upward trend (mean 124% rise, minimum 53% rise in 2 days)[10] will be seen in serial quantitative beta hCG values. If an ectopic pregnancy continues to evolve after medication or surgical abortion, beta hCG values can behave erratically; these patterns are discussed in more detail in the section, Managing Problems in Early Pregnancy.

HORMONE STRUCTURE AND PREGNANCY TEST DESIGN

hCG is closely related in molecular structure to the pituitary hormones LH (luteinizing hormone), FSH (follicle stimulating hormone), and TSH (thyroid stimulating hormone). Each is composed of an alpha and a beta subunit. The alpha subunits of LH, FSH, TSH, and hCG are virtually identical, but the beta subunits are unique. Therefore, only a test that selectively identifies the beta subunit of hCG or its unique molecular conformation is specific for hCG.

Highly sensitive urine pregnancy tests commonly used for office or home tests are specific for hCG, and so is the quantitative serum hCG determination in the laboratory. Less sensitive urine pregnancy tests, however, detect whole molecule hCG rather than the beta subunit and therefore show at least some cross-reactivity with LH since their beta units are almost identical.

PREGNANCY TEST OPTIONS

It is important to understand every test used in your setting, including the sensitivity of the test, the correct procedure for performing the test, and the number of minutes required for the test to register positive or negative results.

HIGHLY SENSITIVE URINE PREGNANCY TESTS

- For home or office use
- Clinical Laboratory Improvement Amendment (CLIA) waived

Table 23–4 Examples of pregnancy tests

Type of test	Level of Sensitivity (mIU/ml)	Manufacturer
Highly sensitive urine pregnancy tests	*20–25 mIU/ml*	
Examples:		
• ICON 25 hCG	25	ICON
• Quick Vue One Step hCG	25	Quidel
• One Step dBest Strip & Casette		
3 min	20	Ameritek
3–5 min	10	
Less sensitive urine pregnancy tests		
Examples:		
CLIA moderate-complexity tests:		
• Pregnicol 2000	1500–2000	Immunostics
• UCG-Slide Test	2000	Wampole
• Pregna-Cert	2000	Diagnostic Specialties
CLIA-waived tests:		
• DTG-2000	2000	Diagnostic Test Group

Highly sensitive urine pregnancy tests are specific for the beta subunit of hCG, so cross-reaction with other hormones is not a problem. Some test kits, which may also be suitable for clinic use, are available without prescription for home use.

Specificity and sensitivity. Highly sensitive urine pregnancy tests provide accurate qualitative (positive/negative) results with hCG levels as low as 5 to 50 mIU/ml, depending on the specific test kit. With a urine test kit with a sensitivity of 25 mIU/ml, results are positive for some women as early as 24 days LMP; test results are positive for 98% of women within 28 days LMP.[16] This is generally true for those women with 28-day cycles and who have normal intrauterine pregnancies. By the time the patient does not menstruate on the first day of the anticipated menses, the pregnancy test is usually positive.

Women's cycle lengths vary from month to month as well as from individual to individual. If ovulation is delayed for some reason, a test on the day the woman thought her period was due could easily be "falsely" negative because the cycle events—implantation and subsequent rising production of hCG—are all a week or two behind schedule.[17] In this situation, a test repeated a week or two later will be positive. One researcher found that sensitivity and accuracy varied for different test kit brands.[18]

Uses. Highly sensitive urine pregnancy tests can be used to confirm pregnancy, or to "rule out" the diagnosis of pregnancy. These tests are appropriate for screening prior to procedures, such as biopsy or x-ray, or prior to prescribing a drug that would be contraindicated during pregnancy. They are also appropriate in screening for possible ectopic pregnancy. Only 1% of patients with ectopic pregnancy would be missed (falsely negative) with a urine test sensitivity of 50 mIU/ml.[12]

LESS SENSITIVE URINE PREGNANCY TESTS

- Most are designated as CLIA moderate complexity although for example the DGT 2000 test is CLIA-waived.

Inexpensive less sensitive urine pregnancy tests, widely used for the last 20 years, depend on binding of hCG in the patient's urine with an anti-hCG antibody in the test solution. Binding of the test antibody prevents clumping (agglutination) of latex particles in the test solution.

Specificity and sensitivity. Because antibodies used in most agglutination tests are not specific for the beta subunit of hCG, cross-reactions are possible. To minimize problems of cross-reaction with LH, agglutination slide-test sensitivity is set so that high levels of hCG are required to give a positive test result. A cross-reaction, therefore, is unlikely to be a source of clinical confusion. However, a test specimen obtained during the brief surge of LH just before ovulation or during the perimenopausal years may cause false positive results in an agglutination pregnancy test because of LH cross-reaction.

The sensitivity of available less sensitive pregnancy tests range from 200 to 2,000 mIU/ml. The clinician should be aware of the sensitivity of the less sensitive urine pregnancy test used in his/her setting.

Uses. Less sensitive tests are inexpensive, fast, easy to perform, and appropriate for confirming pregnancy ≥ 6 weeks LMP. In very early pregnancy, hCG levels may be below the level detected by the less sensitive urine pregnancy tests. In rare cases, the hCG level later in pregnancy (after 16 to 20 weeks) may also decline below the sensitivity for these tests. Less sensitive tests are not appropriate to "rule out" pregnancy because early pregnancy, ectopic pregnancy, and impending spontaneous abortion may be missed. If the initial less sensitive test is negative, a more sensitive test should be used. In very early pregnancy, the quantity of pregnancy tissue produces enough beta hCG for the highly sensitive urine pregnancy test to be positive but not enough for the less sensitive urine pregnancy test to turn positive.

A negative pregnancy test result may be helpful to document disappearance of hCG after induced aspiration or medication abortion. However, the highly sensitive urine pregnancy test is so sensitive that positive results may persist up to 60 days after abortion, whereas the less sensitive test with a sensitivity of 1500 to 2000 mIU/ml is usually negative by two weeks after a uterine aspiration abortion or medication abortion. After medication abortion, a negative less sensitive test or highly sensitive test is 98% accurate in detecting expulsion of the gestational sac.[83] A negative pregnancy test after medication abortion is reassuring, but a positive test may not mean much. In one study, a false positive test occurred in 60% of patients, meaning that they were no longer pregnant and no intervention was required, but the beta hCG level had not fallen below the sensitivity of the 1500–2000 mIU test.[83]

Serum Quantitative Beta hCG Radioimmunoassay (RIA) or Immunometric Assay

Use of a serum quantitative beta hCG as a qualitative (positive/negative) pregnancy test does not have any advantage over sensitive urine tests. Highly sensitive urine pregnancy kits are equally specific for hCG and provide sensitivity that is completely satisfactory for clinical evaluation, with immediate results, and at much lower cost. Only certain clinical situations justify the additional expense of serum hCG testing.

Specificity and sensitivity. Serum quantitative beta hCG tests provide accurate quantitative results with hCG levels as low as 5 mIU/ml; they reliably detect pregnancy soon after implantation occurs or around 21 days LMP. Tests are usually performed in batches because of expense; test processing requires 1 to 2 hours.

Uses. Serum hCG tests can provide a quantitative as well as a qualitative result; serial test specimens can be used to check doubling time or disappearance time when ectopic pregnancy, impending spontaneous abortion, or possible retained placental fragments are being evaluated. High levels are associated with molar pregnancy.

When evaluating the viability of a pregnancy and ruling out spontaneous abortion or ectopic pregnancy, a single beta hCG result alone isn't meaningful. It's really the *pattern* of beta hCG rise, fall, or plateau, in conjunction with other diagnostic tests such as sonography, clinical evaluation of the patient, and consideration of risk factors that leads to a diagnosis of normal or abnormal intrauterine pregnancy or ectopic pregnancy.

Be sure to specify *quantitative* beta hCG when ordering this test. It is optimal to use the same laboratory for serial beta hCG tests in order to limit the possibility of inter-assay variation between laboratories. However, virtually all laboratories now use the Third International Standard for hCG quantitation, limiting variation between laboratories. Given that some patients often have to travel significant distances for a repeat beta hCG test, it may be difficult to have all samples sent to the same laboratory. In this case, as long as the patient is stable, and the clinician has confirmed that all laboratories are using the Third International Standard, it is acceptable to use different laboratories for beta hCG testing.

Home Pregnancy Testing

Home pregnancy test kits offer the advantages of privacy, anonymity, and convenience. Moreover, they are popular. In a national survey, approximately 33% of pregnant women reported using them.[19] Most women chose home testing because results can be obtained quickly and confidentially.[20] Because home pregnancy tests are easily accessible, a woman may identify pregnancy early and thus be more able to be an active manager of her own health care.

Accuracy. Test accuracy can be affected by the techniques and experience of the user, and by the user's ability to follow the test instructions precisely.[21] The most common error with home pregnancy tests is a negative result that occurs because the test was performed too early in pregnancy. An incorrect result could mislead a woman, causing her to delay in getting a clinical evaluation.

Uses. If a home test result is positive, positive results may prompt a woman to seek pregnancy confirmation earlier than she otherwise might and to change her lifestyle earlier than were she to wait for a clinical evaluation. Clinical evaluation is needed to confirm the pregnancy, determine the length of gestation, and identify any possible risk for ectopic or abnormal pregnancy. If the home test result is negative, clinical evaluation also may be needed to determine the cause of menstrual delay or of the other symptoms that have prompted the test, especially if the woman does not resume normal menses soon.

AVOIDING PREGNANCY TEST INTERPRETATION ERRORS

Correctly interpreting pregnancy test results is not entirely straightforward because:

1. hCG levels change drastically over the course of pregnancy, especially during the first 8 to 10 weeks (Figure 23–2).

2. Both positive and negative test results must be interpreted in relation to the sensitivity, specificity, and characteristics of the particular test being used and the clinical evaluation findings, including ultrasound examination when appropriate.

If pregnancy test results do not agree with other clinical signs, consider the possible reasons for the discrepancy. Plan appropriate follow-up or further evaluation to protect the patient against possible consequences of an incorrect test result:

1. Any test result can be wrong. Laboratory errors do occur, including specimen mix-up and incorrectly performed test procedures. For accurate results, instructions for the kit must be followed meticulously and timed with a stopwatch. Use control solutions to verify accuracy. Observe test-kit and reagent expiration dates.

2. Know exactly what kind of pregnancy test was performed and what sensitivity the test has. Without this information, it is not possible to assess the clinical significance of a negative result or to evaluate the possibility of a false positive result.

3. Do not base clinical management on the results of a home pregnancy test. Although home kits have excellent theoretical accuracy, their use even by trained personnel may not reliably provide the sensitivity or specificity needed for optimal clinical management.[22,23] Be careful about accepting the results of a pregnancy test performed in another facility, especially in critical clinical situations such as ectopic pregnancy.

4. False negative results are common with less sensitive urine pregnancy tests. False negative results frequently occur because the test is performed too early or too late in pregnancy. Abnormal pregnancy, urine that is too dilute, and medication that interferes with the test result may all be responsible. Use a highly sensitive urine pregnancy test to "rule out" pregnancy.

5. False negative results are rare with sensitive urine tests but can occur if test procedures are performed incorrectly or if the test reader has red-green color blindness.[24] A highly sensitive urine pregnancy test also may be negative if the test is performed too early in the cycle, before implantation occurs. In this situation, the result is a "true" negative, which could be misleading if not repeated a few days later. Elevated lipids, high immunoglobulin levels, and elevated urine proteins associated with severe kidney disease also can interfere with a test result. If a false negative result is suspected, order a serum quantitative beta hCG.

6. It is rare but known in the literature that urine and serum pregnancy tests may yield false negative results when hCG is present at extreme concentrations. This is known as the "high-dose hook effect." The secondary antibody binding sites become saturated with free hCG so that the primary antibody complex is unable to bind, preventing detection of the antigen.[25] In one case of molar pregnancy, only after multiple dilutions of the serum was a beta hCG of 1.5 million mIU/ml detected.[26] The important thing to re-

member is that laboratory test results should be questioned if they are discordant with clinical findings.

7. False positive pregnancy test results are not common, but they can cause perplexing dilemmas:

— False positive results with highly sensitive urine pregnancy tests are very rare, but laboratory error is always possible. An "accurate" false positive result could occur if the woman has had treatment involving hCG injection within the preceding 14 days, and faint false positive results have been reported with urine samples contaminated by blood or recent use of Chinese herbal medication.[27] If a false positive result is suspected, obtain a serum quantitative beta hCG.

— If a less sensitive urine pregnancy test is positive, but the uterus is not enlarged, perform a confirmatory highly sensitive urine pregnancy test. The positive result could be caused by LH cross-reaction, in which case the highly sensitive urine pregnancy test will be negative because it is specific for beta hCG.

— Less sensitive urine pregnancy tests (agglutination slide tests) also can yield false positive results because of protein or blood in the urine specimen. Consider obtaining a confirmatory highly sensitive urine pregnancy test if the urine specimen shows 1+ proteinuria or more. A highly sensitive urine pregnancy test is likely to give an accurate (negative) result. When a positive pregnancy test is not confirmed by the presence of a pregnancy in the uterus, do not assume the test result is false. Seriously consider the possibility of an ectopic pregnancy.

8. In very rare cases, pregnancy test results are positive even though the patient is not pregnant, because hCG actually is present and originating from a source other than pregnancy. hCG levels persist after a recent pregnancy or after hCG treatment. Low levels of hCG (5 to 30 mIU) may be associated with tumors of the pancreas, ovaries, breast, and many other sites.[28] Some normal postmenopausal women also have low levels of circulating hCG-like substance of pituitary origin.[12]

9. For follow-up after molar pregnancy or choriocarcinoma, use serum quantitative beta hCG testing. The hCG protein produced by tumor cells may be abnormal and in some cases may be missed by other test methods. If persistent hCG levels are found, the condition must be managed by an expert, and hCG levels in both blood and urine should be checked, because false-positive blood results are possible.[29,30]

ULTRASOUND IN VERY EARLY PREGNANCY

Many centers providing gynecological, prenatal, or abortion care routinely use ultrasound for screening. In general, targeted ultrasound in the clinic setting when a woman has a positive pregnancy test has several purposes:

1. Identify that the pregnancy is intrauterine, thereby virtually ruling out an ectopic pregnancy

2. Date the pregnancy

When a highly sensitive urine pregnancy test is positive but no evidence of intrauterine pregnancy is visualized on ultrasound, the patient is assumed to be pregnant but the location of the pregnancy is unknown. When sonography is performed very early in pregnancy, the findings are not always conclusive in either identifying an intrauterine gestation or in excluding an ectopic pregnancy, even with transvaginal ultrasound.

When a patient's highly sensitive urine pregnancy test is positive but no intrauterine pregnancy is visualized by transvaginal sonography, there are several possible explanations:

- Elevated hCG due to reasons other than pregnancy

- Patient is very early in pregnancy; too early for gestational sac to be visualized

- Intrauterine pregnancy is not growing at the normal rate; may be an anembryonic pregnancy or impending spontaneous pregnancy loss

- Ectopic pregnancy

In addition, certain things delay the visualization of a normal gestational sac at the appropriate time. Body habitus (i.e., obesity), the presence of fibroids, uterine anomalies, such as bicornuate uterus, or a severely retroverted uterus can make visualization impossible even though a normal gestation is ongoing. Abnormal or delayed growth of a pregnancy can prevent visualization. The presence of twins or more could also preclude identification of a gestational sac at the normal landmark time.

Correlation of beta hCG, Ultrasound Findings and Clinical Picture

When an intrauterine pregnancy cannot be visualized by transvaginal ultrasound, the clinician must evaluate the ultrasound findings, the pregnancy test results, knowledge of expected beta hCG values, and the patient's clinical picture in conjunction with risk factors of ectopic pregnancy.

The landmarks for timing of findings by transvaginal ultrasound (Table 23–5) are:

Table 23–5 Timing of landmarks in early pregnancy[6] (with transvaginal ultrasound based on 28-day cycle)

20–32 days gestation from LMP	positive highly sensitive urine pregnancy test
35 days LMP (5 weeks)	gestational sac can usually be visualized
40 days LMP (5½ weeks)	yolk sac virtually always is seen
48 days LMP (6½ weeks)	embryonic pole with cardiac motion is seen

Since the amount of beta hCG measurable in early pregnancy directly correlates with the quantity of pregnancy tissue growing, the level of beta hCG at which a gestational sac, the first sign of an intrauterine gestation, *should* be seen on transvaginal ultrasound has been determined. The level of beta HCG at which the gestational sac of a normal intrauterine pregnancy should seen on ultrasound is called the "discriminatory zone." The accepted discriminatory zone of hCG is 1500 to 2000 mIU/ml with ultrasound performed transvaginally.[31]

The sensitivity of the less sensitive urine pregnancy tests discussed in this chapter is 1500 to 2000 mIU/ml (2 IU). This means that when one of these tests is positive, there is enough pregnancy tissue that a gestational sac *should* be seen within the uterus with transvaginal ultrasound.

Knowledge of the discriminatory zone and pregnancy test results is useful in determining whether the pregnancy is not visualized on ultrasound simply because the patient is very early in pregnancy or whether there should be a higher index of suspicion for ectopic pregnancy. If a patient has a positive highly sensitive urine pregnancy test and her LMP was < 5 weeks ago and the less sensitive pregnancy test is negative, the following is true: 1) she is very early in pregnancy, 2) it is too early in pregnancy to expect to be able to visualize a pregnancy by ultrasound, 3) it is too early to determine the location of the pregnancy, and 4) although the pregnancy may be ectopic, the most likely possibility is that it is intrauterine, since only approximately 2% of pregnancies are reported to be ectopic.[32] If the patient is not at high risk for ectopic pregnancy and is deemed to be compliant, she can be given information about the signs and symptoms of ectopic pregnancy with warnings to seek emergency care should they occur, and told to return in 3–7 days for a repeat ultrasound. Most likely, an intrauterine pregnancy will be seen on transvaginal ultrasound at that time. If no intrauterine pregnancy is visualized at the follow-up scan, even if the less sensitivity pregnancy test is negative, the patient should be worked up for ectopic pregnancy.

If, on the other hand, the highly sensitive urine pregnancy test is positive and the 2000 mIU/ml test is also positive, regardless of the patient's

LMP, visualization of intrauterine gestation by transvaginal sonogram is expected. Because the 2000 mIU/ml agglutination test is positive, the patient's hCG is at the level of the discriminatory zone. If no gestational sac is visualized in the uterus, this patient should be presumed to have an ectopic pregnancy, which, if the patient is asymptomatic, may be determined by following serial quantitative beta hCGs and/or by referral for a diagnostic ultrasound.

If patients have risk factors for ectopic pregnancy, bleeding, or free fluid in the cul-de-sac visualized by sonogram, especially if the 2000 mIU/ml test is positive and there is no intrauterine gestational sac visualized by transvaginal ultrasound, they should be presumed to have ectopic pregnancy until proven otherwise. Any patient with acute symptoms of ectopic pregnancy should be referred to the emergency department for definitive treatment.

Ectopic pregnancy will be discussed in more detail later in the chapter in the section Managing Problems in Early Pregnancy.

Earliest Ultrasound Visualization of Pregnancy

The first indication of pregnancy by transvaginal ultrasound is the gestational sac. A true gestational sac can be challenging to distinguish from a "pseudosac." A pseudosac is the sloughing of decidua that produces a fluid collection in the endometrial cavity.[33] Approximately 20% of patients with ectopic pregnancy have a pseudosac visualized on ultrasound.[6]

The transvaginal ultrasound should include evaluation both in the longitudinal and transverse views. The longitudinal view captures the uterus in its long axis, making visualization of the cervix and endometrial cavity up to the fundus possible and orienting the viewer in the pelvis. The papaya in Figure 23–4 resembles a uterus in the longitudinal plane.

The adnexae and uterus should then be viewed in the transverse position. The image of the papaya shown in Figure 23–5, represents the uterus in the transverse plane.

The adnexae, uterus, and cul-de-sac should then be viewed in transverse position. Unless a complete pelvic scan is done, there is a higher possibility of missing a multiple gestation, ectopic pregnancy, uterine anomalies, fibroids, and fluid in the cul-de-sac. Since transvaginal ultrasound allows for visualization of the entire pelvis, identification of the uterus, ovaries, presence or absence of ovarian cysts, and presence or absence of fluid in the cul-de-sac should be noted.

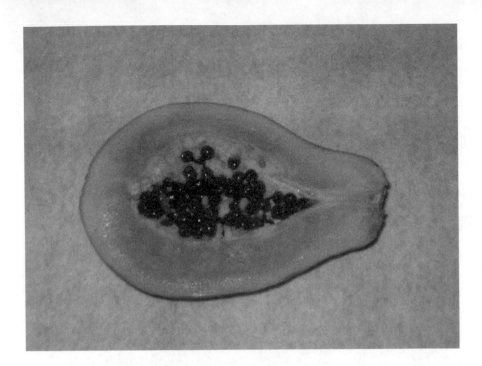

Figure 23–4 Papaya (cut) resembling the shape of the uterus shown in the longitudinal view

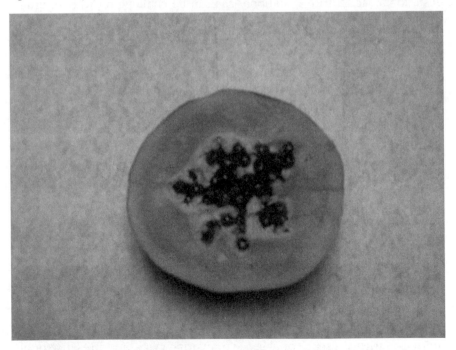

Figure 23–5 Papaya (cut) resembling the shape of the uterus shown in the transverse view

When the clinician/sonographer visualizes all the characteristics of a true gestational sac in the uterus, the likelihood of ectopic pregnancy is remote. In constrast, presence of an actual pseudosac is a harbinger of ectopic pregnancy. Therefore it is vital to assess the sac in multiple planes (longitudinal and transverse) and to be assured that the sac has all the characteristics of a true sac.

To distinguish a true gestational sac from a pseudosac, ascertain that the characteristics of a normal gestational sac are present:

1. Round or oval shape in both longitudinal and transverse views

2. Surrounded completely by a multi-layered echogenic choriodecidual reaction, known as the double decidual reaction. The appearance is of a multi-layered fluffy white cloud surrounding the gestational sac, whiter near the sac and at the outer edge of the reaction. Another description of the appearance of the choriodecidual reaction is that of an orange rind (see Figure 23–6A and 6B).

3. A true gestational sac is a three-dimensional round or oval structure, implanted off-center to the midline, and normally grows about 1 mm/day.[31]

The illustration (Figure 23–7) and the ultrasound image (Figure 23–8) demonstrate a true gestational sac.

In contrast, the illustration (Figure 23–9) and ultrasound images (Figure 23–10) and (Figure 23–11) demonstrate a pseudosac.

Small amounts of free pelvic fluid can be seen in intrauterine pregnancies, as well as in ectopic pregnancies. The presence of a moderate to large amount of fluid in the cul-de-sac has a 96% specificity for diagnosing ectopic pregnancy. Echolucent fluid in the cul-de-sac was the only extrauterine finding in 15% of confirmed ectopic pregnancies. In other words, ectopic pregnancy itself was not visualized directly in the adnexa; fluid in the cul-de-sac was the only visual sonographic clue of ectopic pregnancy, along with absence of intrauterine gesational sac.[35]

In the ultrasound image (Figure 23–12), free fluid in the cul-de-sac is seen.

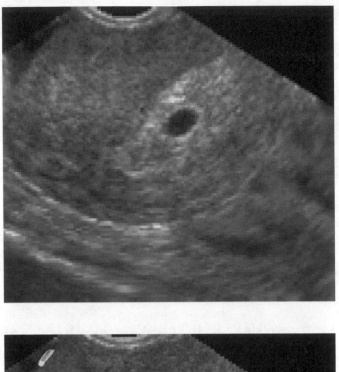

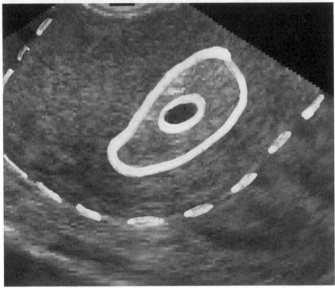

Figure 23–6 A. Intrauterine gestational sac with choriodecidual reaction. The double decidual reaction is seen in which the ring closest to the sac is bright white (echogenic), somewhat faded in the middle of the reaction, and then brighter again at the edge of the choriodecidual reaction. In view B, the inner and outer rings of the reaction are outlined with solid white lines and the uterus is outlined with a broken white line.

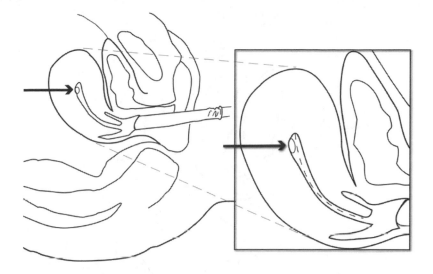

Figure 23–7 Illustration of eccentric implantation. The pregnancy implants into the thickened endometrium. In effect, it burrows into the endometrial lining; it does not float in the endometrial cavity. That's why the gestational sac is off-center to the midline of the endometrial cavity (arrow).

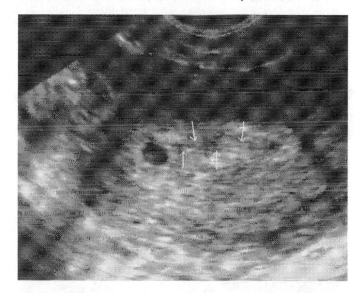

Figure 23–8 Longitudinal view of an intrauterine gestational sac, choriodecual Reaction and endometrial cavity line. Note the thin black line that extends longitudinally through the endometrial cavity, sometimes referred to as the endometrial cavity line (arrows). The gestational sac is adjacent to, but does not displace, the endometrial cavity line, thereby demonstrating an eccentric implantation.[34] In addition, the double decidual reaction (multi-layered echogenicity) surrounding the gestational sac is seen. (Courtesy of Mary Andrews, NP

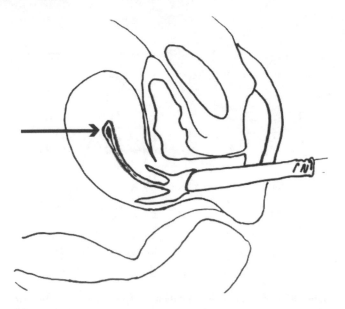

Figure 23–9 Illustration of a pseudosac. This is a fluid collection within the endometrium; the fluid collection can be large or small, irregular shaped or round (at least when viewed in one plane), but it is not implanted; it is midline in the cavity, not eccentric to the midline.

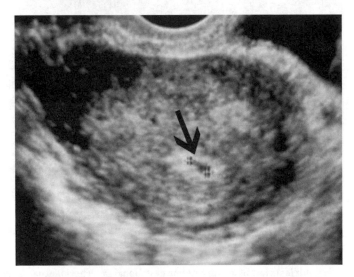

Figure 23–10 Pseudosac Note that the choriodecidual reaction is not multi-layered; it is a thin, homogenous echogenic rim. Note also that the fluid-filled sac (arrow) is mid-line in the uterine cavity, not eccentrically implanted as would be a true gestational sac. Also note that the fluid-filled sac is irregularly-shaped. Another view taken at the same session demonstrates that the sac lost all semblance of roundness when it was viewed in a different plane (Figure 23–11)

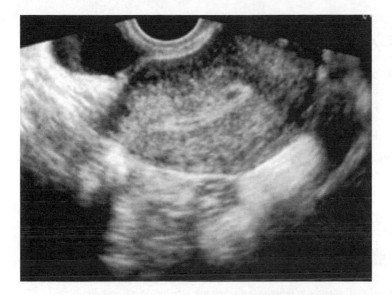

Figure 23–11 Another view of the pseudosac. This image is of the same patient at the same session as Figure 23–10, showing the sac in a different plane. In this plane, the sac is flattened and doesn't resemble a normal round or oval gestational sac at all. These two images emphasize the importance of performing a systematic scan in both the longitudinal and transverse planes and the importance of recognizing red flags when the sac does not match all the characteristics of a normal gestational sac. This patient had an ectopic pregnancy.

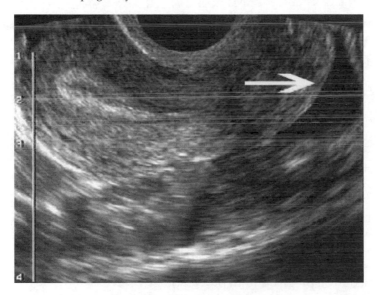

Figure 23–12 Free fluid in the cul-de-sac (Courtesy of NAF)

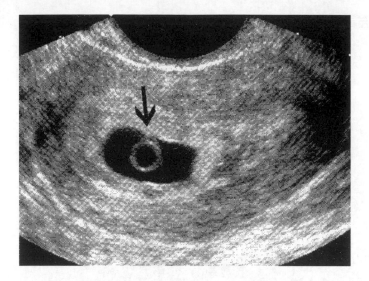

Figure 23–13 Yolk sac appears within the intrauterine gestational sac (arrow).

Visualization of the yolk sac within the gestational sac. Because the yolk sac derives from embryonic tissue, when a sac is seen in the uterus, the presence of a yolk sac within the gestational sac confirms an intrauterine pregnancy (Figure 23–13). When a yolk sac is seen within the intrauterine gestational sac via transvaginal ultrasound, intrauterine pregnancy can be diagnosed with virtually 100% accuracy.[36]

Managing Problems in Early Pregnancy

Consider the possibility of pregnancy, spontaneous abortion, or ectopic pregnancy whenever a woman in the reproductive years has symptoms such as abdominal pain, abnormal bleeding, or irregular or missed menstrual periods. The patient's history, as well as her own assessment of pregnancy risk, may be helpful. For example, in a study of women undergoing evaluation at a hospital emergency department, 63% of the women who thought they might be pregnant, were pregnant; however 10% of women were found to be pregnant even though they reported a normal last menstrual period and stated that there was no chance they could be pregnant.[37] A sensitive pregnancy test is a prudent precaution to take, no matter what the woman's history indicates. An old adage in gynecology and obstetrics is that every woman of reproductive age is presumed to be pregnant until proven otherwise.

Rh screening is a standard recommendation for any pregnant woman, especially when she presents with bleeding. The risk of Rh sensitization resulting from bleeding in early pregnancy is low, and during the early days of development before fetal blood cells are present, the risk should be negligible or absent. The available research to document risk, however, is limited and is based primarily on studies to detect the presence of fetal cells in maternal blood detected by the Kleihauer-Betke (KB) test rather than on the later development of maternal Rh(D) antibodies. Positive KB test results have been reported for non-bleeding women both before and after abortion with gestation as early as 5 to 6 weeks.[38] Because the risks associated with Rh testing and Rh prophylaxis are low, Rh prophylaxis has been widely accepted as a precaution in the United States even though the risk of sensitization is also low. Although Rh prophylaxis is recommended in the United Kingdom following a first-trimester induced abortion or the diagnosis of an ectopic gestation, it is no longer recommended at the time of complete spontaneous miscarriage during the first 12 weeks of pregnancy unless the bleeding is heavy, recurrent, or associated with abdominal pain.[39]

A hemoglobin or hematocrit also is indicated at the time of initial evaluation. The results may help assess the cumulative extent of bleeding and may provide an important baseline for later comparison.

Abnormal bleeding, cramping, and abdominal pain can occur with threatened abortion, complete or incomplete spontaneous abortion, and ectopic pregnancy. However, these symptoms also can occur in an early pregnancy that subsequently progresses to a normal outcome. When these symptoms occur, perform an evaluation immediately: exclude the presence of ectopic pregnancy, and arrange appropriate care for possible spontaneous abortion.

POSSIBLE ECTOPIC PREGNANCY

During the history-taking of a pregnant woman, the risk factors for ectopic pregnancy should be assessed, although more than half of identified ectopic pregnancies occur in women without known risk factors.[40] Table 23–6 outlines the risk factors for ectopic pregnancy.

A woman who has clinical evidence of a possible ruptured ectopic pregnancy, such as hypotension or postural hypotension, fainting, falling hemoglobin or hematocrit, severe abdominal pain, guarding, or rebound tenderness requires immediate referral for emergency management where surgery is available if needed. A highly sensitive urine pregnancy test is almost certain to be positive (false-negative rate is less than 1%),[12] but less sensitive are not sensitive enough to detect the lower hCG levels associated with ectopic gestation in about 50% of cases.[44] Because intervention should not be delayed for the patient who has clinical evidence of possible ruptured ectopic pregnancy, further nonsurgical evaluation is not prudent.

Table 23–6 Risk factors for ectopic pregnancy

Factor	Odds Ratio (and 95% Confidence Interval)		
	Ankum et al.[42] (1996)	Mol et al.[43] (1995)	Dart et al.[41] (1999)
Previous tubal surgery	21 (9.3–47)	–	–
Previous ectopic	8.3 (6.0–11.5)	–	–
In utero DES exposure	5.6 (2.4–13)	–	–
History of PID	2.5 (2.1–3.0)	–	–
History of infertility	2.5–21*	– 5.0 (1.1–28)	
History of chlamydial or gonococcal cervicitis	2.8–3.7*		
Documented tubal abnormality	3.4–25*		
Tubal ligation	–	9.3 (4.9–18)	19 (3.0–139)
Current IUD use	–	4.2–45*	5.0 (1.1–28)

* Range: summary OR not calculated owing to significant heterogenieity between studies.

Source: Murray et al. (2005)[40] with permission.

More commonly, the clinician considers the possibility of ectopic pregnancy because the woman has less serious and nonspecific symptoms such as bleeding in early pregnancy, uterine enlargement that does not correlate with dates (uterus is too small), an ultrasound that fails to demonstrate an intrauterine gestation, or an early uterine aspiration abortion that has failed to recover identifiable products of conception from the uterine cavity. Often the patient is completely asymptomatic. These situations may allow time for further outpatient evaluation if the patient is willing and able to monitor her own symptoms carefully, she has access to emergency intervention and she is by all indications early in her pregnancy. While the evaluation is pending, the patient must be warned to watch for ectopic pregnancy danger signs (Table 23–7) and to return immediately for emergency care if danger signs occur. Further steps in evaluation might include the following:

1. **Quantitative serum beta hCG assay.** Although test results probably will not be available until the next day, an initial level can be compared with the beta hCG level 2 days (48 hours) later if the diagnosis is still uncertain.

   There is no single predictable hCG pattern in ectopic pregnancy. Table 23–8 depicts the expected range of beta hCG rise with viable intrauterine pregnancy, the fall expected with complete spontaneous abortion, and the various patterns seen in ectopic pregnancy.

Table 23–7 Early pregnancy danger signs

Possible Ectopic Pregnancy

Sudden intense pain, persistent pain, or cramping in the lower abdomen, usually localized to one side or the other

Irregular bleeding or spotting with abdominal pain when period is late or after an abnormally light period

Fainting or dizziness persisting more than a few seconds. These may be signs of internal bleeding. (Internal bleeding is not necessarily associated with vaginal bleeding.).

Possible Miscarriage

Late last period and bleeding heavy, possibly with clots or clumps of tissue; cramping more severe than usual

Period is prolonged and heavy—5 to 7 days of "heaviest" days

Abdominal pain or fever

Contact your clinician immediately or go to a hospital emergency room if you develop any of these signs.

Source: Stewart et al. (1987)[45] with permission.

Table 23–8 Rise or fall in sequential quantitative beta hCG values in early IUP, complete SAB and ectopic pregnancy[10,46,47]

Intrauterine pregnancy (IUP):	
Mean increase in 2 days	124%
Minimum expected rise in 2 days	53%
Complete spontaneous abortion:	
Minimum expected decline, depending on initial hCG value	21–35%
Ectopic pregnancy:*	
Group A: *had rising hCGs*	60%
1st two hCG values consistent with IUP	35%
Median increase in 2 days	75%
Group B: *had falling hCGs*	40%
1st two hCG values consistent with complete SAB	20%
Median decline in 2 days	27%
All ectopics combined	
1st two hCG values out of range for IUP or complete SAB	71%
1st two hCG values consistent with range for IUP	21%
1st two hCG values consistent with range for complete SAB	8%

* 200 ectopic pregnancies, hCG pattern in first two beta hCG tests taken at least 24 hours but no more than 7 days apart

Sources: Barnhart et al (2004), Seeber and Barnhart (2006), Silva et al (2006) with permission.

The rate of rise of beta hCG in ectopic pregnancy generally is lower than for intrauterine pregnancies and the drop is usually not as steep as it is for complete spontaneous abortion. In the majority of patients with ectopic pregnancy (71%), the first two beta hCG levels either will not increase as expected for intrauterine pregnancy or won't fall as sharply as expected with completed spontaneous abortion.[46] But the curves of hCG rise or fall in ectopic, normal intrauterine and spontaneously aborting pregnancies overlap. The main point is that there is no characteristic hCG pattern for ectopic pregnancy; in 20% of ectopic pregnancies, the first two hCG values rise as expected in intrauterine pregnancy.[46,48] In 8% of ectopic pregnancies, the hCG decline is as fast or faster than the decline seen with complete spontaneous abortion.[46] Until the location and status of the pregnancy are confirmed, hCG should be followed until the curve is outside of that expected, a definite diagnosis is made by ultrasound, the patient becomes symptomatic or the hCG values fall to non-pregnant levels.

2. **Tissue evaluation, pathology phone report and serial beta hCG testing.** If no intrauterine pregnancy is visualized by transvaginal ultrasound when the beta hCG is 1500–2000 mIU/ml (the discriminatory cut-off), some experts advocate evacuating the contents of the uterus to differentiate a spontaneous abortion from an ectopic pregnancy.[47] If a uterine evacuation has been performed, products of conception should be identified in the fresh tissue aspirate; this confirms an intrauterine pregnancy and virtually rules out ectopic pregnancy. Examination of the fresh specimen has been found to be as accurate as a pathology examination in determining that the abortion was complete[49] although tissue examinations by both the surgeons and the pathologists had poor validity for identifying abnormal abortion outcomes. The histological result (pathology report) is sometimes inconsistent with the diagnosis of the provider who cared for the patient and examined the fresh tissue specimen, and this may result in unnecessary further investigation and treatment.[50] Nonetheless, if products of conception are not identified by examination of the fresh tissue aspirate, send the tissue for microscopic tissue evaluation and a pathology report by phone. Placental villi identified in the specimen evacuated in most instances can rule out an ectopic pregnancy.[51]

If products of conception are not identified in the examination of the fresh tissue aspirate, the first quantitative beta hCG should be drawn immediately after the procedure and again in 48 hours to be sure that the values are halving every 48 hours as expected following successful termination of intrauterine pregnancy. If an ectopic pregnancy is still evolving, hCG levels typically will not be halving—they will typically plateau or rise.

3. **Ultrasound evaluation.** The diagnosis of ectopic pregnancy can be made conclusively if a gestational sac and fetal heartbeat are detected outside of the uterine cavity. Unless an intrauterine gestation (gestational sac with yolk sac) can be identified with certainty or an extrauterine gestation is visible, ultrasound results do not provide a definite diagnosis. As explained previously in the chapter, an intrauterine pregnancy *should* be visualized on transvaginal ultrasound by the time the 1500 to 2000 mIU/ml pregnancy test is positive (or the serum quantitative beta hCG is $\geq$ 2000 mIU/ml).

If after completing these diagnostic steps, ectopic pregnancy cannot be excluded, arrange for additional evaluation. Refer the patient immediately if she becomes symptomatic during the process of evaluation. Laparoscopy may be needed to ascertain the diagnosis.

4. **Expectant management.** If the initial beta hCG is low (<1500 mIU/ml), up to 83% of ectopic pregnancies will resolve spontaneously, and one study of 180 women showed that fertility after expectant management was similar to that after surgery.[52–54]

However, if you choose to manage the patient expectantly, note that ectopic pregnancies have ruptured at very low hCG levels. As many as 10% of women with a ruptured ectopic pregnancy may have a serum hCG level less than 100 mIU/ml[55] and clinically significant internal bleeding has been reported even at levels below the 25 mIU/ml sensitivity of highly sensitive urine pregnancy tests.

Alternatively, some centers treat asymptomatic, early ectopic pregnancy with methotrexate,[56,57] to induce dissolution of tro phoblast tissue. Success rates reported with a single or multiple dose treatment with methotrexate range from 85% to 95%.[56–58]

Early diagnosis is very important in ectopic pregnancy. Although early diagnosis and intervention have helped to reduce ectopic pregnancy mortality, ectopic pregnancy is still the leading cause of pregnancy-related death during the first trimester.[59] Also, early diagnosis allows more time for conservative management, which also may help to preserve the woman's future fertility.

HETEROTOPIC PREGNANCY

Heterotopic pregnancy is the simultaneous occurrence of two or more implantation sites, most commonly a concomitant intrauterine pregnancy and an ectopic pregnancy. The incidence of heterotopic pregnancy in the general population is reported as 1:4,000 in recent literature.[47] Clinicians should be aware of the possibility of heterotopic pregnancy if, following surgical or medication abortion, miscarriage, or progressing intrauterine pregnancy, women exhibit the signs and symptoms of ectopic pregnancy.

Keep in mind the increased risk of heterotopic pregnancy in patients treated with fertility drugs and reproductive assistance. The risk of heterotopic pregnancy in women undergoing in vitro fertilization is 1 in 100,[60] and in women treated with fertility drugs, the incidence is 1 in 3,880.[61]

EARLY PREGNANCY LOSS

Spontaneous Abortion

Approximately 15% of clinically recognized pregnancies end spontaneously in early pregnancy.[62] Missed abortion (failure of pregnancy growth) is also fairly common, but it is unlikely to cause symptoms that would prompt the woman to seek care early in pregnancy. Often the diagnosis is not suspected until prenatal exams reveal that uterine enlargement is not keeping pace with pregnancy dates or an ultrasound evaluation fails to detect an expected fetal pole or cardiac activity at an appropriate time.

In some cases, the diagnosis of spontaneous abortion may be made on the basis of a pelvic examination. If the cervix is dilated and products of conception are visible in the cervix or vagina, then an abortion is inevitable. An ultrasound evaluation may help determine whether the uterine cavity is already empty. In other cases, the diagnosis is suspected on the basis of abnormal bleeding or ultrasound findings. Once the possibility of ectopic pregnancy is excluded, if the woman's bleeding is not heavy and she is stable, then uterine aspiration may not be necessary. One study of expectant management ('waiting and watching') found that most women with a diagnosis of incomplete spontaneous abortion preferred this option to uterine aspiration and that 81% had a successful outcome without surgical intervention, especially when the abortion occurred early in the pregnancy.[63] A recent meta-analysis reported that the overall success rate of expectant management for miscarriage was 78%.[63]

If bleeding and cramping are severe, manual vacuum aspiration (MVA) can empty the uterus; aspiration is indicated if bleeding is so

Table 23–9 Efficacy of misoprostol treatment for early pregnancy loss

(800 μg misoprostol vaginally with a second dose administered on day 3 if expulsion was incomplete)	
Success with one treatment of misoprostol	71%
Success with misoprostol repeated in 48 hours	84%
Efficacy according to types of pregnancy loss	
Embryonic or fetal death	88%
Anembryonic pregnancy	81%
Incomplete or inevitable abortion	93%

Source: Zhang et al. (2005)[64] with permission.

heavy that it is life-threatening. Use of manual vacuum aspiration equipment in the office or emergency room, with a local paracervical block to provide appropriate pain relief, may offer a simple and effective approach.

Alternatively, if bleeding is not severe and the patient is stable, consider treatment with misoprostol. Misoprostol causes cervical softening and increased uterine contractility, thereby facilitating the expulsion of the remaining pregnancy tissue. Treatment of early pregnancy loss with 800 μg of misoprostol vaginally, with the dose repeated after 48 hours when necessary, is safe and has an overall efficacy of 84%.[64] Misoprostol treatment has higher efficacy for certain types of early pregnancy loss—such as incomplete or inevitable abortion and embryonic or fetal death—than for other types of loss such as anembryonic pregnancy. (See Table 23–9). Uterine aspiration is 97% effective for treatment of early pregnancy loss. Educating and informed consent require an explanation of the advantages and disadvantages of uterine aspiration, medical treatment, and expectant management; respect the patient's preference in conjunction with weighing all medical considerations. (See Chapter 24, Abortion, Spontaneous or Induced.)

If the pregnancy is wanted and the patient's condition is stable, you can delay intervention while further evaluating whether the pregnancy may be viable. Serial quantitative beta hCG levels and an ultrasound evaluation are likely to document the diagnosis. When the woman desires to continue her pregnancy, take time for a careful and thorough evaluation. Intervention on the basis of an initial exam or ultrasound will seem abrupt and shocking as the woman first begins to acknowledge the possibility of her loss and grief.

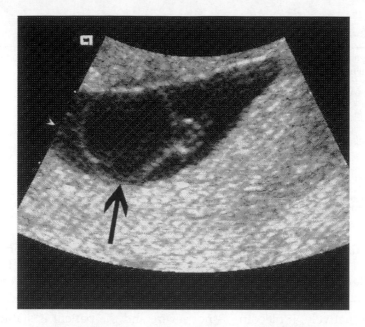

Figure 23–14 **Anembryonic pregnancy.** The amnion can be seen but there is no yolk sac or embryonic structure within it (arrow). (Courtesy of Matthew Reeves MD)

Anembryonic Pregnancy

Anembryonic pregnancy, formerly known by the now outdated term 'blighted ovum,' refers to a pregnancy in which a gestational sac is present but development stopped before formation of the embryo or before it was detectable. Trophoblastic tissue continues to function, resulting in continued growth of the gestational sac, although at a slower than normal rate.[6] An anembryonic pregnancy is diagnosed when a transvaginal ultrasound reveals a mean sac diameter (MSD) of 8 to 10 mm or greater with no visible yolk sac, or an MSD exceeding 16 to 18 mm with no detectable cardiac activity or embryo.[6,25]

Anembryonic pregnancy may be managed expectantly, with MVA, or medically with mifepristone and misoprostol,[66] or with misoprostol alone.

Figure 23–14 demonstrates the classic empty amnion sign; this is the most obvious form of anembryonic pregnancy. The embryo normally essentially fills the entire amnion, so if it is not found easily, it is either not there or not normal.

Embryonic or Fetal Demise

Early pregnancy loss is confirmed when no embryonic heartbeat is seen on transvaginal ultrasound and either 1) the sonogram demon-

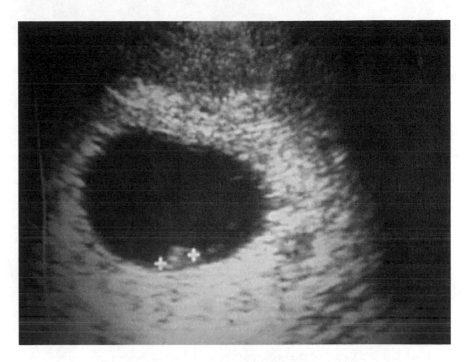

Figure 23–15 Embryonic demise. The embryo (marked) has not grown in proportion to the size of the gestational sac. The caliper placement represent measurement of early embryonic length (courtesy of NAF).

strates an embryo of at least 5 mm in length or 2) the gestational age is known with certainty and is at least 6.5 weeks. Since most women do not know with certainty exactly when conception occurred, it is best to be conservative in estimating gestational age. Repeating the ultrasound study in 3 to 7 days can usually be definitive; under normal circumstances, growth would be about 0.8mm/day. Slow embryonic heart rates at 6 to 7 weeks LMP are associated with embryonic demise. If the embryonic length is 5 mm (6.3 weeks), and the heart rate is less than 80 beats per minute, subsequent demise is very likely within 1 to 2 weeks.[67] At this gestation, the heart rate of a developing embryo should be more than 100 beats per minute. At 6.3 to 7.0 weeks, the heart rate should be 120 beats per minute or more. Without a Doppler recorder on the ultrasound equipment, estimating the heart rate can be difficult, but exact calculation is rarely necessary. If there is any confusion between the fetal and maternal heartbeat, measure the woman's pulse and check the fetal heart rate- the fetal heart rate should be faster. Embryonic or fetal demise may be managed by expectant management, MVA, or medical treatment with misoprostol.

Figure 23–15 shows early embryonic demise. There is no cardiac activity (which can only be assessed in real-time, not on a still image).

Whenever there is a great deal of discrepancy between the gestational sac size and fetal growth, the state of the fetus (sac contents) will usually be a harbinger of the outcome.

EDUCATION AND COUNSELING

The issues surrounding personal fertility are complex, and a pregnancy diagnosis visit should provide the client an opportunity to clarify and articulate her feelings. Before beginning the physical exam and conducting the pregnancy test, find out what the woman hopes her result will be. When presenting the test results, elicit the client's reaction and allow time for her to express her feelings. Assess the woman's support system. Provide referrals if the patient feels counseling would be helpful. This is especially important if her own support system is not adequate. Emphasize that no decision based on the test results need be made that day. Encourage the woman to talk with her partner, family, or friends. Outline all the options available.

- If the client is pregnant and plans to continue her pregnancy, review precautions for optimal pregnancy and be certain she has an appropriate resource for prenatal care. Remind her about danger signs of possible problems in pregnancy (Table 23–7).

- If the client plans to continue her pregnancy, but does not want to parent the child, refer her to a resource that can help with adoption.

- If the client is pregnant but does not plan to continue her pregnancy, refer her for abortion services. In this case, the sooner the decision is made and acted upon, the safer the procedure will be. (see Chapter 24 on Abortion.)

- If the client is not pregnant and wishes she were, counsel her about her own fertility. (see Chapter 25, Impaired Fertility.) If appropriate, refer her for fertility evaluation and help. Remind her about precautions for optimal pregnancy and about taking a daily vitamin that includes folic acid (0.4 mg daily) before and during the first trimester of pregnancy.[68] (See Preconception Care section in this chapter.)

- If the client is not pregnant, plans to continue being sexually active, and is happy with the negative test result, then birth control counseling is appropriate. A pregnancy scare can be a good bridge from risk-taking to effective, ongoing contraceptive use.

Possible Early Pregnancy Exposure to Teratogens

Women who discover they are pregnant may have used or be using prescription or over-the-counter medications, herbal products, illicit substances and other products that may have teratogenic potential. Sixty five percent of women use over-the-counter medications at some point in pregnancy,[69] and use of a potentially teratogenic drug among women of childbearing age has been documented in one out of every 13 visits to ambulatory care practices in the United States.[70] The Organization of Teratology Information Services provides up-to-date resources and fact sheets about both maternal and paternal exposures to medications, herbal products, infectious agents, vaccines, medical conditions, and illicit substances. The organization's website at www.otispregnancy.org includes a map that lists the Teratology Information Service sites.

Domestic Violence Screening and Referral

A review of 13 studies found a prevalence of domestic violence against pregnant women ranging from 0.9% to 20.1%.[71] One study showed that domestic abuse accounted for 22.3% of pregnancy-related trauma.[72] Domestic violence can lead to uterine contractions, preterm labor, placental abruption, and maternal or fetal death. In a Maryland study, homicide was the leading cause of death during pregnancy in a 5-year period.[73] Even after controlling for demographic characteristics such as poverty, abuse during pregnancy has been found to be a risk factor for subsequent homicide or attempted homicide.

The relationship between intimate partner violence and unintended pregnancy has been established.[74] A strong relationship between physical violence and unintended pregnancy was found among women in four U.S. states (Alaska, Maine, Oklahoma, and West Virginia) from 1990–1991. Almost 70% of women reporting domestic violence reported unwanted and/or mistimed pregnancies.[75] The prevalence of domestic violence may be higher among women seeking abortion, although the mechanism through which this relationship occurs is not clearly understood. Women who do not disclose to their partners that they are having an abortion are more likely to be victims of abuse than women who do disclose that they are having an abortion. In an ethnically and racially diverse population of women presenting for pregnancy termination in Houston, physical or sexual abuse or both within the last year was twice as common among women who did not disclose their abortion to their partners.[76] A subset of these women reported that the direct fear of personal harm was the primary reason for nondisclosure.

Because of the prevalence of domestic violence in society, and particularly among women in the prenatal and postpartum period, clinicians providing gynecologic care, pregnancy screening and prenatal care are in a unique position to screen for, recognize, and intervene. Women who have experienced domestic violence often report that a question by a health care worker was the first step in disclosure and recognition.[77]

Screening for domestic violence should be routine. Clinicians may fail to screen for domestic violence due to a lack of confidence in the ability to diagnose it, perceived lack of resources to offer victims, fear of offending victims, lack of time, personal discomfort, and a sense of powerlessness because they believe they have nothing to offer the patient.[78,79] Although screening protocols and training for recognition of domestic violence are valuable, screening through direct and open-ended questions is more important than actual content. A victim may not volunteer information unless a clinician asks about domestic violence. One approach suggests that clinicians would have more success if they changed their role from problem solver to listener and advisor.[80]

Patients should be questioned alone in a supportive, confidential, and nonjudgmental environment. Ask simple, targeted questions. Screening can begin with an opening statement, such as, "Because domestic violence is so common, I routinely ask all my patients if they have been hurt by someone close to them."[81] There are many screening tools for partner violence, which ask the woman if she has ever been slapped or hit by a partner or if a partner has threatened her with violence. Another approach is to ask open-ended questions, such as, "How does your partner treat you? Do you ever feel afraid of your partner?"

The first step toward intervention is screening. The next steps in intervention are: 1) obtain history, 2) diagnose and treat injuries, 3) evaluate the emotional safety of the patient, 4) determine the risk to the victim, 5) determine the need for legal information, 6) develop a follow-up plan, and 7) document the findings.[82] Physical findings that indicate abuse include recurrent or frequent injuries, or multiple injuries in various stages of healing.

Documentation is crucial because even years after injuries have healed, the medical record can substantiate abuse. Include the patient's statements about how the injuries were caused and by whom. Document direct quotations or phrases. Describe the type, number, size, and location of injuries; a body map is helpful visual documentation.

In many states, health care workers are mandated to report domestic violence to state authorities. Clinicians should become familiar with the requirements in their state; training by domestic violence units of local police or district attorney offices are very useful. It is reassuring to have established lines of communication with local police or the district attorney's office prior to an emergency. If a patient fears she is in imminent danger, ask questions about her safety before she leaves the medical facility: "Will you be safe if you leave the facility? Where is your partner? Does he have access to weapons? Are your children in danger?" can assess the immediate risk.[81] If the patient is not at immediate risk, contact a social worker, advocate or local domestic violence hotline. If the patient is in imminent danger without a safe haven, call the police. Occasionally, a violent abuser may threaten the patient and staff. In this case, call 911 and keep staff, the victim, and other patients in a secure area with telephone communication until police get the situation under control.

Clinicians should be aware of community-based resources such as local domestic violence hotlines, shelters, advocacy organizations and support groups for victims of domestic violence. National resources include the National Domestic Violence Hotline (1–800–799-SAFE) and the National Sexual Violence Center (1–877–739–3895). Internet sites include the National Domestic Violence Hotline (www.ndvh.org), the Family Violence Prevention Fund (www.endabuse.org), the National Coalition against Domestic Violence (www.ncadv.org), and local domestic violence hotlines (www.usdoj.gov/ovw/).

Prenatal Care Referral

Encourage early entry into prenatal care so that the patient can take advantage of early prenatal testing and, if indicated, ultrasound. Early care will also give her time to anticipate and complete, if indicated, chorionic villus sampling, amniocentesis, or other recommended tests.

Emphasize the importance of prenatal care, and review the signs and symptoms that may signal problems during early pregnancy: bleeding, spontaneous abortion, and ectopic pregnancy. Because there is often a delay of weeks or longer until the patient actually has her first prenatal appointment with the referral provider, tell the patient whom to contact if a problem or an emergency arises in the interim. If a sexually transmitted infection is diagnosed prior to entry into prenatal care, treat it with an antibiotic regimen recommended for pregnant women. The CDC 2006 STD Treatment Guidelines are available on the web at www.cdc.gov/std/treatment/default.htm and in Chapter 21 on Reproductive Tract Infections.

Have available a list of providers if it is necessary to refer the patient to another provider for prenatal care, because of a high-risk condition, insurance coverage, lack of insurance, or because prenatal services are not offered at your site. In making a referral, consider factors such as the patient's primary language, indications for high-risk perinatal care, distance to the prenatal clinic from her home, the hospital at which she will deliver, and her desire for epidural anesthesia or natural birth.

REFERENCES

1. ACOG. ACOG technical bulletin. Preconceptional care. Number 205-May 1995. American College of Obstetricians and Gynecologists. Int J Gynaecol Ostet 1995;50(2):201–207.
2. Cefalo R, Moos, M-K. Preconceptional health care: a practical guide. 2nd ed. St. Louis, MO: Mosby-Year Book, Inc., 1995.

3. Zabin LS, Emerson MR, Ringers PA, Sedivy V. Adolescents with negative pregnancy test results. An accessible at-risk group. JAMA 1996;275(2):113–117.

4. ACOG. ACOG Practice Bulletin. Clinical Management Guidelines for Obstetrician-Gynecologists. Prenatal diagnosis of fetal chromosomal abnormalities: Am Coll Obstet Gyn, May 2001.

5. Spandorfer SD, Barnhart KT. Role of previous ectopic pregnancy in altering the presentation of suspected ectopic pregnancy. J Reprod Med. Mar 2003;48(3):133–136.

6. Callen PW. Ultrasonography in obstetrics and gynecology. 4th ed. Philadelphia PA: WB Saunders Company, 2000.

7. Soto-Wright V, Bernstein M, Goldstein DP, Berkowitz RS. The changing clinical presention of complete molar pregnancy. Obstet Gynecol 1995;86(5): 775–779.

8. Braunstein GD, Rasor J, Danzer H, Adler D, Wade ME. Serum human chorionic gonadotropin levels throughout normal pregnancy. Am J Obstet Gynecol 1976: 126:678–681.

9. Batzer FR, Weiner S, Corson S, Schlaff S, Otis C. Serial β-subunit human chorionic gondaotropin doubling time as a prognosticator of pregnancy outcome in an infertile population. Fertil Steril 1981;35(3): 307–312.

10. Barnhart KT, Sammel MD, Rinaudo PF, Lan Zhou, Hummel AC, Wensheng Guo. Symptomatic patients with an early viable intrauterine pregnancy: hCG curves redefined. Obstet Gynecol July 2004, 204(1): 50–54.

11. Steier JA, Bergsjo P, Myking OL. Human chorionic gondaotropin in maternal plasma after induced abortion, spontaneous abortion, and removed ectopic pregnancy. Obstet Gynecol 1984;64: 391–394.

12. Braunstein G. hCG testing: a clinical guide for the testing of human chorionic gonadotropin. Abbott Park, IL: Abbott Diagnostics, 1992.

13. Marrs RP, Kletzky OA, Howard WF, Mishell DR, Jr. Disappearance of human chorionic gonadotropin and resumption of ovulation following abortion. Am J Obstet Gynecol 1979;135(6):731–736.

14. Rørbye C, Morgaard M, Nilas L. Prediction of late failure after medical abortion from serial beta hCG measurements and ultrasonography 2004. Hum Reprod;19(1): 85–89.

15. Fiala C, Safar P, Bygdeman M, Gemzell-Danielsson K. Verifying the effectiveness of medical abortion; ultrasound versus hCG testing. Europ J Obstet Gynecol Reprod Biol 2003;109:190–195.

16. Chard T. Pregnancy tests: a review. Hum Reprod 1992;7(5):701–710.

17. Wilcox AJ, Baird DD, Dunson D, McChesney R, Weinberg CR. Natural limits of pregnancy testing in relation to the expected menstrual period. JAMA 2001;286(14):1759–1761.

18. Cole LA, Khanlian SA, Sutton JM, Davies S, Rayburn WF. Accuracy of home pregnancy tests at the time of missed menses. Am J Obs Gyn 2004;190:100–105.

19. Jeng LL, Moore RM, Jr., Kaczmarek RG, Placek PJ, Bright RA. How frequently are home pregnancy tests used? Results from the 1988 National Maternal and Infant Health Survey. Birth. 1991;18(1):11–13.

20. Coons SJ, Churchill L, Brinkman ML. The use of pregnancy test kits by college students. J Am Coll Health 1990;38(4):171–175.

21. Lee C, Hart LL. Accuracy of home pregnancy tests. DICP. 1990;24(7–8):712–713.

22. Doshi ML. Accuracy of consumer performed in-home tests for early pregnancy detection. A J Publ Health 1986;76(5):512–514.

23. Hicks JM, Iosefsohn M. Reliability of home pregnancy-test kits in the hands of laypersons. N Engl J Med 1989;320(5):320–321.

24. Bluestein D. Monoclonal antibody pregnancy tests. American Family Physician. 1988;38(1):197–204.

25. Kazemi MR, Vargas JE, Lo JC. Hyperthyroidism and a negative hCG test in molar pregnancy (Letter to the editor). Am J Med 2004;117:889–890.

26. Tabas JA, Strehlow M, Isaacs E. A false negative pregnancy test in a patient with hydatidiform molar pregnancy (correspondence). N Engl J Med 2003;249(22):2172–2173.

27. IPAS. Pregnancy test trouble shooting guide. Product Literature. Chapel Hill, North Carolina: IPAS, 300 Market Street Suite 200;2003.

28. Bandi ZL, Schoen I, Waters M. An algorithm for testing and reporting serum chorio-gonadotropin at clinically significant decision levels with use of "pregnancy test" re-agents. Clin Chem 1989;35(4):545–551.

29. Rotmensch S, Cole LA. False diagnosis and needless therapy of presumed malignant disease in women with false-positive human chorionic gonadotropin concentrations. Lancet. 2000;355(9205):712–715.

30. Cole LA, Shahabi S, Butler SA, et al. Utility of commonly used commercial human chorionic gonadotropin immunoassays in the diagnosis and management of tropho-blastic diseases. Clin Chem 2001;47(2):308–315.

31. Timor Tritsch IE, Rottem S. (Eds.) Transvaginal sonography. 2nd ed. New York: Else-vier Science Publishing Co., Inc, 1995

32. Centers for Disease Control. Current trends in ectopic pregnancy: United Sates, 1990–92. MMWR 1995;44;46–8.

33. Paul M, Schaff E, Nichols M. Early medical abortion: the roles of clinic assessment, human chorionic gonadotropin assays and ultrasonography in medical abortion practice. Am J Obstet Gynecol 2000;183(2Suppl):S34–43.

34. Yeh, II. Efficacy of the intradecidual sign and fallacy of the double decidual sign in the diagnosis of early intrauterine pregnancy. (Letter to the editor). Radiology 1999;210: 579–582.

35. Della-Giustina D, Denny M. Ectopic pregnancy. Emerg Med Clinics North Am. 2003;21, 565–584.

36. Gracia CR and Barnhart KT. Diaganosing ectopic pregnancy: decision analysis com-paring six strategies. Obstet Gynecol 2001;97(3): 464–470.

37. Ramoska EA, Sacchetti AD, Nepp M. Reliability of patient history in determining the possibility of pregnancy. Ann Emerg Med 1989;18(1):48–50.

38. Jabara S and Barnhart, KT. Is Rh immune globulin needed in early first-trimester abortion? A review. Am J Obstet Gynecol. 2003;188(3):623–627.

39. Weinberg L. Use of anti-D immunoglobulin in the treatment of threatened miscar-riage in the accident and emergency department. Emerg Med J. 2001;18:444–447.

40. Murray H, Baakdah H, Bardell T, Tulandi T. Diagnosis and treatment of ectopic pregnancy. Canadian Medical Association Journal 2005;173(8).

41. Dart IG, Kaplan B, Varaklis K. Predictive value of history and physical examination in patients with suspected ectopic pregnancy. Ann Emerg Med 1999;33: 283–90.

42. Ankum WM, BOL BW, van der Veen F., Bossuyt PM. Risk factors for ectopic preg-nancy: a meta-analysis. Fertil Steril 1996;65:1093–1099.

43. Mol BW, Ankum WM, Bossuyt PM, van der Veen F. Contraception and the risk of ec-topic pregnancy: a meta-analysis. Contraception 1995;52: 337–341.

44. ACOG. Ectopic pregnancy: The American College of Obstetricians and Gynecolo-gists; March 1989. 126.

45. Stewart F, Guest F, Stewart G, Hatcher R. Understanding your body. Every woman's guide to gynecology and health. Figure 8.3, p. 128. New York: Bantam Books, 1987.

46. Silva C, Sammel MD, Zhou L, Gracia C, Hummel AC and Barnhart K. Human cho-rionic gonadotripin profile for women with ectopic pregnancy. Obstet Gynecol March 2006;107(3):605–610.

47. Seeber BE, Barnhart KT. Clinical expert series: suspected ectopic pregnancy. Obstet Gynecol 2006;107:399–413.

48. Kadar N, Caldwell BV, Romero R. A method of screening for ectopic pregnancy and its indications. Obstet Gynecol 1981;58: 641–649.

49. Paul M, Lecklc, E, Mitchell C, Rogers A, Fox M. Is pathology examination useful after surgical abortion? Obstet Gynecol 2002;99(4): 567–571.

50. Heath V, Chadwick V, Cooke I, Manek S, MacKenzie IZ. Should tissue from preg-nancy termination and uterine evacuation routinely be examined histologically? Br J Obstet Gynecol 2000;107(6):727–730.

51. Dart R, Dart L, Mitchell P, O'Rourke N. The utility of a dilatation and evacuation procedure in patients with symptoms suggestive of ectopic pregnancy and indeterminate transvaginal ultrasonography. Acad Emerg Med 1999;6(10):1024–1029.

52. Banerjee S, Aslam N, Woelfer B, Lawrence A, Elson J, Jurkovic D. Expectant management of early pregnancies of unknown location: a prospective evaluation of methods to predict spontaneous resolution of pregnancy. Bri J Obstet Gynaecol 2001;108(2):158–163.

53. Hajenius PJ, Mol WJ, Ankum WM, van der Veen PM, Bossyut M and Lammes FB. Suspected ectopic pregnancy: expectant management in patients with negative sonographic findings and low serum hCG concentrations. Early Pregn: Biol Med (1995):258–262.

54. Strobelt N, Mariani E, Ferrari L, Trio D, Tiezzi A, Ghidini A. Fertility after ectopic pregnancy. Effects of surgery and expectant management. J Reprod Med. 2000;45(10):803–807.

55. Saxon D, Falcone T, Mascha EJ, Marino T, Yao M, Tulandi T. A study of ruptured tubal ectopic pregnancy. Obstet Gynecol 1997;90(1):46–49.

56. Stovall TG, Ling FW. Single-dose methotrexate: an expanded clinical trial. Am J Obstet Gynecol 1993;168(6 Pt 1):1759–1762.

57. Lipscomb GH, Stovall TG, Ling FW. Nonsurgical treatment of ectopic pregnancy. N Engl J Med 2000;343(18):1325–1329.

58. Barnhart KT GG, Ashby R, Sammel M. The medical management of ectopic pregnancy: a meta-analysis comparing "single dose" and "multidose" regimens. Obstet Gynecol. 2003;101(4):778–784.

59. Centers for Disease Control and Prevention. Ectopic pregnancy—United States, 1990–1992. MMWR 1995;44(3):46–48.

60. Beyer DA, Dumesic DA. Heterotopic pregnancy: an emerging diagnostic challenge. OBG Management, 2002, October: 36–46.

61. Yee B, Rosen G, Cassidenti D. 1995. Transvaginal Sonography in Infertility. Lippincott-Raven

62. Sotiriadis A, Makrydimas G, Paptheodorou S, Ioannidis J. Expectant, medical or surgical management of first-trimester miscarriage: a meta-analysis. Obstet Gynecol 2005;105(5):1104–1113.

63. Luise C, Jermy K, May C, Costello G, Collins WP, Bourne TH. Outcome of expectant management of spontaneous first trimester miscarriage: observational study. BMJ Apr 13 2002;324(7342):873–875.

64. Zhang J, Giles JM, Barnhart K, Creinin MD, Westhoff C, Frederick MM. A comparison of medical management with misoprostol and surgical management for early pregnancy failure. N Engl J Med 2005;353(8), 761–769.

65. Moore C, Promes SB. Ultrasound in pregnancy. Emerg Med Clinics N Am 2004;22: 697–722.

66. Grønlund A, Grønlund L, Clevin L, Andersen B, Palmgren N, LidegaardØ. Management of missed abortion: comparison of medical treatment with either mifepristone + misoprostol or misoprostol alone with surgical evacuation. A multi-center trial in Copenhagen county, Denmark. Acta Obstet Gynecol Scand 2002;81: 1060–1065.

67. Doubilet PM, Benson CB. Atlas of Ultrasound in Obstetrics and Gynecology 2003. Lippincott Williams & Wilkins.

68. Erickson JD. Folic acid and prevention of spina bifida and anencephaly. 10 years after the U.S. Public Health Service recommendation. MMWR Recomm Rep. Sep 13 2002;51(RR-13):1–3.

69. Werler MM, Mitchell AA, Hernandez-Diaz S, Honein MA and the National Birth Defects Prevention Study. Use of over-the-counter medications during pregnancy. Am J Obstet Gynecol 2005;193: 771–777.

70. Schwarz EB, Maselli J, Morton M, Gonzales R. Prescription of teratogenic medications in United States ambulatory practices. Am J Med 2005;118: 1240–1249.

71. Gazmararian JA, Lazorick S, Spitz AM, Ballard TJ, Saltzman LE, Marks JS. Prevalence of violence against pregnant women. JAMA 1996 275: 1915–1920.
72. Connolly A, Katz VL, Bash KL, MacMahon MJ, Hansen WF. Trauma and pregnancy. Am J Perinatol 1998, 14(6): 331–336.
73. Horon IL, Cheng D. Enhanced surveillance for pregnancy-associated mortality—Maryland, 1993–1998. JAMA 2001, 285(11): 1455–1459.
74. Pallitto CC, O'Campo P. Is intimate partner violence associated with unintended pregnancy? A review of the literature. Trauma, Violence & Abuse 2005;6(3): 217–235.
75. Gazmararian JA, Adams MM, Saltzman LE, Johnson CH, Bruce, FC, Marks JS et al. The relationship between pregnancy intendedness and physical violence in mothers of newborns (PRAMS Working Group). Obstet Gynecol 1995, 85(6): 1031–1038.
76. Woo J, Fine P, Goetzl, L. Abortion disclosure and the association with domestic violence. Obstet Gynecol 2005;105(6): 1329–1334.
77. Rodriguez M, Quiroga S, Bauer H. Breaking the silence: battered women's perspectives on medical care. Arch Fam Med 1996;5: 153–158.
78. Elliot L., Nerney M, Jones T, Friedmann P. Barriers to screening for domestic violence. J Gen Intern Med 2002;17: 112–116.
79. Gremillion D, Kanof E. Overcoming barriers to physician involvement in identifying and referring victims of domestic violence. Ann Emerg Med 1996;27: 769–773.
80. Director TD, Linden JA. Domestic violence: an approach to identification and intervention. Emerg Med Clinics N Am 2004;22: 1117–1132.
81. Liebschutz JU, Paranjape A. How can a clinician identify violence in a woman's life? In: Liebschutz J, Frayne S., Saxe G, editors. Violence against women: a physician's guide to identification and management. Philadelphia: American College of Physicians-American Society of Internal Medicine, 2003. p.39–69.
82. McLeer S, Anwar T. The role of the emergency physician in the prevention of domestic violence. Ann Emerg Med 1987: 16: 1155–1161.

LATE REFERENCE

83. Godfrey EM, Anderson A, Fielding SL, Creinin MD, Schaff EA. Utility of low-sensitivity and high-sensitivity urine pregnancy tests and indicators of gestational sac expulsion after medical abortion. Contraception 2005;72: 244–245.

Abortion

Maureen Paul, MD, MPH
Felicia H. Stewart, MD

- Regard as urgent any request a woman makes for pregnancy confirmation and provide her with information about all her options, including prompt services or referral if she plans to consider abortion.

- Access to legal, safe abortion is a critical part of women's primary reproductive health care.

- Approximately 88% of all abortions in the United States occur during the first trimester; nearly 60% take place at or before 8 weeks following the onset of the woman's last normal menstrual period.

- Medication methods (most commonly mifepristone followed by misoprostol) are effective and safe options for women seeking abortion during the early weeks of pregnancy.

Women have abortions for many interrelated reasons. In a recent large U.S. survey,[1] women most frequently cited financial concerns, relationship problems, or work, school, or family responsibilities as reasons for their decision to have an abortion. Approximately 12% of the women reported concerns about their own health or that of the fetus as reasons for the abortion, and 1% reported that they were ending a pregnancy that resulted from coerced sex. In another study,[2] women who presented for second-trimester abortions were more likely to have had a delayed diagnosis of pregnancy and to have encountered logistical difficulties in accessing services, such as finding a provider, obtaining public insurance, and arranging transportation.

A woman's decision to terminate her pregnancy is based on her unique situation, and it often involves complex moral considerations regarding her responsibilities to herself and others. Each woman deserves to feel respected and supported as she makes her decision; it is not appropriate or logical to treat abortion as a regrettable human "failure".

In the past, many clinicians delayed scheduling an abortion until 7 weeks following a woman's last menstrual period, because pregnancy tests lacked the sensitivity to confirm early pregnancy and uterine aspiration resulted in slightly higher rates of incomplete abortion. Today, highly sensitive pregnancy tests and ultrasonography (see Chapter 23 on Pregnancy Testing and Management of Early Pregnancy) allow clinicians to diagnose pregnancy and offer safe and effective abortion options during the earliest weeks of pregnancy. Several excellent reviews describe the various clinical abortion techniques in more detail.[3-9] This chapter provides an overview for clinicians who evaluate and refer women for abortion services, as well as those who offer early medication or aspiration abortion in their practices.

LEGAL STATUS OF ABORTION

On January 22, 1973, the U.S. Supreme Court decided two landmark cases—*Roe v. Wade* [410 U.S. 113 (1973)] and *Doe v. Bolton* [410 U.S. 179 (1973)]—that legalized abortion nationwide. In brief, these decisions established the following "trimester framework":

1. In the first trimester, the abortion decision and procedure must be left to the judgment of the pregnant woman and her physician. States have little scope to interfere.

2. In the second trimester, each state may choose to regulate abortion procedures in ways that are reasonably related to the pregnant woman's health.

3. In the third trimester, when a fetus is already viable, the state may choose to promote its interest in potential human life by limiting, or even prohibiting, abortion. It may not, however, impose restrictions that interfere with the life or health of the pregnant woman.

As legal abortion became one of the most commonly performed procedures in the United States, abortion opponents introduced legislation at the local, state, and national levels to curtail access to abortion services. Passage of the Hyde Amendment in 1976 restricted federal funding for abortion, and numerous states regulated abortion through provisions for parental involvement, mandatory waiting periods, biased counseling requirements, and burdensome requirements for facilities.[10] The Supreme Court's 1992 landmark decision in *Planned Parenthood of Southeastern Pennsylvania v. Casey* [505 U.S. 833 (1992)] bolstered this approach by upholding state restrictions on abortion as long as they do not impose an "undue burden" on a woman's ability to choose abortion.[11,12]

The erosion of women's reproductive rights in the United States and globally has accelerated in recent years. On his first day in office in January 2001, President George W. Bush reinstated the "global gag rule" that prohibits foreign non-governmental organizations that receive U.S. family planning funds from engaging in abortion-related activities, resulting in the loss of critical reproductive health services worldwide.[13] In a sweeping 5–4 decision issued in April 2007, the U.S. Supreme Court upheld the federal "Partial-Birth Abortion Ban Act of 2003"[14] which criminalizes a certain safe second-trimester abortion procedure even when a physician believes that the procedure is necessary to preserve a woman's health.[15,16] This decision paves the way for further abortion restrictions by promoting state interest in protecting "fetal life" while dismissing decades of Supreme Court precedent that held women's health paramount. The increasingly conservative make-up of the Supreme Court reflective of this decision combines with recent federal court appointments to undermine women's right to choose abortion.

Notwithstanding these considerable challenges, public support for *Roe v. Wade* remains strong.[17] Passage of the Freedom of Access to Clinic Entrances (FACE) Act in 1993 has provided some protection for clinics and providers from harassment and violence directed against them,[18,19] and nearly all facilities affected by violence remain open. In addition, the availability of mifepristone regimens for medication abortion has prompted increasing numbers of primary care clinicians to offer this service, thereby enhancing women's access to early abortion care.[20-22]

THE PUBLIC HEALTH IMPACT OF LEGAL ABORTION

The *Roe v. Wade* decision ushered in a new era in women's health, producing immediate public health benefits; rates of abortion complications and deaths plummeted because abortion was more readily available closer to home, earlier in pregnancy, and at lower cost.[23] Abortion practices became safer after studies revealed that vacuum aspiration had less morbidity than sharp curettage, local anesthesia was safer than general anesthesia, abortions performed in freestanding clinics were safer than those performed in hospitals, and D&E was safer than labor induction for early second-trimester abortions. In the midst of strident debate over the abortion issue, the foundation of objective public health data has helped guide, or at least inform, judicial rulings and legislative actions.

CHARACTERISTICS OF WOMEN WHO OBTAIN ABORTIONS

Legal abortion statistics are currently reported by 47 states (excluding Alaska, California, and New Hampshire) to the Centers for Disease Control and Prevention (CDC), and they also have been studied through independent surveys. Between 1973 and 1980, the number of legal abortions reported to the CDC increased dramatically from about 600,000 to 1.3 million per year[24] (Table 24–1). During the 1980s, the number of reported legal abortions and the legal abortion rate (number of abotions per 1,000 women ages 15 to 44) remained remarkably stable, varying each year by less than 5%. After peaking in 1990 at 1.4 million, the number of legal abortions reported to the CDC decreased to 853,485 in 2001. This decline, however, in part reflects the CDC's decision in 1997 to stop including the estimated rates for non-reporting states, including California, which accounted for 23% of the 1997 total.[24] Historically, the number of legal abortions reported by the CDC has been 15% lower than the estimated number based on independent surveys by the Guttmacher Institute (GI). Using data from its 13th national survey, GI estimated that the number of abortions performed in 2000 was 1.31 million—having declined from a peak of 1.61 million in 1990.[25]

Nearly 60% of all reported abortions occur during the first 8 weeks following the onset of the LMP, and 88% are performed in the first trimester. The proportion of all abortions provided very early in pregnancy (6 weeks gestation or less) has increased from approximately 14% in 1992 to 25% in 2001.[24]

In the United States, approximately 1 in every 4 pregnant women chooses to terminate her pregnancy.[25] The proportion of pregnancies that end in elective abortion is highest for adolescents and women over age 40; for women who are poor, unmarried, or non-white; and for those who have had either no or 3 previous live births.[24,25] Although the U.S. abortion rate declined among most population subgroups between 1994 and 2001, the rate rose among economically disadvantaged women.[25] Younger women tend to obtain abortions later in pregnancy than do older women. Although 54% of women who obtain abortions report using contraception during the month that they became pregnant,[26,27] they may rely on less-effective methods, use methods inconsistently or incorrectly, or become pregnant despite using the methods perfectly.

How Many Abortions Occur Each Year in the United States?

Because some states do not report their abortion data, statistics published by the CDC on the annual number of abortions performed in the United States are underestimated. More accurate data derive from independent surveys conducted by the Guttmacher Institute (GI). The GI reports that 1.31 million abortions occurred in the United States in 2000.[25]

DECIDING WHETHER TO CONTINUE A PREGNANCY

The process of deciding whether to continue a pregnancy commonly begins as soon as a woman suspects she is pregnant. Some women will have made a firm decision by the time they seek pregnancy confirma-

Table 24–1 Characteristics of women who obtained legal abortions—United States, selected years, 1973 to 2001

Characteristics	1973 %	1980 %	1990 %	1995 %	2001 %
Residence					
In-state	74.8	92.6	91.8	91.5	91.3
Out-of-state	25.2	7.4	8.2	8.5	8.7
Age (years)					
≤ 19	32.7	29.2	22.4	20.1	18.1
20–24	32.0	35.5	33.2	32.5	33.4
> 25	35.3	35.3	44.4	47.4	48.5
Race					
White	72.5	69.9	64.8	59.6	55.4
Black and other	27.5	30.1	35.2	40.4	44.6
Marital Status					
Married	27.4	23.1	21.7	19.7	18.4
Unmarried	72.6	76.9	78.3	80.3	81.6
Weeks of Gestation					
≤ 8	36.1	51.7	51.6	54.0	59.1
9–10	29.4	26.2	25.3	23.1	19.0
11–12	17.9	12.2	11.7	10.9	10.0
13–15	6.9	5.1	6.4	6.3	6.2
16–20	8.0	3.9	4.0	4.3	4.3
≥ 21	1.7	0.9	1.0	1.4	1.4
Reported No. of Legal Abortions	615,831	1,297,606	1,429,247	1,210,883	853,485*

* Excludes AK, CA, and NH

Source: Strauss LT et. al. (2004).[24]

tion; others may need to explore their options further. Providing prompt and convenient pregnancy confirmation services has important benefits, including the following:

- Allows the woman ample time to consider her options
- Facilitates the initiation of pregnancy precautions and prenatal care
- Increases the likelihood that a woman will be eligible for the full range of early abortion options
- Decreases both the risks and the costs of complications if the woman chooses abortion
- Expedites the diagnosis of pregnancy abnormalities, such as ectopic pregnancy

Provide a supportive, nonjudgmental setting so the woman can explore her feelings concerning pregnancy, abortion, her partner, her future life plans, and her ability to provide for a child at present and in the future. Ambivalence is common, and for many women the decision is complicated.[8] Basic factual information and discussion will meet the needs of most women; some patients may desire more extensive education, evaluation, or counseling to ensure that they are making an informed decision without coercion. Depending on the scope of services that your practice provides, you may need to refer patients for financial assistance, further counseling, first- or second-trimester abortions, prenatal care, adoption services, or other necessary care.

METHODS OF ABORTION

A number of options are available for pregnancy termination. Aspiration remains a venerable, safe, and effective method for women seeking abortion during the first trimester. Early medication abortion using mifepristone and misoprostol is available in the United States and many other countries. Other early medication abortion options include methotrexate-misoprostol or misoprostol-only regimens. After the first trimester, the most common method for abortion in the United States is dilation and evacuation (D&E), typically preceded by cervical preparation using osmotic cervical dilating devices or misoprostol. Medical induction using prostaglandins or other agents accounts for a small proportion of abortions after the first trimester.

SELECTING A METHOD

More than any other factor, the duration of pregnancy determines which abortion method the woman may choose (Figure 24–1). She may opt for medication abortion during the first 7 to 9 weeks of pregnancy (depending on the medication regimen), or aspiration throughout the first trimester. Although second-trimester abortion methods include D&E and medical induction, women's options may be limited by cost or by a lack of skilled abortion providers in their communities.[19] The patient will need information about the abortion procedures available; how they are done; their safety, success rates, risks, costs, and time required; and follow-up care. Although the woman may want her partner or other supportive persons involved in the counseling, she also will need a chance to talk privately with you so you can be sure that her decision is not coerced.

There are no evidence-based contraindications to abortion *per se*, although some medical conditions or problems, such as severe anemia, may influence the decision about which abortion method or clinical setting would be safest for the woman. No data are available about the use of medication abortion regimens while breastfeeding. The drug label for mifepristone advises against its use in the following circumstances:

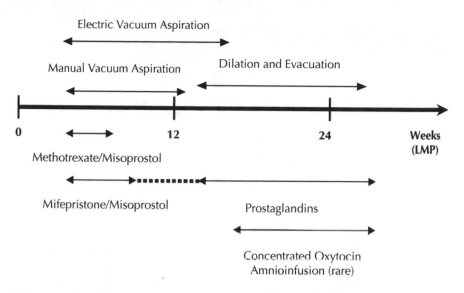

Figure 24–1 Options for terminating pregnancy, by duration of pregnancy

- Confirmed or suspected ectopic pregnancy or undiagnosed adnexal mass
- IUD in place (must be removed before treatment)
- Chronic adrenal failure
- Current long-term systemic corticosteroid therapy
- History of allergy to mifepristone, misoprostol, or other prostaglandin
- Hemorrhagic disorders or concurrent anti-coagulant therapy
- Inherited porphyrias

Although single-dose methotrexate therapy for medication abortion or ectopic pregnancy has little, if any, systemic toxicity, it should not be administered to women with chronic renal or hepatic disease. Methotrexate is a known human teratogen when given in high doses; moreover, congenital abnormalities including limb defects, skull defects, and Mobius sequence have been reported after first-trimester exposure to misoprostol—the prostaglandin used in mifepristone and methotrexate medication abortion regimens.[9] Although data are insufficient to determine teratogenic risk with the doses used for medication abortion, these regimens are not advised for women who would be unwilling to have an aspiration abortion should the medications fail to terminate the pregnancy.[7]

In helping the early-abortion patient decide between medication abortion and aspiration, explain the important features of each method (Table 24–2). Most women will express a clear preference and be highly satis-

Table 24–2 Characteristics of Early Abortion Methods

Aspiration Abortion	Medication Abortion
Highly effective	Highly effective
Procedure brief	Abortion process takes one to several days to complete (sometimes longer)
Involves invasive procedure	Avoids invasive procedure (aspiration) if successful
Allows option of sedation or general anesthesia	Avoids anesthesia
Usually requires only 1 visit	Involves at least 2 visits
Lighter perceived bleeding	Heavier perceived bleeding
Requires clinical setting	May occur in privacy of home

fied with the method they choose.[28] The main advantages of aspiration are its speed and predictability and the option for sedation or general anesthesia. The drawbacks are the procedure's invasiveness and the small risk of uterine perforation. Reasons commonly cited for choosing medication abortion include that it is non-invasive and more "natural" and that it affords women greater privacy and control over the abortion process.[29,30] Disadvantages of medication methods include the length of time required to complete the abortion process (one to several days, or in the case of methotrexate abortion, possibly longer) and the longer period of bleeding and cramping that commonly accompanies passage of the pregnancy.

Since the introduction of mifepristone in Europe over a decade ago, its use for abortion has risen gradually each year to reach over 50% of early abortions in some countries[31] (Figure 24–2). The U.S. Food and Drug Administration (FDA) approved mifepristone in September of 2000, and medication abortion accounted for 6% of all abortions (approximately 10% of early abortions) that occurred in the United States during the first 6 months of 2001.[25] Since then, the proportion of eligible women choosing medication abortion has continued to grow. Most members of the National Abortion Federation, including Planned Parenthood affiliates, currently offer early medication abortion services, and efforts are underway to expand provision by primary care practitioners, including family practice physicians and advanced practice clinicians.[20,22]

Aspiration and D&E Abortion Methods

Introduced in the United States in 1967, aspiration (suction or vacuum curettage) is the method used for virtually all first-trimester instrumental abortions in the United States.[24] Aspiration is a safe and simple way to empty the uterus completely and quickly using modest cervical dilation

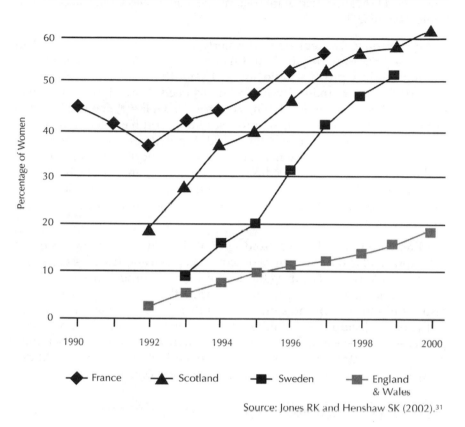

Source: Jones RK and Henshaw SK (2002).[31]

Figure 24 2 Percentage of women eligible for early medical abortion who were prescribed mifepristone, four European countries, 1990–2000

and an electric vacuum pump or hand-held syringe (manual vacuum aspiration).

D&E procedures are used for almost all second-trimester abortion procedures in the United States.[24] Although D&E requires surgical expertise, it is safer than older "instillation" methods of medical induction that involved infusion or injection of prostaglandins, hypertonic saline, or urea into the amniotic cavity.[32,33] Most women prefer D&E to induction methods that typically entail hospitalization, higher costs, and a prolonged period of labor.[34]

Early Medication Abortion Methods

Medication regimens are currently available in the United States for abortion during the first 7–9 weeks of pregnancy, depending on the regimen used. Use of the methotrexate-misoprostol regimen has decreased since the FDA approved mifepristone for early medication abortion in September of 2000.

Mifepristone. Mifepristone (formerly known as RU 486) is sold in the United States under the brand name Mifeprex. Widely used in conjunction with a prostaglandin for early abortion in several European countries for more than 15 years,[35,36] it has been shown to be safe, effective, and acceptable in developing countries as well.[37-40] The combination of mifepristone and misoprostol for early abortion has been used safely by millions of women around the world. Limited research suggests that mifepristone regimens also may be effective for abortion performed later in the first trimester, but bleeding may be heavier, and its safety outside of hospital settings has not been tested.[41] If hospitalization would be necessary for medication options, aspiration abortion is a quicker and less costly alternative.

Mifepristone is a 19-norsteroid with a high affinity for progesterone receptors; it also binds to glucocorticoid receptors and (to a lesser extent) androgen receptors. The drug blocks the action of progesterone, which is necessary to establish and maintain placental attachment. Mifepristone also softens the cervix and stimulates synthesis of prostaglandins by cells of the early decidua.[9] In addition to its use for inducing abortion, mifepristone has been investigated for other medical applications including emergency contraception (in low doses) and treatment of conditions such as uterine leiomyomata, endometriosis, and certain cancers.

Methotrexate. Methotrexate is a folic acid analogue that competitively inhibits dihydrofolate reductase, an enzyme necessary for DNA synthesis. Methotrexate causes abortion by its action on the rapidly dividing cells of the early placenta (cytotrophoblast); when used with misoprostol, it effectively terminates early intrauterine pregnancy during the first 7 weeks dated from the onset of the LMP.[42] Methotrexate is also effective in treating early ectopic pregnancy.[43,44] The drug is marketed for treatment of choriocarcinoma, severe psoriasis, and rheumatoid arthritis. Although early abortion and ectopic pregnancy are not included in the labeling for methotrexate, these uses are supported by published evidence accumulated over many years.

Misoprostol. Misoprostol is a prostaglandin E1 analogue that is used in mifepristone and methotrexate regimens for early abortion. Misoprostol softens the cervix and stimulates uterine contractions, thereby facilitating expulsion of the pregnancy. It can cause mild, short-term systemic prostaglandin effects, including nausea, vomiting, diarrhea, and temporary elevation of body temperature—side effects that women commonly report with all medication abortion regimens. Sold under the brand name Cytotec in the United States, misoprostol is a widely available, inexpensive medication marketed for prevention of gastrointestinal ulcer disease. The FDA has approved an early abortion regimen using mifepristone in combination with misoprostol for early abortion. Extensive evidence also supports the use of misoprostol to manage early pregnancy loss,[45] prepare the cervix before aspiration or D&E abortion, and induce labor.[46]

Misoprostol's effect depends on the route of administration. An oral dose (swallowed) results in more rapid and higher peak blood levels with more intense uterine contractility and side effects, while a vaginal or buccal dose (tucked between the cheek and gum) is absorbed more slowly and has lower peak blood levels, fewer side effects, and a less intense but more sustained uterine effect.[47-49] Sublingual (under the tongue) administration appears to act similarly to oral administration.[49,50] Because the sensitivity of the uterus to misoprostol increases as pregnancy advances, doses used to induce labor in the second or third trimester of pregnancy are lower than those required for early abortion.[41]

Mifepristone-misoprostol regimens. Although use of mifepristone alone results in abortion in some cases, the addition of misoprostol increases efficacy. The early abortion regimen approved by the FDA in 2000 was based on studies conducted more than a decade ago that used 600 mg of mifepristone followed 2 days later by misoprostol, 400 μg administered orally. The patients took both medications at the clinic and returned in approximately 2 weeks for follow-up. The success rate (complete abortion without the need for aspiration) of the FDA-approved regimen is approximately 92% in women with pregnancies of 49 days' duration or less.[51]

Subsequent research has shown that a lower dose of mifepristone, 200 mg, is equally effective[52,53] and that misoprostol at a dose of 800 μg self-administered vaginally at home extends high efficacy through 63 days gestation, has fewer side effects, and is more convenient and private for women.[9,54-57] This evidence-based regimen also provides women flexibility in the time of administration of misoprostol, ranging from as early as 6 hours to 72 hours after mifepristone[55,57-59] (See Table 24–3). Buccal misoprostol is an effective and acceptable alternative to the vaginal route. A randomized trial found that misoprostol 800 ug taken buccally (placed between cheek and gum) 24 to 48 hours after mifepristone is as effective as vaginal misoprostol through 56 days from onset of the LMP[60] (Table 24–3). Studies are ongoing to determine the efficacy of the buccal route through 63 days gestation.

Most U.S. abortion providers use an evidence-based mifepristone regimen in lieu of the original protocol delineated on the product label for mifepristone.[19,61] The FDA permits off-label use of any therapeutic medication,[62] which allows clinicians to offer patients new and improved treatments based on accumulating scientific research.

Table 24–3 Comparison of mifepristone regimens

	FDA-approved Regimen	Evidenced-based Regimen (Vaginal Misoprostol)	Evidenced-based Regimen (Buccal Misoprostol)
Recommended gestational age (dated from onset of the LMP)	49 days or less	63 days or less	56 days or less*
Mifepristone dose	600 mg orally	200 mg orally	200 mg orally
Misoprostol dose	400 μg orally administered during second office visit	800 μg vaginally; supplied during first office visit and administered at home	800 μg buccally; supplied during first office visit and administered at home
Misoprostol timing	48 hours after mifepristone	6 to 72 hours after mifepristone**	24 to 48 hours after mifepristone
Minimum office visits	3	2	2
Approximate cost to patient	$270 for mifepristone $2 for misoprostol 3 office visits	$90 for mifepristone $4 for misoprostol 2 office visits	
Advantages	Some women prefer the oral route of misoprostol administration	• Extends gestational age eligibility • Higher complete abortion rates • Fewer side effects • Fewer clinic visits • Greater flexibility in timing of misoprostol administration • Lower cost	

Adapted from Stewart FH, et. al. (UCSF 2001).[7]

* Research is ongoing to assess the efficacy of the mifepristone-buccal misoprostol regimen through 63 days LMP.

** A mifepristone-vaginal misoprostol interval longer than 48 hours has not been studied in women with pregnancies 57 to 63 days LMP.

Methotrexate-misoprostol regimens.   Prior to the availability of mifepristone in the United States, U.S. researchers developed other regimens for early medication abortion using methotrexate and misoprostol. Because these drugs are widely available and inexpensive, they offer an important alternative when mifepristone is unaffordable or unavailable. Used in combination with misoprostol, methotrexate is 92% to 96% successful in terminating pregnancy through 7 weeks (49 days) of gestation dated from the first day of the LMP.[9,63–65] However, in 15% to 25% of women, the abortion process can take up to a month.[42,64]

Most protocols use intramuscular methotrexate at a dose of 50 mg per square meter of body surface, but a 50 mg dose taken orally (dissolved in orange juice to disguise the taste) is comparably effective.[66,67] Three to 7 days after methotrexate treatment, the woman inserts misoprostol 800 μg vaginally. She may repeat the dose if bleeding does not occur after 24 hours or if she has not aborted by the time of the one-week follow-up visit. Most women will abort successfully by 4 weeks following initiation of treatment.

Misoprostol-only regimens. Misoprostol alone can induce abortion, but combining it with mifepristone is more effective.[68] A variety of early abortion regimens using misoprostol alone has been studied; most involve multiple doses and therefore higher rates of side effects than occur with combined mifepristone regimens.[9] Complete abortion rates in studies using 800 μg vaginal misoprostol (usually pre-moistened before insertion) every 24 hours for two to three doses in pregnancies up to 56 days from the onset of the LMP range from 83% to 92% in various studies.[68-72] The optimal misoprostol regimen for second-trimester abortion has not been established, and regimens may vary by gestational age.[41]

Misoprostol is widely employed by women outside of clinical settings in countries where abortion is illegible or inaccessible. Anecdotal evidence suggests that some women in the United States are using misoprostol to self-induce abortion.[73] This practice may grow as word spreads through informal information networks, and women may present for follow-up treatment after self-administration. Women who seek care due to problems, such as heavy bleeding or incomplete abortion, may not acknowledge use of misoprostol unless the provider specifically requests this information. In addition to following guidelines for problem management and referral used for other medication abortion patients (see below), the clinician may need to: (1) treat or refer for management of side effects, particularly if the woman used large doses of misoprostol; (2) strongly advise aspiration abortion if the pregnancy is ongoing to avoid the potential teratogenic effects of misoprostol; and (3) help the patient obtain the information, family planning care, and other health services that she may need on an ongoing basis.

PROVIDING ABORTION SERVICES
PRE-ABORTION PROCEDURES

Because most women who request abortion are young and healthy, the pre-abortion medical evaluation is usually straightforward. The goals of the evaluation include the following:

- Confirm pregnancy and estimate gestational age

- Identify possible problems that require further evaluation or emergency intervention, such as ectopic gestation or spontaneous abortion.

- Screen as appropriate for infection.

- Identify medical or gynecologic conditions that might influence the choice of appropriate abortion options.

History-Taking

- Recent menstrual history, including the regularity of the menstrual cycle and the onset of the last normal menstrual period

- Prior obstetric and gynecologic history, including previous surgery involving the cervix or uterus, (e.g., conization of the cervix, cesarean delivery, history of leiomyomata [fibroids]) and any complications of previous abortions

- Contraceptive history, including current IUD use, and future contraceptive plans

- Allergies to latex, local anesthetics, antiseptic solutions, analgesics, antibiotics, anti-progestins, prostaglandins, and other drugs

- Current drug use (legal, illicit, or over-the-counter) including anti-coagulants or systemic corticosteroids

- Acute or chronic illnesses that might require more evaluation, adjunctive therapy, or special care in the provision of the abortion or that might preclude one or more methods of abortion

Clinical Examination

Perform a brief physical assessment that includes vital signs and a pelvic examination or ultrasound to determine uterine size and position and to estimate gestational age. Note the presence of any abnormality, such as such as large uterine fibroids or cervical stenosis, that might indicate the need for further evaluation or influence the selection of a procedure. An ultrasound evaluation is indicated if pelvic examination findings are not clear or if you suspect pregnancy beyond the first trimester or an adnexal mass, ectopic pregnancy, or other abnormality.

Laboratory Tests

Recommended laboratory screening includes the following procedures:

- Urine pregnancy test* (unless pregnancy already has been confirmed by ultrasound)

- Hemoglobin or hematocrit, if indicated. (Offer iron supplementation to anemic women [hemoglobin < 10g/dl or hematocrit < 30%].)

---

* A serum pregnancy test is logical only when serial, quantitative hCG levels are needed to monitor a possible ectopic pregnancy or to evaluate a missed or incomplete spontaneous abortion. For confirming pregnancy, a urine pregnancy test performed in a clinical setting is simple, inexpensive, fast (results are available immediately), and has high accuracy. (See Pregnancy Testing and Management of Early Pregnancy, Chapter 23.)

- Rh$_o$(D) determination

- Screening for reproductive tract infection as appropriate. (If Chlamydia, gonorrhea, or bacterial vaginosis is suspected or identified, initiate treatment prior to or at the time of the abortion.)

FIRST-TRIMESTER MEDICATION ABORTION

With its emphasis on patient education, support, and follow-up, medication abortion can be provided appropriately within the scope of practice of most primary care providers, including nurse practitioners, nurse midwives, and physician assistants. The FDA stipulates that medication abortion providers must be able to assess the duration of pregnancy, diagnose ectopic pregnancy, and provide or refer for vacuum aspiration or emergency treatment when necessary; personal expertise in ultrasound or aspiration is not required. These capabilities do not differ from those needed by any clinician caring for reproductive-aged women who may present for diagnosis or evaluation of early pregnancy. Laws in many states, however, restrict the extent to which non-physicians can practice medication abortion,[62] so check with legal experts in your state before initiating the service. The Abortion Access Project (www.abortionaccess.org) may be helpful in providing information and in putting you in touch with a lawyer in your state.

Providing medication abortion does not require specialized facilities; a typical medical office with space for private consultation, physical examination, equipment and medication for handling a medication allergic reaction, and arrangements for a urine pregnancy test and Rh typing suffices. In addition, you need to plan for emergency back-up or referral, 24-hour telephone emergency accessibility, and staff training. Other practical issues to consider include state regulations, if any, specific to the provision of abortion services such as requirements for parental consent or notification, mandatory waiting periods, or counseling. Several organizations can provide additional information about these issues, including the National Abortion Federation (www.prochoice.org).

In the United States, mifepristone is not available through pharmacies; rather, it is sold directly to licensed physicians who meet the aforementioned qualifications after they sign and return a Prescriber's Agreement provided by the drug's distributor. Prescribers agree to report adverse events and to give each patient a Medication Guide to read and a Patient Agreement to read and sign. Information and forms necessary to enroll as a mifepristone provider are available at the distributor's website, www.earlyoptionpill.com. If you plan to use an evidence-based alternative regimen, ask patients to sign an additional consent or addendum that provides information about the alternative regimen, how it differs from the FDA protocol, and its benefits and risks.

Clinical Management

A woman undergoing medication abortion needs detailed information about the regimens, how to use the medications, what to expect during the process, possible side effects and complications, and what to do if she has questions or concerns (Table 24–4). Emphasize that she may need an aspiration procedure if the medication abortion fails or if she has excessive bleeding. Approximately 1% to 3% of women using a mifepristone and misoprostol regimen will require vacuum aspiration for these reasons.[9,51,61]

Medication abortion usually involves two to three office visits (Table 24–5). With the evidence-based regimens commonly used in the United States, 2 visits are required: the first to evaluate the patient and provide the medications, and a follow-up visit to assess whether the medications ended the pregnancy. An additional visit is necessary if the FDA-approved regimen is used, or if state regulations require a separate counseling visit before the patient has an abortion.

The FDA-approved mifepristone regimen requires women to return to the clinic 2 days after mifepristone administration to receive 2 tablets (400 μg) of misoprostol as a single oral dose. Patients who choose the evidence-based regimens with home-use of misoprostol receive four 200 μg-tablets (800 μg) with instructions for vaginal or buccal administration at the appropriate time. All protocols necessitate a follow-up visit to assess the abortion outcome. If a viable pregnancy persists for 2 weeks after treatment, aspiration abortion is recommended because of the potential risk of birth defects following early exposure to methotrexate or misoprostol. If the pregnancy has stopped growing, then the woman may choose to wait for expulsion to occur (Table 24–5).

Table 24–4 Patient education for early medication abortion (see text)

1. Discuss the woman's decision to have an abortion, and confirm that her decision is certain and voluntary.

2. Discuss the treatment alternatives (medication abortion or aspiration), and explain the benefits and risks of each method.

3. Describe the medication regimens available and their FDA status. For mifepristone-misoprostol abortion, explain the differences between the FDA-approved regimen and evidence-based regimens. For methotrexate-misoprostol abortion, explain that the FDA has approved these drugs for other uses, but not for medication abortion.

4. Explain what to expect in regard to bleeding and cramping. These symptoms typically intensify during expulsion of the pregnancy (usually 2–4 hours) and then gradually subside. Passage of clots is common during expulsion. Lighter bleeding or spotting typically lasts about 2 weeks, but may be longer.

5. Explain that the patient is unlikely to see products of conception unless she is close to 9 weeks of pregnancy, in which case the embryo will be very small and often obscured by blood clots.

6. Discuss known side effects of the medication abortion regimen including mild gastrointestinal symptoms; short-term fever, warmth or chills; or oral ulcers (methotrexate only).

7. **Explain that the drugs used for medication abortion may increase the risk of birth defects if the pregnancy were to continue. Emphasize that aspiration abortion is advised if the medication abortion method fails.**

8. Discuss possible complications including failed abortion, incomplete abortion, hemorrhage, or infection. Emphasize that atypical infections have occurred rarely after use of mifepristone combined with vaginal misoprostol (see text).

9. Provide medication instructions, including how to insert the misoprostol vaginally (deep into the vagina after washing hands) or buccally (tucked between cheek and gum) and how to use pain medications.

10. Explain the time commitment and expected number of visits.

11. Provide 24-hour emergency contact information, and emphasize warning signs that may warrant evaluation, including the following:
    a. Prolonged or heavy bleeding (≥2 soaked maxipads for 2 consecutive hours);
    b. Fever (≥100.4° F) lasting more than 4 hours or beginning in the days after misoprostol administration;
    c. Abdominal pain or discomfort or 'feeling sick' (including weakness, nausea, vomiting or diarrhea, with or without fever) more than 24 hours after using misoprostol.

12. Provide information about available contraceptive methods and when to initiate the chosen method, if any.

13. Address issues of confidentiality.

14. Review all required consent forms, which must be signed before administration of the medications.

Table 24-5 Clinical protocols for early medication abortion

Visit	Mifepristone (FDA-Approved Regimen)	Mifepristone (Alternative Evidence-Based Regimens)	Methotrexate Regimen
One	Give 600 mg mifepristone orally	Give 200 mg mifepristone orally Provide four 200-μg tablets misoprostol (800 μg) to take home with instructions for: • vaginal administration in 6–72 hrs (6–48 hrs if 50–63 days since onset of LMP), OR • buccal administration in 24–48 hours	Administer 50 mg/m² body surface area IM or 50 mg orally Provide four 200-μg tablets (800 μg) misoprostol with instructions for vaginal administration at home in 3–7 days
	Administer Rh₀(D)-immune globulin 50-μg to Rh₀(D)-negative women. Provide analgesics and instructions for their use.		
Two	*Day 3* Administer two 200-mg tablets misoprostol orally.	**Optional** *Day 2–7* (at least 24 hrs after misoprostol administration)	*Day 5–9* (at least 24 hrs after misoprostol insertion)
		Assess outcome • If abortion complete, offer contraceptive counseling • If abortion has not occurred, offer repeat dose of vaginal or buccal misoprostol (800 μg) unless patient prefers aspiration. • If ongoing viable pregnancy, follow-up at about Day 14. • If persistent non-viable pregnancy, follow up in about 4 weeks.	Assess outcome • If abortion complete, offer contraceptive counseling. • If abortion has not occurred, provide repeat dose of vaginal misoprostol (800 μg) unless patient prefers aspiration. • If ongoing viable pregnancy, follow-up at about Day 14. • If persistent non-viable pregnancy, follow up in about 4 weeks.
Three	*Day 14* Assess outcome. Schedule aspiration abortion if viable pregnancy.	*Day 14* (if viable pregnancy on previous visit). Schedule aspiration abortion if viable pregnancy persists.	*Day 14* (if viable pregnancy on previous visit). Schedule aspiration abortion if viable pregnancy persists.
Four	Approximately 4–5 weeks after initiation of treatment for patients who are awaiting resolution of a non-viable pregnancy. Offer aspiration if non-viable pregnancy persists.		

No matter which drug combination or regimen they use, women undergoing medication abortion are likely to experience cramping and bleeding. Women may describe the experience as similar to an early miscarriage. In most cases, pain can be managed with acetaminophen (Tylenol), a non-steroidal anti-inflammatory such as ibuprofen, or acetaminophen with codeine phosphate (300 mg/30 mg). Non-steroidal anti-inflammatory agents such as ibuprofen do not interfere with the effectiveness of misoprostol.[74]

Although bleeding may seem abundant to those experiencing it, the amount of bleeding is rarely clinically significant. One study that used mifepristone with oral or vaginal misoprostol through 63 days gestation found median blood losses ranging from 83 to 89 ml,[75] compared with the 50 ml typically lost during menses or the nearly 500 ml typically given in a blood donation. Although the range of bleeding varies widely among women, significant changes in hemoglobin seldom occur.[75] Bleeding is usually heaviest during expulsion of the pregnancy; lighter flow or spotting lasts about 2 weeks on average, but may be longer.[76] Use of combined oral contraceptives does not alter bleeding patterns after medication abortion.[76,77]

Providing patients with parameters for excessive bleeding enhances safety. Advise the patient to call if she soaks two or more large pads per hour for 2 consecutive hours. If the patient feels otherwise well, monitoring periodically by telephone for another 2 hours is acceptable. Patients whose bleeding does not slow after this interval warrant prompt in-person evaluation. Some providers treat excessive bleeding with an ergot alkaloid such as methylergonovine maleate (Methergine) before resorting to aspiration. Bleeding significant enough to require aspiration occurs in less than 1% of patients, and it may be delayed until 3 to 5 weeks after taking mifepristone.[78] Fewer than 1 in 1000 women will need a blood transfusion for heavy bleeding.[9,61]

Side effects common with all medication abortion regimens include nausea, headache, vomiting, diarrhea, dizziness, fever, and chills.[9] These side effects typically subside within a few hours and seldom require treatment. Temperature elevation (100.4° F or more) that lasts more than 4 hours or that begins in the days after misoprostol administration, however, warrants clinical assessment.

Methods used to confirm abortion include a history of bleeding with evidence of uterine involution on follow-up examination, appropriately falling serum quantitative hCG determinations, or ultrasonography.[79] Although most medication abortion researchers in the United States relied on ultrasonography to assess gestational age and clinical outcomes, providers in many countries offer safe medication abortion services without routine use of ultrasound. Whatever method you choose to follow patients, remember these important guidelines:

- If a woman has a gestational sac on initial ultrasound examination and no sac on follow-up, then her abortion is complete. Aspiration for "debris" in the uterus is not indicated unless the patient is bleeding heavily or has symptoms or signs of infection.

- If you are following serum hCGs in a woman who did not have an intrauterine pregnancy confirmed by pre-abortion ultrasound, draw an initial quantitative hCG test on the day of mifepristone or methotrexate administration and a second test about 24 to 72 hours after she uses misoprostol (no later than 1 week following the start of treatment). If the hCG values fall by at least 50%, the abortion is most likely complete.[9,79] Rapidly rising hCG values usually signal a continuing pregnancy, while a slow rise, plateau, or slow fall may indicate ectopic pregnancy (see Pregnancy Testing and Management of Early Pregnancy, Chapter 23).

- Absent or minimal bleeding after taking misoprostol is a warning sign for possible ectopic pregnancy, unless pre-abortion ultrasonography showed a definitive intrauterine pregnancy.

- Sensitive urine pregnancy tests are not useful at the follow-up visit to confirm that the abortion was successful, because hCG may not clear from the body for a month or more following complete abortion (see Pregnancy Testing and Management of Early Pregnancy, Chapter 23).

Ongoing research seeks to simplify the process of medication abortion.[80] For example, one study evaluated the accuracy of using patient history to predict complete abortion; when both patients and providers agreed that expulsion had occurred, ultrasonography showed that they were correct 99% of the time.[81] If further research confirms these results, home-based assessment of outcome may eventually replace in-person follow-up for many women.

First-Trimester Aspiration Abortion

Aspiration using local anesthesia with or without mild oral or intravenous sedation can be provided safely and appropriately in a medical office setting equipped with the same emergency back-up equipment and supplies needed to provide injectable medications (drugs and resuscitation equipment to manage allergic reaction, seizure, or cardiac arrest). In addition, the facility should have available the medication needed to treat uterine atony and a plan for transferring a woman to a surgical facility if she needs an evaluation for uterine perforation. General anesthesia also is available in specialized facilities, but it increases slightly the risk of complications and involves a longer post-procedure recovery time. Most states limit abortion provision to physicians; however, in a few states without such restrictions, advanced practice clinicians have provided aspiration abortions for years with an impressive safety record.[82]

As the first step in an aspiration procedure, perform a bimanual examination to determine the size and position of the uterus. Insertion of a short-bladed speculum, such as a Moore Graves design, permits the clinician to draw the cervix close to the perineum for adequate visualization and to straighten a flexed uterus. Although vaginal cleansing with an antiseptic solution is a common practice, its efficacy in preventing postabortal infection has not been established.[83] Of greater importance is the use of a "no touch" technique (not touching the parts of instruments that will enter the sterile uterine cavity) to help assure asepsis during the abortion procedure.

Administer a local anesthetic such as 0.5% to 1% lidocaine amide (limiting the amount to 200 mg or less) to the cervix to reduce pain. While the patient's cervix is anesthetized, place a tenaculum to keep the cervix stabilized. Using Pratt or Denniston dilators, dilate the cervix gently and incrementally as needed to accommodate an aspiration cannula of appropriate size for the gestation. Typically, the diameter of the cannula in millimeters corresponds to the duration of the pregnancy in weeks (for example, 7 mm cannula for pregnancy at 7 weeks). Insert a cannula connected to a vacuum source (either an electric vacuum pump or a manual vacuum syringe) through the dilated cervix, and evacuate the products of conception by a combination of rotary and back-and-forth motions. Detection of a "gritty" sensation as the cannula moves across the endometrial surface typically indicates that the uterus is empty. Examining the removed tissue helps to confirm complete evacuation and may assist in the diagnosis of ectopic pregnancy, hydatidiform mole, or incomplete spontaneous pregnancy loss. Evaluation is facilitated by suspending the tissue in water, saline, or white vinegar and checking with backlighting.

SECOND-TRIMESTER DILATION AND EVACUATION

D&E, which combines vacuum aspiration with use of forceps,[32] is quite widely available for procedures performed between 13 and 16 weeks' gestation, and experts use this method through 24 weeks or more. Accurate estimation of gestational age is crucial, and intraoperative sonography may be helpful. The cervix requires more dilation for a second-trimester D&E than for a first-trimester aspiration to permit evacuation of the larger products of conception. Preoperative cervical preparation using osmotic dilating devices or misoprostol is recommended as part of the D&E process. After administering anesthesia, the clinician removes the osmotic dilators and empties the uterus using appropriate instruments. Intact D&E, a variant in which the fetus is extracted as intact as possible,[84] is prohibited by law unless a fetocidal agent such as digoxin is administered before the abortion (see Legal Status of Abortion).

SECOND-TRIMESTER INDUCTION ABORTION

A variety of newer techniques, used alone or in combination, has largely replaced instillation methods in the United States.[24] Misoprostol alone, when administered in multiple doses, is effective for second-trimester abortion, but the optimal regimen has yet to be established.[41] Pretreatment with mifepristone enhances efficacy and shortens the time required to induce abortion. The Royal College of Obstetricians and Gynaecologists (RCOG) in the United Kingdom has endorsed the mifepristone-misoprostol combination for abortion at 15 weeks gestation or more when providers with specialized skills for D&E are not available.[85] The regimen recommended by RCOG includes mifepristone, 200 mg orally, followed 36 to 48 hours later by misoprostol 800 μg vaginally, then misoprostol 400 μg orally every 3 hours to a maximum of four oral doses. Success rates as high as 97% have been reported with this protocol.[86] Other methods include vaginal administration of dinoprostone, a prostaglandin approved by the FDA for second-trimester abortion, and intravenous administration of high-dose oxytocin.[87] All second-trimester induction methods have side effects specific to the medications used, and curettage for retained placenta is not uncommon. The relative safety of modern induction methods compared to D&E has not been established, although one limited study reported a higher complication rate with misoprostol induction than with D&E, based solely on the greater need for curettage to remove retained placenta.[88]

ADJUNCTIVE TECHNIQUES

Several adjunctive techniques are used commonly for second-trimester abortions, and they may be used for first-trimester aspiration abortion as well.

Osmotic dilating devices. Dried seaweed of the genus *Laminaria japonica* is highly hygroscopic (absorbs water and expands) and can, over a period of time, dilate the cervix. Synthetic hygroscopic dilators—Lamicel, a magnesium sulfate-impregnated cellulose sponge or Dilapan, a polyacrylonitrile (plastic) rod—produce faster cervical dilation than laminaria, although Lamicel is not as effective when wide dilation is needed. Use of osmotic dilators decreases the risk of cervical laceration or perforation,[89,90] although the small risk of uterine injury in first-trimester abortion may not justify their routine use. Place osmotic dilators (at least one or two for procedures at 14 to 16 weeks; more for later procedures) the day before D&E abortion, or 2 to 4 hours beforehand if you intend to provide a one-day procedure for early second-trimester abortion. Several serial insertions of an increasing number of dilators may be used for procedures later in pregnancy. Place the dilators so they extend through the endocervical canal and dilate both the internal os and the external os. Following placement of laminaria, most of the cervical expansion occurs by 6 hours, but maximum dilation occurs in 12 to 24 hours; dilation occurs in a shorter interval with use of Dilapan or Lamicel.[8]

Misoprostol. Treatment with misoprostol prior to abortion causes cervical softening and dilation (called ripening) that can reduce the need for additional mechanical dilation or make it easier. Vaginal insertion of misoprostol has greater efficacy and fewer side effects than oral administration.[91] Numerous studies suggest that an optimal regimen for first-trimester cervical preparation is 400 µg administered vaginally 3 hours prior to the procedure.[41] This regimen is as effective as overnight laminaria for first-trimester cervical preparation.[92] Preliminary evidence suggests that sublingual administration of misoprostol may prime the cervix as well as vaginal misoprostol, but with a higher incidence of side effects.[93] Buccal misoprostol also may represent an effective alternative route of administration.[94]

Although misoprostol use is common prior to D&E abortion in the United States, optimal regimens are not yet well-defined. One randomized trial of women having abortions at 13 to 16 weeks of pregnancy found that overnight preparation with 3 to 6 laminaria resulted in greater dilation and faster procedure times than vaginal misoprostol 400 µg administered 3 to 4 hours before evacuation.[95] However, most procedures were completed without difficulty, and women expressed strong preference for a one-day procedure. Misoprostol carries the potential problem of inducing contractions that can result in delivery of the fetus, so it may not be acceptable for home administration after the first trimester. Side effects include nausea, vomiting, diarrhea, and fever or shivering. Rare cases of uterine rupture, primarily in women who had a scar from a previous uterine surgery, have been reported following misoprostol use in the second trimester.[41]

Uterotonic agents. Agents such as vasopressin, oxytocin, prostaglandins, and ergotamines (e.g., methylergonovine maleate or Methergine) strengthen uterine contractility, and they may constrict blood vessels as well. Providers use these agents to help reduce the amount of bleeding during and after abortion. Adding vasopressin or oxytocin to the cervical anesthetic solution provides a simple means of administration, as does direct injection of Methergine or oxytocin into the cervix at the end of the procedure. Many providers give patients oral Methergine to use at home for a few days, particularly following second-trimester abortions.[8]

Managing Post-Abortion Complications

Take seriously any complaint or problem after an abortion procedure. Inform all abortion patients to watch for warning signs (Table 24–4), and tell them how to contact you in case they have questions or problems. Prompt recognition and management can be critical in preventing a serious outcome.

The Safety Of Abortion

Modern methods of abortion are remarkably safe. Since the nationwide legalization of abortion in the United States, abortion-related mortality has decreased by 90%, with most of the decline occurring from 1973 to 1976.[96] Recent data indicate that the risk of dying from a legal abortion in the United States is less than 1 in 100,000 procedures, which represents the lowest mortality risk of all pregnancy outcomes. Pregnancy-related death rates are twice as high for spontaneous abortion and 8 times higher for continuing pregnancy and childbirth.[97] In the two largest studies of legally induced first-trimester abortions reported to date, the rate of major complications was less than 1 in 200 cases.[6,98] The single greatest factor influencing the safety of abortion is gestational age. Abortions are safer when performed early in pregnancy, which emphasizes the importance of access for women seeking abortion.[96]

Medication abortion using mifepristone regimens has proven safe and effective. A review of reports from the 202 Planned Parenthood sites that provided early medication abortions using mifepristone and vaginal misoprostol during 2001 to early 2004 found 99.7% efficacy in terminating pregnancy. Only 206 adverse events were reported among 95,163 patients—a rate of 2 adverse events per 1000 abortions.[61] Heavy bleeding was the most common complication, occurring in 2 per 1000 procedures, and few women required blood transfusions (0.5 transfusions per 1000 abortions). Infections requiring parenteral antibiotics were reported at a rate of 0.2 per 1000 mifepristone abortions.

From the time of FDA approval of mifepristone in September of 2000 to mid-2006, 6 fatalities have been reported among the more than half a million U.S. women estimated to have used mifepristone in combination with misoprostol for early abortion, for a mortality rate of approximately 1 per 100,000 procedures. One woman died from hemorrhage resulting from a ruptured ectopic pregnancy,[99] and 5 women died of pelvic infection complicated by septic shock. The causative agent in 4 cases of infection occurring in California (and one additional case from Canada) was *Clostridium sordellii*,[100] a toxin-producing bacterium that has been associated with rare, serious infections following childbirth, spontaneous abortion (miscarriage), gynecological procedures, or other clinical events.[101] The clinical manifestations of *Clostridium sordellii* infections may differ from those typically seen in women with endometritis[100] (see below). Intensive investigations by health authorities have not established a causal relationship between the medications used for early abortion and these adverse events, and contamination of mifepristone and misoprostol tablets has been ruled out. Updated labeling for mifepristone reminds providers to remain aware of the possibility of unrecognized ectopic pregnancy or infection throughout the treatment period.

IMMEDIATE AND SHORT-TERM COMPLICATIONS

Abortion complications, while not common, include the following immediate and short-term problems:

Bleeding. Regardless of whether they have undergone medication or aspiration methods, almost all women have at least some bleeding during and after an abortion. Typically, bleeding persists for at least several days, with light bleeding or spotting continuing for as long as 2 to 4 weeks. In medication abortion patients, the absence of bleeding after misoprostol administration may indicate possible ectopic pregnancy (unless initial ultrasound confirmed intrauterine pregnancy).

Promptly evaluate the source of bleeding that is excessive or prolonged. The most common causes of hemorrhage after aspiration abortion are uterine atony and retained placental or fetal tissue. Atony, which typically occurs immediately after the procedure, almost always responds to uterotonic agents and uterine massage. Women with retained tissue may present with heavy bleeding several days to a few weeks post-abortion (see Incomplete Abortion, below). After a medication abortion, less than 1% of women require aspiration or curettage to stop bleeding, and in rare cases, transfusion (0.1%).[9] Heavy bleeding that requires treatment is often not due to immediate, catastrophic hemorrhage but rather persistent or delayed bleeding that occurs 3–5 weeks following mifepristone administration.[78] Medication abortion patients and providers, therefore, need to remain vigilant for bleeding even if findings appear "normal" on the follow-up examination.

Incomplete abortion. When part of the pregnancy tissue remains in the uterus, the abortion procedure is "incomplete." This problem occurs following approximately 0.3% to 2% of aspiration procedures.[8] Retained pregnancy tissue is likely to cause continued bleeding and cramping that prompt women to seek care. Treatment with misoprostol or vacuum aspiration is appropriate. Medication abortion regimens take a longer time to empty the uterus than does aspiration, and an ultrasound examination may show residual tissue after the pregnancy sac has passed. This normal finding does not require intervention unless the patient is bleeding excessively or has symptoms or signs of an infection.

Continuing pregnancy. In rare cases, an attempt to terminate pregnancy fails altogether (about 0.03% to 0.05% of aspiration procedures and 0.2% to 1% of early medication abortions).[8,9,61] A woman with a continuing pregnancy may have ongoing symptoms of pregnancy and a soft or enlarged uterus. Ultrasound or a low-sensitivity pregnancy test may help to identify this problem (see Pregnancy Testing and Management of Early Pregnancy, Chapter 23). Providing or referring the patient for an effective means to terminate the pregnancy is appropriate treatment.

Meticulous tissue examination after an aspiration abortion minimizes the risk of a continuing pregnancy. Failure to visualize products of conception in the aspirate warrants further investigation for a continuing intrauterine pregnancy or an ectopic pregnancy. Failed aspiration abortion occurs more often in women with uterine abnormalities, such as a bicornuate urterus or cavity distorted by fibroids. Treatment options include medication abortion (if the patient is still within an eligible gestational age limit) or reaspiration using ultrasound guidance as needed. Ongoing pregnancy due to failed medication abortion potentially involves an increased risk for fetal malformation, so the woman should be encouraged to consider carefully before deciding to continue the pregnancy to term.[9]

Intrauterine blood clots. Intrauterine blood clots can occur immediately or as long as a few days after an aspiration abortion; their presence may cause severe cramping and pain. Sometimes called the "postabortal" or "redo" syndrome, this problem occurs after approximately 0.02% of first-trimester vacuum aspiration abortion procedures.[8] Typical findings on the pelvic examination include a large, tense, and tender uterus with little or no bleeding from the cervix. A simple vacuum aspiration remedies the problem; pain and cramping resolve within a few minutes.

Cervical, uterine, or abdominal organ trauma. External cervical tears can occur if the tenaculum detaches from the cervix; in most cases, management involves only pressure and observation, application of ferrous subsulfate (Monsel's) solution, or suture. Similarly, a small midline uterine perforation in the first trimester can be managed safely with careful observation for 2 to 4 hours, and hospitalization may not be necessary if there is no evidence of internal bleeding, abdominal pain, or rebound tenderness. More severe cervical or uterine trauma, and perforation with damage to nearby abdominal vessels or other organs, are rare; reported rates range from 0.01% to 0.2%.[8] Depending on their severity, these complications may require exploratory surgery to identify and repair the uterus or abdominal organ injury, or even hysterectomy. Providers typically prepare the cervix with osmotic dilating devices or misoprostol before second-trimester abortion to decrease the risk of uterine trauma. The risk of perforation also may be reduced by avoiding routine use of a uterine sound or sharp curet during aspiration abortion.[8]

Uterine rupture has been reported with use of misoprostol for induction of labor at term and in conjunction with other uterotonic agents in second-trimester medical abortion. This catastrophic complication is very rare; an incidence estimate based on 14 cases reported in the United States is 2 ruptures per 100,000 second-trimester induction procedures; the incidence may be higher for women who have had a previous cesarean section delivery.[41]

Infection. Infection rates reported in U.S. studies following first-trimester aspiration abortion range from 0.1% to 1.3%; rates are slightly higher, 0.4% to 2.0%, following second-trimester D&E or induction.[8] A systematic review of infectious complications reported in studies that used various medication regimens for first- and second-trimester abortion found an overall infection rate of 0.9%.[102]

Minimize the risk of postabortal infection by screening for pre-existing reproductive tract infections (with treatment before or at the time of the abortion), by emptying the uterus completely during aspiration or D&E abortion, and by administrating prophylactic antibiotics at the time of these procedures.[103] Common regimens include 100 to 200 mg of doxycycline taken as a single dose, or 100 mg taken twice daily for 3 to 7 days.[104] Because patients may experience nausea and vomiting, many providers wait until after the procedure to begin the antibiotics. Although some providers use additional antibiotic prophylaxis for women who may be at increased risk for subacute bacterial endocarditis, neither the American College of Obstetricians and Gynecologists nor the American Heart Association recommends this practice for uninfected therapeutic abortion procedures.[105,106]

Common symptoms of post-abortal pelvic infection include persistent cramping, abdominal pain, fever, discharge, and malaise. Treatment of uncomplicated pelvic infection includes broad spectrum antibiotics and aspiration of retained tissue, if present. Hospitalization for intravenous antibiotic therapy is warranted in patients with severe illness or suspected pelvic abscess and in those who are immunocompromised, unable to tolerate oral medications, or fail to respond to outpatient therapy.

The few patients who developed toxic shock from *Clostridium sordellii* infection presented with atypical findings, including flu-like symptoms and absence of fever.[100] Suspect an atypical infection if a patient manifests the following symptoms or signs in the days following misoprostol use for medication abortion:

- Nausea, vomiting, diarrhea, weakness with or without abdominal pain
- Tachycardia or hypotension
- Lack of fever with little tenderness on pelvic examination
- High hemoglobin or hematocrit value
- Marked leukocytosis (unusually high white blood cell count)

If you suspect atypical infection, refer the patient immediately to the emergency room with a copy of the mifepristone Medication Guide, which has been updated to reflect information about these infections. Because hospital personnel may know little about medication abortion or *Clostridiium sordelli*, call the emergency room to explain why you are making the referral.

OVERALL HEALTH EFFECTS AND LONG-TERM SEQUELAE

Once pregnant, a woman can decide to terminate or continue her pregnancy. One key question with regard to long-term effects is whether a woman who decides to terminate her pregnancy faces greater risk of future adverse outcomes than she would were she to decide to continue the pregnancy. Because the immediate risks of death and serious medical complications are so much lower for abortion than for full-term pregnancy, the *overall* health risks are much lower for abortion. The risk of death associated with pregnancy and childbirth (excluding deaths from miscarriage and ectopic pregnancy) is 7 to 8 per 100,000 live births,[97] and nearly 43% of women who give birth have some kind of maternal morbidity (including cesarean delivery).[107] The risk of death related to abortion is less than 1 in 100,000 cases,[97] and serious morbidity risk is less than 1%.[6,98]

Women who seek abortion services appropriately ask about possible long-term health effects. Public debate about long-term effects has been used as a rationale for limiting women's access to legal abortion services. Several thoughtful and reassuring reviews of this topic have been published,[8] including the conclusion by Surgeon General Everett Koop in 1989 that he found no evidence of medical or psychological harm. As new research findings are published, pay attention to the quality of study design and the criteria for determining causality. Conclusions in three key areas are briefly summarized below.

Future Reproductive Health and Fertility

First-trimester aspiration abortion is not associated with a measurable increased risk for impaired fertility or subsequent spontaneous abortion.[108] A few European reports have suggested an increased risk of preterm birth after first-trimester vacuum aspiration,[109] but methodological problems make the conclusions difficult to draw; other excellent studies have found no association.[108,110,111] Although studies of ectopic pregnancy risk following first-trimester aspiration abortion have shown variable results, none has found a statistically significant association.[8] Although increased risks for spontaneous abortion and preterm or low birthweight delivery have been reported after second-trimester D&E abortion, adequate preparation of the cervix before the procedure may mitigate these risks.[112] Few data are available regarding subsequent reproductive outcomes among women who have had medication abortions, but the fact that a medication abortion is less invasive than an aspiration provides reassurance. One large prospective study of nulliparous women in China found no association between mifepristone-misoprostol abortion and an increased risk of preterm delivery or low birth weight delivery.[111]

Psychological Health

Transient feelings of stress, loss, or sadness may follow what is sometimes a difficult decision to terminate a pregnancy.[113] A large body of sound scientific evidence, however, consistently shows no psychological harm from abortion; in fact, many studies document benefits such as enhanced self-esteem.[114–116] Relief is a predominant emotion after abortion, and long-term follow-up studies confirm that most women remain satisfied with their decision to have had an abortion.[115,117] Major psychiatric problems following abortion are rare,[114,118,119] and they are more likely to occur among women with preexisting mental health conditions.[114,115] Although "abortion trauma syndrome" has been described in materials distributed by lay groups, no such syndrome is defined in peer-reviewed scientific literature or in the professional diagnostic codes.[119] The characteristics described—such as persistent guilt and sadness—are conclusions of self-selected groups of women, in some cases linked to religious groups. If abortion caused incapacitating dysphoric emotional responses frequently, this association would be evident because abortion is a very common procedure.

Breast Cancer

The question of whether induced abortion has any effect on subsequent breast cancer risk has received intense scrutiny. Full-term pregnancy has a dichotomous influence on breast tissue: during early pregnancy there is an increase in growth of breast tissue due to the stimulus of estrogens; later in pregnancy, differentiation of mammary tissue occurs. The differentiation effect is apparently related to a decrease in a future risk for breast cancer among women who have at least one full-term pregnancy.[120]

Epidemiologic research on this topic is complex because of study design problems that could lead to spurious association. For example, recall bias may explain some of the positive associations found in case-control studies that compare abortion histories of healthy women with those of women who have breast cancer, because healthy women are less likely than women with cancer to report sensitive events such as prior abortion.[121] Prospective studies that collect data on reproductive events *before* the diagnosis of breast cancer have found no association between induced abortion and breast cancer. A recent comprehensive reanalysis of the worldwide research on abortion and breast cancer, including 53 studies from 16 countries, confirms this conclusion.[122] Moreover, the National Cancer Institute's (NCI) board of scientific advisers has concluded that no evidence supports a true association between induced abortion and subsequent breast cancer risk.[123]

ROUTINE POST-ABORTION CARE AND CONTRACEPTION

Fertility returns quickly following abortion. Ovulation, and with it the possibility of another pregnancy, may occur as soon as 10 days after abortion. Helping a woman initiate an effective method of contraception is an essential task in providing abortion care, and it should not be deferred to a follow-up visit. If the unplanned pregnancy occurred while the woman was using a contraceptive, help her identify any personal, situational, or method-related factors that may have contributed to the contraceptive failure. Also, explain the availability of emergency contraception and provide a supply she can have on hand at home in case of future need.

The woman may start a hormonal method of contraception immediately after an aspiration or D&E abortion or as soon as she wishes after using misoprostol in medication abortion regimens. Many providers initiate the hormonal method on the same day as the abortion, or any time within the first 7 days for oral contraceptives and injectables, or any time within the first 5 days for the patch or ring. An IUD can safely be inserted at the conclusion of an aspiration procedure or at the time pregnancy expulsion is confirmed following medication abortion.

REFERENCES

1. Finer LB, Frahwirth LF, Dauphinee LA, Singh S, Moore AM. Reasons U.S. women have abortions: quantitative and qualitative perspectives. Perspect Sex Reprod Health 2005;37:110–118.
2. Drey EA, Foster DG, Jackson RA, Lee SJ, Cardenas LH, Darney PD. Risk factors associated with presenting for abortion in the second trimester. Obstet Gynecol 1006;107:128–135.

3. Edwards J, Carson SA. New technologies permit safe abortion at less than six weeks' gestation and provide timely detection of ectopic gestation. Am J Obstet Gynecol 1997;176:1101–1106.

4. Baird DT, Grimes DA, Van Look PFA. Modern methods of inducing abortion. Oxford; Cambridge, Ma: Blackwell Science, 1995.

5. Darney P, Morbuch P, Korn A. Protocols for office gynecologic surgery. London, UK: Blackwell Science; 1996.

6. Grimes DA. Management of abortion. In: Rock JA, Jones HW III (eds). TeLinde's operative gynecology. 9th ed. Philadelphia: Lippincott Williams & Wilkins; 2003.

7. Stewart FH, Wells ES, Flinn SK, Weitz TA. Early medical abortion: issues for practice. San Francisco, CA: University of California San Francisco, Center for Reproductive Health Research & Policy; 2001.

8. Paul M, Lichtenberg ES, Borgatta L, Stubblefield P, Grimes DA (eds). A clinician's guide to medical and surgical abortion. New York: Churchill Livingstone; 1999.

9. American College of Obstetricians and Gynecologists (ACOG). Medical management of abortion. ACOG Practice Bulletin No. 67. Obstet Gynecol 2005;106:871–882.

10. Stewart FH, Shields WC, Hwang AC. Keeping abortion legal: a look beyond Roe v. Wade. Contraception 2003;68:307–308.

11. Anonymous. Court reaffirms Roe but upholds restrictions. Family Plann Perspect 1992;24:174–177,185.

12. Cates W Jr, Grimes DA, Hogue LL. Topics for our times: Justice Blackmun and legal abortion–a besieged legacy to women's reproductive health. Am J Public Health 1995;85:1204–1206.

13. Crane BB, Dusenberry J. Power and politics in international funding for reproductive health: the US Global Gag Rule. Reprod Health Matters 2004;12:128–137.

14. Partial Birth Abortion Ban Act. Public Law 108–105, HR760, S3, 18 U.S. Code 1531.

15. Stewart FH, Shields WC, Hwang AC. The federal abortion ban: a clinical and moral dilemma and international policy setback. Contraception 2004;69:433–435.

16. Greene MF, Ecker L. Abortion, health, and the law. New Engl J Med 2004;350: 184 186.

17. Pew Research Center. Abortion, the court and the public. Washington DC: Pew Research Center; October 3, 2005.

18. Grimes DA, Forrest JD, Kirkman AL, Radford B. An epidemic of antiabortion violence in the United States. Am J Obstet Gynecol 1991;165:1263–1268.

19. Henshaw SK, Finer LB. The accessibility of abortion services in the United States, 2001. Perspect Sex Reprod Health 2003;35:16–24.

20. Prine LW, Lesnewski R. Medication abortion and family physicians' scope of practice. J Am Board Fam Pract 2005;18:304–306.

21. Kruse B. Advanced practice clinicians and medical abortion: increasing access to care. J Am Womens Assoc 2000;55:167–168.

22. Hwang AC, Koyama A, Taylor D, Henderson JT, Miller S. Advanced practice clinicians' interest in providing medical abortion: results of a California survey. Perspect Sex Reprod Health 2005;37:92–97.

23. Cates W, Jr., Grimes DA, Schulz KF. The public health impact of legal abortion: 30 years later. Perspect Sex Reprod Health 2003;35:25–28.

24. Strauss LT, Herndon J, Parker WY, et al. Abortion surveillance—United States, 2001. MMWR Surveill Summ Nov 26 2004;53:1–32.

25. Finer LB, Henshaw SK. Abortion incidence and services in the United States in 2000. Perspect Sex Reprod Health 2003;35:6–15.

26. Jones RK, Darroch JE, Henshaw SK. Contraceptive use among U.S. women having abortions in 2000–2001. Perspect Sex Reprod Health 2002;34:294–303.

27. Finer LB, Henshaw SK. Disparities in rates of unintended pregnancy in the United States, 1994 and 2001. Perspect Sex Reprod Health 2006;38:90–96.

28. Henshaw RC, Naji SA, Russell IT, Templeton AA. Comparison of medical abortion with surgical vacuum aspiration: women's preferences and acceptability of treatment. BMJ 1993;307:714–717.
29. Winikoff B. Acceptability of medical abortion in early pregnancy. Fam Plann Perspect 1995;27:142–148, 185.
30. Fielding SL, Edmunds E, Schaff EA. Having an abortion using mifepristone and home misoprostol: a qualitative analysis of women's experiences. Perspect Sex Reprod Health 2002;34:34–40.
31. Jones RK, Henshaw SK. Mifepristone for early medical abortion: experiences in France, Great Britain and Sweden. Perspect Sex Reprod Health 2002;34:154–161.
32. Drimes DA, Schulz KF, Cates W Jr, Tyler CW Jr. Mid-trimester abortion by dilation and evacuation: a safe and practical alternative. N Engl J Med 1977;296:1141–1145.
33. Grimes DA, Schulz KF. Morbidity and mortality from second-trimester abortions. J Reprod Med 1985;30:505–514.
34. Grimes DA, Smith SM, Witham AD. Mifepristone and misoprostol versus dilation and evacuation for midtrimester abortion: a pilot randomized controlled trial. BJOG 2004;111:148–153.
35. Peyron R, Aubeny E, Targosz V, et al. Early termination of pregnancy with mifepristone (RU 486) and the orally active prostaglandin misoprostol. N Engl J Med 1993;328:1509–1513.
36. Urquhart DR, Templeton AA, Shinewi F, et al. The efficacy and tolerance of mifepristone and prostaglandin in termination of pregnancy or less than 63 days gestation; UK multicentre study–final results. Contraception 1997;55:1–5.
37. Winikoff B, Sivin I, Coyaji KJ, et al. Safety, efficacy, and acceptability of medical abortion in China, Cuba, and India: a comparative trial of mifepristone-misoprostol versus surgical abortion. Am J Obstet Gynecol 1997;176:431–437.
38. Coyaji K, Elul B, Krishna U, et al. Mifepristone abortion outside the urban research hospital setting in India. Lancet 13 2001;357:120–122.
39. Elul B, Hajri S, Ngoc NTN, et al. Can women in less-developed countries use a simplified medical abortion regimen? Lancet 2001;357:1402–1405.
40. Ngoc NTN, Nhan VQ, Blum J, Mai TT, Durocher JM, Winikoff B. Is home-based administration of prostaglandin safe and feasible for medical abortion? Results from a multisite study in Vietnam. BJOG 2004;111:814–819.
41. Goldberg A, Greenberg MB, Darney PD. Drug therapy: misoprostol and pregnancy. New Engl J Med 2001;344:38–47.
42. Creinin MD, Vittinghoff E, Keder L, Darney PD, Tiller G. Methotrexate and misoprostol for early abortion: a multicenter trial. I. Safety and efficacy. Contraception 1996;53:321–327.
43. Lipscomb GH, Stovall TG, Ling FW. Nonsurgical treatment of ectopic pregnancy. N Engl J Med 2000;343:1325–1329.
44. Barnhart KT, Gosman G, Ashby R, Sammel M. The medical management of ectopic pregnancy: a meta-analysis comparing "single dose" and "multidose" regimens. Obstet Gynecol 2003;101:778–784.
45. Zhang J, Gilles JM, Barnhart K, Creinin MD, Westhoff C, Frederick MM. A comparison of medical management with misoprostol and surgical management for early pregnancy failure. N Engl J Med 2005;353:761–769.
46. Blanchard K, Clark S, Winikoff, Gaines G, Kabani G, Shannon C. Misoprostol for women's health: a review. Obstet Gynecol 2002;99:316–332.
47. Zieman M, Fong SK, Benowitz NL, Bankster D, Darney PD. Absorption kinetics of misoprostol with oral or vaginal administration. Obstet Gynecol 1997;90:88–92.
48. Danielsson KG, Marions L, Rodriguez A, Spur BW, Wong PY, Bygdeman M. Comparison between oral and vaginal administration of misoprostol on uterine contractility. Obstet Gynecol 1999;93:275–280.
49. Tang OS, Schweer H, Seyberth HW, Lee SW, Ho PC. Pharmacokinetics of different routes of administration of misoprostol. Hum Reprod 2002;17:332–336.

50. Schaff EA, DiCenzo R, Fielding SL. Comparison of misoprostol plasma concentrations following buccal and sublingual administration. Contraception 2005;71:22–25.
51. Spitz IM, Bardin CW, Benton L, Robbins A. Early pregnancy termination with mifepristone and misoprostol in the United States. N Engl J Med 1998;338:1241–1247.
52. World Health Organisation Task Force on Post-Ovulatory Methods of Fertility Regulation. Comparison of two doses of mifepristone in combination with misoprostol for early medical abortion: a randomized trial. BJOG 2000;107:524–530.
53. Shannon CS, Winikoff B, Hausknecht R, et al. Multicenter trial of a simplified mifepristone medical abortion regimen. Obstet Gynecol 2005;105:345–351.
54. El-Refaey H, Rajasekar D, Abdalla M, Calder L, Templeton A. Induction of abortion with mifepristone (RU 486) and oral or vaginal misoprostol. N Engl J Med 1995;332:983–987.
55. Schaff EA, Fielding SL, Westhoff C. Randomized trial of oral versus vaginal misoprostol 2 days after mifepristone 200 mg for abortion up to 63 days of pregnancy. Contraception 2002;66:247–250.
56. Schaff EA, Stadalius LS, Eisinger SH, Franks P. Vaginal misoprostol administered at home after mifepristone (RU486) for abortion. J Fam Pract 1997;44:353–360.
57. Schaff EA, Fielding SL, Westhoff C, et al. Vaginal misoprostol administered 1, 2, or 3 days after mifepristone for early medical abortion: A randomized trial. JAMA 2000;284:1948–1953.
58. Schaff EA, Fielding SL, Westhoff C. Randomized trial of oral versus vaginal misoprostol at one day after mifepristone for early medical abortion. Contraception 2001;64:81–85.
59. Creinin MD, Fox MC, Teal S, Chen A, Schaff EA, Meyn LA; MOD Study Trial Group. A randomized comparison of misoprostol 6 to 8 hours versus 24 hours after mifepristone for abortion. Obstet Gynecol 2004;103:851–859.
60. Middleton T, Schaff E, Fielding SL, et al. Randomized trial of mifepristone and buccal or vaginal misoprostol for abortion through 56 days of last menstrual period. Contraception 2005;72:328–332.
61. Henderson JT, Hwang AC, Harper CC, Stewart FH. Safety of mifepristone in clinical use. Contraception 2005;72:175–178.
62. Borgmann CE, Jones BS. Legal issues in the provision of medical abortion. Am J Obstet Gynecol 2000;183:S84–S94.
63. Creinin MD, Carbonell JL, Schwartz JL, Varela L, Tanda R. A randomized trial of the effect of moistening misoprostol before vaginal administration when used with methotrexate for abortion. Contraception 1999;59:11–16.
64. Wiebe E, Dunn S, Guilbert E, Jacot F, Lugtig L. Comparison of abortions induced by methotrexate or mifepristone followed by misoprostol. Obstet Gynecol 2002;99: 813–819.
65. Kahn JG, Becker BJ, MacIsaac L, et al. The efficacy of medical abortion: a meta-analysis. Contraception 2000;61:29–40.
66. Creinin MD, Vittinghoff E, Schaff E, Klaisle C, Darney PD, Dean C. Medical abortion with oral methotrexate and vaginal misoprostol. Obstet Gynecol 1997;90:611–616.
67. Wiebe ER. Oral methotrexate compared with injected methotrexate when used with misoprostol for abortion. Am J Obstet Gynecol 1999;181:149–152.
68. Jain JK, Dutton C, Harwood B, Meckstroth KR, Mishell DR Jr. A prospective randomized, double-blinded, placebo-controlled trial comparing mifepristone and vaginal misoprostol to vaginal misoprostol alone for elective termination of pregnancy. Hum Reprod 2002;17:1477–1482.
69. Jain JK, Harwood B, Meckstroth KR, Mishell DR. Early pregnancy termination with vaginal misoprostol combined with loperamide and acetaminophen prophylaxis. Contraception 2001;63:217–221.
70. Jain JK, Meckstroth KR, Park M, Mishell DR. A comparison of tamoxifen and misoprostol to misoprostol alone for early pregnancy termination. Contraception 2000;60:353–356.

71. Esteve JL, Varela L, Velazco A, Tanda R, Cabezas E, Sanchez C. Early abortion with 800 micrograms of misoprostol by the vaginal route. Contraception 1999;59: 219–225.

72. Borgatta L, Mullally B, Vragovic O, Gittinger E, Chen A. Misoprostol as the primary agent for medical abortion in a low-income urban setting. Contraception 2004;70:121–126.

73. Rosing MA, Archbald CD. The knowledge, acceptability, and use of misoprostol for self-induced medical abortion in an urban US population. JAMWA 2000;55:183–185.

74. Creinin MD, Shulman T. Effect of nonsteroidal anti-inflammatory drugs on the action of misoprostol in a regimen for early abortion. Contraception 1997;56:165–168.

75. Tang OS, Lee SWH, Ho PC. A prospective randomized study on the measured blood loss in medical termination of early pregnancy by three different misoprostol regimens after pretreatment with mifepristone. Hum Reprod 2002;17:2865–2868.

76. Davis A, Westhoff C, de Nonno L. Bleeding patterns after early abortion with mifepristone and misoprostol or manual vacuum aspiration. JAMWA 2000;55:141–144.

77. Tang O, Gao P, Cheng L, Lee SW, Ho PC. A randomized double-blind placebo-controlled study to assess the effect of oral contraceptive pills on the outcome of medical abortion with mifepristone and misoprostol. Hum Reprod 1999;14:722–725.

78. Allen RH, Westhoff C, DeNonno L, Fielding SL, Schaff EA. Curettage after mifepristone-induced abortion: frequency, timing, and indications. Obstet Gynecol 2001;98:101–106.

79. Paul M, Schaff E, Nichols M. The roles of clinical assessment, human chorionic gonadotropin assays, and ultrasonography in medical abortion practice. Am J Obstet Gynecol 2000;183:S34-S43.

80. Harper C, Ellertson C, Winikoff B. Could American women use mifepristone-misoprostol pills with less medical supervision? Contraception 2002;65:133–135.

81. Rossi B, Creinin MD, Meyn LA. Ability of the clinician and patient to predict the outcome of mifepristone and misoprostol medical abortion. Contraception 2004;70:313–317.

82. Goldman MB, Occhiuto JS, Peterson LE, Zapka JG, Palmer H. Physician assistants as providers of surgically induced abortion services. Am J Public Health 2004;94:1352–1357.

83. Lundh C, Meirik O, Nygren K-G. Vaginal cleansing at vacuum aspiration abortion does not reduce the risk of postoperative infection. Acta Obstet Gynecol Scand 1983;62:275–277.

84. Chasen ST, Kalish RB, Gupta M, Kaufman JE, Rashbaum WK, Chervenak FA. Dilation and evacuation at $\geq$ 20 weeks: comparison of operative techniques. Am J Obstet Gynecol 2004;190:1180–1183.

85. Royal College of Obstetricians and Gynaecologists. The care of women requesting induced abortion. London: Guideline Development Group; 2000.

86. Ashok PW, Templeton A, Wagaarachchi PT, Flett GMM. Midtrimester medical termination of pregnancy: a review of 1002 consecutive cases. Contraception 2004;69:51–58.

87. Winkler CL, Gray SE, Hauth JC, Owen J, Tucker JM. Mid second trimester labor induction: concentrated oxytocin compared with prostaglandin E2 vaginal suppositories. Obstet Gynecol 1991;77:297–300.

88. Autry AM, Hayes EC, Jacobson GF, Kirby RS. A comparison of medical induction and dilation and evacuation for second-trimester abortion. Am J Obstet Gynecol 2002;187:393–397.

89. Schutz KF, Grimes DA, Cates W Jr. Measures to prevent cervical injury during suction curettage abortion. Lancet 1983;1:1182–1184.

90. Grimes DA, Schulz KF, Cates WJ Jr. Prevention of uterine perforation during curettage abortion. JAMA 1984;251:2108–2111.

91. Lawrie A, Penney G, Templeton A. A randomized comparison or oral and vaginal misoprostol for cervical priming before suction termination of pregnancy. BJOG 1996;103:1117–1119.

92. MacIsaac L, Grossman D, Balistreri E, Darney P. A randomized controlled trial of laminaria, oral misoprostol, and vaginal misoprostol before abortion. Obstet Gynecol 1999;93:766–770.

93. Vimala N, Mittal S, Kuman S, Dadhwal V, Sharma Y. A randomized comparison of sublingual and vaginal misoprostol for cervical priming before suction termination of first-trimester pregnancy. Contraception 2004;70:117–120.

94. Patel A, Talmont E, Morfesis J, et al. Adequacy and safety of buccal misoprostol for cervical preparation prior to termination of second-trimester pregnancy. Contraception 2006;73:420–430.

95. Goldberg AB, Drey EA, Whitaker AK, Kang MS, Meckstroth KR, Darney PD. Misoprostol compared with laminaria before early second-trimester surgical abortion: a randomized trial. Obstet Gynecol 2005;106:234–241.

96. Bartlett LA, Berg CJ, Shulman HB, et al. Risk factors for legal induced abortion-related mortality in the United States. Obstet Gynecol 2004;103:729–737.

97. Grimes DA. Estimation of pregnancy-related mortality risk by pregnancy outcome, United States, 1991 to 1999. Am J Obstet Gynecol 2006;194:92–94.

98. Hakim-Elahi E, Tovell HM, Burnhill MS. Complications of first-trimester abortion: a report of 170,000 cases. Obstet Gynecol 1990;76:129–135.

99. Shannon C, Brothers LP, Philip NM, Winikoff B. Ectopic pregnancy and medical abortion. Obstet Gynecol 2004;104:161–167.

100. Fischer M, Bhatnagar J, Guarner J, et al. Fatal toxic shock syndrome associated with Clostridium sordellii after medical abortion. N Engl J Med 2005;353:2352–2360.

101. McGregor JA, Soper DE, Lovell G, Todd JK. Maternal deaths associated with Clostridium sordellii infection. Am J Obstet Gynecol 1989;161:987–995.

102. Shannon C, Brothers P, Philip NM, Winikoff B. Infection after medical abortion: a review of the literature. Contraception 2004;70:183–190.

103. Sawaya GF, Grady D, Kerlikowske K, Grimes DA. Antibiotics at the time of induced abortion: the case for universal prophylaxis based on a meta-analysis. Obstet Gynecol 1996;87:884–890.

104. Lichtenberg ES, Shott S. A randomized clinical trial of prophylaxis for vacuum abortion: 3 versus 7 days of doxycycline. Obstet Gynecol 2003;101:726–731.

105. American College of Obstetricians and Gynecologists (ACOG). ACOG Practice Bulletin. Antibiotic prophylaxis for gynecologic procedures. Washington, DC: ACOG; 2001:23.

106. Dajani AS, Taubert KA, Wilson W, et al. Prevention of bacterial endocarditis. Recommendations by the American Heart Association. JAMA 1997;277:1794–1801.

107. Danel I, Berg C, Johnson CH, Atrash H. Magnitude of maternal morbidity during labor and delivery: United States, 1993–1997. Am J Public Health 2003;93:631–634.

108. Hogue CJR. Impact of abortion on subsequent fertility. Clin Obstet Gynaecol 1986;13:95–103.

109. Moreau C, Kaminski M, Ancel PY, et al. Previous induced abortions and the risk of very preterm delivery: results of the EPIPAGE study. BJOG 2005;112:430–437.

110. Henshaw SK. Studying the health effects of induced abortion (letter). Fam Plann Perspect 2000;32:305–306.

111. Chen A, Yuan W, Meirik O, et al. Mifepristone-induced early abortion and outcome of subsequent wanted pregnancy. Am J Epidemiol 2004;160:110–117.

112. Kalish RB, Chasen ST, Rosenzweig LB, Rashbaum WK, Chervenak FA. Impact of midtrimester dilation and evacuation on subsequent pregnancy outcome. Am J Obstet Gynecol 2002;187:882–885.

113. Adler NE, David HP, Major BN, Roth SH, Russo NF, Wyatt GE. Psychological responses after abortion. Science 1990;248 (4951):41–44.

114. Adler NE. Abortion and the null hypothesis. Arch Gen Psychiatry 2000;57:785–786.

115. Major B, Cozzarelli C, Cooper L, et al. Psychological responses of women after first-trimester abortion. Arch Gen Psychiatry 2000;57:777–784.

116. Henshaw R, Naji S, Russell I, Templeton A. Psychological responses following medical abortion (using mifepristone and gemeprost) and surgical vacuum aspiration: a patient-centered, partially randomized prospective study. Acta Obstet Gynecol Scand 1994;73:812–818.

117. Kero A, Hogberg U, Lalos A. Wellbeing and mental growth–long-term effects of legal abortion. Social Sci Med 2004;58:2559–2569.

118. Urquhart DR, Templeton AA. Psychiatric morbidity and acceptability following medical and surgical methods of abortion. Br J Obstet Gynaecol 1991;98:396–399.

119. Stotland NL. The myth of the abortion trauma syndrome. JAMA 1992;268: 2078–2079.

120. Michels KB, Willett WC. Does induced or spontaneous abortion affect the risk of breast cancer? Epidemiology 1996;7:521–528.

121. Bartholomew LL, Grimes DA. The alleged association between induced abortion and risk of breast cancer: biology or bias? Obstet Gynecol Survey 1998;53:59–65.

122. Collaborative Group on Hormonal Factors in Breast Cancer. Breast cancer and abortion: collaborative reanalysis of data from 53 epidemiological studies, including 83,000 women with breast cancer from 16 countries. Lancet 2004;363:1007–1016.

123. Couzin J. Review rules out abortion-cancer link. Science 2003; 299(5612):1498.

Impaired Fertility

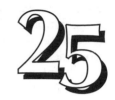

Anita L. Nelson, MD
John R. Marshall, MD

- Helping individuals develop their reproductive life plans and providing them the information and skills necessary to achieve those plans is the mission of family planning.

- Maximizing a couple's ability to become pregnant until the man and woman reach their desired family size is essential to helping them achieve their goals.

- Basic education and fertility assessment for couples with impaired fertility can take place in the primary reproductive health care setting; couples who require more extensive assessment and treatment should be referred.

- Contraception can provide protection against frequent causes of infertility. Condoms reduce the risk of tubal infertility. Hormonal contraceptives can reduce the risk of endometriosis, ectopic pregnancy, and endometrial and ovarian cancer.

While contraception is designed to prevent pregnancy and infertility treatment is designed to enable pregnancy, both processes allow couples to prepare for the pregnancies they want. Pregnancy preparation provides an opportunity to optimize the outcome of pregnancy for the mother, and her infant and, hopefully, the family unit. Preconceptional care should be an integral part of every infertility workup (See Chapter 23).

On average, 80% to 85% of couples trying to become pregnant will conceive within 1 year, and an additional 5% to 10% will conceive in the second year. *Infertility* is diagnosed if a couple has no conception despite having had unprotected vaginal intercourse for 12 months. *Primary infertility* is the diagnosis when the couple has never conceived. *Secondary infertility* is the term used for couples that have previously conceived but are now not able to conceive despite at least 12 months of unprotected intercourse.

PROBABILITY OF PREGNANCY

For the average *fertile* couple, the probability of conception has historically been estimated to be about 20% each cycle, which means that there is an 80% probability that conception will *not* occur. Multiplying that 20% probability by the 13 cycles in a year determines that only 5% of fertile couples will still not have conceived by the end of 1 year.[1,2] With more time, the number of couples who have not conceived decreases spontaneously, even without intervention. Couples with pregnancy potential but with a lower per-cycle fertility rate (*subfertility*) will have lower cumulative pregnancy rates for a given period of time. For example, it might take 18 months for subfertile couples to achieve the same cumulative pregnancy rate that the more fertile couples achieve in 12 months.

Therefore, those who are not pregnant after 1 year of trying fall into three groups: normal but unlucky, subfertile, or sterile. It is clear that the 12-month rule is arbitrary and that some couples are labeled as being infertile when they are not. However, because today many men and women have often delayed parenthood, they may not tolerate undue delays in conception. Therefore, evaluation and targeted interventions are often started before the rules of probability have had a chance to reveal all fertile couples. This observation also reminds us of the importance of using a placebo control group for comparison whenever new infertility therapies are being tested. New interventions must demonstrate not only that they produce pregnancies, but that they produce *more* pregnancies than would occur without any intervention.

Because the fertile couples conceive and drop out of the group of people who are still trying to become pregnant, it is clear that the longer couples have been infertile, the lower the likelihood that they will ultimately conceive without treatment. This is illustrated in Table 25–1. However, the prognosis is not as bad as it first appears. Although the fecundity of a couple that has been infertile for 5 years is only 0.04 (i.e., 20% of normal), 37% of these couples will conceive within the next 12 months.[3]

However, looking at the aggregate of couples, time to pregnancy also seems to have implications for pregnancy outcomes. The longer it takes for couples to conceive, the greater are the risks for spontaneous abortion, ectopic pregnancy, and preterm delivery. These risks may reflect the underlying fertility problems the couples face (e.g., older age, tubal damage), but the mechanisms are not clear.[4]

The prevalence of subfertility and infertility has been recalculated based on two newer prospective studies.[5,6] These researchers show that single cycle fertility is greater than had been previously estimated. In a study of 518 Chinese textile workers who were trying to conceive, about

Table 25–1 Incidence of spontaneous conception over time among non-sterile couples with mean fecundability of 0.2 (pregnancy rate = 20% per month)

No. Months Without Conception	Proportion (%) Couples Not Yet Having Conceived	Mean Fecundability of Couples Not Yet Having Conceived	Proportion (%) Couples Who Will Conceive Within 12 Months Among Couples Not Yet Having Conceived
0	100	0.20	86
6	32	0.14	77
12	14	0.11	69
24	4	0.08	57
36	2	0.06	48
48	1	0.05	42
60	0.6	0.04	37

Source: Lobo RA (1997).[3]

50% became clinically pregnant in the first 2 cycles and more than 90% achieved that status by 1 year. Monthly fecundity varied between 30% to 35%. In a second study, pregnancy rates at 1, 3, 6, and 12 cycles were 38%, 68%, 81%, and 92%.[7] This suggests that workup and treatment might be appropriate to start after 6 months without conception. Of the subfertile couples with a year without conception, 52.6% had a live birth by 36 months.[8]

Impacts of Age

Fertility rates change dramatically as women age. After age 37, women tend to recruit follicles at much faster rates and reduce their ovarian reserves rapidly.[9] The remaining follicles are less sensitive to gonadotropin stimulation, which means that a smaller cohort of follicles is recruited each cycle, which reduces pregnancy rates. In addition, older women have a marked increase in the risk of spontaneous abortion. Due to a higher incidence of abnormalities (aneuploidy) in older eggs, spontaneous abortion rates are 7% to 15% for women under 30 but rise to 34% to 52% in women over 40[10,11] These influences are reflected in the success rates with assisted reproductive technologies (ART). Pregnancy and live birth rates for ART cycles clearly vary by age. Per embryo transfer, the live birth rate was 36.9% for women younger than 35 but plummeted to 10.7% for women age 41 to 42.[12] Advanced paternal age does not seem to carry the same risk for trisomy as advanced maternal age, but the incidence of autosomal dominant disorders and X-linked recessive disease does seem to increase with paternal age.

REQUIREMENTS FOR FERTILITY

An efficient approach to the workup of the infertile couple begins with an understanding of the requirements for fertility. There are requirements that relate exclusively to the woman, those that relate exclusively to the man, and the remaining requirements that relate to the couple.

Requirements for Female Fertility

- Reasonably good health and nutrition to permit ovulatory cycling and support of a pregnancy
- Functioning reproductive anatomy and physiology
  - An introitus and vagina that permit penile entry
  - A vagina capable of capturing sperm
  - A patent cervix with cervical mucus that periodically permits passage of sperm into the upper genital tract
  - Ovulatory cycling with extrusion of the ovum
  - Fallopian tubes that permit the sperm to fertilize the ovum and that facilitate migration of the conceptus into the uterus
  - A uterus capable of permitting implantation and developing and sustaining the conceptus to term
  - Adequate hormonal status to maintain pregnancy
- Normal immunologic responses to accommodate sperm, fertilization, and fetal health
- Absence of genetic causes of recurrent losses (e.g., balanced translocations, etc.)

Requirements for Male Fertility

- Normal spermatogenesis of functional sperm
- Functioning ductal system
- Ability to transmit the sperm into the woman's vagina
  - Ability to maintain an erection until coital ejaculation
  - Ability to achieve a normal ejaculation within the vaginal vault
- Absence of genetic causes of recurrent losses (e.g., balanced translocations, etc.)

Requirements for a Couple's Fertility

- Ability and desire for intravaginal, penile coital activity
- Correct timing of intercourse within a woman's cycle

OVERVIEW OF CAUSES OF INFERTILITY

As can be anticipated, couples present with a variety of causes for their fertility challenges. Overall, the causes for infertility are distributed as indicated in Table 25–2.

INITIAL INFERTILITY WORKUP

Infertility evaluation is traditionally offered to couples who fail to conceive after 1 year of unprotected intercourse. However, prompt infertility evaluation is indicated for women over 35, women with oligomenorrhea or amenorrhea, women with histories of endometriosis or past PID, and men with known poor quality semen. For women who are concerned about the fertility potential but not seeking pregnancy at this time, an abbreviated panel of tests can provide important information about ovarian reserve, semen quality and/or ovulation.

A workup for infertility begins with a comprehensive medical, social, reproductive, and genetic history for each partner. A family pedigree may help identify inherited disorders such as Down syndrome, neural tube defects, cystic fibrosis, and hemoglobinopathies. Ethnic background is important to guide in testing for conditions that are more concentrated in certain groups. Computer data bases such as OMIM (Online Mendelian Inheritance in Man; www.ncbi.nlm.nih.gov) and Gene Tests (www.genetests.org) can provide clinicians up-to-date information about syndromes and recommended screening tests.[13] Encourage all women to optimize their physical condition and to avoid alcohol or tobacco exposure.

Table 25–2 Causes of infertility

Category	Cases Attributed To (%)
Sperm and other male problems	30–40%
Ovarian dysfunction	10–15%
Tubal and pelvic pathology	30–40%
Unexplained infertility (including time)	10%
Unusual problems	5%

Table 25–3 Normal reference values for semen analysis

Volume of ejaculate	≥ 2 ml
Liquefaction: conversion into a liquid	≤ 60 months
pH	≥ 7.2
Viscosity	< 3 (range 0–4)
Sperm concentration	≥ 20 million sperm/cc
Total sperm count	≥ 40 million sperm/ejaculate
Percent motile	≥ 50% at one hour
Frward progression	> 2 (range 0–4)
Normal morphology	≥ 30% have normal shape (oval heads, single tail, etc)

Source: ASRM (2001).[14]

INITIAL EVALUATION OF THE MAN

Abnormalities in the male partner completely explain the problems of 20% of infertile couples, but male abnormalities contribute to infertility in an additional 20% to 40% of couples. Therefore, a *semen analysis* should be performed even if the woman has an obvious, treatable problem, such as anovulation. Treating the woman for a few cycles is not in her best interests when her partner may have a problem that leaves little or no possibility of conception. A history of having previously fathered children does not obviate the need for a semen analysis.

The semen analysis provides information about the quality of the sperm and the ejaculation process. Experts recommend that at least 2 properly performed semen analyses be obtained at least 4 weeks apart. Specimens should be collected after 2 to 3 days of abstinence. Shorter periods of abstinence can reduce semen volume and density. Longer periods increase the proportion of abnormal sperm. The specimen should be evaluated within 1 hour of collection. Occasionally, cultural proscriptions preclude collection of a specimen. In those cases, a *post-coital test* (see below) may be helpful to obtain semen for analysis.

WHO standards for normal reference values (Table 25–3) for semen analysis have changed in recent years, both as a reflection of lowered sperm counts in modern men and the recognition that even in fertile men, only a small portion of the sperm have normal morphology.

The semen can be classified into three groups: fertile, indeterminate, and subfertile (see Table 25–4). Although sperm concentration, motility, and morphology are all important, morphology appears to be slightly but significantly more discriminating. If a single parameter falls into the subfertile, the odds ratio for infertility is between 2 and 3. If two parameters are in the subfertile range, the odds ratio for infertility is between

Table 25–4 Fertile, indeterminate, and subfertile ranges for sperm measurements

| Variable | Semen Measurement | | |
	Concentration (10^6/ml)	Motility (%)	Morphology (% normal)
Fertile range	> 48.0	> 63	> 12
Indeterminate range	13.5–48.0	32–63	9–12
Subfertile range	< 13.5	< 32	< 9

Source: Guzick D, et al. (2001).[15]

5.5 and 7.2. If all three are in the subfertile range, the odds ratio for infertility is 15.8.[15]

If the results of the semen analysis fall within the fertile range, no additional evaluation of the sperm is required. If the results persistently fall in the subfertile range, conduct a further evaluation to identify any treatable causes of the abnormality. Ask about childhood illnesses and developmental health, systemic medical conditions, tobacco use, a history of surgeries or sexually transmitted infections (STIs), gonadal exposure to toxins, including heat and use of steroid alpha or beta androgenic agents. Physical findings of excessive muscle mass, hypospadias, testicular irregularities, varicocele, or vas deferens abnormalities may warrant a further workup.[16] Kleinfelter Syndrome may occur in up to 8% of azoospermic men. Other tests that may be indicated by specialists include vital staining, antisperm antibodies, semen fructose, peroxidase staining, culture and biochemical analysis.[14] In special cases, serum FSH levels may be informative, as may be a post-ejaculate urinalysis.

INITIAL EVALUATION OF THE WOMAN

The initial infertility evaluation of the woman includes a history, a physical examination, and laboratory testing.

Medical History

The history can be very informative and can guide in the selection of appropriate laboratory tests. Critical elements include a detailed menstrual history, general health history, medications, history of abdomino-pelvic surgery, STIs (especially pelvic inflammatory disease), fertility with different partners, outcomes of any pregnancies, duration of unprotected intercourse, and coital activity (type, frequency, and timing in relation to the menstrual cycle). Obtaining family history of genetic problems, endocrinopathies and fertility problems is also helpful.

Menstrual cycle factors. Ovulatory dysfunction accounts for 40% of infertility in women,[17] but is increasing in frequency because more women are delaying childbearing and because obesity is becoming more common among reproductive-aged women. Chronic anovulation can be diagnosed if the woman's cycles are longer than 35 days or if she has fewer than 8 spontaneous cycles a year. In women with more regular menses, it is important to learn if she has moliminal symptoms such as premenstrual bloating, breast tenderness, or lower back pain suggest ovulatory cycling. Excessive weight gain commonly leads to anovulation. Eating disorders create hypoestrogenemic amenorrhea as can excessive exercise patterns. Noting the patient's weight and menstrual patterns at different ages can help pinpoint the role that weight (inadequate or excessive) may have played in the etiology of her infertility. Thyroid dysfunction, prolactin excess, and other endocrine problems can compromise fertility. Testing for diabetes prior to conception is very important since abnormally high glucose levels are associated with higher rates of pregnancy loss and serious fetal malformations. A history of menstrual changes following ovarian surgery can also raise the issue of limited ovarian reserve.

Tubal factors. Suspect tubal factors if the infertile woman has regular monthly menses (especially if she experiences Mittelschmerz or moliminal symptoms) or has a history of chronic pelvic pain, endometriosis, PID, pelvic surgery, or cervical infections.

Uterine factors. Suspect endometrial scarring (Asherman's Syndrome) if a woman has had amenorrhea following a dilation and curettage (D&C).

Cervical factors. Consider that cervical factors may be contributed to a woman's infertility if she has a history of having had a cone biopsy, LEEP, or a cervical laceration with childbirth or with a D&C. Rarely is a cervical factor the only cause of problems with conception.

Physical Examination

The physical examination can be very targeted. Except for women with primary amenorrhea (see Chapter 20 on Menstrual Disorders and Menstrually-Related Concerns) or women with indications of genetic conditions that can cause infertility (such as Turner's syndrome or premature ovarian failure), the examination of obviously healthy women includes inspection for clinical signs of hypoestrogenism (dry vagina) or hyperandrogenism (acne, hirsutism, etc.), a thyroid exam, a breast exam, and a careful and complete pelvic exam. During the pelvic exam, pay attention to the presence of tenderness or any anatomical anomalies such as vaginal septa, uterine or ovarian masses, cul-de-sac tenderness, or immobility of the pelvic structures.

Table 25–5 Initial laboratory studies for evaluating fertility

All patients	Complete blood count, Chlamydia trachomatis antibody titers
If > 35 yrs of age, prior ovarian surgery, multiagent chemotherapy, or pelvic irradiation	FSH on cycle day 3 or clomiphene citrate challenge test
If anovulatory	>TSH, prolactin. Consider 2H-GTT, especially if family history of DM
If amenorrheic	FSH, E2 (interpret only after 14 days)
If obese	Diabetes screening
If hirsute	Total or free testosterone and 17-hydroxyprogesterone specimen collected in the morning during the follicular phase

Laboratory Testing

Routine laboratory tests are outlined in Table 25–5 by indication.

FURTHER EVALUATION OF THE WOMAN

The problems identified by the initial workup should drive the followup evaluations. There is no standard "infertility panel." Many tests have been used over the years, but not all of them are appropriate in all cases. Furthermore, the utility of some tests has been questioned and many older tests have been replaced. For a test to be useful, it must identify an abnormality, which, when treated, results in improved fecundability. Below is a discussion of appropriate follow-up tests to perform, organized by cause of infertility. It should be noted that couples can have multiple challenges to their fertility and, therefore, may require tests in different categories to identify all their problems. Available tests are listed in Table 25–6.

OVULATORY DYSFUNCTION

Ovulatory dysfunction most commonly presents as oligomenorrhea, but can also be found in women with polymenorrhea and those with normal cycles and hirsutism. Obviously, ovulatory dysfunction may exist if there is amenorrhea. If there is any question about the accuracy of the patient's menstrual history, ask her to fill in a menstrual calendar for 3 months to provide a prospective record of her menses, to document her condition and also to serve as a guide for making recommendations about timed coitus. Withdrawal bleeding in response to a *progestin challenge test* can demonstrate estrogen production and a responsive endo-

Table 25–6 Tests for further evaluation of the woman

To evaluate ovulation

Progestin challenge test

Home ovulation kits

Luteal phase serum progesterone

To identify tubal obstruction or peritoneal adhesions

Hysterosalpingogram (HSG)

Laparoscopy with chromotubation

To identify uterine (including endometrial) structural abnormalities

Pelvic ultrasound

Saline infusion sonography (SIS)

Hysteroscopy

Hysterosalpingogram

Tests no longer used routinely

Postcoital test

Antisperm antibody

Basal body temperatures (BBTs)

Biopsy for endometrial dating

---

metrium in women who have not recently menstruated. Typically MPA 5–10 mg or Norethindrone 2.5 mg can be given daily for 10–12 days.

For women with menstrual histories consistent with chronic anovulation (< 8 cycles a year or cycle length > 35 days), perform appropriate tests to identify correctable etiologies such as hyperandrogenemia (*total testosterone, 17-hydroxyprogesterone*), thyroid dysfunction (*thyroid stimulating hormone*), pituitary tumor (*prolactin*), and extremes of weight or excessive exercise. Women with less obvious ovulatory defects benefit from documentation of their anovulation. Measure serum *progesterone* during the mid-luteal phase. Progesterone levels less than 3 ng/mL confirm the diagnosis of anovulation, whereas levels greater than 10 ng/mL correlate well with normal "in phase" endometrial changes and generally confirm ovulation. The timing of this midluteal progesterone test is critical. Draw the sample about 7 days prior to the onset of the next menses (estimated from the cycle length documented in the *menstrual calendar*) or 7 days after the LH surge (identified by *home ovulation detection kits*). These kits can predict ovulation in about 90% of women. Ovum release generally occurs 36 hours after initiation of the LH rise and 24 hours after the LH peak. Women often use ovulation detection kits to time intercourse. Evening urine specimens are particularly predictive. Salivary tests have also been approved by the FDA.

In the past, women used graphs of their *basal body temperatures* (BBTs) to determine if ovulation occurred. The woman took her temperature immediately after awakening at the same time each day and before getting out of bed. Ovulation was confirmed if her BBTs showed a biphasic pattern, with luteal phase temperatures being about 0.7° F higher than the follicular phase temperatures. This temperature increase is due to progesterone. However, BBTs have largely been abandoned because of the greater accuracy of the hormonal measurements mentioned previously.

OVARIAN RESERVE

Tests of ovarian reserve can predict the success of ovulation induction and are particularly important for women over 35, women with prior ovarian surgery, and those with a history of multi-drug chemotherapy or pelvic irradiation. It is generally thought that women with abnormal test results will have a greater probability of pregnancy if they use one of the assisted reproductive technologies (ART) with eggs donated by younger women.

The most common test of functional reserve is an FSH level drawn on cycle day 3 (CD_3 FSH). An elevated level (> 15 MIU/ml) suggests a decreased probability of pregnancy, especially in women over age 40. Early studies showed that no fertilizations occurred with eggs aspirated from women who had CD_3 FSH values greater than 24 MIU/mL.[18,19] Even if repeat tests demonstrate lower FSH levels, the potential for pregnancy remains low.[20] Elevated cycle day 3 estradiol levels (> 80 pg/mL) can also identify women with low fecundability.

Another test used to identify problems not revealed by the CD_3 FSH test is a *clomiphene citrate challenge test*. Women are given clomiphene citrate 100 mg daily on cycle days 5 to 9. FSH and estradiol (E_2) levels are drawn on cycle days 3 and 10. If CD_3 FSH is elevated and CD_3 E_2 is low, conception is highly unlikely. If CD_3 values are normal but CD_{10} FSH is elevated, the chance of fertility is low. The positive predictive value of these tests is about 90%. However, their sensitivity is only 7% to 26%.[21] Other tests (GnRH agonist test, inhibin B levels, Müllerian inhibiting substance levels or numbers of antral follicles) have also been proposed as indicators of oocyte quality and the likelihood of pregnancy following ovulation induction.

POLYCYSTIC OVARIAN SYNDROME (PCOS)

About 70% of women with ovulatory dysfunction have polycystic ovarian syndrome (PCOS). It is important to try to identify women with PCOS, because the therapies used for PCOS with women are different from treatment for other anovulatory causes of infertility. The criteria for

Table 25–7 Clinical criteria for PCOS

1990 NICHHD Criteria	2003 Rotterdam Criteria	Modified 1990 NIH/NICHHD Criteria	
• Clinical evidence of hyperandrogenism[a] and/or biochemical signs of hyperandrogenism[b] • Oligo-ovulation (i.e. cycle duration > 35 days or < 8 cycles per year) • Exclusion of related disorders[d]	• Two of the following three features: —Oligo-ovulation or anovulation —Clinical[a] and/or biochemical signs of hyperandrogenism[b] —Polycystic ovaries • Exclusion of other etiologies[d]	**Criterion** Androgen excess Ovarian Dysfunction Exclusion	**Description** Clinical[a] and/or biochemical hyperandrogenism[b] Oligo-anovulation and/or polycystic appearing ovaries on ultrasound[c] Other androgen excess or ovulatory disorders[d]

[a] Such as hirsutism, acne, androgenic alopecia.

[b] Hyperandrogenemia, such as elevated levels of total or free testosterone.

[c] Defined by either the number of intermediate follicles (> 8–12 follicles each 2 to 8–9 mm in diameter) and/or increased ovarian volume (e.g., > 10 ml[3]).

[d] Including, but not limited to, 21-hydroxylase deficient nonclassic adrenal hyperplasia, thyroid dysfunction, hyperprolactinemia, neoplastic androgen secretion, Cushing syndrome, or drug-induced androgen excess.

Sources: Zawadski JK (1992);[22] Rotterdam ESHRE/ASRM-Sponsored PCOS Consensus Workshop Group (2004)[23]; Azziz R (2005).[24]

the diagnosis of PCOS are in flux. The criteria from the 1991 NIH Consensus Conference[22] (see Table 25–7) have been very helpful, particularly in general practice, but many reproductive endocrinologists found them to be too restrictive. Many regularly cycling patients, especially those with hirsutism, had fertility problems similar to PCOS women, but were excluded by the NIH definition. Therefore, in an attempt to broaden the definition of PCOS, the Rotterdam criteria were developed in 2003[23] (see Table 25–7). Although the two PCOS definitions differ, they both emphasize that the most important step in the diagnosis is to rule out other pathologies as a cause of the patient's problems. A clinically useful compromise[24] between these two definitions recommends that most women be diagnosed using the NIH criteria; the Rotterdam criteria are applied only for the ovulating patients with polycystic ovaries and evidence of androgen excess. This means that most anovulatory women will need only TSH, prolactin and testosterone measurements to diagnose PCOS. Hirsute women with regular cycles will also need 17-hydroxyprogesterone testing and pelvic ultrasound. Other tests may be needed in more complicated cases. However, measurement of gonadotropins, their ratios, or estradiol is not required.

TUBAL DAMAGE

Suspect tubal damage and/or peritoneal factors in infertile women who ovulate and who have histories of sexually transmitted infections (especially Chlamydia, gonorrhea or PID) or elevated anti-Chlamydia antibodies. Such women warrant early evaluation of tubal patency.[25] Women with known or suspected endometriosis or a history of a prior abdominopelvic infection or surgery also deserve evaluation.

There are several tests to investigate tubal damage. Unfortunately, these tests are used only to describe tubal structure (patent or obstructed). They provide little information about the tubal function.

Hysterosalpingogram (HSG). Hysterosalpingography is the traditional method for evaluating the endometrial cavity and tubal patency. Women should be tested in the follicular phase of their menstrual cycles. Antibiotic prophylaxis is generally warranted. Contrast medicine is infused into the endometrial cavity under pressure with fluoroscopic monitoring and x-ray recording. Submucous fibroids and endometrial polyps appear as filling defects in the endometrial cavity. Tubal patency is confirmed when the dye pools in crescent-shaped collections between loops of bowel.

Laparoscopy. Laparascopy provides direct visualization of the pelvic structures and can identify endometriosis, adnexal adhesions, and significant tubal disease. Tubal patency is confirmed when a dilute solution of a sterile dye (methylene blue or indigo carmine) introduced through the cervix (chromotubation) is seen flowing out the fimbriae. Laparoscopy also provides the opportunity for adhesolysis or fulguration or excision of endometriotic implants.

UTERINE ABNORMALITIES

Pelvic ultrasound. If a pelvic exam suggests a pelvic mass, ultrasound can help distinguish a uterine from an ovarian mass. Ultrasound can distinguish leiomyomas with minimal effects on fecundity (pedunculated, subserosal, intramural) from those with more potential for blocking implantation (submucosal).[26,27] Ovarian masses can be characterized as solid or cystic. Endometrial polyps, septa, and submucosal fibroids are best visualized with saline infusion sonography. A narrow catheter is threaded through the cervix into the endometrial cavity and a small balloon is inflated to occlude the cervical os. A few tablespoons of sterile fluid are introduced through the catheter to separate the walls of the cavity and allow for clear imaging of polyps, synechia, septa, and fibroids.

Hysteroscopy. Diagnostic hysteroscopy can be performed in the office or clinic under local anesthesia and sedation. However, most hysteroscopy is performed under anesthesia in an operating room. Following cervical dilation, the hysteroscope is introduced into the endometrial cavity. Distending medium separates the uterine walls and permits direct visualization of the endometrial cavity. With an operative hysteroscope, therapeutic polypectomy and resection of submucous fibroids are possible.

PROGNOSIS

All couples seeking infertility services need a clear, accurate estimate of their prognosis. Studies show that many women want to participate in fertility treatment decisions, but they lack the information necessary to making informed choices.[28]

Couples who seek pregnancy relatively late in their reproductive lives face special problems. These couples have only few remaining ovulations; their fecundity decreases over time; they have higher rates of spontaneous abortions and fetal chromosomal abnormalities; they face obstacles to adoption; and they may need to use donated eggs if they opt for in vitro fertilization. Consequently, rapid evaluation and prompt initiation of therapy become very important. Prognosis is determined by the therapy applied, the underlying cause(s) of the infertility, and the length of time the couple has been attempting to conceive. See Table 25–8.

Success rates have been compared across many techniques,[29] but comparison is difficult because success rates are also dependent upon the skill and experience of the provider.

TARGETING THERAPIES FOR INFERTILITY

Today, virtually all therapy is targeted toward overcoming five categories of infertility: 1) male infertility, 2) ovulation disorders, 3) tubal abnormalities, 4) endometriosis, and 5) unexplained infertility. The number of therapeutic options and the effectiveness of these options have increased greatly. New medications can enhance ovulation. The assisted reproductive technologies (ARTs) in which both the eggs and sperm are manipulated in the laboratory have resulted in over a million births. ARTs include in vitro fertilization and intracytoplasmic sperm injection (ICSI) (see Table 25–9). Various techniques can be combined with ovulation induction to enhance outcomes. Adoption is an option that should be discussed with all couples, as should the psychological stresses that arise in conjunction with infertility and its treatment.[31]

TREATMENT OF MALE INFERTILITY

Azoospermia (no sperm) in men with inadequate gonadotrophin levels can be treated with injections of FSH and LH or GnRH pulses. Vas deferens reanastomosis can reverse surgical sterilization, or sperm obtained from the portion of the vas proximal to the interruption can be used with IVF (in-vitro fertilization). Varicocele repair can sometimes

Table 25–8 Distribution of primary diagnosis in 2198 infertile couples and live birth rate by diagnoses

	No. (%)	Live Birth Rates of Patients in Group %*
Female factors		
Ovulation disorders	386 (17.6)	41.5
Oligomenorrhea	294 (13.4)	42.5
Amenorrhea	40 (1.8)	47.5
Hyperprolactinemia	52 (2.4)	30.8
Tubal disease	509 (23.1)	21.8
Complete obstruction	212 (9.6)	14.2
Other	297 (13.5)	27.3
Endometriosis	146 (6.6)	29.5
Stage I and II	93 (4.2)	36.6
Stage III and IV	53 (2.4)	17.0
Male factors		
Oligospermia	369 (16.8)	29.8
Azoospermia	156 (7.1)	34.6
Unexplained	562 (25.6)	32.2
Other†	70 (3.2)	41.4

* Live birth rate includes treatment-related and treatment-independent conceptions

† Luteal phase defect (n=38), cervical defect (n=17), and uterine defect (n=15)

Source: Smith S (2003).[30]

improve oligospermia or abnormalities of sperm form or motility. Men whose sperm are unable to fertilize the egg can be offered intra-cytoplasmic sperm injection (ICSI).

However, most male infertility requires treatment using *donor sperm*, either alone or mixed with the patient's sperm. Because of the potential for transmission of human immunodeficiency virus (HIV), virtually all donor semen now comes from large, commercial frozen-semen banks that provide HIV-negative semen with a known ability to fertilize and known donor physical characteristics. Fecundity is about 10% per cycle using thawed donor semen placed in the vagina.[34] *Intrauterine insemination (IUI)* is more effective than vaginal or endocervical placement of semen, and two IUIs performed just prior to ovulation are more effective than one.[31]

Table 25–9 Assisted reproductive technologies: definitions

Intrauterine insemination (IUI). IUI is the insemination, directly into the endometrial cavity, of washed and concentrated sperm, which can come from the husband, a donor, or a mixture.

IUI with controlled hyperstimulation. IUI used in conjunction with ovulation induction improves fecundity in almost all clinical situations.[31] Two studies examining determinants of success[32,33] found that the overall pregnancy rate was 10% to 15% per cycle, with most pregnancies occurring within the first 3 to 4 cycles. Determinants of success were the number of follicles ovulated and the motility and morphology of the sperm in the ejaculate. Factors such as older female age, a diagnosis of endometriosis or tubal factor, duration of infertility, and a number of cycles previously treated without pregnancy were associated with less success.

In vitro fertilization (IVF). IVF is the process whereby oocytes, usually matured by controlled gonadotropin hyperstimulation, are aspirated from the ovary under ultrasonic guidance or laparoscopy and further matured and artificially fertilized in the laboratory. Following fertilization and development for 2 to 4 days (morula stage), the zygotes are transferred to the endometrial cavity via a catheter inserted through the cervix. Because of the gonadotropin stimulation, multiple oocytes are usually harvested. In order to diminish the likelihood of multiple pregnancies, no more than 3 or 4 fertilized eggs are placed in the endometrial cavity. Extra zygotes can be cryopreserved for later transfer. If the subfertile woman is older than 35 to 39 years, most programs require that she accept oocytes from a younger donor.

Gamete intrafallopian transfer (GIFT). Oocytes are matured and aspirated from the ovary, as in IVF. Sperm from the partner is washed and concentrated. Both oocytes and sperm are then placed directly into the fallopian tube where fertilization takes place. This method is used in women with no tubal damage.

Zygote intra-fallopian transfer (ZIFT). ZIFT uses the early steps of IVF; however, immediately following fertilization, the zygotes are placed into the fallopian tube to mature (with IVF, the zygotes are placed into the endometrial cavity during the morula stage). This method is also used in women with no tubal damage.

Intra-cytoplasmic sperm injection (ICSI). ICSI is useful when sperm are not able to penetrate the egg and fertilize it in vivo. Oocytes are matured and aspirated from the ovary as in IVF. Using micro-manipulative instruments under microscopic visualization, fertilization is accomplished by introduction of a single washed sperm into the cytoplasm of the oocyte. Following development to the morula stage, the zygote is transferred to the endometrial cavity as in IVF, although ZIFT is also possible.

TREATMENT OF FEMALE INFERTILITY

Treatment of Infertility Caused By Anovulation

Therapy is best targeted to treat the underlying cause of the woman's anovulation. Correction of thyroid dysfunction or suppression of hyperprolactinemia will generally result in resumption of ovulatory cycling in affected women. Women with extremes of weight can benefit by normalization of their weight; for women whose anovulation is associated with excessive weight, loss of as little as 10% to 15% of body weight is often associated with return of fertility.[35,36] Women with hypothalamic amenorrhea due to eating disorders or excessive exercise need to resolve those lifestyle problems. In one study in which 26 underweight women underwent counseling and gained weight, there was a 73% pregnancy rate.[37]

Clomiphene citrate. The first line therapy for women with anovulation or oligo-ovulation who do not have PCOS is clomiphene citrate. It is an antiestrogen that competitively binds to hypothalmic estrogen receptors. With its estrogen receptors blocked, the hypothalamus senses a drop in circulating estrogen levels and increases GnRH pulses, which triggers FSH and LH release and induces follicular maturation and ovulation. Clomiphene is most effective in patients who have normal gonadotropin levels, oligo-ovulation or anovulation, and withdrawal bleeding following a progestin challenge. Clomiphene treatment, given orally for 5 days early in the cycle starting at 50 mg per day induces ovulation in 70% of such patients. If the treatment is successful, ovulation usually occurs on the 12th or 13th day following the start of the clomiphene. Sperm are made available just prior to ovulation. If ovulation does not occur, clomiphene doses are increased each month up to a limit of 150 to 200 mg each treatment day until ovulation is induced. Anovulatory women who are responsive to clomiphene citrate should be treated for at least 6 cycles, but the treatment should probably be limited to a maximum of 12 cycles. In the absence of other causes of infertility, pregnancy rates among women who take clomiphene are comparable to pregnancy rates of women who have spontaneous ovulations. The overall pregnancy rate is 70% to 75% after 6 to 9 ovulatory cycles. Ovulation induction with clomiphene is associated with a modest increase in the occurrence of multiple pregnancy (8%) and ovarian cysts (> 1%).[38] Many newer protocols call for pretreating women with GnRH agonists, or aromatase inhibitors in the cycle prior to clomiphene use.

Gonadotropins. Injections of *gonadotropins* such as FSH (with or without LH), provide direct stimulation to the ovaries. This therapy is best suited to patients who are not responsive to clomiphene. The gonadotropins are given by daily injection for 7 to 12 days. Ovarian response is monitored by measuring serum estrogen daily and ultrasound. When the follicles are in the right size range (> 16mm), ovulation will be induced with an injection of hCG, the LH surrogate. If too many follicles are stimulated, hCG should be withheld in order to avoid hyperstimulation syndrome. Sperm are provided just prior to ovulation. In women who have no other causes of infertility, pregnancy rates with gonadotropin therapy are about the same as those in women with spontaneous ovulations. However, even with close monitoring, multiple pregnancy rates with gonadotropin therapy are increased (20% of cases), as is the risk of ovarian cysts (1% to 3%).

Pulsatile GnRH administered by infusion pump also stimulates the pituitary to release FSH and LH. In a number of ways, pulsatile GnRH and gonadotropin therapy are similar in effectiveness, patient selection, and how their use is monitored. However, the rate of high order multiple pregnancies may be lower and episodes of hyperstimulation may be reduced.

Metformin. Metformin currently is the first line therapy for anovulatory cycling in women with PCOS.[39] Because metformin should be used regardless of the patient's insulin resistance status, routine testing for insulin resistance is unwarranted. Metformin reduces the concentration of insulin within the ovaries, which reduces ovarian androgen production and increases ovulation and pregnancy rates. In a Cochrane review, women with PCOS treated with metformin were 3.88 times more likely to ovulate than were women taking placebo (95% CI=2.25–6.69).[39] Side effects such as nausea, vomiting, and other gastrointestinal problems occur in up to 20% of women taking the drug, but serious adverse events, such as lactic acidosis, are rare. In one study, metformin use continued through the first trimester in women with PCOS who had histories of recurrent losses reduced spontaneous abortion rates in the first trimester from 42% to 9%.[40] Other researchers have shown that metformin continued into second- and third-trimesters helped reduce the development of gestational diabetes (23% vs. 3%). Ovulation rates are higher when metformin is combined with clomiphene citrate (see below) compared to metformin as a single agent (76% vs 46%). Similarly, the odds ratio for pregnancy was 4.40 (CI 1.96–9.85) for combined therapy compared to the use of clomiphene citrate alone.[39] However, the safety of this combined regimen is not as well established as single-agent metformin, so combined therapy is reserved for women who fail first-line therapy.[39] If the patient has excessive adrenal production of androgens (e.g., DHEAS > 2 mcg/ml), a *glucocorticoid* agent can be added to improve success rates.[41]

Aromatase inhibitors. Aromatase inhibitors such as letrozole or anastrozole block conversion of androstenedione to estrogen. The drop in circulating estradiol causes an increase in FSH secretion and spurs growth of follicles. In one small trial, PCOS women who had not conceived with clomiphene were given letrozole 2.5 mg daily on cycle days 3 to 7; their ovulation rate was 84% and the pregnancy rate rose to 27%.[42] Women who use aromatase inhibitors have lower rates of multiple gestations and spontaneous abortion than do women who use clomiphene.[43,44] However, letrozole contains a new product warning about the potential for congenital anomalies. Canadian researchers reported that higher dose therapy (5 mg/d) was associated with higher rates of poor outcomes. This concern may temper enthusiasm for the use of this agent, at least until there are more reassuring reports in the literature. Gonadotrophin therapy is generally used if patients do not ovulate with these medications.

Surgery. Surgical therapies, such as laparoscopic ovarian drilling using diathermy or laser, have also shown clinical promise in restoring ovulation to PCOS patients resistant to clomiphene and unable or un-willing to undergo gonadotrophin therapy.[45]

Treatment of Infertility Caused by Tubal Abnormalities

The most effective treatment of infertility caused by tubal abnormal-ities is in-vitro fertilization (IVF), which bypasses the tubal abnormality. To increase intrauterine pregnancy rates, some experts recommend bilat-eral salpingectomy prior to performing IVF in women with tubal damage due to PID or endometriosis. Older surgical techniques, such as tuboplasty, are less effective than IVF, except in cases of tubal ligation re-versal. Pregnancy rates with IVF now equal or exceed those with GIFT or ZIFT, which now are rarely used.[77]

Treatment of Infertility Associated With Endometriosis

Conservative management is often recommended for Stage I and II (mild to moderate) endometriosis.[46] A meta-analysis of large-scale studies has shown that none of the available medical therapies resulted in greater fertility than placebo, and many of the therapies may delay fertility.[47] Laparoscopic treatment of minimal and mild endometriosis may improve success rates.[48,49] IUI and controlled hyperstimulation may improve fertility rates after laparoscopic ablation.[50,51] A sobering note is that only one pregnancy will occur in every 7.7 women treated.[52] IVF has a role only if simpler therapy is unsuccessful.

The preferred treatment of infertility associated with severe endome-triosis is surgical ablation followed by IVF. There are no randomized trials to support this recommendation; however, the pregnancy rates in untreated advanced (Stage III, IV) endometriosis approach zero, and case reports of pregnancies after surgical repair suggest a benefit.

Treatment for Unexplained Infertility

In the absence of a correctable abnormality, the therapy of unex-plained infertility is always empiric. Expectant management is the op-tional strategy for couple with a 35% probability of conception in the next year.[78] After a trial of conservative management to rule out simple subfertility, the preferred treatment of unexplained infertility is IUI with controlled hyperstimulation.[53,54] IVF is considerably more costly than clo-miphene citrate and IUI.[79] ICSI is not superior to IVF.[55] The roles of em-pirical use of clomiphene without IUI in the treatment of unexplained in-fertility is debatable and present data are inconclusive.[56]

LONGER TERM IMPACTS OF ASSISTED REPRODUCTIVE TECHNOLOGIES

In 2002, in the United States alone, 115,392 ART procedures were reported to the CDC. They resulted in over 45,000 deliveries, which represented 1% of all births. Conflicting study results raise questions about the short and longer term consequences of these technologies in three areas: impact on the pregnancy outcome, risks of anomalies and other effects on the infant, and long-term effects on maternal health.

Adverse Pregnancy Outcomes. ART is associated with a 10-fold increased risk of multifetal pregnancies (32% vs. 3%). Multifetal pregnancy increases the risks of prematurity, low and very low birthweight, malpresentation, placenta previa and abruption, premature rupture of membranes, intrauterine growth retardation, and umbilical core prolapse. Most studies also show that even the singleton births in ART are at almost a 2 times higher risk for low and very low birthweight.[57] When the birth weight of singletons born after ART were compared to the birth weights of couples who were evaluated for infertility but who spontaneously conceived in the same practice during the same time period, those who achieved pregnancy with ART (mainly IVF and ICSI) had shorter pregnancy and lower mean birth weight.[58] CDC studies also concluded that in the U.S. experience, there has been no increase in the risk of spontaneous abortion associated with most ARTs, except with cycles stimulated with clomiphene citrate and use of thawed embryos.[59]

Risk of Anomalies with ART. It is very difficult to assess the risk of major malformations attributable to ART itself. Infertile couples who use ART have health issues that make them different from the general population and increase their baseline risks of fetal anomalies. Women undergoing ART are generally older than spontaneously conceiving women. Because women undergoing ART are very closely monitored for pregnancy, it would be expected that their rates of reported early pregnancy losses (so called "chemical pregnancies") would be higher than those of women in the general population. In addition, the ART registries follow the offspring long term to identify delayed anomalies, while in the general population birth defect rates generally reflect only those anomalies identified at birth.

There are biologically plausible reasons why ART offspring could be at higher risk. In the 1980s, the NIH found that the risk of anomalies was low and not higher than in the control population.[60] Most registries in Europe have also been reassuring. U.K. researchers report one or more congenital anomalies in the first week of life in 2.2% to 2.7% of ART offspring, which was within the range expected.[61,62] In France, the IVF anomaly rate was 2%[63] and longer term follow up found that height, weight and scholastic performance of IVF children was comparable to the general population.[64] On the other hand, Scandinavian studies raised concerns about specific syndromes with IVF infants: neural tube defects, alimentary atresia and omphalocele.[65] Cardiac malformations were reported in other studies in the region.[66] Australian studies also report higher rates of malformation.[67] Imprinting disorders, in which recessive conditions can be expressed even if only one parent carries the mutation, appear to be higher in ART;[68] therefore, disorders such as Beckwith-Wiedeman Syndrome, Prader-Willi Syndrome, and Angelman Syndrome appear in higher numbers in ART.

Because the background rate of these specific anomalies is very low, and most of them can generally be detected easily in pregnancy, the slightly increased rates associated with these ART techniques are not worrisome. However, there are specific concerns about ICSI offspring. In several studies ICSI infants have demonstrated higher rates of anomalies (such as hypospadias and some chromosomal abnormalities, including translocation) than the rates among spontaneously conceived infants.

Several analyses comparing the risk of abnormalities among offspring of women undergoing ART compared with women who conceived spontaneously have reported conflicting conclusions. In its review of the issue, the ART Children's Health Panel stated that "the evidence is suggestive of no association between ART and overall serious malformations". The panel found that there was not adequate evidence to determine if ART caused an increase in hypospadias. The panel also concluded that the evidence was suggestive but not conclusive that ART increased imprinting disorders, but emphasized how very rare these conditions are.[69] In contrast, a second meta-analysis of pooled results from all suitable published studies suggested that children born following ART are at increased risk of birth defects. The authors advised that couples seeking ART treatment should be informed of the risk.[70] More recently, another large-scale study found no increased incidence of fetal chromosome or structural abnormalities in women who used any form of ART.[71] A recent U.S. evaluation comparing IVF children to naturally conceived children found major birth defects rates of 6.2% and 4.4%, respectively.[80] In light of the confusion, advise couples seeking ART that controversy exists and that there may be a slight increase in the risk of some anomalies. However, the baseline risks are so small that these increases will only rarely result in problems.

Long-Term Maternal Health Risks. The current consensus, based on several epidemiologic studies, is that the use of fertility drugs (ovulation induction) with or without ART does not increase the risk of breast cancer, once an adjustment has been made for low parity. The National Cancer Institute agreed with this conclusion, but called for more studies, particularly about the effect multi-fetal pregnancies and multiple births might have on breast cancer.[72] The use of fertility drugs and ART does not increase a woman's risk of getting ovarian cancer when her risks are compared to other infertile women who do not receive infertility treatments.[73] The use of clomiphene citrate does not increase the risk of melanoma, thyroid or cervical cancer.[74]

OTHER OPTIONS: ADOPTION

Many couples faced with infertility choose to adopt. Licensed adoption agencies may or may not allow communication between the birth parents and adopting parents, and they generally involve a longer wait than do independent adoptions. Couples may seek the help of providers who have contact with women with unwanted pregnancies. Attorneys, clergy, friends, and independent adoption centers can also aid in matching couples with birth parents. Adopting children from other countries, older children, or children with special needs may minimize the waiting period, but may be associated with other challenges. Present these options to infertile clients, along with referrals to adoption resources.

EMOTIONAL ASPECTS OF COPING WITH INFERTILITY

Many couples who seek help for infertility eventually achieve pregnancy, often in the course of the preliminary investigation. However, some couples must eventually confront the reality of probable sterility. The impact of this, coupled with the stresses of fertility evaluation and treatment, may damage a couple's relationship or an individual's self-concept. Normal reactions to the diagnosis include processes similar to other grieving processes: surprise, denial, isolation, anger, guilt, sorrow, and, finally, resolution. Frustration, isolation, depression, and prolonged stress are also common. Couples suffer a loss of privacy, a disruption of spontaneity, and the stresses that accompany sexual performance on demand. The monthly menses is a painful mark of yet another cycle of failure.[75]

Remember how disruptive infertility diagnosis and treatment can be for couples. Recognize also that stress may affect the success of fertility treatments.[76] Take an active and complementary role in helping infertile couples to cope:

- Refer couples for psychological counseling if their depression or anxiety appears serious.

- Refer couples to infertility networks and support groups specifically designed to help people with infertility problems. One such group is RESOLVE, www.resolve.org.

- Remain sensitive to the heightened vulnerability of infertility patients.

References

1. American College of Obstetricians and Gynecologists: Infertility (ACOG Technical Bulletin Number 125). Washington, DC, ACOG, 1989.
2. Hull M, Glazener C, Kelly J, et al. Population study of causes, treatment, and outcome of infertility. BMJ 1985; 291:1693–1697.
3. Lobo RA, Mishell DR Jr, Paulsen RJ, Shoupe D. Mishell's Textbook of infertility, contraception, and reproductive endocrinology, 4th Edition. Malden MA: Blackwell Science, 1997. Adapted from Leridon H, Spira A. Problems in measuring the effectiveness of infertility therapy. Fertil Steril 1984; 41:580–586.
4. Axmon A, Hagmar L. Time to pregnancy and pregnancy outcome. Fertil Steril 2005;84:966–974.
5. Wang X, Chen C, Wang L, et al. Conception, early pregnancy loss, and time to clinical pregnancy: a population-based prospective study. Fertil Steril 2003;79:577–584.
6. Gnoth C, Frank-Herrmann P, Freundl G. Opinion: natural family planning and the management of infertility. Arch Gynecol Obstet 2002;267:67–71.
7. Gnoth C, Godehardt E, Frank-Herrmann P, et al. Definition and prevalence of subfertility and infertility. Hum Reprod 2005;20:1144–1147.
8. Snick HK, Snick TS, Evers JL, Collins JA. The spontaneous pregnancy prognosis in untreated subfertile couples: the Walcheren primary care study. Hum Reprod 1997;12(7):1582–1588.
9. Lobo RA. Potential options for preservation of fertility in women. N Engl J Med 2005;353:64–73.
10. Wilcox AJ, Weinberg CR, O'Connor JF, et al. Incidence of early loss of pregnancy. N Engl J Med 1988;319:189–194.
11. Warburton D. Reproductive loss: how much is preventable? N Engl J Med 1987;316:158–160.
12. Centers for Disease Control and Prevention (CDC). 2003 Assisted reproductive technology (art) report: national summary and fertility clinic results. Atlanta: Centers for Disease Control and Prevention, 2005. Accessed 03/03/06 at www.cdc.gov/ART/ART2003/index.htm
13. Practice Committee of the American Society for Reproductive Medicine. Aging and infertility in women. Fertil Steril. 2004 Sep;82 Suppl 1:S102–S106.
14. ASRM. Patient's Fact Sheet: Diagnostic testing for male factor infertility. Birmingham AL: American Society for Reproductive Medicine, 2001. Accessed 2/25/06 at www.asrm.org/Patients/FactSheets/Testing_Male-Fact.pdf
15. Guzick D, Overstreet J, Factor-Litvak P, et al. Sperm morphology, motility and concentration in fertile and infertile men. N Engl J Med 2001;345:1388–1393.
16. AUA and ASRM. Report on optimal evaluation of the infertile male. Baltimore MD and Birmingham AL: American Urological Association and American Society for Reproductive Medicine, 2001.
17. Mosher WD, Pratt WF. Fecundity and infertility in the United States: incidence and trends. Fertil Steril 1991;56:192–193.
18. Toner JP, Philput CB, Jones GS, Muasher SJ. Basal follicle-stimulating hormone level is a better predictor of in vitro fertilization performance than age. Fertil Steril 1991;55:784–791.
19. van Montfrans JM, Hoek A, van Hooff MH, et al. Predictive value of basal follicle-stimulating hormone concentrations in a general subfertility population. Fertil Steril 2000;74:97–103.
20. Scott RT, Opsahl MS, Leonardi MR, et al. Life table analysis of pregnancy rates in a general infertility population relative to ovarian reserve and patient age. Hum Reprod 1995;10:1706–1710.
21. Jain T, Soules MR, Collins JA. Comparison of basal follicle-stimulating hormone versus the clomiphene citrate challenge test for ovarian reserve screening. Fertil Steril 2004;82:180–185.

22. Zawadski JK, Dunaif A. Diagnostic criteria for polycystic ovary syndrome: towards a rational approach. In: Dunaif A, Givens JR, Haseltine F, eds. Polycystic ovary syndrome. Boston: Blackwell Scientific, 1992:377–384.

23. Rotterdam ESHRE/ASRM-Sponsored PCOS Consensus Workshop Group. Revised 2003 consensus on diagnostic criteria and long-term health risks related to polycystic ovary syndrome. Fertil Steril 2004;81:19–25.

24. Azziz R. Diagnostic criteria for polycystic ovary syndrome: a reappraisal. Fertil Steril 2005;83:1343–1346.

25. Dabeekausen Y, Evers J, Land J, Stals F. Chlamydia trachomatis antibody testing is more accurate than hysterosalpingography in predicting tubal factor infertility. Fertil Steril 1994;61:833–837.

26. Donnez J, Jadoul P. What are the implications of myomas on fertility? A need for a debate? Hum Reprod 2002;17:1424–1430.

27. Oliveira FG, Abdelmassih VG, Diamond MP, et al. Impact of subserosal and intramural uterine fibroids that do not distort the endometrial cavity on the outcome of in vitro fertilization-intracytoplasmic sperm injection. Fertil Steril 2004;81:582–587.

28. Stewart DE, Rosen B, Irvine J, et al. The disconnect: infertility patients' information and the role they wish to play in decision making. Medscape Womens Health 2001;6(4):1.

29. Duckitt K. Infertility and subfertility. In Clinical evidence. London: BMJ Publishing Group, 2001:5:1279–1302.

30. Smith S, Pfeifer SM, Collins JA. Diagnosis and management of female infertility. JAMA 2003;290:1767–1770.

31. Cohlen BJ, Vandekerckhove P, te Velde ER, Habbema JD. Timed intercourse versus intra-uterine insemination with or without ovarian hyperstimulation for subfertility in men. Cochrane Database Syst Rev 2000;(2):CD000360.

32. Montanaro Gauci M, Kruger TF, Coetzee K, et al. Stepwise regression analysis to study male and female factors impacting on pregnancy rate in an intrauterine insemination programme. Andrologia 2001;33(3):135–141.

33. Nuojua-Huttunen S, Tomas C, Bloigu R, et al. Intrauterine insemination treatment in subfertility: an analysis of factors affecting outcome. Hum Reprod 1999;14:698–703.

34. Cooke ID. Donor insemination - timing and insemination method. In: Templeton A, Cooke ID, O'Brien PMS, eds. 35th RCOG study group evidence-based fertility treatment. London: RCOG Press, 1998.

35. Kiddy DS, Hamilton-Fairley D, Bush A, et al. Improvement in endocrine and ovarian function during dietary treatment of obese women with polycystic ovary syndrome. Clin Endocrinol (Oxf) 1992;36:105–111.

36. Pasquali R, Casimirri F, Vicennati V. Weight control and its beneficial effect on fertility in women with obesity and polycystic ovary syndrome. Hum Reprod 1997;12 Suppl 1:82–87.

37. Bates GW, Bates SR, Whitworth NS. Reproductive failure in women who practice weight control. Fertil Steril 1982;37:373–378.

38. Nasseri S, Ledger WL. Clomiphene citrate in the twenty-first century. Hum Fertil (Camb) 2001;4(3):145–151.

39. Lord JM, Flight IH, Norman RJ. Insulin-sensitising drugs (metformin, troglitazone, rosiglitazone, pioglitazone, D-chiro-inositol) for polycystic ovary syndrome. Cochrane Database Syst Rev 2003;(3):CD003053.

40. Jakubowicz DJ, Iuorno MJ, Jakubowicz S, et al. Effects of metformin on early pregnancy loss in the polycystic ovary syndrome. J Clin Endocrinol Metab 2002;87:524–529.

41. ACOG Committee on Practice Bulletins-Gynecology. ACOG Practice Bulletin. Clinical management guidelines for obstetrician-gynecologists number 34, February 2002. Management of infertility caused by ovulatory dysfunction. Obstet Gynecol 2002;99:347–358.

42. Al-Omari WR, Sulaiman WR, Al-Hadithi N. Comparison of two aromatase inhibitors in women with clomiphene-resistant polycystic ovary syndrome. Int J Gynaecol Obstet 2004;85:289–291.
43. Mitwally MF, Biljan MM, Casper RF. Pregnancy outcome after the use of an aromatase inhibitor for ovarian stimulation. Am J Obstet Gynecol 2005;192:381–386.
44. Al-Fozan H, Al-Khadouri M, Tan SL, Tulandi T. A randomized trial of letrozole versus clomiphene citrate in women undergoing superovulation. Fertil Steril 2004;82:1561–1563.
45. Farquhar C, Lilford RJ, Marjoribanks J, Vandekerckhove P. Laparoscopic 'drilling' by diathermy or laser for ovulation induction in anovulatory polycystic ovary syndrome. Cochrane Database Syst Rev 2005:CD001122.
46. Parazzini F. Ablation of lesions or no treatment in minimal-mild endometriosis in infertile women: a randomized trial. Gruppo Italiano per lo Studio dell'Endometriosi. Hum Reprod 1999;14:1332–1334.
47. Hughes E, Fedorkow D, Collins J, Vandekerckhove P. Ovulation suppression for endometriosis. Cochrane Database Syst Rev 2003;(3):CD000155.
48. Jacobson TZ, Barlow DH, Koninckx PR, Olive D, Farquhar C. Laparoscopic surgery for subfertility associated with endometriosis. Cochrane Database Syst Rev 2002;(4):CD001398.
49. Kennedy S, Bergqvist A, Chapron C, D'Hooghe T, Dunselman G, Greb R, Hummelshoj L, Prentice A, Saridogan E; on behalf of the ESHRE Special Interest Group for Endometriosis and Endometrium Guideline Development Group. ESHRE guideline for the diagnosis and treatment of endometriosis. Hum Reprod 2005;20(10): 2698–2704.
50. Adamson GD. Treatment of endometriosis-associated infertility. Semin Reprod Endocrinol 1997;15:263–271.
51. Ledger WL. Endometriosis and infertility: an integrated approach. Int J Gynaecol Obstet 1999;64 Suppl 1:S33-S40.
52. Olive DL, Pritts EA. Treatment of endometriosis. N Engl J Med 2001;345:266–275.
53. Hughes EG. The effectiveness of ovulation induction and intrauterine insemination in the treatment of persistent infertility: a meta-analysis. Hum Reprod 1997;12:1865–1872.
54. Singh M, Goldberg J, Falcone T, et al. Superovulation and intrauterine insemination in cases of treated mild pelvic disease. J Assist Reprod Genet 2001;18:26–29.
55. Ruiz A, Remohi J, Minguez Y, et al. The role of in vitro fertilization and intracytoplasmic sperm injection in couples with unexplained infertility after failed intrauterine insemination. Fertil Steril 1997;68:171–173.
56. Nasseri S, Ledger WL. Clomiphene citrate in the twenty-first century. Hum Fertil (Camb) 2001;4(3):145–151.
57. Schieve LA, Meikle SF, Ferre C, et al. Low and very low birth weight in infants conceived with use of assisted reproductive technology. N Engl J Med 2002;346:731–737.
58. De Geyter C, De Geyter M, Steimann S, Zhang H, Holzgreve W. Comparative birth weights of singletons born after assisted reproduction and natural conception in previously infertile women. Hum Reprod 2006;21(3):705–712.
59. Schieve LA, Tatham L, Peterson HB, et al. Spontaneous abortion among pregnancies conceived using assisted reproductive technology in the United States. Obstet Gynecol 2003;101:959–967.
60. Morin NC, Wirth FH, Johnson DH, et al. Congenital malformations and psychosocial development in children conceived by in vitro fertilization. J Pediatr 1989;115: 222–227.
61. MRC Working Party on Children Conceived by In Vitro Fertilisation. Births in Great Britain resulting from assisted conception, 1978–87. BMJ 1990;300:1229–1233.
62. Rizk B, Doyle P, Tan SL, et al. Perinatal outcome and congenital malformations in in-vitro fertilization babies from the Bourn-Hallam group. Hum Reprod 1991;6(9): 1259–1264.

63. FIVNAT (French In Vitro National). French National IVF Registry: analysis of 1986 to 1990 data. Fertil Steril 1993;59:587–595.
64. Olivennes F, Kerbrat V, Rufat P, et al. Follow-up of a cohort of 422 children aged 6 to 13 years conceived by in vitro fertilization. Fertil Steril 1997;67:284–289.
65. Ericson A, Kallen B. Congenital malformations in infants born after IVF: a population-based study. Hum Reprod 2001;16:504–9.
66. Koivurova S, Hartikainen AL, Gissler M, et al. Neonatal outcome and congenital malformations in children born after in-vitro fertilization. Hum Reprod 2002;17:1391–1398.
67. Lancaster PA. Registers of in-vitro fertilization and assisted conception. Hum Reprod 1996;11:89–104; discussion 105–109.
68. Schieve LA, Rasmussen SA, Buck GM, Schendel DE, Reynolds MA, Wright VC. Are children born after assisted reproductive technology at increased risk for adverse health outcomes? Obstet Gynecol 2004;103:1154–1163.
69. Hudson C, Robinson KA, Ananthakrishman A, et al. A comprehensive review of the health and developmental outcomes of children conceived through assisted reproductive technologies [abstract]. Am J Hum Genet 2004:75
70. Hansen M, Bower C, Milne E, et al. Assisted reproductive technologies and the risk of birth defects–a systematic review. Hum Reprod 2005;20:328–338.
71. Shevell T, Malone FD, Vidaver J, et al. Assisted reproductive technology and pregnancy outcome. Obstet Gynecol 2005;106:1039–1045.
72. National Cancer Institute. Summary Report: Early Reproductive Events and Breast Cancer Workshop. 2003. Accessed 2/27/06 at www.cancer.gov/cancerinfo/ere-workshop-report.
73. Kashyap S, Moher D, Fung MF, Rosenwaks Z. Assisted reproductive technology and the incidence of ovarian cancer: a meta-analysis. Obstet Gynecol 2004;103:785–794.
74. Althuis MD, Scoccia B, Lamb EJ, et al. Melanoma, thyroid, cervical, and colon cancer risk after use of fertility drugs. Am J Obstet Gynecol 2005;193:668–674.
75. Greil AL. Infertility and psychological distress: a critical review of the literature. Soc Sci Med 1997;45:1679–1704.
76. Klonoff-Cohen H, Chu E, Natarajan L, Sieber W. A prospective study of stress among women undergoing in vitro fertilization or gamete intrafallopian transfer. Fertil Steril 2001;76:675–687.

LATE REFERENCES

77. Van Voorhis BJ. Outcomes from assisted reproductive technology. Obstet Gynecol 2006;107(1):183–200.
78. Steures P, van der Steeg JW, Hompes PG, Habbema JD, Eijkemans MJ, Broekmans FJ, Verhoeve HR, Bossuyt PM, van der Veen F, Mol BW; Collaborative Effort on the Clinical Evaluation in Reproductive Medicine. Intrauterine insemination with controlled ovarian hyperstimulation versus expectant management for couples with unexplained subfertility and an intermediate prognosis: a randomised clinical trial. Lancet 2006;368(9531):216–221.
79. Nelson HP, Adamson GD. Effective empiric treatment of infertility. Sexuality Reprod Menopause 2006;4(2):48–51.
80. Olson CK, Keppler-Noreuil KM, Romitti PA, Budelier WT, Ryan G, Sparks AE, Van Voorhis BJ. In vitro fertilization is associated with an increase in major birth defects. Fertil Steril 2005;84(5):1308–1315.

Menopause and Perimenopausal Health

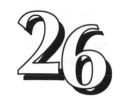

Anita L. Nelson, MD
Felicia H. Stewart, MD

- Perimenopause is a clinical diagnosis. Tests of levels of gonadotrophins and/or estradiol are at best unnecessary, but at worst may lead to a misdiagnosis.

- Many perimenopausal women need effective contraception. Although women over age 40 have significantly lower fertility potential than do women in their 20s, an unintended pregnancy at this time in life can be particularly disturbing.

- The most important therapeutic recommendation for postmenopausal women is to adopt healthy lifestyles.

- Routine "replacement" of hormones for postmenopausal women is not warranted. Hormone treatment can, however, be offered as a targeted therapy to treat specific conditions, such as hot flashes, urogenital atrophy and osteoporosis prevention. Provide treatment at the lowest doses for the shortest duration needed.

DEFINITIONS: PERIMENOPAUSE, MENOPAUSE, POST-MENOPAUSE

A woman's reproductive years often have an intriguing symmetry. Just as menarche is the first menses, menopause marks the end of menstruation. The anovulatory cycling characteristic of the first 2 to 5 years of a woman's reproductive life following menarche is mirrored in the anovulatory cycling and hormonal fluctuations that occur during the 2 to 8 perimenopausal years approaching menopause.

Menopause is the cessation of menstruation following loss of ovarian function. Generally, it is a retrospective diagnosis; women are postmenopausal one year after their last menses, unless there are other causes of their amenorrhea. Menopause occurs regardless of a woman's age when the number of ovarian follicles she has left drops below the critical level of about 1,000.

Perimenopause is the time in a woman's life from the onset of her first symptom of loss of ovarian cycling until 1 year after her last menses. Perimenopause is a relatively new concept; the word was not even listed in Stedman's Medical Dictionary 25th edition in 1989.

Menopausal transition is the term used to define the years from the onset of the loss of ovarian cycling to her last menses.

These terms have been formally defined in the STRAW recommendations (see Figure 26–1).[1] Climacterium, is an older term, which is less precise, and refers to the period of endocrinologic, somatic and transitory physiologic changes occurring in the transition to the menopause.

Most women entering menopause today are healthy. However, health challenges during this time of life are important. There are so many women (baby boomers) now moving into and through these years that the public health implications and financial implications are enormous. From both the medical and societal perspectives, this is uncharted water. Never in history has there been an expectation that women on average would spend one third of their lives after menopause. The health habits established during the perimenopausal and early post-menopausal years can determine the woman's health status and quality of life for her crit-

Recommendations of Stages of Reproductive Aging Workshop (STRAW), Park City, Utah, USA. July 2001.

Stages:	-5	-4	-3	-2	-1	0	+1	+2
Terminology:	Reproductive			Menopausal Transition		FMP	Postmenopause	
	Early	Peak	Late	Early	Late*		Early*	Late
				Perimenopause				
Duration of Stage:	Variable			Variable		Final Menstrual Period	1 yr	4 yrs	Unit demise
Menstrual Cycles:	Variable to regular	Regular		Variable cycle length (≥ 7 days; different from normal)	≥2 skipped cycles and an interval of amenorrhea (≥ 60 days)		Amenorrhea x 12 months		None
Endocrine:	Normal FSH		↑ FSH	↑ FSH			↑ FSH		

* Stages most likely to be characterized by vasomotor symptoms   ↑ = elevated

* Stages most likely to be characterized by vasomotor symptoms, ↑ = elevated

Source: Soules MR, et al. (2001).[1]

Figure 26–1 STRAW Regime *Recommendations of Stages of Reproductive Aging Workshop (STRAW), Park City, Utah, USA. July 2001.*

ical elderly years after 75, when serious health problems (and costs) are greatest.

PERIMENOPAUSE

PERIMENOPAUSAL PHYSIOLOGY

Each woman travels her own unique course through perimenopause. Women who experienced regular cycling in their 20s and 30s often notice subtle changes in their menstrual cycles starting in their late 30s and early 40s. At first, they may note a reduction in the interval between their menstrual periods and, later, an irregular and longer spacing between menses, as more cycles are anovulatory. Because of anovulation, menses can become irregular, heavy, and prolonged enough to require evaluation, intervention, and occasionally, surgical therapy.

The earliest manifestations of functional ovarian changes begin by age 35 to 40; fertility per cycle starts to decline in this age group, usually even before menstrual disorders or hot flashes develop. In Hutterite populations with unregulated fertility, 11% of women had their last pregnancy before age 34, and 33% completed childbearing before age 40; only about 13% had any pregnancies after age 45.[2] In donor insemination programs, women under age 31 had annual pregnancy rates of 74%; women over age 35 had rates of 54%.[3] In a U.S. study, women over age 35 required 9 to 10 cycles to conceive, rather than the average 6 cycles for younger women.

Early in a woman's life, her ovarian follicles are very responsive to stimulation by follicle-stimulating hormone (FSH). By age 35 to 40, remaining follicles require higher gonadotropin levels to stimulate maturation. FSH levels are able to increase to stimulate remaining follicles because ovarian follicle production of inhibin B decreases, which reduces negative feedback from the ovary to the hypothalamus and pituitary.

The hormonal hallmark of perimenopause is not low estrogen levels. It is fluctuating or "irregularly irregular" estrogen levels.[4] For some women, these hormonal and gonadotrophin fluctuations are so extreme that the perimenopausal period can best be described as "hormonal chaos."[5]

PERIMENOPAUSE SYMPTOMS AND DIAGNOSIS

At least 15% to 40% of menstruating women in their 40s experience hot flashes, which are often as disturbing as those that occur after menopause.[6] Hot flashes in this age group do not necessarily result from low serum estrogen levels, but occur in the context of dramatically fluctuating estrogen levels.[5] Although we do not completely understand the etiology of hot flashes, women (and men) tend to become symptomatic when their estrogen levels decline rapidly. Absolute estrogen levels in themselves do not explain hot flashes: there is no difference in average estrogen levels between symptomatic and asymptomatic women.[7] The trough estradiol levels can be associated with poor sleep, hot flashes, higher anxiety and depression, even in cycling reproductive-age women.[8] Menstrual cycle lengthening becomes apparent only in the last 2 years of cycling. Mean cycle lengths in the last 4 years for healthy U.S. women were 30.48, 35.02, 45.15 and 80.22 days.[177]

Outside the context of fertility prediction, the only reason to diagnose a woman as perimenopausal is to provide her with an understanding of the symptoms she is experiencing. The diagnosis of perimenopause is a clinical one. When she notes changes in her menstrual cycling or experiences vasomotor symptoms, she may be confidently diagnosed as perimenopausal unless other etiologies (such as thyroid disease or medication) can explain her complaints. No one symptom or laboratory test is accurate enough to rule perimenopause in or out.[9] Sex steroid measurements using either serum or salivary specimens are not only unnecessary and costly, but because of the dramatic fluctuations in circulating levels that women experience during those years, may falsely suggest that a woman is menopausal when she is not.

PERIMENOPAUSAL SYMPTOM TREATMENT

Perimenopausal women with persistent or severe vasomotor symptoms can be treated with combined hormonal contraception[10] or with postmenopausal doses of estrogen/progestin treatments, although the latter can worsen the menstrual abnormalities that often accompany perimenopause. If a woman becomes symptomatic during the hormone-free week of combined hormonal contraceptive use, she can try reducing or eliminating the placebo period. Other approaches include combining postmenopausal estrogen therapy with either depot medroxyprogesterone acetate (DMPA) or the levonorgestrel-releasing intrauterine system. Non-hormonal treatment options, such as those discussed below for postmenopausal women, are also helpful for treating symptomatic perimenopausal women.

PERIMENOPAUSAL HEALTH PROMOTION

Most women in their perimenopausal years consider themselves to be in reasonably good health; however, they may need to make significant changes prior to menopause to optimize their health after menopause. Encourage them to adopt or maintain long-term healthy lifestyles. Obesity is a major health problem: 56% of women age 20 to 34 and 75% of those age 35 to 44 are overweight or obese. Obesity in older women is most often due to inadequate exercise and/or overeating. A decrease in ovulatory cycling may make it more challenging for women in their 40s and 50s to lose weight. During the luteal phase, a woman's resting metabolic rate increases. Without that change in metabolism in the second half of the menstrual cycle, caloric intake is stored as fat rather than burned as energy. Promote exercise, not only to contribute to weight control and to improve cardiovascular health, but also to enhance bone remodeling and muscle strength for balance. As many as 70% to 80% of older U.S. women have physical activity levels that are lower than recommended.[11] Screen for signs of stress and depression.

CONTRACEPTIVE OPTIONS FOR PERIMENOPAUSAL WOMEN

Many perimenopausal women need effective contraception. Although women over age 40 have significantly lower baseline fertility than do women in their 20s, an unintended pregnancy at this time in life can be disturbing. In the United States, nearly one-third of pregnancies among women aged 40 or older are electively terminated; this proportion approximates that for adolescents younger than age 14.[12]

The most common method of contraception used by U.S. couples over age 30 is sterilization. For women still at risk for pregnancy, the full range of contraceptive choices is available. Long-term efficacy and convenience are critical features to consider, as are the women's health problems. Remind women who still have menses that menopausal hormone regimens used for hot flash treatment do not prevent ovulation. Provide all at-risk women with emergency contraception (EC). (See Chapter 6 on Emergency Contraception.)

Intrauterine Contraception (IUC). The copper IUD provides convenient and excellent long-term pregnancy protection without hormones. The levonorgestrel intrauterine system (LNG IUS) is a particularly attractive alternative for women in the perimenopause, because the endometrial suppression offered by the LNG IUS prevents erratic, anovulatory perimenopausal bleeding and reduces the risk for endometrial hyperplasia that can present at this time of life.

Combined hormonal contraceptives. When non-contraceptive benefits are factored into the equation, combined hormonal contraceptives (pills, patches, and vaginal rings) may be appropriate and appealing options for healthy, nonsmoking, nonobese perimenopausal women. Used cyclically, combined hormonal methods cause predictable withdrawal bleeding and prevent the endometrial consequences of unopposed endogenous estrogen, such as hyperplasia and endometrial cancer. Combined hormonal contraceptives also stabilize (at least 3 out of every 4 weeks) the woman's hormone levels and reduce her hot flashes. There is also evidence that use of low-dose OCs may slow some of the bone loss characteristic of these years. Extended cycle or continuous use of combined oral contraceptives or vaginal contraceptive rings achieves all of these objectives and eliminates menses, dysmenorrhea, and hormonal fluctuations that occur during the placebo pill week.

In the wake of the Women's Health Initiative (WHI) studies, women are often confused by the apparently conflicting information they hear about hormones. On the one hand, perimenopausal women are being reassured that long-term use of pharmacologic doses of estrogen and progestin in contraceptives does not increase their risk of breast cancer or significantly increase their risk of cardiovascular disease if they are healthy and normotensive. On the other hand, women are told that use of estrogen-progestin therapy (EPT) after the menopause increases the risk of myocardial infarction (MI) in the short run (first year of use) and of breast cancer in the long run. The answer is not the formulation (OCs versus EPT), but it is the woman. Healthy reproductive-aged women are not affected by low-dose OCs because they are already exposed to endogenous hormones. In postmenopausal women, EPT extends the years of hormone exposure and may increase the risk for breast cancer. Previously established atherosclerosis may be destabilized by initiating EPT in older women.

Progestin-only contraceptives. For perimenopausal women who have contraindications to the pharmacologic doses of estrogen found in combined hormonal contraceptives, a progestin-only contraceptive, such as the levonorgestrel-releasing intrauterine system (LNG-IUS), progestin-only pills, or progestin injections (DMPA), can be used for contraception. Menopausal treatment doses of estrogen may be added to DMPA to reduce losses in bone mineralization and to help control hot flashes as well as to reduce breakthrough bleeding induced by DMPA. This combination may also be continued through the early menopausal years until it is reasonably likely that the woman is no longer at risk for pregnancy. Estrogen should not be combined with progestin-only pills for contraception because the estrogen may soften the cervical mucus and permit sperm entry into the upper genital track.

Barrier methods. Barrier methods may be an appropriate choice for a woman who is willing to accept a lower efficacy rate, especially considering that her baseline pregnancy risk is low. Condoms can be combined with other methods if she is at risk for sexually transmitted infections (STIs).

Sterilization. Female sterilization of perimenopausal women is feasible but costly. It also subjects women to operative risks generally for only a few years of contraceptive protection. Male sterilization may be a more appropriate option.

MENOPAUSE

Menopause means permanent cessation of menses following or in association with loss of ovarian follicular activity. Menopause can be diagnosed in women in the following circumstances:

- Women who have had surgical removal of their ovaries

- Women with intact ovaries who have been amenorrheic for 1 year with no other cause

- Women who had a hysterectomy with ovarian preservation when ovarian estradiol production has decreased to a menopausal level

After menopause, women are no longer at risk for pregnancy since they have no more recruitable follicles, but this lack of follicles also results in decreased ovarian production of estrogen. The median age of menopause is 51.3 years. Approximately 1% of women undergo menopause before age 40; at the other extreme, 2% of women are still not menopausal at age 55. Menopause before age 30 can be associated with chromosomal abnormalities (e.g., gonadal dysgenesis), so a genetic evaluation is appropriate in this situation.[13] *Premature menopause* (< 40 years old) and *early menopause* (< 45 years old) are strongly influenced by family history,[14] but otherwise, the age of menopause does not follow a clear familial pattern and is generally not predictable. Women who smoke, have type-1 diabetes, live at high altitudes, or are undernourished or vegetarian undergo menopause at younger ages than do women without these risk factors. Premature menopause is a risk factor for significant medical problems, including osteoporosis and cardiovascular disease, and can be a personal tragedy for a woman who has not yet completed her desired childbearing.

DIAGNOSIS OF MENOPAUSE

There are no blood tests to diagnose menopause early and reliably enough to guarantee a woman that she is no longer at risk for pregnancy.[15,178] As a recent editorial said, "No test for menopause exists, and clinicians should stop acting as if one does."[179]

During the perimenopausal years (STRAW Stages -3 to 0), day-to-day fluctuations of both gonadotropins and hormones can be quite extreme:[16] FSH levels can temporarily crest to very high levels, and estradiol (E_2) levels can plunge into the menopausal range. There is no need to measure FSH or luteinizing hormone (LH) levels to test for menopause in a woman with hot flashes who is still menstruating; her cycling verifies that she still has ovarian steroidogenesis (she is not menopausal) and her symptoms classify her as perimenopausal. At best, tests of gonadotropins could confirm her premenopausal state; at worst, they could confuse the picture and put her at risk for unintended pregnancy with a false diagnosis of menopause. In some situations, it may be helpful to determine her thyroid stimulating hormone (TSH) level, and to rule out other causes of menstrual disorder. For the same reason, hormone tests also are not reliable indicators of when to discontinue hormonal contraceptive methods that may mask the symptoms of menopause. Fortunately, the diagnosis of menopause need not be made precisely. Some experts recommend that healthy women continue to use hormonal contraceptives until age 53 to 55, when the likelihood of pregnancy is very slight.[10] The only clinical reasons to make the diagnosis is to provide women reassurance that they are no longer at risk for pregnancy and to know if any vaginal bleeding should be characterized as "postmenopausal bleeding", which would require evaluation.

The diagnosis of menopause is made when a patient has been amenorrheic for 12 months with no other etiology. However, it is not necessary to wait for 1 year of amenorrhea to initiate treatment for symptomatic women. The women who chose not to use hormonal contraception should not be required to suffer hot flashes and related symptoms or to undergo accelerated loss of bone mineralization for 12 months to formally diagnose menopause before any therapy is initiated. It is quite feasible to provide symptomatic women who have had less than a year of amenorrhea with postmenopausal hormonal treatments or other therapies listed below, along with the advice that they continue to use nonhormonal contraception until the diagnosis of menopause is secure.

HEALTH RISKS IN THE MENOPAUSE

Most women over age 50 are not well informed about their long-term health risks. In a telephone survey of U.S. women, 34% reported that breast cancer is the greatest health problem confronting women, while less than 8% reported that cardiovascular disease or stroke was a major concern.[17] Cardiovascular disease caused 34% of all deaths in women over age 65 in 1999, whereas breast cancer accounted for only 4%.[18]

In fact, at every age after 55, more women die of heart disease than of any other cause. The distortion in women's perceptions of their real health hazards can be dangerous. Health care provider recommendations for smoking cessation, exercise promotion, and dietary changes may be ignored because they have no impact on the woman's breast cancer susceptibility and because they may require profound, and often challenging, lifestyle modifications. On the other hand, women may be reluctant to use EPT even in the short term, because they harbor an inflated estimate of their baseline risk of developing breast cancer. Inform women of their true health risks, design appropriate interventions, and make referrals as needed.

Because cardiovascular disease (CVD) is such an enormous health problem,[19] it is important to identify risk factors for CVD, including diabetes, hypertension, dyslipidemia, smoking, obesity, and a family history of CVD. Diabetic women enter menopause with the same probabilities for heart attack and stroke as similarly aged men and should be treated a *priori* as if they have coronary artery disease (CAD).[19]

Many women have risk factors for CVD. In the United States, 25% of women are sedentary, 20% smoke, 52% over age 45 have hypertension, and 40% over age 55 have elevated cholesterol.[17] Guidelines have been published for estimating the 10-year risk of CAD in women and for controlling those risks.[20,21] For example, blood pressure control is critical in forestalling premature myocardial infarction (MI) and stroke; the upper limit for normal blood pressures in healthy women is now 120 mm Hg systolic and 80 mm Hg diastolic. Statins have been shown to improve life expectancy in women with dyslipidemia. For every 2-point drop in low-density lipoprotein (LDL) cholesterol, the risk of heart attack in men decreases by 1%. The data for women appear to be similarly impressive.

Women at high risk for breast cancer ($\geq$ 1.7% risk of developing breast carcinoma in the next 5 years) may wish to use chemoprophylaxis with appropriate selective estrogen receptor modulators (SERMs), such as tamoxifen or raloxifene, or to enroll in trials testing aromatase-inhibiting agents. Osteoporotic women and osteopenic women with risks factors can combine exercise, calcium, and Vitamin D with prescription therapies to reduce their risk of future fracture.

The most important therapeutic recommendation for menopausal women to help them improve both the quantity and the quality of their remaining years is to adopt healthy lifestyles. Smokers should be provided realistic estimates of the effects that their smoking will have on their health. All women should avoid second-hand smoke exposure. Overweight women need to learn the impact that their excess pounds may have on their risk for CVD diabetes and cancer. Controlled weight and avoidance of visceral obesity contribute greatly to reducing a woman's risk for fatal and non-fatal MI. Similarly, women should be told that exercise could improve their quality of life. Women who exercise have an extended CVD-free life and a reduced risk of respiratory disease.[22] However, providers must recognize that almost 1 out of every 5 women age 40 to 55 reports some limitation in physical functioning (e.g., hypertension, arthritis, cancer, obesity, stress, or poverty)[23] and should tailor individual health promotion programs to meet the individual constraints of their patients.

POSTMENOPAUSAL SYMPTOMS

Surveys show that most women have positive or neutral feeling about the menopause.[24] Because women age as they move into menopause, it is difficult to assess which symptoms are due to ovarian senescence, to aging or to life changes commonly occurring in midlife. However, the most common clinical symptom of the "menopausal syndrome" is the hot flash, but many symptomatic women report being troubled by fatigue, moodiness, depression, difficulty sleeping, decreased libido and orgasmic response, anxiety, changes in memory and cognition, weight gain, joint pain, scalp hair loss, hair growth or acne on face, skin changes, palpations, nausea, headaches, and urinary tract infections. Hot flashes may occur because without estrogen, there is a constriction in the thermoregulatory zone in symptomatic women, making them need to radiate off heat at lower temperatures than other women.

Hot flashes affect 68% to 90% of recently menopausal women in the United States;[25] these flashes can be quite uncomfortable and embarrassing. During a flash, women radiate heat from all parts of their bodies; toe temperatures have been observed to increase by up to 7 degrees Fahrenheit.[26] At night, the flashes can disrupt a woman's normal sleep cycle. Even if a woman is not completely awakened, the quality of her sleep may be diminished by hot flashes. Studies with laboratory polysonographs have not always supported this observation. Some have reported no decrease in sleep quality between postmenopausal women and premenopausal women or between symptomatic women and asymptomatic women, although the postmenopausal women reported increased dissatisfaction with their sleep.[27,28] The 2005 NIH State-of-the-Science Conference Statement concluded that there is moderate evidence that menopause is the cause of sleep disturbances in some women, but it is unclear whether difficulty sleeping is due solely to vasomotor symptoms.[29] Chronic sleep deprivation has been linked to mood disturbances, irritability, anxiety, and tearfulness.[30,31] The prevalence of mood symptoms in premenopause is 8–37%; in the perimenopause 11–21%, and in postmenopause (natural or surgical) 8–38%.[29] Sleep disruptions also can significantly reduce a woman's ability to concentrate and remember. In one study of reproductive-aged women who were tested prior to bilateral oophorectomy and again 2 months postoperatively, those given placebo demonstrated significantly decreased scores in immediate and delayed recall of paired association compared to those given hormonal therapies, who retained their abilities in those areas.[32] The biological plausibility of this functional impairment is supported by perfusion studies, which clearly demonstrate significantly reduced blood flow to the brain during the 20 to 30 minutes that each hot flash lasts.[33]

THERAPEUTIC APPROACHES TO CONTROLLING VASOMOTOR SYMPTOMS

Today many women prefer to try to control their vasomotor symptoms with non-hormonal approaches. There are many possible interventions, including lifestyle management, some herbal therapies, non-hormone prescription drugs, and estrogen or estrogen/progestin therapies and other hormonal therapies. Many of these approaches can be combined, if necessary, to achieve adequate symptomatic relief. Unfortunately, several therapies continue to be extensively advertised to women even though appropriately controlled trials have shown that they offer no more relief than placebo pills. It should be noted that placebo treatments for vasomotor symptoms have very strong effects; a 30% to 60% reduction in hot flash frequency and a 10% to 30% reduction in severity has been reported in placebo arms of several studies. For this reason, it is not appropriate to endorse or prescribe any therapy that has not proven itself superior to placebo in independent clinical trials, even if the mechanism of action sounds appealing or the testimonials offered are persuasive.

Lifestyle Measures for Hot Flashes

The following recommendations should be offered to symptomatic women:

- Smoking cessation reduces hot flashes and is imperative for good overall health.

- A woman may notice that certain things (such as spicy foods, computer screens, or chocolate) spark her symptoms. Have her avoid those triggers.

- Layered clothing may help. Removing a jacket during a hot flash may reduce heat discomfort, and the jacket can be put back on if a post-flash chill occurs.

- Control room temperature and, more importantly, humidity. This helps some women reduce discomfort during hot flashes.

- Relaxation techniques and self-hypnosis reduce the number hot flashes by up to 50%.[34,35]

- Exercise may not alter the frequency or intensity of hot flashes, but it improves sleep quality (and cardiac and bone health).

Over-the-Counter Agents for Hot Flashes

Nearly 1 out of every 3 Americans uses complementary therapies. In the United States, annual expenditures for such treatments total $5 billion to $6 billion each year. Although few clinical studies exist, data are becoming more available about the effectiveness of these treatments.[36,37] The following over-the-counter therapies have been evaluated in clinical trials that included placebo arms. However, little information is available about possible adverse effects or long-term risks of any of these therapies. These agents are not tested for content, purity or safety. Black cohosh and soy products have estrogenic effects and should be used with extreme caution in women with contraindications to estrogen.

- *Soy isoflavones.* Phytoestrogens are derived from soy, garbanzo beans, and legumes. The active ingredients in many isoflavones are genistein and daidzein. Early studies found short-term reduction in hot flash frequency with isoflavones of 45%,[38,39] although a long-term study showed a return of symptoms on therapy after 12 weeks of use.[40,43] One randomized trial with 100 mg of soy isoflavones taken daily for 4 months showed a statistically significant improvement above the placebo arm,[41] but other studies with 72 mg and 114 mg did not show improvement.[42,43] A meta-analysis found early strong reduction in hot flashes that decreased over time but still remained more effective than placebo.[44] If plant proteins are substituted for animal proteins, there can be a beneficial effect on lipid profiles, but soy protein that is added to regular diets do not show beneficial effects.[45] In addition, if soy supplements are used, the woman must be advised to significantly decrease her routine dietary intake to accommodate the soy calories. Modest intake of soy supplements throughout the day is better than a larger single dose.[46]

- *Red clover isoflavones.* Two placebo-controlled studies of 40 mg/d of red clover isoflavones showed a 54% to 75% reduction of hot flashes vs. a 30% reduction with placebo, but two other placebo-controlled studies showed no effect above that provided by placebo.[47–49] A meta-analysis of all six studies found no statistically significant difference compared to placebo.[44]

- *Black cohosh* (20 to 40 mg/day). One large study reported a reduction in "menopausal symptoms" in 80% of women by 4 weeks of treatment. Five other studies reported improvements in symptoms but did not include placebo controls. Some placebo-controlled studies suggested that black cohosh was more effective, but more recent studies question that finding.[50,51] In one study, an isopropanolic extract of black cohosh root 40 mg per day decreased hot flashes more than placebo especially in newly menopausal women; although the frequency of hot flashes was not reported.[52] The German Commission E recommends limiting use of black cohosh to 6 months because that is the extent of the longest study they evaluated. Caution has been raised about adverse effects of black cohosh on the liver, but impurities in the preparations may have been responsible.[53] In combination with St. John's Wort, black cohosh reduced hot flashes by 53% vs. 24%.[180]

Non-hormonal Prescription Drug and Acupuncture Therapies for Control of Vasomotor Symptoms

- *Clonidine.* Applying one patch (0.05 to 0.1 mg) each week reduced hot flashes by 46% in one clinical trial, but 40% of women discontinued clonidine because of side effects such as dizziness and dry mouth.[54] As with other alpha adrenogenic agonists (lofexidine and methyldopa) that alter neurotransmitters in the hypothalamus to regulate the neuroregulatory center, clonidine reduces hot flashes about 20% to 65%,[55–57] but appears to be most effective in women with tamoxifen induced hot flashes.[44] Clonidine is particularly attractive for women with hypertension requiring medical intervention, because clonidine may be used to help both control hypertension and hot flashes. Clonidine raises the sweating threshold in symptomatic, but not asymptomatic, postmenopausal women.[58]

- *Selective serotonin reuptake inhibitors (SSRIs).* Venlafaxine 37.5 to 75 mg daily, paroxetine 10 to 20 mg daily, or fluoxetine 20 mg daily, have demonstrated significantly larger reductions in hot flashes than placebo in small scale studies.[59–61] Using venlafaxine 37.5 mg daily for one week followed by 75 mg per day, 46% of women had greater than a 50% reduction in their hot flashes compared to baseline.[62] Paroxetine 10 mg daily reduced hot flash frequency and severity scores by 40.6% and 45.6% compared to 13.7% responses for the placebo. Women also reported subjective improvements in sleep. At higher doses, paroxetine 20 mg daily reduced both scores by over 50%, but the placebo effect also doubled to over 26%.[63] These study outcomes were impressive because the SSRIs were often given to breast cancer survivors using tamoxifen and, therefore, experiencing severe vasomotor symptoms. The SSRIs are particularly useful as first line therapy for menopausal women who have significant mood disorders associated with their vasomotor symptoms. However, women should be counseled that 2% to 23% of SSRI users experience sexual dysfunction.

- *Bellergal-S.* This is a combination of belladonna alkaloids, ergotamine tartrate, and phenobarbital. As an "autonomic system stabilizer," Bellergal-S inhibits the sympathetic-parasympathetic pathway. Early studies showed a 66% reduction in menopausal symptoms with Bellergal-S compared to a 24% reduction with placebos.[64] A more recent study showed that all benefits were seen at 2 and 4 weeks of treatment, but that by 8 weeks, there was no difference in the frequency of hot flashes experienced by women using Bellergal and placebos.[65] Bellergal often sedates, which may be helpful if it is used only at night. There is some potential for addiction. Bellergal should *not* be prescribed to women with hypertension, because it continues to be a potent vasoconstrictor (ergotamine).

- *Gabapentin.* In one small study, gabapentin 900 mg reduced hot flashes by 45% compared with a 29% placebo effect.[66] In a later study, more than 400 women with two or more hot flashes were randomly assigned to placebo, gabapentin 300 mg daily, or gabapentin 300 mg 3 times a day. At 8 weeks, the placebo group had a 15% reduction in hot flash severity scores whereas the high-dose gabapentin groups experienced a 46% reduction in these hot flash severity scores.[67] Higher doses of gabapentin (2400 mg/d) relieved hot flashes as well as estrogen but use was associated with significantly more side effects.[181] Gabapentin has been associated with anorgasmia.

- *Soy Prescription* capsules (60 g of soy protein) taken daily reduced hot flashes 45% vs. a 30% placebo effect.[68] These capsules are not available in the United States.

- Accupuncture significantly reduced the severity but not the frequency of nocturnal hot flashes when compared to placebo.[182]

Hormonal Prescription Therapies for Control of Vasomotor Symptoms

Estrogen-containing Therapies

The most effective therapy currently available for hot flashes is *hormonal therapy (HT)—estrogen therapy (ET)* for hysterectomized women and *estrogen-progestin therapy (EPT)* for women with an intact uterus. Well-designed, randomized, prospective, placebo-controlled, cross-over trials comparing estrogen treatment to placebo indicate the following:[69–72]

- Estrogen shows a significantly greater clinical effect than placebo for treatment of hot flashes. Depending upon the dose used, ET and EPT reduced hot flash frequency by 80% to 96% compared to a 50% reduction observed with placebo use.

- HT may have a relatively slow onset of action. Decreases in hot flash intensity and frequency can be observed within 1 week of HT initiation, but the maximal effect is generally not achieved for at least 1 month of use. Do not rush to increase HT doses in the short term, unless the woman experiences no improvement.

- An abrupt discontinuation in estrogen-containing treatments can cause in a return of symptoms. Often, within 1 to 3 months, a rebound occurs in which the woman experiences more frequent hot flashes than she had prior to starting therapy.

New studies have found that EPT and ET with 50% to 75% of the doses previously considered "conventional" can reduce hot flash frequency and severity almost as well as the conventional doses.[72] Given these results, it would be prudent to start with the lowest dose and increase the dose only if needed. For women using older conventional doses, consider lowering their doses slowly over time. There is no arbitrary limit to the number of years a woman may use hormone therapy to control bothersome symptoms as long as the overall benefits of ET/EPT use outweigh its health risks. For more on health risks, read the following section on impacts of hormone therapies on other aspects of postmenopausal health.

Tibolone. This compound, with estrogenic, progestogenic, and androgenic properties, has been used by an estimated 8 million menopausal women worldwide for treating vasomotor symptoms, sexual dysfunction and osteoporosis over the last 20 years.[73] A comparative trial of tibolone 2.5 mg versus conjugated equine estrogen 0.625/MPA 5 mg found that tibolone users had less vaginal bleeding during cycles 4 to 6, and much less breast tenderness. Hot flash control was better with HT. Both therapies improved quality of life. Tibolone does not cause withdrawal bleeding when used in women with at least 1 year of amenorrhea.[29] Tibolone was not approved by the FDA for use in the United States.

Androgens (with estrogen). Preparations with low-dose estrogen plus androgen may provide more relief than low-dose estrogen alone.[74] Some small studies with estrogen and androgen showed that the combination reduced lack of concentration, depressive moods, and fatigue more than did estrogen alone,[75] and found positive effects for improving libido.[29] Androgens reduce sex hormone binding globulin (SHBG) and may alter lipids or increase acne and hirsutism.

Bioidentical (and "natural") hormones. Treatments with compounded mixtures of a variety of sex steroids (estrone, estradiol, estriol, DHEA, progesterone, pregnenolone, testosterone) with composition and doses based on the patient's salivary concentration or empirically on clinical response to initial doses have little data to support their benefits or to counsel about short- or long-term adverse events, because they are not FDA tested or regulated.

Non-estrogen Containing Hormonal Prescription Therapies for Control of Vasomotor Symptoms

Other hormones used without estrogen may be helpful in treating women with hot flashes.

- **Progestin compounds.** Depot medroxyprogesterone acetate (DMPA) 150 mg IM or MPA 10 mg daily led to an 85% to 87% reduction in hot flashes in postmenopausal women. Side effects can include mastalgia, mood changes, bloating, and weight gain. Few women can sustain these doses of MPA for long-term use. Micronized progestin, off-label, has also been recognized to reduce hot flashes.

- **Megestrol acetate.** One study showed that 74% of women had ≥ 50% reduction in hot flashes compared to 20% of women who used placebo.[76]

Treatments with No Evidence of Efficacy in Treatment of Hot Flashes

Women may be attracted to claims made by over-the-counter therapies. Advise women that there is no scientific evidence that any of these agents will help them better than sugar pills.

- **Evening primrose oil.** One randomized, double-blinded 6-month clinical trial showed no significant benefit.[77] In addition, the agent causes gas and bloating and may increase the activity of anticoagulants.

- **Chasteberry.** No clinical studies have been conducted in menopausal women.

- **Dong quai.** One double-blinded placebo-controlled study using 4.5 g dong quai root as monotherapy showed no difference from placebo.[78] It may increase bleeding in patients using warfarin.

- **Ginseng.** One randomized, double-blinded, placebo-controlled study of Ginsana (200 mg) for 16 weeks found no significant improvement in 3 out of 3 quality-of-life scales.[79] Ginseng may improve mood and sleep, but it does not appear to reduce hot flashes.[29]

- **Vitamin E.** A 4-week trial found no difference in hot flashes in women using 800 IU compared to placebo.[80,81]

- **Kava.** Kava has been shown to be effective in reducing anxiety, but there is no evidence that it is effective in reducing hot flashes. Kava has been associated with liver damage and the FDA has issued a warning about potential harm.[29]

GENITOURINARY ATROPHY

With time, most postmenopausal women who do not use estrogen-containing therapies will develop genitourinary atrophy. This is a particularly true of postmenopausal women who do not have sexual intercourse. The vagina, the trigone of the bladder, and the urethra have the highest concentrations of estrogen receptors in the body. Atrophy of the cervix can be responsible for mild Pap smear abnormalities such as ASC-US.

Vagina. The most common problems that result from urogenital atrophy are dyspareunia and vaginal infections and atrophy. Women with low estrogen levels (especially those who do not engage in vaginal intercourse) experience a thinning of the vaginal epithelium. As its rugations flatten, the vagina becomes considerably less elastic. There is breakdown of the collagen, smooth muscle and elastin in the vagina. The underlying local vessels and lymphatic supply disappear, resulting in decreased transudation during sexual arousal.[82] Vaginal dryness is reported as a frequent sexual problem by 44% of postmenopausal women compared to 14% of premenopausal women.[83] Vaginal atrophy is an important issue today as the male partners of postmenopausal women are being successfully treated for erectile dysfunction; the women may not be physically prepared for coitus. Water-soluble and silicone-based lubricants can provide coital lubrication but do not increase tissue elasticity. However, tissue elasticity and thickening generally is evident within 6 weeks of initiating therapy with topical estrogens such as creams, suppositories, and rings. There is some systemic absorption of the estrogen, although serum levels resulting from intravaginal therapies are significantly lower than those associated with oral or transdermal HT agents. More prolonged treatment (up to 12 months) may be required to restore underlying vascular and lymphatic structures, which provide coital lubrication. Oral estrogen therapies are also beneficial for urogenital symptoms, but the results of studies are mixed concerning the effectiveness of transdermal estradiol.[29] Atrophy of the vagina also decreases natural vaginal defenses against infection. Vaginal fluid loses its protective acidity; the rise in vaginal pH (pH = 6.5–7.5) results from the loss of glycogen in the vaginal epithelium transudate. Glycogen is needed to support lactobacillus in the vaginal ecosystem. Studies have shown that estrogen creams placed on the outer third of the vagina minimizes endometrial stimulation.[84] However, in women who have a uterus, there is a possibility that long term use of unopposed estrogen in the vagina may induce endometrial hyperplasia. Many experts recommend that these estrogen therapies be supplemented by periodic progestin challenges, especially in women with other risk factors for endometrial carcinoma.

Urinary tract. After menopause, bladder infections also increase. Constriction of the estrogen-sensitive vaginal tissues causes the urethral meatus to rotate downward, closer to the vagina. Estrogen may effectively treat resultant irritative urinary symptoms, such as frequency and urgency, and reduce the risk of recurrent urinary tract infections.[85]

Dysuria in postmenopausal women can be due to the increased incidence of cystitis, to the thinned tissue surrounding the urethral tissue, or to the development of urethral caruncles. Caruncles form when tissues surrounding the urethral meatus contract and evert the distal portion of the urethral tissue externally. This creates a red, tender, fleshy halo surrounding the meatus. The caruncle tissue may not sufficiently epithelialized to tolerate external exposure and can be easily irritated, although many women with caruncles are asymptomatic. Topical estrogen cream can reverse these changes in symptomatic women.

Pelvic Relaxation.   Earlier investigators hypothesized that problems such as cystoceles, rectoceles, and uterine prolapse might be caused or worsened by lack of estrogen. Similarly, since genuine stress incontinence tends to worsen after menopause, low estrogen levels were blamed for this problem. Today, however, we recognize that estrogen deficiency does not cause these problems. Postmenopausal hormone therapy does not cure incontinence,[86] and may even increase the risk.[87]

However, topical estrogen is often used in conjunction with other therapies to treat the *consequences* of pelvic relaxation. For example, a cystocele that protrudes from the vagina can become easily eroded as it rubs against the labia when a woman walks. Locally applied estrogen can help thicken the affected epithelium and reduce erosion. Estrogen used with vaginal pessaries can also reduce the incidence of friction erosions in the vault. Finally, pre-treatment of the vagina with local estrogen is used to improve the outcome of postmenopausal incontinence surgery.

OSTEOPENIA, OSTEOPOROSIS AND FRACTURE

In the 5 to 6 years following a woman's last menses, she loses her bone mineral density (BMD) at the fastest rate in her life. Each year, a recently menopausal woman loses up to 4% to 8% of her trabecular BMD and 1% to 2% of her cortical BMD. The rate of bone loss slows over time. However, unless measures are taken, most women are at risk for becoming osteopenic or even osteoporotic if they live long enough. Lifetime bone loss is about 35% of cortical bone and 50% of trabecular bone.[88] According to the NHANES III study, over half of women in the United States over age 50 had osteoporosis or osteopenia.[89] The prevalence of low bone mineralization varies by ethnicity. African-American women have the lowest rates of osteopenia and osteoporosis (28% and 8%), while non-Hispanic white women have the highest rates (42% and 17%), and Mexican-American women are intermediate (37% and 13%).

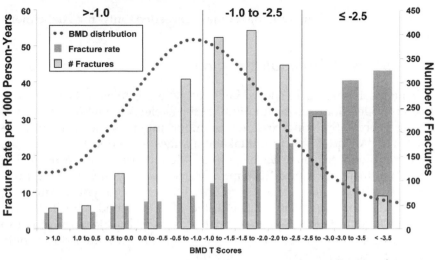

Source: Siris ES et al. (2005).[91]

Figure 26–2 National osteoporosis risk assessment: fracture rates, population T score distribution, and number of fractures

Low BMD puts a woman at a higher risk for bone fracture. Approximately one-third to one-half of women will have at least one osteoporotic fracture during their lifetimes.[90] Every standard deviation in bone mineral density below normal is associated with more than a doubling of the risk of fracture. However, because there are significantly more women with osteopenia than with osteoporosis, more fractures occur in women with osteopenia (see Figure 26–2).[91] The most common fractures among women under 65 are wrist or forearm fractures, which usually result when women extend their arms to try to break their falls. Later in life, women frequently experience spontaneous vertebral crush fractures, which not only create painful spinal deformities, but also result in the loss of mobility, loss of height, and increases in respiratory problems as well as abdominal protrusion which causes dyspepsia. The average American woman loses more than 1 inch of height after menopause; each inch represents 2.5 vertebral fractures.

The most serious fracture site is the hip. Women with osteopenia have a doubled risk for hip fracture compared to women with normal BMD, and women with osteoporosis have a nearly 9-fold increased risk.[91] A 70-year-old woman who suffers a hip fracture faces an 8% to 18% increase in her baseline risk of dying during the 6 months following fracture. One year after the hip fracture, only 50% of the survivors that age are completely healed; 25% are dependent on family members for care, and the remaining 25% are living in nursing homes. Older women have even worse outcomes. Hip fracture is the second most common reason older women are placed in nursing homes, exceeded only by Alzheimer's disease.

Osteoporosis Prevention Measures

Bone health measures should begin early in life. Weight-bearing exercise in moderation is critical to initiate the skeletal modeling and remodeling process. Smoking cessation is important, as is moderation in alcohol use. Adequate calcium intake at all ages is needed to provide the building blocks to construct new bone. Menopausal women not using hormonal therapy require 1,200 mg of calcium a day; those taking postmenopausal hormone therapy need only 1,000 mg. The typical American diet is deficient in calcium. (See Table 26–1 for food sources.) Most women require daily supplements, which should be taken with food to maximize absorption. Calcium should be taken in divided doses; only 500 or 600 mg can be absorbed at any time.

Adequate vitamin D can be obtained from 10 to 15 minutes of sun exposure 2 to 3 times per week. However, because of extensive use of sunscreen for skin cancer prevention, vitamin D deficiencies are now widespread. People who live above latitude 52°, where the ultraviolet B radiation is filtered by the earth's atmosphere in the winter months, require vitamin D supplementation with 400 to 800 IU/day from at least October to March. Elderly women and women who are housebound or unable to synthesize vitamin D may routinely need vitamin D supplementation. Smoking worsens the state of vitamin D in postmenopausal women.[93] Studies show that even in Miami, many reproductive-aged women had vitamin D deficiency at the end of winter. One placebo-controlled, British trial in which people age 15 to 85 were mailed 100,000 IU Vitamin D every 4 months for 5 years showed a 22% overall reduction in all fracture risk and a 33% lower rate for fracture of the hip, wrist or forearm, or vertebra compared to placebo users.[94] The WHI study of calcium 1,000 mg with vitamin D3 400 IU daily found that bone density increased in the treatment group compared to placebo users. The women who took the study medication had a reduced risk of hip fracture (RR=0.71; 0.52–0.97), but there was no statistically consistent reduction of fracture at other sites. The risk of renal calculi increased by 17% (95% CI=1.02–1.34).[95]

Offer prophylactic measures to all menopausal women, even women who enter menopause with robust bone. Therapies to prevent osteoporosis are most effective when initiated early in menopause, because the goal is to preserve the maximum bone density and strength to prevent later fractures.[96,97] In addition to recommending adequate intake of calcium and vitamin D and smoking cessation, encourage exercise to increase muscle strength, balance, and bone architecture. To help prevent older women from falling, recommend home safety improvements such

Table 26–1 Dietary sources of calcium

Food	Serving	Calcium (mg)	% DV
Cheddar cheese, shredded	1.5 oz.	306	31%
Milk, nonfat	8 fl oz.	302	30%
Yogurt, plain, low fat	8 oz.	300	30%
Milk, reduced fat (2% milk fat)	8 fl oz.	297	30%
Milk, whole (3.25% milk fat)	8 fl oz.	291	29%
Cottage cheese, 1% milk fat	2 cups	276	28%
Mozzarella, part skin	1.5 oz.	275	28%
Tofu, firm, with calcium	1.5 cups	275	28%
Orange juice, calcium fortified	6 fl oz.	200 260	20 26%
Salmon, pink, canned, solids with bone	3 oz.	181	18%
Tofu, soft, with calcium	0.5 cups	138	14%
Frozen yogurt, vanilla, soft serve	0.5 cup	103	10%
Turnip greens, boiled	0.5 cup	99	10%
Kale, cooked	1 cup	94	9%
Ice cream, vanilla	0.5 cup	85	8.5%
Soy beverage, calcium fortified	8 fl oz.	80–500	8–50%
Chinese cabbage, raw	1 cup	74	7%
Tortilla, corn, ready to bake/fry	1 medium	42	4%
Sour cream, reduced fat, cultured	2 tbsp.	32	3%
Broccoli, raw	0.5 cup	21	2%
Cream cheese, regular	1 tbsp.	12	1%

Source: Surgeon General's Report (2004).[92]

as removing loose rugs, rerouting wiring out of their pathways, installing lights over all stairways, and ensuring that porches, tubs and showers, and stairways have guardrails. Recommend vision correction. If possible, avoid prescribing treatments that create problems such as hypotension or dizziness. The role of hip protectors is questionable but may be important in certain clinical situations. Home safety guides are offered in English, Spanish, and Chinese at www.cdc.gov/ncipc/duip/preventadultfalls.htm.

Osteoporosis Screening

There is no clear consensus about screening recommendations for osteoporosis. The National Osteoporosis Foundation (NOF) recommends screening all Caucasian women over age 65, women who have experienced at least one atraumatic fracture, and post-menopausal women with other risk factors (see Table 26–2).[98] Few data are available for other groups of women. Medical conditions (Table 26–3) and medications (Table 26–4) can contribute to osteoporosis. More extensive lists of risk factors have been recommended and are slightly superior to the NOF list in predicting bone mineral loss.[99] However, regardless of the list of risk factors used, only half of women with osteoporosis will be identified on the basis of risk factors.[100]

Table 26–2 National Osteoporosis Foundation (NOF) Risk factors for osteoporosis and related fractures in Caucasian postmenopausal women

Major Risk Factors
- Personal history of fracture as an adult
- History of fragility fracture in a first-degree relative
- Low body weight (< 127 lbs)
- Current smoking
- Use of oral corticosteroid therapy for more than 3 months

Additional Risk Factors
- Impaired vision
- Estrogen deficiency at an early age (< 45 yrs)
- Dementia
- Poor health/frailty
- Recent falls
- Low calcium intake (lifelong)
- Low physical activity
- Alcohol in amounts > 2 drinks per day

Table 26–3 Medical conditions that may be associated with an increased risk of osteoporosis

AIDS/HIV	hypogonadism	rheumatoid arthritis
amyloidosis	primary and secondary	severe liver disease
ankylosing spondylitis	amenorrhea	biliary cirrhosis (especially
chronic obstructive	hypophosphatasia	primary)
pulmonary disease	idiopathic scoliosis	spinal cord transsection
congenital porphyria	inadequate diet	sprue
Cushing's syndrome	inflammatory bowel disease	stroke (CVA)
eating disorders (e.g.	insulin-dependent diabetes	thalassemia
anorexia nervosa)	mellitus	thyrotoxicosis
female athlete triad	lymphoma and leukemia	tumor secretion of parathyroid
gastrectomy	malabsorption syndromes	hormone-related peptide
Gaucher's disease	mastocytosis	weight loss
hemochromatosis	multiple myeloma	
hemophilia	multiple sclerosis	
hyperparathyroidism	pernicious anemia	

Table 26–4 Drugs that may be associated with reduced bone mass in adults

aluminum	gonadotropin-releasing	thyroxine (long-acting
anticonvulsants	hormone agonists	supraphysiologic doses)
(phenobarbital, phenytoin)	immunosuppressants	tamoxifen (premenopausal use)
cytotoxic drugs	lithium	total parenteral nutrition
glucocorticosteroids and	heparin (long-term use)	
adrenocorticotropins	DMPA	

Source: Physician's Guide to Prevention and Treatment of Osteoporosis (2003).[98]

There are only a few imaging studies that are effective in screening for bone mineral density. Dual-energy X-ray absorptiometry (DEXA) is the most specific and sensitive screening approach. Ultrasound scans of the calcaneus also play a role in screening of women who are not at high risk.[101] Women found to have osteopenia or osteoporosis on ultrasound should be referred for DEXA scans to confirm of their diagnoses. CT scans are more accurate than DEXA but are too expensive to use in mass screening. X-ray films are not sensitive enough to detect early signs of bone loss. Generally a woman must lose 40% of her BMD for X-rays to detect bone thinning.

The DEXA T score compares a woman's BMD to the average BMD of healthy women in their peak years of BMD (usually 30 year olds). If a postmenopausal woman's T score is between 1 and 2.5 standard deviations below normal (-1 to -2.5), she has *osteopenia*. If her T score is more than 2.5 standard deviations below normal (less than -2.5), she has *osteoporosis*. The T score is intended for use in post-menopausal women, it is not appropriate for testing young women who have not yet achieved their maximal BMD.

On the other hand, the DEXA Z score compares a given woman's BMD to the BMD of her age-matched controls. A low Z score requires a work-up for acute (secondary) bone loss (e.g. hyperparathyroidism, Paget's disease, etc.). A normal Z score should not be reassuring to a postmenopausal woman, it only means that she has lost as much bone as other women her age, not that she has healthy bone.

Medical Therapies for Osteopenia/Osteoporosis

The medications listed in Table 26–5 have proven effective in preserving bone mineral density. There is no consensus about when to initiate such therapy to prevent fractures. Different organizations advocate different thresholds of BMD and recognize different risk factors. The WHO is currently revamping its treatment guidelines. Age and other risk factors are expected to play important roles in the new guidelines in deciding if and when therapy should be started. The therapies for treatment of osteopenia include estrogen; those for the treatment of osteoporosis do not. The US Preventive Services Task Force found that good evi-

Table 26–5 Drug therapies for osteoporosis prevention

Drug for prophylaxis
• Estrogens with or without progestin
• Alendronate (daily or once-a-week)
• Risedronate (off label use) (once-a-week)
• Ibandronate (once a month)
• Raloxifene daily

dence that the use of combined estrogen and progestin results in reduced risk for fractures.[102] The National Osteoporosis Foundation (NOF) recommends treatment for postmenopausal women with no risk factors whose T scores are below −2.0 and for post-menopausal women with one or more risk factors with T scores below −1.5,[98] as well as for post-menopausal women with vertebral or hip fracture, regardless of their T scores. Treatment is also indicated for steroid-induced osteoporosis in women of any age. Estrogens, bisphosphonates, and SERMs have been clearly shown to reduce fractures. All three work as anti-resorptive agents: they slow the activity of the osteoclast cells, which break down old stressed bone.

Hormone therapies.   In the WHI, 5 years of *estrogen* therapy, with or without progestins, reduced the risk of vertebral fractures by 50% to 80% and reduced the incidence of non-vertebral fracture by 25%. What is particularly significant about the WHI findings was that it is the only prospective study ever conducted that was able to show a reduction in the risk of fracture in the general population. All other agents have been tested in populations with established osteopenia or osteoporosis or prior fractures. In other studies, 10 years of EPT reduced hip fracture rates by nearly 75%.[103] Although one analysis found that the EPT impact on fracture was greatest in women under age 60, the WHI, which had a mean entry age of 63 years, demonstrated a 39% reduction in hip fractures with EPT[104] and ET.[105] Most clinical trials of postmenopausal hormonal therapies for osteoporosis prevention have been oral therapies using relatively higher doses of formulations, such as 0.625 mg of conjugated equine estrogen. The NIH, the FDA and the WHI Writing Group concluded that estrogen should be used for postmenopausal osteoporosis prevention for women at significant risk of osteoporosis and for whom non-estrogen medications are not considered appropriate. However, since that time, the FDA has approved a small estrogen patch whose only clinical application is the prevention of osteoporosis. Intriguingly, serum levels of estradiol with this product may be raised only minimally (7 to 9 pg/mL), and therefore remain well within the post menopausal range, but distinct improvement is seen in BMD. Oral products with only

0.3 mg conjugated equine estrogen have also been found to prevent loss of BMD.

Tibolone also is an effective antiresorptive agent. In 2-year trials, tibolone 2.5 mg daily increased mean BMD from baseline in the lumbar spine, total hip, and femoral neck compared to the placebo arm, which lost BMD at each of these sites.[106] Tibolone is not available in the United States.

Bisphosphonates. *Alendronate* is a bisphosphonate, which prevents vertebral and non-vertebral (including hip) fractures in women with established osteoporosis or osteopenia. It is generally taken once per week. Risedronate is a newer bisphosphonate that has proven to be effective in reducing both vertebral and non-vertebral fractures in osteoporotic postmenopausal women.[107] Ibandronate is available as a once-a-month oral therapy and is available by injection once every 3 months. All three bisphosphonates reduce vertebral fractures by over 40% and non vertebral fractures by 40% to 50% in three-year clinical trials. Safety and efficacy of alendronate have been shown for up to 10 years of use. Alendronate has been demonstrated to reduce hip fractures.[108] After 7 years of alendronate use, discontinuation for up to 1 year did not result in any loss of BMD. *Risedronate* 5 mg daily reduced radiographically detected vertebral fractures in osteoporotic postmenopausal women by 45% in 3 years.[109] One study showed that risedronate 2.5 or 5 mg daily reduced hip fractures in elderly women with osteoporosis by 40% in 3 years.[110] Another study showed a trend toward improvement in joint structure and symptoms in patients with primary knee osteoarthritis.[111] *Ibandronate* given 2.5 mg a day reduced vertebral fractures in osteoporotic women by 52% in 3 years of treatment. Monthly dosing appeared to have equal efficacy compared to daily dosing in a 1-year study.[112] Ibandronate prevents both vertebral and "non-vertebral" fractures significantly. In a comparison trial between alendronate and risedronate, the effect on BMD was greater with the former treatment, but the study was not intended to test for fracture reduction (both groups had similar fracture reduction).[113] In a recent review of 368 cases of non-healing lesions of the jaw, 95% of the women were receiving both intravenous biphosphonates and chemotherapy. Fewer than 20 cases have been reported with oral biphosphonates.[183]

Other treatments. The SERM, *raloxifene*, increases BMD, decreases bone turnover, and reduces vertebral fracture rates by 49% in 4 years of use by osteopenic women without inducing any increase in the risk of endometrial cancer as had been seen with other SERMs.[114] Although hip BMD measurements improve with its use, raloxifin does not reduce hip fracture rates.[115,116]

Androgens added to estrogen not only decrease osteoclast activity (decreasing bone reabsorption), but they also stimulate osteoblast activity to promote more bone mineralization. Therapy with testosterone alone increased bone strength and resistance to mechanical stress as well as increasing BMD. DHEA 50 mg daily increased total and lumbar spine BMD.[117] Calcitonin, parathyroid hormone, and zoledronic acid and pamidronate infusions are used only for the treatment, not prevention, of osteoporosis.[118]

EFFECT OF HORMONE THERAPIES ON OTHER ASPECTS OF POSTMENOPAUSAL HEALTH

MOOD DISORDERS

Many women (especially those with hot flashes) complain of difficulties with sleep around the time of menopause[119] even though formal sleep studies show that sleep length and architecture are not adversely affected by menopause.[27,28] Recognizing that the issue here is one of perception of sleep quality, it is interesting that a randomized controlled trial (RCT) found that women on ET reported significant improvement in sleep and fewer awakenings; they also reported feeling less tired the next day.[120] Women both with and without hot flashes reported significant improvement in sleep quality with hormonal therapy. In the WHI, symptomatic women were found to have a small but significant improvement in their perceived sleep quality for the first 3 years of study on EPT.[121] Women who suffer hot flashes in the menopausal period may develop depressive symptoms that cause significant morbidity, even though they may not be due to clinical depression. In one RCT, ET lowered depression symptom scores more than placebo and also lowered menopausal-related symptoms.[122] In another study, EPT given to reduce vasomotor symptoms improved mood, as measured by the Kupperman Index, more than did placebo.[70] As outlined above, another approach to treating women with menopausal mood disorders due to estrogen deficiency is to use SSRIs, which will directly address their depressive symptoms and reduce vasomotor symptoms.

Testosterone patches (300 mg) have been shown to improve the sense of well being and sexual pleasure (libido, sexual activity and orgasm) of hypoandrogenic, oophorectomized women.[123] The North American Menopause Society concludes that postmenopausal women with decreased sexual desire associated with personal distress and not other identifiable causes may be candidates for testosterone therapy.[124] Testosterone patches were not approved by the FDA in recent hearings because of potential adverse effects.

Table 26–6 Women's Health Initiative (WHI) results

	EPT		ET	
	Hazard Ratio	**95% CI**	**Hazard Ratio**	**95% CI**
CHD	1.29	1.02–1.63	0.91	0.75–1.12
Stroke	1.31*	1.02–1.68*	1.39	1.10–1.77
Thrombosis	2.11	1.58–2.82	1.33	0.99–1.79
DVT	2.07	1.44–2.87	1.47	1.08–2.08
PE	2.13	1.39–3.25	1.34	0.87–2.06
Invasive breast cancer	1.26†	1.00–1.59†	0.77	0.59–1.01
Colorectal cancer	0.63	0.43–0.92	1.08	0.75–1.53
Hip fractures	0.66	0.45–0.96	0.61	0.41–0.91
Vertebra fractures	0.66	0.44–0.96	0.62	0.42–0.93
Total mortality	0.90	0.02–1.18	1.04	0.88–1.22

* Estimate updated Wassertheil Smoller S, et al (2003).[125]

† No increase in risk was seen in women who had never used HT prior to study enrollment

Modified from: Rossouw JE (2002),[104] WHI Study Group (2004).[108]

PREVENTION OF CHRONIC CONDITIONS

The US Preventive Services Task Force (USPSTF) found that the use of estrogen and the use of combined estrogen and progestin results in both benefits and harms, and it recommends against the routine use of combined estrogen and progestin for the prevention of chronic conditions in postmenopausal women (grade D recommendation).[102] The Task Force concluded that a shared decision-making approach to preventing chronic disease in perimenopausal and postmenopausal women involves "consideration of individual risk factors and preferences in selecting effective interventions for reducing the risk for fracture, heart disease and cancer". The USPSTF did not evaluate the use of hormone therapy for the management of menopausal symptoms.[102]

The WHI studied the impact of postmenopausal hormone therapy on many different health outcomes, beyond the traditional labeled indications. It was designed to answer questions about the efficacy and safety of HT, especially used in older women not experiencing hot flashes. The findings of both the EPT and ET arms are summarized in Table 26–6. It should be noted that the mortality rates in both treatment arms were the same as those in the placebo arm. See the following discussions for more details.

Colorectal Cancer

Colon cancer is the third leading cause of cancer deaths in U.S. women. Screening with 3 fecal occult blood samples annually and colonoscopy every 5 to 10 years is important for early detection. High-risk women may need more frequent tests. The Nurses Study suggested that current users of hormone therapy had a statistically significant reduction in the risk of colorectal cancer and large adenoma development.[126] In the WHI, EPT users had a hazard ratio of 0.63 (0.43 – 0.92) for developing colorectal carcinoma but there was no reduction in mortality from colorectal carcinoma. ET users had no protection.[104]

Cognition

Cognition requires multiple mental processes, including attention, perception, working memory, executive function, learning, and memory. Over time, the function of each of these processes is affected by natural aging, disease, drugs, sleep deprivation, and hormonal changes. Dementia is a significant decline in memory accompanied by a decline in at least one other cognitive domain (aphasia, apraxia, agnosia, or disruption in the ability to abstract) that is significant enough to interfere with occupational or social functioning.[127]

Postmenopausal women given estrogen in prospective nonrandomized trials had better regional perfusion to the hippocampus and performed better on memory tests.[128,129] On the other hand, reproductive-aged women who had estrogen production halted by treatment with leuprolide acetate depot for 3 months had significant declines in their verbal memory functioning; this decline was reversed when estrogen was added to the GnRH agonist.[130] The effect of ET on older women is more complex. When estrogen was given to women with Alzheimer's Disease (AD), it did not slow the progression of the disease.[131,132] In older women (mean age 72) tested at baseline and 6 years later, those who were past users of hormone therapy had less decline in scores over time, but current users experienced the same declines as never users.[133]

A prospective study done in Cache County, Utah, similarly showed that women who had previously used hormone therapy for 10 years had the lowest risk of developing AD, but current hormone therapy users, even women who had used hormone therapy for more than a decade, showed no protection against AD.[134]

In the largest RCT to date, the Women's Health Initiative Memory Studies (WHIMS), women who used HT over age 65 had a doubling of their risk of developing probable dementia. However, all the statistically significant increased risk was confined to women over age 75.[135] This finding verified that starting EPT in elderly women increases the risk of all-cause dementia, especially vascular dementia. In a parallel study, WHIMS showed that EPT given to women over age 65 did not improve global cognitive function as measured by the Modified Mini Mental Status Exam (MMMSE). In fact, twice as many EPT users as placebo users suffered a significant decline (> 2 standard deviations) in their scores.[136] However, there was no evidence that EPT increased the risk of developing mild cognitive impairment. At this time, we can make the following conclusions:

1. Providing EPT to older (over 75 years) women increases their risk of developing dementia.

2. There is no evidence of any improvement in global cognitive function in older (over 65 years) women started on EPT and some suggestion of adverse effects.

3. Younger women should not take EPT to reduce their risk of developing dementia, but there is no evidence that EPT taken early in menopause increases their risk of developing AD later in life.

During the clinical RCT of fracture rates in women treated for 3 years with raloxifene or placebo, the cognitive test scores of participants were studied in a secondary analysis. The raloxifene group tended to have a lower risk of decline on tests of attention and verbal delayed recall although overall scores of cognition were not different.[137]

Risks and Side Effects of Postmenopausal Hormonal Therapy

There has been discussion about the appropriateness of the population studied in the WHI (mostly older women) and about the applicability of the results of the WHI to younger populations of healthier women.[138,139] Younger women in the WHI had a far different response to hormones than older women.[140] How should the results of WHI be interpreted since only one strength of one estrogen and one estrogen/progestin compound, one route of administration, and one dose was studied? Should the results be applied to lower doses of the same compounds, to different estrogens, to different progestins, and to different routes of administration (e.g., topical gels or transdermal products)? The FDA and WHI have decided that the answers to this question must be yes—unless a product can demonstrate that it is different from the study drugs. The WHI cost over $750 million, so it is unlikely that any company will be able to fund a similarly scaled project to demonstrate that it is substantially different from these studied drug compounds. Providers need to be familiar with the age and health status of the WHI participants to understand how to apply the study results to the individual patients they are caring for. Insight from other studies is also provided in the following sections.

Cardiovascular Effects of Postmenopausal Hormone Therapies

After decades of observational study data demonstrated that ET and EPT use reduced risk of MI, the results of the randomized clinical trials showing an increase in risk of MI during the first 12 to 18 months of EPT use were initially quite surprising.[104] However, subsequent interpretation of the WHI data have suggested that estrogen given to women with established atherosclerosis may initially disrupt pre-existing athersclerotic plaque and increase the risk of arterial occlusion. This was suggested by the fact that it was only in the first year of use that the EPT group had any statistically higher rates of coronary heart disease than the placebo group.[141] All women appeared to be at increased risk for MI with EPT use, but women with elevated LDL-cholesterol were at even higher risk.[141]

Most of the intermediate biomarkers and risk factors for cardiovascular disease improved more with EPT than with placebo. For example, women assigned to EPT had greater reduction in total cholesterol, LDL cholesterol, glucose, and insulin levels and greater increases in the high-density lipoprotein (HDL) cholesterol than did women in the placebo group.[141] This is compatible with the observation that longer term use of ET/EPT by healthy women might reduce the risk of cardiovascular disease, as has been reported by earlier observational studies.

Women studied in the estrogen-only arm of WHI demonstrated *no* increase in the risk of cardiovascular events or mortality, even though this study followed women for 6.8 years. The hazard ratio for CHD showed a slight protective effect (0.91), but it was not statistically significant because the confidence interval crossed 1 (0.75–1.12).[105] In younger ET users (age 50 to 59), there was a suggestion of lower CHD risk.[142] However, because CHD is relatively uncommon in women in their mid-fifties, it would be necessary to treat 1,000 women to prevent one heart attack.[184] A more detailed analysis of these data show a tendency for more cardiovascular protection when younger menopausal women were given ET.[142] However, the numbers of cases were small. Therefore, the NIH, the FDA, the USPSTF, the American Heart Association, and other leading organizations have all advised that clinicians not suggest to patients that using either ET or EPT reduces a woman's risk of CVD.

VTE and Stroke Risk with Postmenopausal Hormone Therapy

The risk of stroke with HT use increased progressively with the duration of use. Over the complete study periods, EPT users had 31% more risk of stroke than non-users, and ET users had a hazard ratio of 1.39 (CI 1.10–1.77).[125] EPT-associated thromboembolic events (deep vein thrombosis and pulmonary embolus) were in the range anticipated from previous studies (RR 2.11). Interestingly, ET use was associated with no statistically significant increased risk in such thromboembolic events (RR=1.32, 95% CI=.99–1.75[185]). Given this observation, it is difficult to suggest that transdermal delivery systems would be associated with fewer venous thromboembolic (VTE) events until a comparative trial can be conducted or larger epidemiologic studies are performed.

Uterine Cancer with Postmenopausal Hormone Therapy

For women with intact uteri, using estrogen *without* progestin significantly increases the risk for endometrial hyperplasia and cancer. In the 3-year PEPI study, women randomized to receive only estradiol were more likely to develop simple, complex, or atypical hyperplasia, compared to women receiving estradiol and micronized progestin.[143] Metaanalysis of long-term epidemiologic studies has found a relative risk of 2.3 (95% CI 2.1 -2.5), about 1 additional woman in 1,000, for endometrial cancer in women with uteri who use ET without progestin.[144] Women who have undergone endometrial ablation are also at risk, because there remain isolated islands of residual endometrial tissue. The increased risk for endometrial cancer can be reduced to baseline if the estrogen is supplemented with cyclic[145] or continuous progestin.[146]

The WHI found no increase in risk for uterine cancer with up to 5 years of EPT use compared to use of placebo.[147] Progestin can be given cyclically (at least 12 to 14 days per month), continuously (with daily estrogen), in a pulsed pattern (combined with estrogen for 3 days, then removed for 3 days),[148] or by an independent route (progestin-releasing IUS). Less frequent dosing of progestin (such as every 3 to 4 months) may not provide the same protective effect on the endometrium as do the more conventional therapies. For example, one study found that women who had withdrawal periods only quarterly had a 1.5% rate of hyperplasia compared to a baseline rate of 0.9%.[149]

Breast Cancer—Risk, Assessment, Prophylaxis and Effects of Postmenopausal Hormone Therapy

Breast cancer is the second most common cancer that occurs in postmenopausal women (after skin cancer) and the second most frequent cause of cancer deaths (after lung cancer). A Caucasian women's risk for developing breast cancer increases every year she lives until she is age 80; her lifetime risk will approach 12.5%. Risks are somewhat lower among African American women. Heavier-set women are at highest risk; the risk increases 3% for every point increase in a woman's BMI.[150]

Risk Assessment and Prophylactic Treatment

Calculate each individual woman's risk for developing breast cancer. In most cases, use the Gail model (available at www.cancer.

gov/bcrisktool/) to estimate the patient's 5-year and lifetime risks. The Gail model is not appropriate for estimating risk in high-risk women or unscreened women because it will underestimate the risk in those groups.

Discuss chemoprophylaxis with high-risk women. Tamoxifen 20 mg per day for 5 years reduced the risk of developing breast cancer by 49% in women with a 5-year risk greater than 1.66%.[151] Prophylaxis with this agent is most appropriate in premenopausal women who are less likely to be at risk for endometrial cancer or venous thromboembolism. The International Breast Cancer Intervention Study (IBIS) raised concerns about prophylaxis in older women if it is used in those women therapy should be stopped 30 days before any major surgery or other immobilization.[152] Raloxifene may be more appropriate to use in older women.[153] Aromatase inhibitors are clearly superior to tamoxifen in preventing a second primary breast cancer in women who have had one episode of breast cancer,[154] but the safety and efficacy of this class of agents in primary prophylaxis has not been established.

Hormone Exposure and Risk of Breast Cancer

Many factors link development of breast cancer to sex steroids. Factors that reduce a woman's lifetime exposure to hormones reduce her risk for breast cancer: early menopause, bilateral oophorectomy, and the use of antiestrogens (tamoxifen or raloxifen). Women who undergo early menarche or late menopause are at higher than average risk for developing breast cancer, as are women with the higher body mass indices. Hormone exposure may act indirectly by increasing cell proliferation or by increasing the chances that a mutant cell line might emerge. It is, therefore, not surprising that continuing a woman's exposure to estrogen and progestin for longer periods of time into the postmenopausal years might increase her risk of breast cancer.

In the WHI study, long-term use (> 5 years) of estrogen with progestins increased a woman's risk of developing invasive breast cancer but not ductal carcinoma in situ (DCIS).[155] In the WHI, EPT users with diagnosed breast cancer were more likely to have more advanced (i.e., regional or metastatic) and larger (1.7 cm vs 1.5 cm) cancers than women using placebo (25.4% vs 16.0%). The observational Million Women Study (England) reported that even a few months of EPT use increased the risk of developing breast cancer as well as dying from breast cancer.[156] Several studies suggest that EPT use, particularly continuous EPT use, blocks the natural decrease in breast density that occurs in the early years of menopause or may even increase density in older women, both of which diminish mammographic sensitivity. The WHI also found that EPT users were more likely to have abnormal mammograms than women taking placebo, thus requiring more follow-up.[155]

The estrogen-only arm of the WHI found that even longer exposure (6.8 years) to CEE was *not* associated with any increase in breast cancer risk. In fact the hazard rate was 0.8, but the confidence interval included 1 (0.62–1.04), so no protection was claimed.[155]

Advise patients considering the use of EPT (note that ET users do not have any of these concerns) that the WHI showed that:

- Short-term use of EPT has not been shown to increase the risk of breast cancer.[157] Only use for more than 5 years has been associated with an increased risk. Estrogen alone does not increase risk for up to 6–8 years of use.

- The absolute risk a woman faces when using EPT depends upon her baseline risk. The 8 excess invasive cancers per 10,000 women per year reported in the WHI reflect the older age of women in that study (63.2 years old on average). Over the same period of use, fewer 50-year-old women would get breast cancer as a result of EPT use because their background risk is lower.

There is no long-term increase in breast cancer risk among former EPT users. Women return rapidly to their baseline risk. In long-term clinical trials, the increase in breast cancer risk induced by EPT had disappeared within 2 to 4 years after the hormone was stopped. Mammographic density returns to baseline within 2 to 4 weeks of stopping EPT.[158] Periodic vacations from EPT prior to mammography may be helpful in maintaining the sensitivity of the screening for women using EPT.

Although early short-term studies of women given EPT after breast cancer did not show any increased risk in the development of a second breast cancer,[159–161] a large prospective study had to be cancelled because the recurrence rates were higher in cancer survivors using hormones.[162] Therefore, use caution when considering ET/EPT for women with a prior history of breast cancer.[163]

In contrast to the increase in mammographic density seen with the use of EPT in menopausal women, tibolone had the same neutral effect on breast images as did the placebo.[164] However, the Million Woman Study found that there was an increased risk of breast cancer associated with tibolone use, which was larger than that seen with ET or EPT.

Other Health Risks of Postmenopausal Hormone Therapy

The current use of hormones increases the risk of gallbladder disease by 2 to 3 times. One observational study indicated an increased risk of ovarian cancer in EPT users compared to non-users,[165] but the WHI has reported no statistically significant increase (RR 1.58; CI 0.77–3.24).[147] After 10 years of EPT use, there might be a light increase in ovarian cancer risk.[184]

SIDE EFFECTS OF POSTMENOPAUSAL HORMONE THERAPY

IRREGULAR SPOTTING AND BLEEDING

Most menopausal women who begin cyclic HT experience regular withdrawal bleeding, which most find undesirable.[166] Combined continuous formulations of hormone treatments were designed to reduce this bothersome event. However, over one-third of women using continuous HT at conventional doses experienced breakthrough bleeding during the first 3 to 12 months. Lower dose HT achieves cumulative amenorrhea faster than the older conventional doses.[167]

OTHER SIDE EFFECTS

Breast tenderness is a common side effect of ET and EPT. Introduce hormones slowly (e.g., one-half dose every 3 days, then increasing frequency of use, and then increasing doses) to reduce this side effect. Generally, mastalgia resolves, but some women may benefit from significantly lower-dose therapy or may need weekend "holidays" to control their breast symptoms. Some women experience nausea; taking estrogen transdermally may help. Headaches, bloating, and fatigue are other issues that can arise in hormone users. Try changing doses, formulations, or route of administration.

CONTRAINDICATIONS TO POSTMENOPAUSAL HORMONE THERAPY

Product labeling lists the following conditions as contraindications to menopausal estrogen treatment:

- Pregnancy
- Unexplained vaginal bleeding
- Active liver disease; chronic, impaired liver function
- Active thrombophlebitis or thromboembolic disorder
- Carcinoma of the breast
- Known or suspected estrogen-dependent neoplasia

Cautions (relative contraindications) to hormone treatment include seizure disorder, hypertension, familial hyperlipidemia, migraine headache, and gallbladder disease. The risk estrogen may pose for a woman with a history of thrombosis is unknown, but will generally preclude her use of ET/EPT. Although a history of estrogen-dependent cancer is listed as a contraindication to estrogen treatment, it is unknown whether EPT use increases a woman's risk for recurrence of endometrial cancer after she has been successfully treated. The risk of squamous cell cervical carcinoma recurrence is believed to be unaffected by postmenopausal hormone therapy. Little is known about the impact on women with a prior history of ovarian cancer.[168] ET could aggravate endometriosis or cause growth of uterine leiomyomata, but in practice, these effects are not commonly clinically significant.

POSTMENOPAUSAL HORMONE THERAPY CHOICES

There is a growing array of products used to provide postmenopausal hormonal therapies—oral, transdermal patches and gels, and intravaginal creams, rings, and suppositories in an impressive array of doses. Oral therapies are most frequently used with different formulations. CEE has been available for over 50 years and was the formulation studied in 0.625 mg daily doses by the WHI. Lower doses of CEE (0.30 mg and 0.45 mg) are now more widely utilized. Estradiol formulations have been available in the United States for decades and have been used even more extensively in Europe. Ethinyl estradiol (EE), the estrogen used in birth control pills, is being used in some combination perimenopausal hormone treatment products.

Both transdermal patches, which provide therapy for 3 to 7 days, and daily applied transdermal gels are available. Transdermal estrogen (estradiol), which avoids first-pass hepatic effects, has been used for more than a decade. Transdermal estradiol patches were found in one study to have less impact on thrombosis.[169] Products containing estrogen (E_1) and estriol (E_3) have been developed, building on the fact that the estrogens are rapidly interconverted, both in the circulation and intracellularly. Compounding pharmacies offer to design specific combinations of the various estrogens for individual women in combinations of two or three of these basic estrogens. However, there is no evidence of either clinical efficacy or safety of these so-called bioidentical products as is routinely required of FDA-approved products, and there is concern that these compounds may be actively promoted for women with known contraindications to ET/EPT.

Topical ET/EPT. Percutaneous estrogen creams and gels are now available for application to various extremities once a day; the slow absorption of estrogen from the reservoir in the skin throughout the day permits control of vasomotor symptoms. Estrogen vaginal cream can be used for treatment of urogenital atrophy—either alone or in combination with systemic hormone therapies. An estradiol-releasing vaginal ring is approved for treating hot flashes as well as urogenital atrophy in hysterectomized women. In the future, estrogen/progestin releasing vaginal rings may be designed for women with intact uteri.

Progesterone.   Progesterone is needed to provide endometrial protection for women with intact uteri, but it also contributes to symptom relief in combination with estrogen or as a sole agent. Oral progestins, such as medroxyprogesterone acetate, have traditionally been used due to their long half-lives. Micronized progesterone can be used daily, orally or vaginally, with a more favorable impact on HDL and glucose tolerance.[170] Some of the progestins from oral contraceptives, such as levonorgestrel, norethindrone, norgestimate, and drospirenone are being used successfully in products for menopause treatment. The levonorgestrel intrauterine system (LNG-IUS) has been used as the progestin source of EPT in postmenopausal women, although this is not an FDA-approved indication and is based on a limited number of small studies.[171] Clinical trials are underway testing the efficacy of percutaneous progestin creams for hot flash control. Compounded progesterone creams have been popularized as sole hormone therapies, with very little scientific testing; the NIH is currently investigating the safety and efficacy of these products in clinical trials.

POSTMENOPAUSAL ANDROGEN THERAPY

Ovarian androgen production slows over the years. A 40-year-old woman has only half the androsteine levels of a 20-year old woman. During the years immediately following menopause, testosterone production varies—a few women have higher levels, most stay relatively stable, and some fall. However, 4 to 5 years into menopause, androgens levels uniformly fall. Much of the early research work on androgens focused on libido. Studies have found that testosterone supplementation often increases sexual fantasies and other measures of libido but has no measurable effect on the frequency of intercourse or orgasm. More recently, however, placebo-controlled studies have shown that androgen treatment may also enhance a woman's sense of well-being and energy as measured by standardized indices.[172] Testosterone is also important for bone preservation. Within the bone, some testosterone is converted to estrogen, which reduces osteoclast activity; testosterone also directly stimulates osteoblasts to rebuild bone. Endogenous testosterone levels are especially likely to be low in oophorectomized women and older menopausal women.[173] Today, only one product is available for testosterone treatment. A matrix transdermal patch for testosterone therapy for postmenopausal women was disapproved by the FDA but may reenter into clinical trials.[174] In prescribing androgens, consider the potential adverse impact on lipids.

Studies of the safety and efficacy of dehydroepiandrosterone (DHEA) and related compounds are also underway. One study found that DHEA replacement in elderly women with very low serum DHEAS levels could reverse age-related changes in fat mass, fat-free mass, and BMD.[175] Unfortunately, DHEA is not subject to FDA regulations, so the potency and purity of any given product is not monitored. However, small clinical studies indicate that the maximum dose of DHEA should be limited to 25 mg/day to minimize adverse effects on lipids.

SUMMARY

Emphasize lifestyle changes in promoting long-term health for all perimenopausal and postmenopausal women. Recommend exercise, weight control, stress management, accident prevention and social connectedness. Women with vasomotor symptoms deserve treatment. Alternatives include some herbal remedies, SSRIs and hormonal therapies. Help the patient make an informed therapeutic choice by weighing the benefits against possible adverse effects and risks. Provide therapy at the lowest dose for the shortest duration of time needed. Other therapy benefits include a reduced risk of osteoporosis and bone fracture. For women with osteoporosis or osteopenia, both SERMs (raloxifene) and bisphosphonates (alendronate, risedronate, ibandronate) provide BMD protection and have variable but a growing body of evidence about fracture protection. Bisphosphonates are more attractive now with more convenient weekly or monthly dosing. Exercise and calcium are also essential for bone health. Vitamin D supplements are also frequently needed.

For women with risk factors for CVD (such as hypertension, diabetes, obesity, hyperlipidemia, or elevated C-reactive protein), directed therapies are most appropriate. Consistent use of antihypertensive agents is challenging, but blood pressure normalization extends years of life. Use of ACE inhibitors in appropriate candidates not only reduces stroke and MI risk, but also protects against renal failure. Statins combined with diet and exercise help reduce cardiovascular events. For diabetic women, good glucose control with diet and oral hypoglycemic agents and/or insulin is the healthiest approach and improves longevity as well as quality of years (delayed onset of blindness, renal failure, etc.).

In a long-term study, dispositional optimism has been shown to be associated with a decreased risk of cardiovascular disease.[176] Mental exercise and social connectedness are key recommendations for the mental activity and psychological health of the patient. Advise all women to keep healthy, get involved, stay alert, and keep in contact with others—sage advice to maintaining long-term vivaciousness and quality of life.

REFERENCES

1. Soules MR, Sherman S, Parrott E, Rebar, Santoro N, Utian W, Woods N. Executive summary: stages of reproductive aging workshop (STRAW). Fertil Steril 2001; 76:874-8.

2. Tietze C. Reproductive span and rate of reproduction among Hutterite women. Fertil Steril 1957;8(1):89–97.
3. van Noord-Zaadstra BM, Looman CW, Alsbach H, Habbema JD, te Velde ER, Karbaat J. Delaying childbearing: effect of age on fecundity and outcome of pregnancy. BMJ 1991;302:1361–5.
4. World Health Organization. Report of a WHO scientific group: Research on the menopause. Geneva: WHO Technical Report Series 670, 1981.
5. Santoro N, Brown JR, Adel T, Skurnick JH. Characterization of reproductive hormonal dynamics in the perimenopause. J Clin Endocrinol Metab 1996;81:1495–1501.
6. Oldenhave A, Jaszmann LJ, Haspels AA, Everaerd WT. Impact of climacteric on well-being. A survey based on 5213 women 39 to 60 years old. Am J Obstet Gynecol 1993;168:772–80.
7. Freedman RR. Menopausal hot flashes. In: Lobo RA, Kelsey J, Marcus R, eds. Menopause: Biology and Pathobiology. San Diego: Academic Press, 2000:219.
8. Hollander LE, Freeman EW, Sammel MD, Berlin JA, Grisso JA, Battistini M. Sleep quality, estradiol levels, and behavioral factors in late reproductive age women. Obstet Gynecol 2001;98:391–7.
9. Bastian LA, Smith CM, Nanda K. Is this woman perimenopausal? JAMA 2003; 289:895–902.
10. Kaunitz AM. Oral contraceptive use in menopause. Am J Obstet Gynecol 2001;185(2 Suppl):S32–7.
11. Buchner DM. Physical activity and quality of life in older adults. JAMA 1997; 277:64–6.
12. Henshaw SK. Unintended pregnancy in the United States. Fam Plann Perspect 1998; 30:24–29, 46.
13. Rebar RW. Premature ovarian failure. In: Lobo RA, Kelsey J, Marcus R, eds. Menopause: Biology and Pathobiology. San Diego: Academic Press, 2000:142.
14. de Bruin JP, Bovenhuis H, van Noord PA, Pearson PL, van Arendonk JA, te Velde ER, Kuurman WW, Dorland M. The role of genetic factors in age at natural menopause. Hum Reprod 2001;16:2014–8.
15. Burger HG, Dudley EC, Hopper JL, Groome N, Guthrie JR, Green A, Dennerstein L. Prospectively measured levels of serum follicle-stimulating hormone, estradiol, and the dimeric inhibins during the menopausal transition in a population-based cohort of women. J Clin Endocrinol Metab 1999;84:4025–30.
16. Santoro N, Brown JR, Adel T, Skurnick JH. Characterization of reproductive hormonal dynamics in the perimenopause. J Clin Endocrinol Metab 1996;81:1495–501.
17. Mosca L, Jones WK, King KB, Ouyang P, Redberg RF, Hill MN. Awareness, perception, and knowledge of heart disease risk and prevention among women in the United States. American Heart Association Women's Heart Disease and Stroke Campaign Task Force. Arch Fam Med 2000;9:506–15.
18. Anderson RN. Deaths: leading causes for 1999. Natl Vital Stat Rep. 2001;49(11):1–87.
19. Centers for Disease Control and Prevention (CDC). Major cardiovascular disease (CVD) during 1997–1999 and major CVD hospital discharge rates in 1997 among women with diabetes-United States. MMWR 2001;50:948–54.
20. Mosca L, Appel LJ, Benjamin EJ, Berra K, Chandra-Strobos N, Fabunmi RP, et al. American Heart Association. Evidence-based guidelines for cardiovascular disease prevention in women. Circulation 2004;109:672–93.
21. Executive Summary of The Third Report of The National Cholesterol Education Program (NCEP) Expert Panel on Detection, Evaluation, And Treatment of High Blood Cholesterol In Adults (Adult Treatment Panel III). JAMA 2001;285:2486–97.
22. Kushi LH, Fee RM, Folsom AR, Mink PJ, Anderson KE, Sellers TA. Physical activity and mortality in postmenopausal women. JAMA 1997;277:1287–92.
23. Pope SK, Sowers MF, Welch GW, Albrecht G. Functional limitations in women at midlife: the role of health conditions, behavioral and environmental factors. Womens Health Issues 2001;11:494–502.

24. Dennerstein L, Smith AM, Morse C, Burger H, Green A, Hopper J, Ryan M. Menopausal symptoms in Australian women. Med J Aust 1993;159:232–6.
25. Tietze C. Reproductive span and rate of reproduction among Hutterite women. Fertil Steril 1957;8(1):89–97.
26. Molnar GW. Body temperatures during menopausal hot flashes. J Appl Physiol 1975; 38:499–503.
27. Young T, Rabago D, Zgierska A, Austin D, Laurel F. Objective and subjective sleep quality in premenopausal, perimenopausal, and postmenopausal women in the Wisconsin Sleep Cohort Study. Sleep 2003;26(6):667–672.
28. Freedman RR. Pathophysiology and treatment of menopausal hot flashes. Semin Reprod Med 2005;23(2):117–125.
29. National Institutes of Health. National Institutes of Health State-of-the-Science Conference statement: management of menopause-related symptoms. Ann Intern Med 2005;142(12 Pt 1):1003–1013.
30. Baker A, Simpson S, Dawson D. Sleep disruption and mood changes associated with menopause. J Psychosom Res 1997;43:359–69.
31. Kronenberg F, Cote LJ, Linkie DM, Dyrenfurth I, Downey JA. Menopausal hot flashes: thermoregulatory, cardiovascular, and circulating catecholamine and LH changes. Maturitas 1984;6:31–43
32. Phillips SM, Sherwin BB. Effects on memory function in surgically menopausal women. Psychoneuroendocrinology 1992;17:485–95.
33. Greene RA. Estrogen and cerebral blood flow: a mechanism to explain the impact of estrogen on the incidence and treatment of Alzheimer's disease. Int J Fertil Womens Med 2000;45:253–7.
34. Freedman RR, Woodward S. Behavioral treatment of menopausal hot flushes: evaluation by ambulatory monitoring. Am J Obstet Gynecol 1992;167:436–9.
35. Wijma K, Melin A, Nedstrand E, Hammar M. Treatment of menopausal symptoms with applied relaxation: a pilot study. J Behav Ther Exp Psychiatry 1997;28:251–61.
36. Taylor M. Alternatives to conventional hormone replacement therapy. Contemp Ob/GYN 1999 May:23–50.
37. Hudson T. Managing perimenopausal symptoms: an integrative medicine approach. The Female Patient 2001;26:33–40.
38. Upmalis DH, Lobo R, Bradley L, Warren M, Cone FL, Lamia CA. Vasomotor symptom relief by soy isoflavone extract tablets in postmenopausal women: a multicenter, double-blind, randomized, placebo-controlled study. Menopause 2000; 7(4):236–42.
39. Brzezinski A, Adlercreutz H, Shaoul R, Rösler A, Shmueli A, Tanos V, and Schenker JG. Short-term effects of phytoestrogen-rich diet on postmenopausal women. Menopause 1997;4:89–94
40. St Germain A, Peterson CT, Robinson JG, Alekel DL. Isoflavone-rich or isoflavonepoor soy protein does not reduce menopausal symptoms during 24 weeks of treatment. Menopause 2001;8:17–26.
41. Han KK, Soares JM Jr, Haidar MA, de Lima GR, Baracat EC. Benefits of soy isoflavone therapeutic regimen on menopausal symptoms. Obstet Gynecol 2002;99:389–94.
42. Penotti M, Fabio E, Modena AB, Rinaldi M, Omodei U, Vigano P. Effect of soy-derived isoflavones on hot flushes, endometrial thickness, and the pulsatility index of the uterine and cerebral arteries. Fertil Steril. 2003;79(5):1112–7.
43. Nikander E, Kilkkinen A, Metsa-Heikkila M, Adlercreutz H, Pietinen P, Tiitinen A, Ylikorkala O. A randomized placebo-controlled crossover trial with phytoestrogens in treatment of menopause in breast cancer patients. Obstet Gynecol. 2003; 101(6):1213–20.
44. Nelson HD, Vesco KK, Haney E, Fu R, Nedrow A, Miller J, Nicolaidis C, Walker M, Humphrey L. Nonhormonal therapies for menopausal hot flashes: systematic review and meta-analysis. JAMA 2006;295(17):2057–2071.

45. Teede HJ, Dalais FS, Kotsopoulos D, Liang YL, Davis S, McGrath BP. Dietary soy has both beneficial and potentially adverse cardiovascular effects: a placebo-controlled study in men and postmenopausal women. J Clin Endocrinol Metab 2001;86:3053–60.

46. Setchell KD, Brown NM, Desai PB, Zimmer-Nechimias L, Wolfe B, Jakate AS, Creutzinger V, Heubi JE. Bioavailability, disposition, and dose-response effects of soy isoflavones when consumed by healthy women at physiologically typical dietary intakes. J Nutr. 2003;133(4):1027–35.

47. Baber R, Templeman C, Morton T, Kelly GE, West L. Randomized, placebo-controlled trial of an isoflavone supplement and menopausal symptoms in women. Climacteric 1999;2:85–92.

48. Knight D, Howes J, Eden J. The effect of Promensil, an isoflavone extract, on menopausal symptoms. Climacteric 1999;2:79–84.

49. Fugh-Berman A, Kronenberg F. Red clover (Trifolium pratense) for menopausal women: current state of knowledge. Menopause 2001;8(5):333–7.

50. Taylor M. Botanicals: medicines and menopause. Clin Obstet Gynecol 2001; 44:853–63.

51. McKenna DJ, Jones K, Humphrey S, Hughes K. Black cohosh: efficacy, safety, and use in clinical and preclinical applications. Altern Ther Health Med 2001;7(3):93–100.

52. Osmers R, Friede M, Liske E, Schnitker J, Freudenstein J, Henneicke-von Zepelin HH. Efficacy and safety of isopropanolic black cohosh extract for climacteric symptoms. Obstet Gynecol 2005;105(5 Pt 1):1074–1083. Erratum in: Obstet Gynecol. 2005 Sep; 106(3):644.

53. Need Note

54. Laufer LR, Erlik Y, Meldrum DR, Judd HL. Effect of clonidine on hot flashes in postmenopausal women. Obstet Gynecol 1982;60:583–6.

55. Clayden JR, Bell JW, Pollard P. Menopausal flushing: double-blind trial of a non-hormonal medication. Br Med J 1974;1(905):409–12.

56. Hammond MG, Hatley L, Talbert LM. J Clin Endocrinol Metab 1984;58:1158–60.

57. Jones KP, Ravnikar V, Schiff I. A preliminary evaluation of the effect of lofexidine on vasomotor flushes in post-menopausal women. Maturitas 1985;7(2):135–9.

58. Freedman RR, Dinsay R. Clonidine raises the sweating threshold in symptomatic but not in asymptomatic postmenopausal women. Fertil Steril 2000;74(1):20–3.

59. Loprinzi CL, Kugler JW, Sloan JA, Mailliard JA, LaVasseur BI, Barton DL, et al. Venlafaxine in management of hot flashes in survivors of breast cancer: a randomised controlled trial. Lancet 2000;356:2059–63.

60. Stearns V, Isaacs C, Rowland J, Crawford J, Ellis MJ, Kramer R, et al. A pilot trial assessing the efficacy of paroxetine hydrochloride (Paxil) in controlling hot flashes in breast cancer survivors. Ann Oncol 2000;11:17–22.

61. Loprinzi CL, Sloan JA, Perez EA, Quella SK, Stella PJ, Mailliard JA, et al. Phase III evaluation of fluoxetine for treatment of hot flashes. J Clin Oncol 2002;20:1578–83.

62. Loprinzi CL, Levitt R, Barton D, Sloan JA, Dakhil SR, Nikcevich DA, et al. Phase III comparison of depomedroxyprogesterone acetate to venlafaxine for managing hot flashes: north central cancer treatment group trial N99C7. J Clin Oncol 2006;Epub

63. Stearns V, Slack R, Greep N, Henry-Tilman R, Osborne M, Bunnell C, et al. Paroxetine is an effective treatment for hot flashes: results from a prospective randomized clinical trial. J Clin Oncol 2005;23:6919–30. Erratum in: J Clin Oncol 2005;23:8549.

64. Lebherz TB, French L. Nonhormonal treatment of the menopausal syndrome. A double-blind evaluation of an autonomic system stabilizer. Obstet Gynecol 1969; 33:795–9.

65. Bergmans MG, Merkus JM, Corbey RS, Schellekens LA, Ubachs JM. Effect of Bellergal Retard on climacteric complaints: a double-blind, placebo-controlled study. Maturitas 1987;9(3):227–34.

66. Guttuso T Jr, Kurlan R, McDermott MP, Kieburtz K. Gabapentin's effects on hot flashes in postmenopausal women: a randomized controlled trial. Obstet Gynecol 2003;101:337–45.

67. Pandya KJ, Morrow GR, Roscoe JA, Zhao H, Hickok JT, Pajon E, Sweeney TJ, Banerjee TK, Flynn PJ. Gabapentin for hot flashes in 420 women with breast cancer: a randomised double-blind placebo-controlled trial. Lancet 2005;366:818–24.

68. Albertazzi P, Pansini F, Bonaccorsi G, Zanotti L, Forini E, De Aloysio D. The effect of dietary soy supplementation on hot flushes. Obstet Gynecol 1998;91:6–11.

69. Coope J, Thomson JM, Poller L. Effects of 'natural oestrogen' replacement therapy on menopausal symptoms and blood clotting. Br Med J 1975;4:139–43.

70. Derman RJ, Dawood MY, Stone S. Quality of life during sequential hormone replacement therapy-a placebo-controlled study. Int J Fertil Menopausal Stud 1995; 40(2):73–8.

71. Greendale GA, Reboussin BA, Hogan P, Barnabei VM, Shumaker S, Johnson S, Barrett-Connor E. Symptom relief and side effects of postmenopausal hormones: results from the Postmenopausal Estrogen/Progestin Interventions Trial. Obstet Gynecol 1998;92:982–8.

72. Utian WH, Shoupe D, Bachmann G, Pinkerton JV, Pickar JH. Relief of vasomotor symptoms and vaginal atrophy with lower doses of conjugated equine estrogens and medroxyprogesterone acetate. Fertil Steril 2001;75:1065–79.

73. Albertazzi P, Di Micco R, Zanardi E. Tibolone: a review. Maturitas. 1998;30:295–305.

74. Simon J, Klaiber E, Wiita B, Bowen A, Yang HM. Differential effects of estrogen-androgen and estrogen-only therapy on vasomotor symptoms, gonadotropin secretion, and endogenous androgen bioavailability in postmenopausal women. Menopause 1999;6:138–46.

75. Sarrel PM. Psychosexual effects of menopause: role of androgens. Am J Obstet Gynecol 1999;180:S319–24.

76. Loprinzi CL, Michalak JC, Quella SK, O'Fallon JR, Hatfield AK, Nelimark RA, et al. Megestrol acetate for the prevention of hot flashes. N Engl J Med 1994;331:347–52.

77. Chenoy R, Hussain S, Tayob Y, O'Brien PM, Moss MY, Morse PF. Effect of oral gamolenic acid from evening primrose oil on menopausal flushing. BMJ 1994; 308(6927):501–3.

78. Hirata JD, Swiersz LM, Zell B, Small R, Ettinger B. Does dong quai have estrogenic effects in postmenopausal women? A double-blind, placebo-controlled trial. Fertil Steril 1997;68:981–6.

79. Wiklund IK, Mattsson LA, Lindgren R, Limoni C. Effects of a standardized ginseng extract on quality of life and physiological parameters in symptomatic postmenopausal women: a double-blind, placebo-controlled trial. Swedish Alternative Medicine Group. Int J Clin Pharmacol Res 1999;19(3):89–99.

80. Emmert DH, Kirchner JT. The role of vitamin E in the prevention of heart disease. Arch Fam Med 1999;8(6):537–42.

81. Barton DL, Loprinzi CL, Quella SK, Sloan JA, Veeder MH, Egner JR, Fidler P, Stella PJ, Swan DK, Vaught NL, Novotny P. Prospective evaluation of vitamin E for hot flashes in breast cancer survivors. J Clin Oncol 1998;16:495–500.

82. Society of Obstetricians and Gynaecologists of Canada. The detection and management of vaginal atrophy. Number 145, May 2004. Int J Gynaecol Obstet 2005; 88:222–8.

83. Rosen RC, Taylor JF, Leiblum SR, Bachmann GA. Prevalence of sexual dysfunction in women: results of a survey study of 329 women in an outpatient gynecological clinic. J Sex Marital Ther 1993;19(3):171–88.

84. Cicinelli E, Di Naro E, De Ziegler D, Matteo M, Morgese S, Galantino P, et al. Placement of the vaginal 17beta-estradiol tablets in the inner or outer one third of the vagina affects the preferential delivery of 17beta-estradiol toward the uterus or periurethral areas, thereby modifying efficacy and endometrial safety. Am J Obstet Gynecol. 2003;189(1):55–8

85. Hextall A, Cardozo L. The role of estrogen supplementation in lower urinary tract dysfunction. Int Urogynecol J Pelvic Floor Dysfunct 2001;12:258–61.

86. Zullo MA, Oliva C, Falconi G, Paparella P, Mancuso S. Efficacy of estrogen therapy in urinary incontinence. A meta-analytic study. Minerva Ginecol 1998;50:199–205.
87. Grodstein F, Lifford K, Resnick NM, Curhan GC. Postmenopausal hormone therapy and risk of developing urinary incontinence. Obstet Gynecol. 2004;103(2):254–60.
88. Riggs BL, Melton LJ 3rd. Involutional osteoporosis. N Engl J Med 1986;314:1676–86.
89. Looker AC, Orwoll ES, Johnston CC Jr, Lindsay RL, Wahner HW, Dunn WL, et al. Prevalence of low femoral bone density in older U.S. adults from NHANES III. J Bone Miner Res 1997;12:1761–8.
90. Jones G, Nguyen T, Sambrook PN, Kelly PJ, Gilbert C, Eisman JA. Symptomatic fracture incidence in elderly men and women: the Dubbo Osteoporosis Epidemiology Study (DOES). Osteoporos Int 1994;4:277–82.
91. Siris ES, Miller PD, Barrett-Connor E, Faulkner KG, Wehren LE, Abbott TA, et al. Identification and fracture outcomes of undiagnosed low bone mineral density in postmenopausal women: results from the National Osteoporosis Risk Assessment. JAMA 2001;286:2815–22.
92. U.S. Department of Health and Human Services. Bone health and osteoporosis: A report of the Surgeon General. Rockville, MD: U.S. Department of Health and Human Services, Office of the Surgeon General, 2004
93. Valimaki MJ, Laitinen KA, Tahtela RK, Hirvonen EJ, Risteli JP. The effects of transdermal estrogen therapy on bone mass and turnover in early postmenopausal smokers: a prospective, controlled study. Am J Obstet Gynecol. 2003;189(5):1213–20
94. Trivedi DP, Doll R, Khaw KT. Effect of four monthly oral vitamin D3 (cholecalciferol) supplementation on fractures and mortality in men and women living in the community: randomised double blind controlled trial. BMJ 2003;326:469.
95. Jackson RD, LaCroix AZ, Gass M, Wallace RB, Robbins J, Lewis CE, et al; Women's Health Initiative Investigators. Calcium plus vitamin D supplementation and the risk of fractures. N Engl J Med 2006;354:669–83.
96. Lindsay R, Cosman F. Estrogen in prevention and treatment of osteoporosis. Ann N Y Acad Sci 1990;592:326–333;discussion 334–45.
97. Torgerson DJ, Bell-Syer SE. Hormone replacement therapy and prevention of nonvertebral fractures: a meta-analysis of randomized trials. JAMA 2001;285:2891–7.
98. Physician's Guide to Prevention and Treatment of Osteoporosis. Washington DC: National Osteoporosis Foundation, 2003. Accessed 3/5/06 at www.nof.org/professionals/clinical/clinical.htm
99. Cadarette SM, Jaglal SB, Murray TM, McIsaac WJ, Joseph L, Brown JP. Evaluation of decision rules for referring women for bone densitometry by dual-energy x-ray absorptiometry. JAMA 2001;286:57–63.
100. Siris ES, Miller PD, Barrett-Connor E, Faulkner KG, Wehren LE, Abbott TA, et al. Identification and fracture outcomes of undiagnosed low bone mineral density in postmenopausal women: results from the National Osteoporosis Risk Assessment. JAMA 2001;286:2815–22.
101. Khaw KT, Reeve J, Luben R, Bingham S, Welch A, Wareham N, Oakes S, Day N. Prediction of total and hip fracture risk in men and women by quantitative ultrasound of the calcaneus: EPIC-Norfolk prospective population study. Lancet. 2004; 363(9404):197–202.
102. U.S. Preventive Services Task Force. Hormone therapy for the prevention of chronic conditions in postmenopausal women: recommendations from the U.S. Preventive Services Task Force. Ann Intern Med 2005;142(10):855–60. Summary for patients in: Ann Intern Med 2005;142(10):I59.
103. Cauley JA, Seeley DG, Ensrud K, Ettinger B, Black D, Cummings SR. Estrogen replacement therapy and fractures in older women. Study of Osteoporotic Fractures Research Group. Ann Intern Med 1995;122:9–16.

104. Rossouw JE, Anderson GL, Prentice RL, LaCroix AZ, Kooperberg C, Stefanick ML, et al. Risks and benefits of estrogen plus progestin in healthy postmenopausal women: principal results from the Women's Health Initiative randomized controlled trial. JAMA 2002;288:321–33.

105. Anderson GL, Limacher M, Assaf AR, Bassford T, Beresford SA, Black H, et al; Women's Health Initiative Steering Committee. Effects of conjugated equine estrogen in postmenopausal women with hysterectomy: the Women's Health Initiative randomized controlled trial. JAMA. 2004;291(14):1701–12.

106. Gallagher JC, Baylink DJ, Freeman R, McClung M. Prevention of bone loss with tibolone in postmenopausal women: results of two randomized, double-blind, placebo-controlled, dose-finding studies. J Clin Endocrinol Metab 2001;86:4717–26.

107. Harris ST, Watts NB, Genant HK, McKeever CD, Hangartner T, Keller M, et al. Effects of risedronate treatment on vertebral and nonvertebral fractures in women with postmenopausal osteoporosis: a randomized controlled trial. Vertebral Efficacy With Risedronate Therapy (VERT) Study Group. JAMA 1999;282:1344–52.

108. Bone HG, Hosking D, Devogelaer JP, Tucci JR, Emkey RD, Tonino RP, et al; Alendronate Phase III Osteoporosis Treatment Study Group. Ten years' experience with alendronate for osteoporosis in postmenopausal women. N Engl J Med 2004;350.1189–99.

109. Adachi JD, Rizzoli R, Boonen S, Li Z, Meredith MP, Chesnut CH 3rd. Vertebral fracture risk reduction with risedronate in post-menopausal women with osteoporosis: a meta-analysis of individual patient data. Aging Clin Exp Res 2005;17:150–6.

110. McClung MR, Geusens P, Miller PD, Zippel H, Bensen WG, Roux C, et al; Hip Intervention Program Study Group. Effect of risedronate on the risk of hip fracture in elderly women. N Engl J Med. 2001 Feb 1;344(5):333–40.

111. Spector TD, Conaghan PG, Buckland-Wright JC, Garnero P, Cline GA, Beary JF, et al. Effect of risedronate on joint structure and symptoms of knee osteoarthritis: results of the BRISK randomized, controlled trial [ISRCTN01928173]. Arthritis Res Ther 2005;7:R625–33.

112. Miller PD, McClung MR, Macovei L, Stakkestad JA, Luckey M, Bonvoisin B, et al. Monthly oral ibandronate therapy in postmenopausal osteoporosis: 1-year results from the MOBILE study. J Bone Miner Res 2005;20:1315–22.

113. Rosen CJ, Hochberg MC, Bonnick SL, McClung M, Miller P, Broy S, et al; Fosamax Actonel Comparison Trial Investigators. Treatment with once-weekly alendronate 70 mg compared with once-weekly risedronate 35 mg in women with postmenopausal osteoporosis: a randomized double-blind study. J Bone Miner Res 2005;20:141–51.

114. Ettinger B, Black DM, Mitlak BH, Knickerbocker RK, Nickelsen T, Genant HK, et al. Reduction of vertebral fracture risk in postmenopausal women with osteoporosis treated with raloxifene: results from a 3-year randomized clinical trial. Multiple Outcomes of Raloxifene Evaluation (MORE) Investigators. JAMA 1999;282(7):637–45.

115. Prestwood KM, Gunness M, Muchmore DB, Lu Y, Wong M, Raisz LG. A comparison of the effects of raloxifene and estrogen on bone in postmenopausal women. J Clin Endocrinol Metab 2000;85:2197–202.

116. Umland EM, Rinaldi C, Parks SM, Boyce EG. The impact of estrogen replacement therapy and raloxifene on osteoporosis, cardiovascular disease, and gynecologic cancers. Ann Pharmacother 1999;33:1315–28.

117. Villareal DT, Holloszy JO, Kohrt WM. Effects of DHEA replacement on bone mineral density and body composition in elderly women and men. Clin Endocrinol (Oxf) 2000;53:561–8.

118. Downs RW Jr, Bell NH, Ettinger MP, Walsh BW, Favus MJ, Mako B, et al. Comparison of alendronate and intranasal calcitonin for treatment of osteoporosis in postmenopausal women. J Clin Endocrinol Metab 2000;85:1783–8.

119. Oldenhave A, Jaszmann LJ, Haspels AA, Everaerd WT. Impact of climacteric on well-being. A survey based on 5213 women 39 to 60 years old. Am J Obstet Gynecol 1993;168(3 Pt 1):772–80.

120. Polo-Kantola P, Erkkola R, Helenius H, Irjala K, Polo O. When does estrogen replacement therapy improve sleep quality? Am J Obstet Gynecol 1998;178(5):1002–9.
121. Hays J, Ockene JK, Brunner RL, Kotchen JM, Manson JE, Patterson RE, et al. Effects of estrogen plus progestin on health-related quality of life. N Engl J Med 2003; 348:1839–54.
122. Soares CN, Almeida OP, Joffe H, Cohen LS. Efficacy of estradiol for the treatment of depressive disorders in perimenopausal women: a double-blind, randomized, placebo-controlled trial. Arch Gen Psychiatry 2001;58(6):529–34.
123. Simon J, Braunstein G, Nachtigall L, Utian W, Katz M, Miller S, Waldbaum A, Bouchard C, Derzko C, Buch A, Rodenberg C, Lucas J, Davis S. Testosterone patch increases sexual activity and desire in surgically menopausal women with hypoactive sexual desire disorder. J Clin Endocrinol Metab 2005;90:5226–33.
124. North American Menopause Society. Estrogen and progestogen use in peri- and postmenopausal women: September 2003 position statement of The North American Menopause Society. Menopause 2003;10:497–506.
125. Wassertheil-Smoller S, Hendrix SL, Limacher M, Heiss G, Kooperberg C, Baird A, et al; WHI Investigators. Effect of estrogen plus progestin on stroke in postmenopausal women: the Women's Health Initiative: a randomized trial. JAMA 2003; 289(20):2673–84.
126. Grodstein F, Martinez ME, Platz EA, Giovannucci E, Colditz GA, Kautzky M, et al. Postmenopausal hormone use and risk for colorectal cancer and adenoma. Ann Intern Med 1998;128:705–12.
127. American Psychiatric Association. Diagnostic and Statistical Manual of Mental Disorders 4th Ed Washington DC APA 1994.
128. Maki PM, Resnick SM. Longitudinal effects of estrogen replacement therapy on PET cerebral blood flow and cognition. Neurobiol Aging 2000;21(2):373–83.
129. Resnick SM, Maki PM, Golski S, Kraut MA, Zonderman AB. Effects of estrogen replacement therapy on PET cerebral blood flow and neuropsychological performance. Horm Behav 1998;34(2):171–82.
130. Sherwin BB, Tulandi T. 'Add-back' estrogen reverses cognitive deficits induced by a gonadotropin-releasing hormone agonist in women with leiomyomata uteri. J Clin Endocrinol Metab 1996;81(7):2545–9.
131. Henderson VW, Paganini-Hill A, Miller BL, Elble RJ, Reyes PF, Shoupe D, et al. Estrogen for Alzheimer's disease in women: randomized, double-blind, placebo-controlled trial. Neurology 2000;54(2):295–301.
132. Mulnard RA, Cotman CW, Kawas C, van Dyck CH, Sano M, Doody R, et al. Estrogen replacement therapy for treatment of mild to moderate Alzheimer disease: a randomized controlled trial. Alzheimer's Disease Cooperative Study. JAMA 2000; 283(8):1007–15.
133. Matthews K, Cauley J, Yaffe K, Zmuda JM. Estrogen replacement therapy and cognitive decline in older community women. J Am Geriatr Soc 1999;47(5):518–23.
134. Zandi PP, Carlson MC, Plassman BL, Welsh-Bohmer KA, Mayer LS, Steffens DC, Breitner JC. Cache County Memory Study Investigators. Hormone replacement therapy and incidence of Alzheimer disease in older women: the Cache County Study. JAMA 2002;288(17):2123–9.
135. Shumaker SA, Legault C, Rapp SR, Thal L, Wallace RB, Ockene JK, et al; WHIMS Investigators. Estrogen plus progestin and the incidence of dementia and mild cognitive impairment in postmenopausal women: the Women's Health Initiative Memory Study: a randomized controlled trial. JAMA 2003;289(20):2651–62.
136. Rapp SR, Espeland MA, Shumaker SA, Henderson VW, Brunner RL, Manson JE, et al; WHIMS Investigators. Effect of estrogen plus progestin on global cognitive function in postmenopausal women: the Women's Health Initiative Memory Study: a randomized controlled trial. JAMA 2003;289(20):2663–72.

137. Yaffe K, Krueger K, Sarkar S, Grady D, Barrett-Connor E, Cox DA, Nickelsen T; Multiple Outcomes of Raloxifene Evaluation Investigators. Cognitive function in postmenopausal women treated with raloxifene. N Engl J Med 2001;344(16):1207–13.

138. Garbe E, Suissa S. Hormone replacement therapy and acute coronary outcomes: methodological issues between randomized and observational studies. Hum Reprod 2004;19:8–13.

139. Ostrzenski A, Ostrzenska KM. WHI clinical trial revisit: imprecise scientific methodology disqualifies the study's outcomes. Am J Obstet Gynecol 2005;193:1599–604; discussion 1605–6.

140. Parker Pope T. In study of women's health, design flaws raise questions. Wall Street Journal. 2006 Feb 28.

141. Manson JE, Hsia J, Johnson KC, Rossouw JE, Assaf AR, Lasser NL, et al; Women's Health Initiative Investigators. Estrogen plus progestin and the risk of coronary heart disease. N Engl J Med 2003;349(6):523–34.

142. Hsia J, Langer RD, Manson JE, Kuller L, Johnson KC, Hendrix SL, et al. Conjugated Equine Estrogens and Coronary Heart Disease: The Women's Health Initiative. Arch Intern Med 2006;166.357–65.

143. PEPI Trial Writing Group. Effects of hormone replacement therapy on endometrial histology in postmenopausal women. The Postmenopausal Estrogen/Progestin Interventions (PEPI) Trial. JAMA 1996;275:370–5.

144. Grady D, Gebretsadik T, Kerlikowske K, Ernster V, Petitti D. Hormone replacement therapy and endometrial cancer risk: a meta-analysis. Obstet Gynecol 1995; 85:304–313.

145. Persson I, Yuen J, Bergkvist L, Schairer C. Cancer incidence and mortality in women receiving estrogen and estrogen-progestin replacement therapy-long-term follow-up of a Swedish cohort. Int J Cancer 1996;67:327–32.

146. Weiderpass E, Adami H-O, Baron JA, Magnusson C, Bergstrom R, Lindgren A, et al. Risk of endometrial cancer following estrogen replacement with and without progestins. J Natl Cancer Inst 1999;91:1131–7.

147. Anderson GL, Judd HL, Kaunitz AM, Barad DH, Beresford SA, Pettinger M, et al; Women's Health Initiative Investigators. Effects of estrogen plus progestin on gynecologic cancers and associated diagnostic procedures: the Women's Health Initiative randomized trial. JAMA 2003;290(13):1739–48.

148. Casper RF. Regulation of estrogen/progestogen receptors in the endometrium. Int J Fertil Menopausal Stud 1996;41:16–21.

149. Ettinger B, Selby J, Citron JT, Vangessel A, Ettinger VM, Hendrickson MR. Cyclic hormone replacement therapy using quarterly progestin. Obstet Gynecol 1994;83(5 Pt 1):693–700.

150. Hankinson SE, Willett WC, Manson JE, Hunter DJ, Colditz GA, Stampfer MJ, et al. Alcohol, height, and adiposity in relation to estrogen and prolactin levels in postmenopausal women. J Natl Cancer Inst 1995;87:1297–302.

151. Fisher B, Costantino JP, Wickerham DL, Redmond CK, Kavanah M, Cronin WM, et al. Tamoxifen for prevention of breast cancer: report of the National Surgical Adjuvant Breast and Bowel Project P-1 Study. J Natl Cancer Inst 1998;90:1371–88.

152. IBIS investigators. First results from the International Breast Cancer Intervention Study (IBIS-I): a randomised prevention trial. Lancet 2002;360:817–824.

153. Vogel VG, Costantino JP, Wickerham DL, Cronin WM, Cecchini RS, Atkins JN, Bevers TB, Fehrenbacher L, Pajon ER Jr, Wade JL 3rd, Robidoux A, Margolese RG, James J, Lippman SM, Runowicz CD, Ganz PA, Reis SE, McCaskill-Stevens W, Ford LG, Jordan VC, Wolmark N; National Surgical Adjuvant Breast and Bowel Project (NSABP). Effects of tamoxifen vs raloxifene on the risk of developing invasive breast cancer and other disease outcomes: the NSABP Study of Tamoxifen and Raloxifene (STAR) P-2 trial. JAMA 2006;295(23):2727–2741.

154. Grana G. Adjuvant aromatase inhibitor therapy for early breast cancer: A review of the most recent data. J Surg Oncol 2006;93(7):585–92.

155. Stefanick ML, Anderson GL, Margolis KL, Hendrix SL, Rodabough RJ, Paskett ED, Lane DS, Hubbell FA, Assaf AR, Sarto GE, Schenken RS, Yasmeen S, Lessin L, Chlebowski RT; WHI Investigators. Effects of conjugated equine estrogens on breast cancer and mammography screening in postmenopausal women with hysterectomy. JAMA 2006;295(14):1647–1657.

156. Beral V; Million Women Study Collaborators. Breast cancer and hormone-replacement therapy in the Million Women Study. Lancet 2003;362(9382):419–27.

157. Li CI, Malone KE, Porter PL, Weiss NS, Tang MT, Cushing-Haugen KL, Daling JR. Relationship between long durations and different regimens of hormone therapy and risk of breast cancer. JAMA 2003;289(24):3254–63.

158. Colacurci N, Fornaro F, De Franciscis P, Mele D, Palermo M, del Vecchio W. Effects of a short-term suspension of hormone replacement therapy on mammographic density. Fertil Steril 2001;76(3):451–5.

159. DiSaia PJ, Grosen EA, Kurosaki T, Gildea M, Cowan B, Anton-Culver H. Hormone replacement therapy in breast cancer survivors: a cohort study. Am J Obstet Gynecol 1996;174:1494–8.

160. O'Meara ES, Rossing MA, Daling JR, Elmore JG, Barlow WE, Weiss NS. Hormone replacement therapy after a diagnosis of breast cancer in relation to recurrence and mortality. J Natl Cancer Inst 2001;93:754–62.

161. Brewster WR, DiSaia PJ, Grosen EA, McGonigle KF, Kuykendall JL, Creasman WT. An experience with estrogen replacement therapy in breast cancer survivors. Int J Fertil Womens Med 1999;44(4):186–92.

162. Holmberg L, Anderson H;HABITS steering and data monitoring committees. HABITS (hormonal replacement therapy after breast cancer-is it safe?), a randomised comparison: trial stopped. Lancet. 2004;363(9407):453–5

163. Chlebowski RT, McTiernan A. Elements of informed consent for hormone replacement therapy in patients with diagnosed breast cancer. J Clin Oncol 1999; 17(1):130–42.

164. Lundstrom E, Christow A, Kersemaekers W, Svane G, Azavedo E, Soderqvist G, et al. Effects of tibolone and continuous combined hormone replacement therapy on mammographic breast density. Am J Obstet Gynecol 2002;186:717–22.

165. Rodriguez C, Patel AV, Calle EE, Jacob EJ, Thun MJ. Estrogen replacement therapy and ovarian cancer mortality in a large prospective study of US women. JAMA 2001; 285:1460–5.

166. den Tonkelaar I, Oddens BJ. Preferred frequency and characteristics of menstrual bleeding in relation to reproductive status, oral contraceptive use, and hormone replacement therapy use. Contraception 1999;59:357–62.

167. Archer DF, Dorin M, Lewis V, Schneider DL, Pickar JH. Effects of lower doses of conjugated equine estrogens and medroxyprogesterone acetate on endometrial bleeding. Fertil Steril 2001;75(6):1080–7.

168. Guidozzi F, Daponte A. Estrogen replacement therapy for ovarian carcinoma survivors: A randomized controlled trial. Cancer 1999;86:1013–8.

169. Scarabin PY, Oger E, Plu-Bureau G. Differential association of oral and transdermal oestrogen-replacement with venous thromboembolism risk. Lancet 2003;362:428–32.

170. The Writing Group for the PEPI Trial. Effects of estrogen or estrogen/progestin regimens on heart disease risk factors in postmenopausal women. The Postmenopausal Estrogen/Progestin Interventions (PEPI) Trial. JAMA 1995;273(3):199–208.

171. Andersson K, Mattsson LA, Rybo G, Stadberg E. Intrauterine release of levonorgestrel—a new way of adding progestogen in hormone replacement therapy. Obstet Gynecol 1992;79:963–7.

172. Shifren JL, Braunstein GD, Simon JA, Casson PR, Buster JE, Redmond GP, et al. Transdermal testosterone treatment in women with impaired sexual function after oophorectomy. N Engl J Med 2000;343:682–8.

173. Simon JA. Safety of estrogen/androgen regimens. J Reprod Med 2001;46:281–90.

174. Mazer NA. Testosterone deficiency in women: etiologies, diagnosis, and emerging treatments. Int J Fertil Womens Med 2002;47(2):77–86.
175. Villareal DT, Holloszy JO, Kohrt WM. Effects of DHEA replacement on bone mineral density and body composition in elderly women and men. Clin Endocrinol (Oxf) 2000;53:561–8.
176. Giltay EJ, Kamphuis MH, Kalmijn S, Zitman FG, Kromhout D. Dispositional optimism and the risk of cardiovascular death: the Zutphen Elderly Study. Arch Intern Med 2006;166:431–6.

LATE REFERENCES

177. Ferrell RJ, Simon JA, Pincus SM, Rodriguez G, O'Connor KA, Holman DJ, Weinstein M. The length of perimenopausal menstrual cycles increases later and to a greater degree than previously reported. Fertil Steril 2006;86(3):619–624.
178. Henrich JB, Hughes JP, Kaufman SC, Brody DJ, Curtin LR. Limitations of follicle-stimulating hormone in assessing menopause status: findings from the National Health and Nutrition Examination Survey (NHANES 1999–2000). Menopause 2006; 13(2):171–177.
179. Santoro N. Doctor, can you order that menopause test? Menopause 2006;13(2): 158–159.
180. Uebelhack R, Blohmer JU, Graubaum HJ, Busch R, Gruenwald J, Wernecke KD. Black cohosh and St. John's wort for climacteric complaints: a randomized trial. Obstet Gynecol 2006;107(2 Pt 1):247–255.
181. Reddy SY, Warner H, Guttuso T Jr, Messing S, DiGrazio W, Thornburg L, Guzick DS. Gabapentin, estrogen, and placebo for treating hot flushes: a randomized controlled trial. Obstet Gynecol 2006;108(1):41–48.
182. Huang MI, Nir Y, Chen B, Schnyer R, Manber R. A randomized controlled pilot study of acupuncture for postmenopausal hot flashes: effect on nocturnal hot flashes and sleep quality. Fertil Steril 2006;86(3):700–710.
183. Woo SB, Hellstein JW, Kalmar JR. Narrative [corrected] review: bisphosphonates and osteonecrosis of the jaws. Ann Intern Med 2006;144(10):753–761.
184. The Practice Committee of the American Society for Reproductive Medicine. Estrogen and progestogen therapy in postmenopausal women. Fertil Steril 2006;86 Suppl 5:S75–S88.
185. Curb JD, Prentice RL, Bray PF, Langer RD, Van Horn L, Barnabei VM, Bloch MJ, Cyr MG, Gass M, Lepine L, Rodabough RJ, Sidney S, Uwaifo GI, Rosendaal FR. Venous thrombosis and conjugated equine estrogen in women without a uterus. Arch Intern Med 2006;166(7):772–780.

Contraceptive Efficacy

James Trussell, PhD

- Pregnancy rates during *perfect use* reflect how effective methods can be in preventing pregnancy when used *consistently and correctly* according to instructions.

- Pregnancy rates during *typical use* reflect how effective methods are for the average person who does not always use methods correctly or consistently.

- Pregnancy rates during typical use of adherence-dependent methods generally vary widely for different groups using the same method, primarily due to differences in the propensity to use the method perfectly.

- Additional empirically-based estimates of pregnancy rates during perfect use are needed.

A general explanation of the sources of evidence and the logic underlying the summary table on contraceptive efficacy (Table 3–2) is provided in Chapter 3 on Choosing a Contraceptive. This chapter more completely explains the derivation of the estimates of the first-year probabilities of pregnancy during typical use (column 2) and perfect use (column 3) in Table 3–2, reproduced as Table 27–1.[1,2,3] The chapter also contains tables summarizing the literature on contraceptive efficacy for each method. These are arranged in the order in which they appear in summary Table 27–1. In these tables, all studies were conducted in the United States unless otherwise noted. In the epidemiology literature, the term *efficacy* refers to how well an intervention (in this case a contraceptive method) works in clinical trials and the term *effectiveness* refers to how well it works in actual practice. We use both sorts of evidence in this chapter, but in this chapter and in Chapter 3 and throughout the book, we use these terms interchangeably in the common everyday sense of how well a method works.

NO METHOD

Our estimate of the percentage of women becoming pregnant among those not using contraception is based on populations in which the use of contraception is rare, and on couples who report that they stopped using contraceptives because they want to conceive. Based on this evidence, we conclude that 85 of 100 sexually active couples would experience an accidental pregnancy in the first year if they used no contraception. Available evidence in the United States suggests that only about 40% of married couples who do not use contraception (but who still wish to avoid pregnancy) become pregnant within 1 year.[4] However, such couples are almost certainly selected for low fecundity or low frequency of intercourse. They do not use contraception because, in part, they are aware that they are unlikely to conceive. The probability of pregnancy of 85%, therefore, is our best guess of the fraction of women now using reversible methods of contraception who would become pregnant within 1 year if they were to abandon their current method but not otherwise change their behavior. Couples who have unprotected intercourse for a year without achieving pregnancy are, by definition, infertile (but by no means are they necessarily sterile—see Chapter 3 and Chapter 25 on Impaired Fertility). Table 27–2 summarizes the studies of the risk of pregnancy among women who are neither using contraception nor breastfeeding.

TYPICAL USE OF SPERMICIDES, WITHDRAWAL, FERTILITY AWARENESS-BASED METHODS, DIAPHRAGM, MALE CONDOM, ORAL CONTRACEPTIVE PILLS, AND DEPO-PROVERA

Our estimates of the probability of pregnancy during the first year of typical use for spermicides, withdrawal, fertility awareness-based methods, the diaphragm, the male condom, the pill, and Depo-Provera are taken from the 1995 National Survey of Family Growth (NSFG), corrected for underreporting of abortion.[5] The characteristics of users of different methods, while reflecting the population actually using each method in the United States, vary greatly. For example, 63% of the intervals of use of the diaphragm were contributed by women aged 30 and older, compared with only 16% for Depo-Provera and 24% for the male condom. Therefore, the estimates are standardized to reflect the estimated probabilities of pregnancy that would be observed if users of each method had the same characteristics (for example, the same age distribution, marital/cohabiting status distribution, and the same fraction living in poverty).

The correction for underreporting of abortion may produce estimates that are too high because women in abortion clinics (surveys of whom provided the information for the correction) tend to overreport use of a contraceptive method at the time they became pregnant. Moreover, women in personal interviews for the NSFG also might overreport use of a contraceptive method at the time of a conception leading to a live birth. Evidence for this suspicion is provided by uncorrected first-year probabilities of pregnancy of 3.7% for the IUD and 2.3% for Norplant (methods with little or no scope for user error) in the 1995 NSFG; these probabilities are much higher than rates observed in clinical trials of these methods, and for this reason we did not base the typical-use estimates for these two methods on the NSFG.[6] We would naturally expect overreporting of contraceptive use in both the NSFG and surveys conducted in abortion clinics, because the woman (couple) can then blame the pregnancy on contraceptive "failure."

Thus, biases in opposite directions affect these estimates. Pregnancy rates based on the NSFG alone would tend to be too low because induced abortions (and contraceptive failures leading to induced abortions) are underreported but would tend to be too high because contraceptive failures leading to live births are overreported. We reason that the former bias is the more important one.

The NSFG does not ask for brand of pill; thus combined and progestin-only pills cannot be distinguished. However, since use of the combined pill is far more common than use of the progestin-only pill, the results from the NSFG overwhelmingly reflect typical use of combined pills. The efficacy of progestin-only pills may be lower than that for combined pills since progestin-only pills are probably less forgiving of nonadherence to the dosing schedule.

PERFECT USE OF THE SPONGE AND DIAPHRAGM

Our estimates of the probabilities of pregnancy during the first year of perfect use of the sponge and diaphragm correspond with results of a reanalysis of data from two clinical trials in which women were randomly assigned to use the diaphragm or sponge and the diaphragm or cervical cap.[7] The results indicate that among parous women who use the sponge perfectly, 19.4% to 20.5% will experience a pregnancy within the first year. The corresponding range for nulliparous women is 9.0% to 9.5%. In contrast, parous users of the diaphragm do not appear to have higher pregnancy rates during perfect use than do nulliparous users; 4.3% to 8.4% of all women experience an accidental pregnancy during the first year of perfect use of the diaphragm. Our revised estimates in the third column of Table 27–1 (and Table 3–2 in Chapter 3 on Choosing a Contraceptive) are obtained from the midpoints of these ranges.

TYPICAL USE OF THE SPONGE

We next faced the problem of whether and how to revise the estimates for the sponge during typical use (the second column). The proportion becoming pregnant during the first year of typical use for parous users of the sponge (27.4%) was about twice as high as for nulliparous users of that method (14.0%). The evidence for the diaphragm is mixed. In the sponge-diaphragm trial, the proportion becoming pregnant in the first year of typical use for parous users of the diaphragm (12.4%) was marginally lower than that for nulliparous users (12.8%). In the cap-diaphragm trial, the proportion becoming pregnant among parous users (29.0%) is almost double that among nulliparous users (14.8%).[8] Faced with this information, we set the estimates for nulliparous users of the sponge equal to the estimate for all users of the diaphragm based on the NSFG (16%). We doubled the estimates for nulliparous users of the sponge to obtain the estimate for parous users.

FEMALE CONDOM

The typical-use estimate for the female condom is based on the results of a 6-month clinical trial of the Reality female condom; 12.4% of women in the United States experienced a pregnancy during the first 6 months of use.[8] The 12-month probability of pregnancy for users of Reality in the United States was projected from the relation between the pregnancy rates in the first 6 months and the pregnancy rates in the second 6 months for users of the diaphragm, sponge and cervical cap.[8] The probability of pregnancy during 6 months of perfect use of Reality by U.S. women who met the adherence criteria stipulated in the study protocol was 2.6%. Those who reported fewer than 4 acts of intercourse during the month prior to any follow-up visit, who did not use Reality at every act of intercourse, who ever reported not following the Reality instructions, or who used another method of contraception were censored at the beginning of the first interval where nonadherence was noted.[9] Under the assumption that the probability of pregnancy in the second six months of perfect use would be the same, the probability of pregnancy during a year of perfect use would be 5.1%.

PERFECT USE OF WITHDRAWAL AND SPERMICIDES

Our estimate of the proportion becoming pregnant during a year of perfect use of withdrawal is an educated guess based on the reasoning that pregnancy resulting from preejaculatory fluid is unlikely.[10–12]

Our estimate of the proportion becoming pregnant during a year of perfect use of spermicides is based on a recent NIH trial of 5 spermicides.[13] We assumed that the pregnancy rate per cycle during perfect use would be constant, extrapolated a one-year probability from the 6-cycle probability reported for each method, and took as our estimate the median (18%) of those 5 estimates. Our estimate is considerably higher than would be expected from the extensive literature on the contraceptive efficacy of spermicides.

Six studies outside the United States,[14-19] in addition to several U.S. studies reviewed earlier,[1] have yielded very low probabilities of pregnancy during the first year of typical use of spermicides, much lower than any estimates for barriers with spermicides. The efficacy literature on spermicides is dominated by studies of suppositories, foams, and film, and high spermicide efficacy is documented only in these studies. There are few studies of creams and gels used alone, and those with the lowest pregnancy rates are more than 30 years old (Table 27-3). We consider it likely that the spermicide studies suffer from flaws in analysis or design that are not apparent in the brief published descriptions. For example, an FDA advisory committee was openly skeptical of one German study:[14] "the way in which the survey was designed and the manner in which the various incentives were offered" (physicians reportedly received a fee for completing survey data forms) "would clearly make the data resulting from the survey unacceptable to any scientific group or regulatory agency."[20,21]

The first clinical trial of Emko vaginal foam is also one of the few studies to compute separate pregnancy rates for cycles in which the product was used at every act of intercourse and for cycles in which unprotected intercourse occurred.[22] The design of that trial was also quite sophisticated. Women were randomly assigned to six groups. Each group used three different spermicidal products for three cycles each. The six groups represented all possible permutations of orders of use of the three products. If the pregnancy rate for three cycles of consistent use of Emko vaginal foam is extrapolated, then the implied proportion becoming pregnant in the first year of consistent use is 8.9%.

A recent randomized clinical trial comparing the efficacy of a film and a foaming tablet—the first trial of spermicides conducted according to modern standards of design, execution, and analysis—supports the conclusion that the contraceptive efficacy of spermicides is considerably lower than was previously thought.[23] In that trial, 6-month probabilities of pregnancy during consistent use were 28% for the tablet and 24% for the film, probabilities that were nearly identical to the risks during typical use in that trial and that are about the same as the 12-month probability of pregnancy during typical use of spermicides in the 1995 NSFG.

PERFECT USE OF FERTILITY AWARENESS-BASED METHODS

The perfect-use estimates for fertility awareness-based methods are based on empirical estimates of 4.8% for the Standard Days method, 3.5% for the TwoDay method, and 3.2% for the ovulation method.[24-26] Published "method failure" rates for other variants of natural family planning are incorrect (see Chapter 3).

PERFECT USE OF THE MALE CONDOM

Our estimate of the proportion becoming pregnant during a year of perfect use of the male condom is based on results from the only three studies of the male condom meeting modern standards of design, execution, and analysis.[27-29] In each study couples were randomly assigned to use either a latex condom or a polyurethane condom. All three studies reported efficacy during consistent use but only one reported efficacy during perfect use;[28] in that study the 6-cycle probability of pregnancy during perfect use (0.7%) was 70% of that (1%) during typical use. We assumed that in the other two studies the 6-cycle probability of pregnancy during perfect use would also be 70% of the 6-cycle probability during typical use, assumed that the pregnancy rate per cycle during perfect use would be constant, extrapolated a one-year probability from the 6-cycle probability reported for the latex condom in each trial, and took as our estimate the median (2%, also the mean) of those 3 estimates. This estimate is consistent with an estimate based on studies of condom breakage and slippage.[30] Under the assumption that 1.5% of condoms break or slip off the penis and that women have intercourse twice a week, then about 1.5% of women would experience condom breaks during the half-week that they are at risk of pregnancy during each cycle. The per-cycle probability of conception would be reduced by 98.5%, from 0.1358 to only 0.0020, if a condom failure results in no protection whatsoever against pregnancy, so that about 2.6% of women would become pregnant each year.[31] Unfortunately, breakage and slippage rates did not accurately predict pregnancy rates during consistent use in one clinical trial of the latex and polyurethane male condom,[27] and estimates of condom breakage and slippage during intercourse or withdrawal vary substantially across studies in developed countries,[30] from a low of 0.6% among commercial sex workers in Nevada's legal brothels[30] to a high of 7.2% among monogamous couples in North Carolina.[32]

PERFECT USE OF THE ORAL CONTRACEPTIVE PILLS, DEPO-PROVERA, AND IMPLANON, AND TYPICAL USE OF IMPLANON

Although the lowest reported pregnancy rate for the combined pill during typical use is 0% (Table 27–11), recent studies indicate that pregnancies do occur, albeit rarely, during perfect use. Hence we set the perfect-use estimate for the pill at the very low level of 0.3%. The lowest reported pregnancy rate for the progestin-only pill exceeds 1% (see Table 27–10). It is likely that the progestin-only pill is less effective than the combined pill during typical use, since the progestin-only pill is probably less forgiving of nonadherence to the dosing schedule. Whether the progestin-only pill is also less effective during perfect use is unknown.

The perfect-use estimate for Depo-Provera is the weighted average of the seven studies of the 150 mg IM dose shown in Table 27–12. These trials yield an estimate of efficacy during perfect rather than typical use because either women late for an injection were discontinued or all pregnancies reported occurred during actual use (after one injection but before the next was scheduled). In two large trials of DMPA-SC, there were no reported pregnancies during perfect use in either study;[33] a typical-use pregnancy rate is not available, since pregnancy was defined as a positive pregnancy test prior to the next scheduled injection. It is unlikely that DMPA-SC never fails, so we set the pregnancy rate during perfect use equal to that of DMPA-IM during perfect use. It is possible that DMPA-SC has higher efficacy than DMPA-IM during prefect use, but the company that markets both products has made no such claim. A review of the contraceptive efficacy of Implanon found no pregnancies in 53,530 cycles of use; Organon later retracted some of the data in that review, but this retraction did not affect the pregnancy rate (0.0%).[34] A second study also found no pregnancies in 15,653 treatment cycles.[35] Likewise, there were no pregnancies in a trial in the United States with 6,186 cycles.[36] However, pregnancies during use of Implanon have been reported in Australia after the product was approved for marketing.[37] We arbitrarily set the perfect-use and typical-use failure rates for Implanon at 0.05%.

EVRA AND NUVARING

The typical- and perfect-use estimates for the Evra patch and NuvaRing were set equal to those for the pill. It is possible that the patch and ring will prove to have better efficacy than the pill during typical use, because of better adherence with the dosing schedule. However, such superior efficacy has not been demonstrated in randomized trials. While in one trial the failure rate was lower among women randomly assigned to use the Evra patch (1.2%) than among those assigned to use the pill (2.2%), the difference was not statistically significant (p=0.6).[38] In a subsequent paper that argues that better adherence to the dosing schedule leads to better contraceptive efficacy of the patch than the pill during typical use, the authors acknowledge that it would require a trial with 24,143 subjects to demonstrate such superiority and conclude that "studies of this size to compare effectiveness may not be practical."[39] In the one study in which women were randomly assigned to the NuvaRing or the pill, the pregnancy rates were identical (1.2 per 100 women-years of exposure).[40]

IUD

The estimate for typical use of the ParaGard (Copper T 380A) IUDs is taken directly from the large study for that method shown in Table 27–13. The estimate for Mirena (LNG-IUS) is the weighted average of the results from the three studies shown in Table 27–13. The estimate for perfect use of the Copper T 380A was obtained by removing the pregnancies that resulted when the device was not known to be in situ,[41] on the perhaps-questionable assumption that these pregnancies should be classified as user failures and the empirically-based assumption that expulsions are so uncommon that the denominator of the perfect-use pregnancy rate is virtually the same as the denominator for the typical-use rate (Table 27–13). The perfect-use estimate for the LNG-IUS was derived analogously. No differences in the typical-use and perfect-use estimates for LNG-IUS are apparent due to the fact that only one significant digit is shown.

STERILIZATION

The weighted average of the results from the eight vasectomy studies in Table 27–16 analyzed with life-table procedures is 0.01% becoming pregnant in the year following the procedure. In these studies, pregnancies occurred after the ejaculate had been declared to be sperm-free. This perfect-use estimate of 0.01% is undoubtedly too low, because clinicians are understandably loath to publish articles describing their surgical failures and journals would be reluctant to publish an article documenting poor surgical technique. The difference between typical-use and perfect-use pregnancy rates for vasectomy would depend on the frequency of unprotected intercourse after the procedure had been performed but before the ejaculate had been certified to be sperm-free. We arbitrarily set the typical- and perfect-use estimates to 0.15% and 0.10%, respectively. For female sterilization, there is no scope for user error. The typical- and perfect-use estimates are the pooled results from the U.S. Collaborative Review of Sterilization, a prospective study of 10,685 women undergoing tubal sterilization.[42] We are less concerned about publication bias with female than with male sterilization because the largest studies of female sterilization are based on prospective, multi-center clinical trials, not retrospective reports from one investigator.

CONTRACEPTIVE CONTINUATION

Contraceptives will be effective at preventing unintended pregnancy only if women or couples continue to use them once they have initiated use. The proportions of women continuing use at the end of the first year for spermicides, withdrawal, fertility awareness-based methods, the diaphragm, the male condom, the pill, Depo-Provera and Norplant were obtained from the 1995 NSFG.[6] Only method-related reasons for discontinuation (changing methods or termination of contraceptive use while still at risk for unintended pregnancy) were counted. Other reasons for discontinuing use of a method (such as attempting to get pregnant or not having intercourse) are not counted in the discontinuation rate because these reasons are unrelated to the method and do not apply to women seeking to avoid pregnancy and at risk of becoming pregnant. For nulliparous users of the sponge, we used the continuation rate for the diaphragm; for parous users, we adjusted the continuation rate for the diaphragm to reflect higher pregnancy rates. For the female condom, we adjusted the continuation rate for the male condom to reflect a higher pregnancy rate.

We set the continuation rates for the Evra patch and NuvaRing equal to that for the pill. We set the continuation rate for Implanon equal to that for Norplant, which was derived from the 1995 NSFG.

Discontinuation rates of the two IUDs (for reasons related to the contraceptive) are based on clinical trials. The estimate for the Copper T 380A IUD was taken directly from the large study for that method shown in Table 27–13. The estimate for the LNG-IUS is the weighted average from the three studies shown in Table 27–13.

EMERGENCY CONTRACEPTION

Typically, if 100 women have unprotected intercourse once during the second or third week of their menstrual cycle, about 8 would become pregnant. If those same women used combined emergency contraceptive pills (ECPs), only 2 would become pregnant (a 75% reduction);[43] if they used the progestin-only ECP, only 1 would become pregnant (an 89% reduction).[44] Copper T IUD insertion is extremely effective, reducing the risk of pregnancy following unprotected intercourse by more than 99%.[45] Moreover, a copper T IUD can be left in place to provide continuous effective contraception for up to 10 years.

THE LACTATIONAL AMENORRHEA METHOD (LAM)

LAM is a highly effective, *temporary* method of contraception. If the infant is being fed only its mother's breastmilk (or is given supplemental non-breastmilk feeds only to a minor extent) and if the woman has not experienced her first postpartum menses, then breastfeeding provides more than 98% protection from pregnancy in the first 6 months following a birth.[46,47] Four prospective clinical studies of the contraceptive effect of this LAM demonstrated cumulative 6-month life-table perfect-use pregnancy rates of 0.5%, 0.6%, 1.0%, and 1.5% among women who relied solely on LAM.[48–51]

REFERENCES

1. Trussell J, Kost K. Contraceptive failure in the United States: a critical review of the literature. Stud Fam Plann 1987;18:237–283.
2. Trussell J, Hatcher RA, Cates W, Stewart FH, Kost K. Contraceptive failure in the United States: an update. Stud Fam Plann 1990;21:51–54.
3. Trussell J. Contraceptive failure in the United States. Contraception 2004;70:89–96.
4. Grady WR, Hayward MD, Yagi J. Contraceptive failure in the United States: estimates from the 1982 National Survey of Family Growth. Fam Plann Perspect 1986; 18:200–209.
5. Fu H, Darroch JE, Haas T, Ranjit N. Contraceptive failure rates: new estimates from the 1995 National Survey of Family Growth. Fam Plann Perspect 1999;31:56–63.
6. Trussell J, Vaughan B. Contraceptive Failure, method-related discontinuation and resumption of use: results from the 1995 National Survey of Family Growth. Fam Plann Perspect 1999;31:64–72 & 93.
7. Trussell J, Strickler J, Vaughan B. Contraceptive efficacy of the diaphragm, the sponge and the cervical cap. Fam Plann Perspect 1993;25:100–105, 135.
8. Trussell J, Sturgen K, Strickler J, Dominik R. Comparative contraceptive efficacy of the female condom and other barrier methods. Fam Plann Perspect 1994;26:66–72.
9. Farr G, Gabelnick H, Sturgen K, Dorflinger L. Contraceptive efficacy and acceptability of the female condom. Am J Public Health 1994;84:1960–1964.
10. Ilaria G, Jacobs JL, Polsky B, Koll B, Baron P, MacLow C, Armstrong D, Schlegel PN. Detection of HIV-1 DNA sequences in pre-ejaculatory fluid. Lancet 1992;340:1469.
11. Pudney J, Oneta M, Mayer K, Seage G, Anderson D. Pre-ejaculatory fluid as potential vector for sexual transmission of HIV-1. Lancet 1992;340:1470.
12. Zukerman Z, Weiss DB, Orvieto R. Does preejaculatory penile secretion originating from Cowper's gland contain sperm? J Assist Reprod Genet 2003;20:157–159.
13. Raymond EG, Chen PL, Luoto J. Contraceptive effectiveness and safety of five non-oxynol-9 spermicides: a randomized trial. Obstet Gynecol 2004;103:430–439.
14. Brehm H, Haase W. Die alternative zur hormonalen kontrazeption? Med Welt 1975; 26:1610–1617.
15. Dimpfl J, Salomon W, Schicketanz KH. Die spermizide barriere. Sexualmedizin 1984; 13:95–98.
16. Florence N. Das kontrazeptive vaginal-suppositorium: ergebnisse einer klinischen fünfjahresstudie. Sexualmedizin 1977;6:385–386.
17. Godts P. Klinische prüfung eines vaginalem antikonzipiens. Ars Medici 1973; 2:589–593.

18. Iizuka R, Kobayashi T, Kawakami S, Nakamura Y, Ikeuchi M, Chin B, Mochimaru F, Sumi K, Sato H, Yamaguchi J, Ohno T, Shiina M, Maeda N, Tokoro H, Suzuki T, Hayashi K, Takahashi T, Akatsuka M, Kasuga Y, Kurokawa H. Clinical experience with the Vaginal Contraceptive Film containing the spermicide polyoxyethylene nonylphenyl ether (C-Film study group). Jpn J Fertil Steril 1980;25:64–68. (In Japanese; translation supplied by Apothecus Inc.)
19. Salomon W, Haase W. Intravaginale kontrazeption. Sexualmedizin 1977;6:198–202.
20. Over-the-Counter Contraceptives and Other Vaginal Drug Products Review Panel (Elizabeth B. Connell, Chairman). Encare Oval. Memorandum to Food and Drug Administration Commissioner Donald Kennedy, February 9, 1978.
21. Stewart FH, Stewart G, Guest FJ, Hatcher RA. My body, my health: the concerned woman's guide to gynecology. New York NY: John Wiley & Sons, 1979.
22. Mears E. Chemical contraceptive trial: II. J Reprod Fertil 1962;4:337–343.
23. Raymond E, Dominik R, the spermicide trial group. Contraceptive effectiveness of two spermicides: a randomized trial. Obstet Gynecol 1999;93:896–903.
24. Arévalo M, Jennings V, Sinai I. Efficacy of a new method of family planning: the Standard Days Method. Contraception 2002;65:333–338.
25. Arévalo M, Jennings V, Nikula M, Sinai I.Efficacy of the new TwoDay Method of family planning. Fertil Steril 2004;82:885–892.
26. Trussell J, Grummer-Strawn L. Contraceptive failure of the ovulation method of periodic abstinence. Fam Plann Perspect 1990;22:65–75.
27. Frezieres RG, Walsh TL, Nelson AL, Clark VA, Coulson AH. Evaluation of the efficacy of a polyurethane condom: results from a randomized controlled clinical trial. Fam Plann Perspect 1999;31:81–87.
28. Walsh TL, Frezieres RG, Peacock K, Nelson AL, Clark VA, Bernstein L. Evaluation of the efficacy of a nonlatex condom: results from a randomized, controlled clinical trial. Perspect Sex Reprod Health 2003;35:79–86.
29. Steiner MJ, Dominik R, Rountree RW, Nanda K, Dorflinger LJ. Contraceptive effectiveness of a polyurethane condom and a latex condom: a randomized controlled trial. Obstet Gynecol 2003;101:539–547.
30. Albert AE, Warner DL, Hatcher RA, Trussell J, Bennett C. Condom use among female commercial sex workers in Nevada's legal brothels. Am J Public Health 1995; 85:1514–1520.
31. Kestelman P, Trussell J. Efficacy of the simultaneous use of condoms and spermicides. Fam Plann Perspect 1991;23:226–227, 232.
32. Steiner M, Piedrahita C, Glover L, Joanis C. Can condom users likely to experience condom failure be identified? Fam Plann Perspect 1993;25:220–223, 226.
33. Jain J, Jakimiuk AJ, Bode FR, Ross D, Kaunitz AM. Contraceptive efficacy and safety of DMPA-SC. Contraception 2004;70:269–275.
34. Croxatto HB, Mäkäräinen L. The pharmacodynamics and efficacy of Implanon. An overview of the data. Contraception 1998;58:91S–97S. Retraction in: Rekers H, Affandi B. Contraception 2004;70:433.
35. Croxatto HB, Urbancsek J, Massai R, Coelingh Bennink H, van Beek A. A multicentre efficacy and safety study of the single contraceptive implant Implanon. Implanon Study Group. Hum Reprod 1999;14:976–981.
36. Funk S, Miller MM, Mishell DR, Archer DF, Poindexter A, Schmidt J, Zampaglione E and for the Implanon℠ US Study Group. Safety and efficacy of Implanon℠, a single-rod implantable contraceptive containing etonogestrel. Contraception 2005; 71:319–326.
37. Harrison-Woolrych M, Hill R. Unintended pregnancies with the etonogestrel implant (Implanon): a case series from postmarketing experience in Australia. Contraception 2005;71:306–308.
38. Audet MC, Moreau M, Koltun WD, Waldbaum AS, Shangold G, Fisher AC, Creasy GW. Evaluation of contraceptive efficacy and cycle control of a transdermal contraceptive patch vs an oral contraceptive. JAMA 2001;285:2347–2354.

39. Archer DF, Cullins V, Creasy GW, Fisher AC. The impact of improved compliance with a weekly contraceptive transdermal system (Ortho Evra® on contraceptive efficacy. Contraception 2004;69:189–195.
40. Oddsson K, Leifels-Fischer B, de Melo NR, Wiel-Masson D, Benedetto C, Verhoeven CH, Dieben TO. Efficacy and safety of a contraceptive vaginal ring (NuvaRing) compared with a combined oral contraceptive: a 1-year randomized trial. Contraception 2005;71:176–82.
41. Sivin I. Personal communication to James Trussell, August 13, 1992.
42. Peterson HB, Xia Z, Hughes JM, Wilcox LS, Tylor LR, Trussell J. The risk of pregnancy after tubal sterilization: findings from the U.S. Collaborative Review of Sterilization. Am J Obstet Gynecol 1996;174:1161–1170.
43. Trussell J, Rodríguez G, Ellertson C. Updated estimates of the effectiveness of the Yuzpe regimen of emergency contraception. Contraception 1999;59:147–151.
44. Task Force on Postovulatory Methods of Fertility Regulation. Randomised controlled trial of levonorgestrel versus the Yuzpe regimen of combined oral contraceptives for emergency contraception. Lancet 1998;352:428–433.
45. Trussell J, Ellertson C. Efficacy of emergency contraception. Fertil Control Rev 1995; 4:8–11.
46. Kennedy KI, Rivera R, McNeilly AS. Consensus statement on the use of breastfeeding as a family planning method. Contraception 1989;39:477–496.
47. Kennedy KI, Labbok MH, Van Look PFA. Lactational amenorrhea method for family planning. Int J Gynaecol Obstet. 1996;54:55–57.
48. Kazi A, Kennedy KI, Visness CM, Khan T. Effectiveness of the lactational amenorrhea method in Pakistan. Fertil Steril 1995;64:717–723.
49. Labbok MH, Hight-Laukaran V, Peterson AE, Fletcher V, von Hertzen H, Van Look PFA. Multicenter study of the Lactational Amenorrhea Method (LAM): I. Efficacy, duration, and implications for clinical application. Contraception 1997;55:327–336.
50. Pérez A, Labbok MH, Queenan JT. Clinical study of the lactational amenorrhoea method for family planning. Lancet 1992;339:968–970.
51. Ramos R, Kennedy KI, Visness CM. Effectiveness of lactational amenorrhea in prevention of pregnancy in Manila, the Philippines: non-comparative prospective trial. Br Med J 1996;313:909–912.

Table 27–1 **Percentage of women experiencing an unintended pregnancy during the first year of typical use and the first year of perfect use of contraception and the percentage continuing use at the end of the first year. United States**

Method (1)	% of Women Experiencing an Unintended Pregnancy within the First Year of Use		% of Women Continuing Use at One Year[3] (4)
	Typical Use[1] (2)	Perfect Use[2] (3)	
No method[4]	85	85	
Spermicides[5]	29	18	42
Withdrawal	27	4	43
Fertility awareness-based methods	25		51
Standard Days method[6]		5	
TwoDay method[6]		4	
Ovulation method[6]		3	
Sponge			
Parous women	32	20	46
Nulliparous women	16	9	57
Diaphragm[7]	16	6	57
Condom[8]			
Female (Reality)	21	5	49
Male	15	2	53
Combined pill and progestin-only pill	8	0.3	68
Evra patch	8	0.3	68
NuvaRing	8	0.3	68
Depo-Provera	3	0.3	56
IUD			
ParaGard (copper T)	0.8	0.6	78
Mirena (LNG-IUS)	0.2	0.2	80
Implanon	0.05	0.05	84
Female sterilization	0.5	0.5	100
Male sterilization	0.15	0.10	100

Emergency Contraceptive Pills: Treatment initiated within 72 hours after unprotected intercourse reduces the risk of pregnancy by at least 75%.[9]

Lactational Amenorrhea Method: LAM is a highly effective, *temporary* method of contraception.[10]

Source: See text.
(continued)

Notes:

1 Among _typical_ couples who initiate use of a method (not necessarily for the first time), the percentage who experience an accidental pregnancy during the first year if they do not stop use for any other reason. Estimates of the probability of pregnancy during the first year of typical use for spermicides, withdrawal, fertility awareness-based methods, the diaphragm, the male condom, the pill, and Depo-Provera are taken from the 1995 National Survey of Family Growth corrected for underreporting of abortion; see the text for the derivation of estimates for the other methods.

2 Among couples who initiate use of a method (not necessarily for the first time) and who use it _perfectly_ (both consistently and correctly), the percentage who experience an accidental pregnancy during the first year if they do not stop use for any other reason. See the text for the derivation of the estimate for each method.

3 Among couples attempting to avoid pregnancy, the percentage who continue to use a method for 1 year.

4 The percentages becoming pregnant in columns (2) and (3) are based on data from populations where contraception is not used and from women who cease using contraception in order to become pregnant. Among such populations, about 89% become pregnant within 1 year. This estimate was lowered slightly (to 85%) to represent the percentage who would become pregnant within 1 year among women now relying on reversible methods of contraception if they abandoned contraception altogether.

5 Foams, creams, gels, vaginal suppositories, and vaginal film.

6 The Ovulation and TwoDay methods are based on evaluation of cervical mucus. The Standard Days method avoids intercourse on cycle days 8 through 19.

7 With spermicidal cream or jelly.

8 Without spermicides.

9 The treatment schedule is one dose within 120 hours after unprotected intercourse, and a second dose 12 hours after the first dose. Both doses of Plan B can be taken at the same time. Plan B (1 dose is 1 white pill) is the only dedicated product specifically marketed for emergency contraception. The Food and Drug Administration has in addition declared the following 22 brands of oral contraceptives to be safe and effective for emergency contraception: Ogestrel or Ovral (1 dose is 2 white pills), Levlen or Nordette (1 dose is 4 light-orange pills), Cryselle, Levora, Low-Ogestrel, Lo/Ovral, or Quasence (1 dose is 4 white pills), Tri-Levlen or Triphasil (1 dose is 4 yellow pills), Jolessa, Portia, Seasonale, or Trivora (1 dose is 4 pink pills), Seasonique (1 dose is 4 light-blue-green pills), Empresse (one dose is 4 orange pills), Alesse, Lessina, or Levlite (1 dose is 5 pink pills), Aviane (one dose is 5 orange pills), and Lutera (one dose is 5 white pills),

10 However, to maintain effective protection against pregnancy, another method of contraception must be used as soon as menstruation resumes, the frequency or duration of breastfeeds is reduced, bottle feeds are introduced, or the baby reaches 6 months of age.

Table 27–2 Summary of studies of pregnancy rates among women neither contracepting nor breastfeeding[a]

Reference	N for Analysis	Life-Table 12-Month % Pregnant	Characteristics of the Sample	LFU (%)[g]	Comments
Grady et al., 1986	1,228	43.1	All married	20.6[r]	1982 NSFG; estimate far too low; see text
Sivin and Stern, 1979	420	75.1	48% nulliparous	?	Following removal of copper-medicated IUD for planned pregnancy
Vessey et al., 1978	779	82	All nulligravid	?	Britain; Oxford/FPA study following cessation of method use for planned pregnancy; conceptions leading to a live birth
Tatum, 1975	553	84.6		17.2	Following removal of copper-medicated IUD for planned pregnancy
Sivin, 1987	96	87	All parous	?	Chile, Dominican Republic, Finland, Sweden, United States; following removal of Norplant for planned pregnancy
Tietze and Lewit, 1970	378	88.2	89% aged 15–29	19.0	Following removal of nonmedicated IUD for planned pregnancy
Sheps, 1965	397	88.8	All married Hutterites	?	Conceptions leading to the first live birth following marriage among women reporting no fetal losses before the first conception
Vessey et al., 1978	1,343	89	All parous	?	Britain; Oxford/FPA study following cessation of method use for planned pregnancy; conceptions leading to a live birth
Belhadj et al., 1986	110	94.0c	All parous; aged 8–36	9.1	Brazil, Chile, Dominican Republic, Singapore, United States; following removal of medicated IUD for planned pregnancy

Notes:

a Updated from Trussell and Kost (1987), Table 1.

c Calculated by James Trussell from data in the article.

g Most of these studies incorrectly report the loss to follow-up probability as the number of women lost at any time during the study divided by the total number of women entering the study. Thus, these are the probabilities presented in the table. However, the correct measure of LFU would be a gross life-table probability. When available, gross 12-month probabilities are denoted by the letter "g."

r Nonresponse rate for entire survey.

For table references, see reference section.

Table 27–3 Summary of studies of contraceptive failure: spermicides[a]

Reference	Method Brand	N for Analysis	Life-Table 12-Month % Pregnant	Index	Total Exposure	Maximum Exposure	Characteristics of the Sample	LFU (%)[g]	Comments
				Risk of Pregnancy — Pearl Index Pregnancy Rate					
Edelman, 1980	S'positive	200		0.0	2,682 Mo.	?		?	Study conducted by Jordan-Simner, Inc., as reported by Edelman
Squire et al., 1979	Semicid Suppository	326	0.3				69% aged 20–34; 55% married; "well educated"; "highly motivated"; 24% prior use of oral contraceptives	0.0[c]	89% reported exclusive use of foam
Soloman and Haase, 1977	Patentex (Encare) Oval	1,652		0.3[c]	34,506 Cy.	54 Mo.	13% aged 15–20, 48% aged 21–30, 33% aged 31–40, 6% aged 41–45, 42% nulliparous	?	Subjects who used for less than one year excluded? Germany
Iizuka et al., 1980	Vaginal Contraceptive Film (C-Film)	168		0.6	2,161 Mo.	?	All women had been pregnant before; 20% aged <25, 64% aged 25–34,17% aged 35+	?	Japan
Brehm and Haase, 1975	Patentex (Encare) Oval	10,017		0.9[c]	63,759 Cy.	?	18% aged <21, 20% aged >35; 46% parity 0	?	Germany; FDA rejected this study because of flawed design (see text)
Florence, 1977	a-gen 53	103		1.2[c]	2,255 Cy.	61 Mo.	17% aged 17–20, 51% aged 21–30, 20% aged 31–40,12% aged 41+	?	Belgium
Dimpfl et al., 1974	Patentex (Encare) Oval	482	1.5				22% aged <21,25% aged >31; 44% parity 0; 60% married	?	Denmark, Germany, Poland, Switzerland
Bushnell, 1965	Emko Vaginal Foam	130		1.8	2,737 Mo.	57 Mo.	Aged 17–51; 76% aged 20–35	?	

(continued)

CONTRACEPTIVE TECHNOLOGY

Table 27-3 Summary of studies of contraceptive failure: spermicides[a]—(cont'd)

Reference	Method Brand	N for Analysis	Life-Table 12-Month % Pregnant	Risk of Pregnancy — Pearl Index Pregnancy Rate			Characteristics of the Sample	LFU (%)[g]	Comments
				Index	Total Exposure	Maximum Exposure			
Godts, 1973	a-gen 53	56		1.9c	1,344 Cy.	32 Mo.	21% aged 18–20, 46% aged 21–30, 18% aged 31–40, 14% aged 41+; all gravid	?	
Carpenter and Martin, 1970	Emko Pre-fil Vaginal Foam	1,778		3.4c	17,200 Cy.	18 Cy.	69% aged 21–35; 24% ≥12 years education; 44% no previous contraceptive experience	14.2c	All women agreed to exclusive use of foam
Brigato et al., 1982	Vaginal Contraceptive Film (C-Film)	37		3.9c	924 Mo.	?		?	Italy
Wolf et al., 1957	Preceptin Vaginal Gel	112		4.2c	1,145 Mo.	?	All aged 13–40; mean age = 25; all married	6.9c	
Bernstein, 1971	Emko Pre-fil Vaginal Foam	2,932		4.3c	28,332 Cy.	20 Cy.	70% aged 21–35; 39% ≥12 years education	16.1c	All women agreed to exclusive use of foam
Tyler, 1965	Delfen Vaginal Foam	672		5.0	9,486 Cy.	≥16 Mo.	Rates for full applicator doses and half doses combined	?	
Apothecus, 1992	Vaginal Contraceptive Film (C-Film)	761		5.5	6,501 Mo.	?			Belgium, Netherlands, Britain, Germany, Switzerland, Denmark, Sweden, Israel, Egypt; results never published; quality of study unknown

(continued)

Table 27–3 Summary of studies of contraceptive failure: spermicides[a]—*(cont'd)*

Reference	Method Brand	N for Analysis	Life-Table 12-Month % Pregnant	Risk of Pregnancy Pearl Index Pregnancy Rate Index	Total Exposure	Maximum Exposure	Characteristics of the Sample	LFU (%)[g]	Comments
Kleppinger, 1965	Delfen Vaginal Foam	138		7.5	1,116 Mo.	19 Mo.	53% aged 21–30; 27% postpartum	0.0[c-g]	
Dubrow and Kuder, 1958	Delfen Vaginal Cream	338		7.6	633 Mo.	12 Mo.	Mean age = 25; 93% ≤12 years education; 39% black; 45% Puerto Rican t	59.5[c]	
Dubrow and Kuder, 1958	Preceptin Vaginal Gel	835		8.1	3,728 Mo.	23 Mo.	Mean age = 25; 93% ≤12 years education; 39% black; 45% Puerto Rican t	45.1[c]	
Wolf et al., 1957	Delfen Vaginal Cream	875		8.9[c]	5,232 Mo.	30 Mo.	All aged 13–40; mean age = 25; all married	13.0[c]	
Frankman et al., 1975	Vaginal Contraceptive Film (C-Film)	237		9.0	1,866 Mo.	23 Mo.		?	Sweden; data included in Apothecus (1992)
Rovinsky, 1964	Delfen Vaginal Cream	251		9.1	2,915 Mo.	67 Mo.	70% aged 20–34; 55% Puerto Rican; 10% ≥13 years education	28.0[c]	
Raymond et al., 2004	100 mg suppository (Encare)	299	10.0[d]				44% aged 18–25	22	Random assignment to 100 mg suppository, 52.5 mg gel, 100 mg gel, 150 mg gel or 100 mg film
Raymond et al., 2004	100 mg film (Ortho Options Contraceptive Film)	295	11.9[d]				43% aged 18–25	24	Random assignment to 100 mg film, 52.5 mg gel, 100 mg gel, 150 mg gel or 100 mg suppository

(continued)

Table 27–3 Summary of studies of contraceptive failure: spermicides^a—(cont'd)

| | | | Life-Table 12-Month % Pregnant | Risk of Pregnancy | | | | | |
| | | | | Pearl Index Pregnancy Rate | | | | | |
Reference	Method Brand	N for Analysis		Index	Total Exposure	Maximum Exposure	Characteristics of the Sample	LFU (%)^g	Comments
Vessey et al., 1982		?		11.9	303 Yr.	?	All white; at recruitment aged 25–39 and married; at enrollment, all women had been using the diaphragm, IUD, or pill successfully for at least 5 months	0.3^{t,v}	Britain; Oxford/FPA study
Jones and Forrest, 1992		267	13.4				Aged 15–44^r	21^r	NSFG 1988; probability when standardized and corrected for estimated underreporting of abortion = 30.2^s
Raymond et al., 2004	150 mg gel (Ortho Options Conceptrol)	300	14.0^{c,d}		43% aged 18–25	21	Random assignment to 150 mg gel, 52.5 mg gel, 100 mg gel, 100 mg film or 100 mg suppository		
Vaughan et al., 1977		596	14.9^a				Aged 15–44; all married^t	19.0^r	NSFG 1973
Trussell and Vaughan, 1999		164	15.3				Aged 15–44^t	21^r	NSFG 1995
Raymond et al., 2004	100 mg gel (Ortho Options Conceptrol)	295	15.5^a				46% aged 18–25	25	Random assignment to 100 mg gel, 52.5 mg gel, 150 mg gel, 100 mg film or 100 mg suppository
Fu et al., 1999		?	16.6					21^r	NSFG 1995; probability when standardized and corrected for estimated underreporting of abortion = 29.0^s

(continued)

Table 27–3 Summary of studies of contraceptive failure: spermicides[a]—(cont'd)

Reference	Method Brand	N for Analysis	Life-Table 12-Month % Pregnant	Pearl Index Index	Total Exposure	Maximum Exposure	Characteristics of the Sample	LFU (%)[g]	Comments
								Risk of Pregnancy	
				Pearl Index Pregnancy Rate					
Grady et al., 1983		1,106	17.5[s,c]				Aged 15–44; all married[18.2[r]	NSFG 1973 and 1976	
Schirm et al., 1982		1,106	17.9[s]				Aged 15–44; all married[t]	18.2[r]	NSFG 1973 and 1976
Mears, 1962	Emko Aerosol Foam (nonoxynol 10–11)	425		18.0[c]	722 Cy.	3 Cy.	Pearl index of 9.3 among consistent and 48.4 among inconsistent users	>20[c,t]	Britain; postal trial; random assignment to foam, foaming tablet, or pessary with crossover design
Kasabach, 1962	Koromex A Jelly	242		21.0[c]	2,058 Mo.	24 Mo.	36% aged 25–35; all married; 68% "had a high school education"; all parous	19.3[c]	
Bracher and Santow, 1992		89	21.5				27% aged <20, 56% aged 20–29, 17% aged 30+; 49% parity 0; 87% married or cohabiting	25[r]	Australian Family Survey; first use of method
Grady et al., 1986		284	21.8[s]				Aged 15–44; all married[t]	20.6[r]	NSFG 1982
Raymond et al., 2004	52.5 mg gel (Advantage S)	296	22.2[d]				43% aged 18–25	20	Random assignment to 52.5 mg gel, 100 mg gel, 150 mg gel, 100 mg film or 100 mg suppository
Dingle and Tietze, 1963	Lactikol	170		23.5	1,789 Mo.	36 Mo.	Median age = 24.5	3.2[t]	
Frank, 1962	Koromex A Jelly	824		24.8[c]	5,767 Mo.	12 Mo.	72% aged 21–35	17.0[c]	

(continued)

Table 27-3 Summary of studies of contraceptive failure: spermicides[a]—*(cont'd)*

Reference	Method Brand	N for Analysis	Life-Table 12-Month % Pregnant	Risk of Pregnancy — Pearl Index Pregnancy Rate — Index	Total Exposure	Maximum Exposure	Characteristics of the Sample	LFU (%)[g]	Comments
Raymond et al., 1999	Vaginal Contraceptive Film	369	24.9[d]				Aged 18–35; 17% nulligravid	5.8	Mexico, Ecuador, Guatemala, Ghana, United States; random assignment to Vaginal Contraceptive Film or Conceptrol foaming tablets
Raymond et al., 1999	Conceptrol foaming tablets	365	28.0[d]				Aged 18–35; 16% nulligravid	7.3	Mexico, Ecuador, Guatemala, Ghana, United States; random assignment to Conceptrol foaming tablets or Vaginal Contraceptive Film
Tietze and Lewit, 1967	Emko Vaginal Foam	779	28.3				86% < age 30; all married; 47% ≥ high school completion; 75% nonwhite	6.9[g]	
Dingle and Tietze, 1963	Durafoam	42[r]		28.5	2,985 Mo.	36 Mo.	Median age = 26.1	3.2[t]	
Mears, 1962	Genexol Pessary (nonoxynol 10–11)	425		30.3	730 Cy.	3 Cy.		>20[c,t]	Britain; postal trial; random assignment to foam, foaming tablets, or pessary with crossover design

(continued)

Table 27–3 Summary of studies of contraceptive failure: spermicides[a]–(cont'd)

Reference	Method Brand	N for Analysis	Life-Table 12-Month % Pregnant	Pearl Index Pregnancy Rate			Characteristics of the Sample	LFU (%)[g]	Comments
				Index	**Total Exposure**	**Maximum Exposure**			
Tietze and Lewit, 1967	Cooper Creme and Creme Jel, Koromex A, Lactikol Creme and Jelly, Lanesta Gel	806	36.8				79% < age 30; all married; 53% ≥ high school completion; 75% nonwhite	3.4[g]	
Mears, 1962	Volpar Foaming Tablets (phenyl mercuric acetate)	425		48.2[c]	728 Cy.	3 Cy.	Pearl index of 44.4 among consistent and 64.1 among inconsistent users	>20[c,t]	Britain; postal trial; random assignment to foam, foaming tablet, or pessary with crossover design
Mears and Please, 1962	Staycept Cream (hexyl resorcinol)	678		49.6[c]	707 Cy.	3 Cy.	Pearl index of 31.4 among consistent and 132.0 among inconsistent users	>41[c,t]	Britain; postal trial; random assignment to cream, foaming tablet, or pessary with crossover design
Mears and Please, 1962	Genexol Pessary (quinine)	678		52.2	647 Cy.	3 Cy.		>41[c,t]	Britain; postal trial; random assignment to cream, foaming tablet, or pessary with crossover design
Smith et al., 1974	Vaginal Contraceptive Film (C-Film)	63[c]		55.7[c]	194[c] Mo.	<15[c]	Aged 16–35	9.5[c]	Britain; trial terminated for ethical reasons

(continued)

Table 27–3 **Summary of studies of contraceptive failure: spermicides**ᵃ—*(cont'd)*

| | | | Risk of Pregnancy | | | | | | |
| | | | Life-Table 12-Month % Pregnant | Pearl Index Pregnancy Rate | | | | | |
Reference	Method Brand	N for Analysis		Index	Total Exposure	Maximum Exposure	Characteristics of the Sample	LFU (%)ᵍ	Comments
Mears and Please, 1962	Volpar Foaming Tablets (phenyl mercuric acetate)	678		59.0c	705 Cy.	3 Cy.	Pearl index of 47.8 among consistent and 106.7 among inconsistent users	>41 c,t	Britain; postal trial; random assignment to cream, foaming tablet, or pessary with crossover design

Notes:

ᵃ Updated from Trussell and Kost (1987), Table 2.

ᶜ Calculated by James Trussell from data in the article.

ᵈ 6-month probability; 12-month probability not available.

ᵍ Most of these studies incorrectly report the loss to follow-up probability (LFU) as the number of women lost at any time during the study divided by the total number of women entering the study. Thus, these are the probabilities presented in the table. However, the correct measure of LFU would be a gross life-table probability. When available, gross 12-month probabilities are denoted by the letter "g." Nonresponse rate for entire survey.

ˢ Standardized: Vaughan et al., (1977) (1973 NSFG)—intention (the average of probabilities for preventers and delayers); Grady et al., (1983) (1973 and 1976 NSFG)—intention. Our calculation (the average of probabilities for preventers and delayers); Schirm et al., (1982) (1973 and 1976 NSFG)—intention, age, and income; Grady et al., (1986) (1982 NSFG)—intention, age, poverty status, and parity; Jones and Forrest, (1992) (1988 NSFG)—age, marital status, and poverty status; Fu et al., (1999) (1995 NSFG)—age, union status, poverty status.

ᵗ Total for all methods in the study.

ᵛ The authors report that LFU for "relevant reasons (withdrawal of cooperation or loss of contact)" was 0.3% per year in the 1982 study. In the 1982 study, women had been followed for 9.5 years on average; if 0.3% are LFU per year, then 2.8% would be LFU in 9.5 years. LFU including death and emigration is about twice as high as LFU for "relevant reasons."

For table references, see reference section.

Table 27-4 Summary of studies of contraceptive failure: withdrawal

| Reference | N for Analysis | Life-Table 12-Month % Pregnant | Risk of Pregnancy — Pearl Index Pregnancy Rate | | | Characteristics of the Sample[w] | LFU (%)[g] | Comments |
			Index	Total Exposure	Maximum Exposure			
Vessey et al., 1982	?		6.7	674 Yr.	?	All white; at recruitment aged 25–39 and married; at enrollment, all women had been using the diaphragm, IUD, or pill successfully for at least 5 months	0.3[t,v]	Britain; Oxford/FPA study
Bracher and Santow, 1992	94	14.2				25% aged <20, 66% aged 20–29, 9% aged 30+; 57% parity 0; 92% married or cohabiting	25[r]	Australian Family Survey; first use of method
Westoff et al., 1961	~74		16.7	1,287 Mo.		All married; all white	5.7[r]	FGMA study
Cliquet et al., 1977	2,316	17.3			?	All aged 30–34 living in Belgium; 93% living as married[t]	22[r]	Belgium; 1971 National Survey on Family Development (NEGO II)
Trussell and Vaughan, 1999	440	18.8				Aged 15–44[t]	21[r]	NSFG 1995
Fu et al., 1999	?	20.1					21[r]	NSFG 1995; probability when standardized and corrected for estimated underreporting of abortion = 27.1[s]

(continued)

Table 27–4 Summary of studies of contraceptive failure: withdrawal—*(cont'd)*

Reference	N for Analysis	Risk of Pregnancy				Characteristics of the Sample^w	LFU (%)^g	Comments
		Life-Table 12-Month % Pregnant	Pearl Index Pregnancy Rate					
			Index	Total Exposure	Maximum Exposure			
Debusschere, 1980	3,561	20.8				Aged 16–44 living in Flanders; 85% married^t	40^r	Belgium; 1975–1976 National Survey on Family Development (NEGO III)
Peel, 1972	62		21.9	1,640 Mo.	60 Mo.	All married	2.9^t	Britain; Hull Family Survey

Notes:

a Updated from Trussell and Kost (1987), Table 1.

c Calculated by James Trussell from data in the article.

g Most of these studies incorrectly report the loss to follow-up probability (LFU) as the number of women lost at any time during the study divided by the total number of women entering the study. Thus, these are the probabilities presented in the table. However, the correct measure of LFU would be a gross life-table probability. When available, gross 12-month probabilities are denoted by the letter "g."

r Nonresponse rate for entire survey.

s Fu et al., (1999) (1995 NSFG) — age, union status, poverty status.

t Total for all methods in the study.

v The authors report that LFU for "relevant reasons (withdrawal of cooperation or loss of contact)" was 0.3% per year in the 1982 study. In the 1932 study, women had been followed for 9.5 years on average; if 0.3% are LFU per year, then 2.8% would be LFU in 9.5 years. LFU including death and emigration is about twice as high as LFU for "relevant reasons."

w Unless otherwise noted, characteristics refer to females.

For table references, see reference section.

Table 27–5 Summary of studies of contraceptive failure: fertility awareness methods[a]

Reference	Method	N for Analysis	Life-Table 12-Month % Pregnant	Risk of Pregnancy — Pearl Index Pregnancy Rate — Index	Total Exposure	Maximum Exposure	Characteristics of the Sample	LFU (%)[g]	Comments
Trussell and Grummer Strawn, 1990	Ovulation	725	3.2				Mean age = 30; proven fertility; agreed to use OM alone; cohabiting; 765 of 869 learned OM to satisfaction of teachers; 725 entered effectiveness study	?	Reanalysis of W.H.O. (1981) trial; probability based on 13 cycles of *perfect* use
Arévalo, et al., 2004	TwoDay	450	3.5				23% aged 18–24; 29% aged 25–29; 26% aged 30–34; 22% aged 35–39; all parous	4.4	Guatemala, Peru, and the Philippines
Rice et al., 1981	Calendar + BBT	723	8.2				Aged 19–44; 9% aged 19–24, 54% aged 25–34, 37% aged 35–44; all parity 1+	3.4[c]	United States, France, Colombia, Canada, Mauritius
Dolack, 1978	Ovulation	329		10.5[c]	3,354 Cy.	?	Aged 19–48; mean age = 28; 40% had used oral contraceptives prior to study	18.0[c]	
Arévalo et al., 2002	Standard Days	478	12.0					7.1	Bolivia, Peru, Philippines
Johnston et al.,	CervicalMucus + BBT + Other Signs	268	13.3[c]				73% aged 22–32; all married or de facto married; 48% ≥12 years education (n = 460)	33.9[c,t]	Australia; probability based on 13 cycles
Wade et al., 1981	Cervical Mucus + BBT + Calendar	239	13.9[c]				Aged 20–39; 78% married	11.4[c,g]	Random assignment to OM or CM + BBT + Cal
Johnston et al., 1978	Calendar + BBT + Other Signs	192	14.3				73% aged 22–32; all married or de facto married; 48% ≥12 years education (n = 460)	33.9[c,t]	Australia; probability based on 13 cycles
Tietze et al., 1951	Calendar	409		14.4	7,267 Mo.	>60 Mo.	57% aged 25–34	13.4[c,t]	

(continued)

Table 27–5 Summary of studies of contraceptive failure: fertility awareness methods[a]—(cont'd)

Reference	Method	N for Analysis	Life-Table 12-Month % Pregnant	Risk of Pregnancy Pearl Index Pregnancy Rate			Characteristics of the Sample	LFU (%)[g]	Comments
				Index	Total Exposure	Maximum Exposure			
Vessey et al., 1982	Rhythm	?		15.5	161 Yr.	?	All white; at recruitment aged 25–39 and married; at enrollment, all women had been using the diaphragm, IUD, or pill successfully for at least 5 months	0.3[v]	Britain; Oxford/FPA study
Klaus et al., 1979	Ovulation	?	15.8[n]				67% aged 18–34; 52% ≥13 years education; some use of concurrent methods	2.9[n]	Probability based on only 12 cycles
Johnston et al., 1978	Cervical Mucus + BBT + Other Signs + Other Methods	94	16.0				78% aged 22–32; all married or de facto married; 53% ≥12 years education ("other" not limited to rhythm)	33.9[c,t]	Australia; probability based on 13 cycles
Grady et al., 1986	Rhythm	167	16.1[s]				Aged 15–44; all marr e[t]	20.6[r]	NSFG 1982
Ball, 1976	Ovulation	124		16.8[c]	1,626 Cy.	22 Cy.	Aged 20–39	1.6[c]	Australia
Bracher and Santow, 1992	Rhythm	137	17.9				14% aged <20, 75% aged 20–29, 11% aged 30+; 46% parity 0; 92% married or cohabiting	25[r]	Australian Family Survey; first use of method
Kambic et al., 1981, 1982	Ovulation or Cervical Mucus + BBT	235	18.2[n]				81% aged 20–34; 83% married; approx. 30% used barrier methods concurrently[t]	6.5[n]	
Grady et al., 1983	Rhythm	412	18.3[s,c]				Aged 15–44; all married[t]	18.2[r]	NSFG 1973 and 1976

Table 27-5 Summary of studies of contraceptive failure: fertility awareness methods[a]—(cont'd)

			Risk of Pregnancy					
				Pearl Index Pregnancy Rate				
Reference	Method	N for Analysis	Life-Table 12-Month % Pregnant	Index	Total Exposure	Maximum Exposure	Characteristics of the Sample	LFU (%)[g]	Comments
Johnston et al., 1978	Ovulation + Other Methods	71	18.8				80% aged 22–32; all married or de facto married; 49% ≥12 years education ("other" not limited to rhythm)	33.9[c,t]	Australia; probability based on 13 cycles
Vaughan et al., 1977	Rhythm	220	19.1[s]				Aged 15–44; all married[t]	19.0[r]	NSFG 1973
W.H.O., 1981	Ovulation	725	19.6				Mean age about 30; proven fertility; agreed to use OM alone; 54% desired no more children; 765 of 869 learned OM to satisfaction of teachers; 725 entered effectiveness study	?	New Zealand, India, Ireland, Philippines, El Salvador; probability based on 13 cycles
Trussell and Vaughan, 1999		250	19.8				Aged 15–44[t]	21[r]	NSFG 1995
Fu et al., 1999		?	20.2					21[r]	NSFG 1995; probability when standardized and corrected for estimated underreporting of abortion = 25.3[s]

(continued)

Table 27-5 Summary of studies of contraceptive failure: fertility awareness methods[a]—(cont'd)

Reference	Method	N for Analysis	Risk of Pregnancy					Characteristics of the Sample	LFU (%)[g]	Comments
			Life-Table 12-Month % Pregnant	Pearl Index Pregnancy Rate						
				Index	Total Exposure	Maximum Exposure				
Jones and Forrest, 1992	Rhythm	289	20.9					Aged 15–44[r]	21[r]	NSFG 1988; probability when standardized and corrected for estimated underreporting of abortion = 31.4[s]
Bartzen, 1967	BBT	335		21.3[c]	4,824 Cy.	58 Mo.		Aged 19–45; mean age = 28	11.6[c]	
Schirm et al., 1982	Rhythm	412	23.7[s]					Aged 15–44; all married[t]	18.2[r]	NSFG 1973 and 1976
Marshall, 1976	Ovulation + BBT	84		23.9[c]	1,195 Cy.	32 Mo.		67% aged 20–34	1.2[c]	Britain
Johnston et al., 1978	Ovulation	586	26.4					59% aged 22–32; all married or de facto married; 44% ≥12 years education	33.9[c,t]	Australia; probability based on 13 cycles

(continued)

Table 27-5 Summary of studies of contraceptive failure: fertility awareness methods[a]—(cont'd)

Reference	Method	N for Analysis	Risk of Pregnancy				Characteristics of the Sample	LFU (%)[g]	Comments
			Life-Table 12-Month % Pregnant	Pearl Index Pregnancy Rate					
				Index	Total Exposure	Maximum Exposure			
Wade et al., 1981	Ovulation	191	37.2[c]				Aged 20–39; 74% married	13.8[c,g]	Random assignment to OM or CM + BBT + Cal

Notes:

[a] Updated from Trussell and Kost (1987), Table 3.

[c] Calculated by James Trussell from data in the article.

[g] Most of these studies incorrectly report the loss to follow-up probability (LFU) as the number of women lost at any time during the study divided by the total number of women entering the study. Thus, these are the probabilities presented in the table. However, the correct measure of LFU would be a gross life-table probability. When available, gross 12-month probabilities are denoted by the letter "g."

[n] Only net probabilities for this study.

[r] Nonresponse rate for entire survey.

[s] Standardized: Vaughan et al., (1977) (1973 NSFG)—intention (the average of probabilities for preventers and delayers); Grady et al., (1983) (1973 and 1976 NSFG)—intention. Our calculation (the average of probabilities for preventers and delayers); Schirm et al., (1982) (1973 and 1976 NSFG)—intention, age, and income; Grady et al., (1986) (1982 NSFG)—intention, age, poverty status, and parity; Jones and Forrest, (1992) (1988 NSFG)—age, marital status, and poverty status; Fu et al., (1999) (1995 NSFG)—age, union status, poverty status.

[t] Total for all methods in the study.

[v] The authors report that LFU for "relevant reasons" (withdrawal of cooperation or loss of contact)" was 0.3% per year in the 1982 study. In the 1982 study, women had been followed for 9.5 years on average; if 0.3% are LFU per year, then 2.8% would be LFU in 9.5 years. LFU including death and emigration is about twice as high as LFU for "relevant reasons."

For table references, see reference section.

Table 27–6 Summary of studies of contraceptive failure: cervical cap and other female barrier methods with spermicide[a]

Reference	Method Brand	N for Analysis	Risk of Pregnancy				Characteristics of the Sample	LFU (%)[g]	Comments
			Life-Table 12-Month % Pregnant	Pearl Index Pregnancy Rate					
				Index	Total Exposure	Maximum Exposure			
Shihata and Trussell, 1991	FemCap	106	4.8					0.0[g]	Probability based on 13 cycles
Denniston and Putney, 1981	Prentif Cavity-rim	110	8.0[a,r]				98% aged 20–35; 70% nulliparous	20.9[c]	
Cagen, 1986	Prentif Cavity-rim	620	8.1[n]				87% aged 20–34; 80% always used spermicide and 14% never did	38.5[c]	LFU = "no response"
Koch, 1982	Prentif Cavity-rim	372	8.4				76% aged 20–29: 65% college graduates	8.0[c]	Women advised also to use condom for the first several cap uses
Mauck et al., 1996	Lea's Shield	79	8.7[b]				Mean age = 29.6, mean education = 14.2 years; 19% nulliparous	6.4[b,g]	
Richwald et al., 1989	Prentif Cavity-rim	3,433	11.3				Mean age 29.0; 91% white non-Hispanic; 80% unmarried; almost 60% college graduates; 64% one or more previous pregnancies; 6.1% failure rate among perfect users, 11.9% among imperfect users	18[g]	Women advised to use extra spermicide or use condoms during first 2 months of use; 15 sites; 14 in Los Angeles, 1 in Santa Fe
Mauck et al., 1999	FemCap	355	13.5[c]				Mean age = 29.1; 23% nulligravid	3.7[c]	Random assignment to FemCap or Ortho All-Flex diaphragm

(continued)

Table 27–6 Summary of studies of contraceptive failure: cervical cap and other female barrier methods with spermicide[a]—(cont'd)

Reference	Method Brand	N for Analysis	Life-Table 12-Month % Pregnant	Pearl Index Pregnancy Rate Index	Total Exposure	Maximum Exposure	Characteristics of the Sample	LFU (%)[g]	Comments
					Risk of Pregnancy				
Powell et al., 1986	Prentif Cavity-rim and Vimule	477	16.6				67% aged 25–34 "about half" unmarried; 97% high school graduates; 17% using the pill when fitted for cap	43.8[c]	Canada; back-up methods encouraged (including the emergency contraceptive pills used by 23 women in cases of cap dislodgement)
Bernstein et al., 1986	Prentif Cavity-rim	687[c]	17.4				95% aged ≤35, 16% married, 96% ≥ high school completion	26.3[c-g]	Random assignment to the diaphragm or cervical cap
Kassell and McElroy, 1981	Prentif Cavity-rim	90		18.1[c]	731 Mo.	12 Mo.	Mean age = 23.6; mean education = 14.7 years	10.0[c]	
Boehm, 1983	Prentif Cavity-rim	47		18.1[c]	397 Mo.	12 Mo.		31.6	All women reported exclusive use of cap
Lehfeldt and Sivin, 1984	Prentif Cavity-rim	130	19.1				37% aged 16–25; 72% college graduates; 91% nulliparous	7.2 [c]	All women agreed to exclusive use of cap

(continued)

Table 27-6 Summary of studies of contraceptive failure: cervical cap and other female barrier methods with spermicide[a]—(cont'd)

			Risk of Pregnancy						
				Pearl Index Pregnancy Rate					
Reference	Method Brand	N for Analysis	Life-Table 12-Month % Pregnant	Index	Total Exposure	Maximum Exposure	Characteristics of the Sample	LFU (%)[g]	Comments
Smith and Lee, 1984	Prentif Cavity-rim and Vimule	33	27.0				80% aged 20–29; clients at university student health service	1.5–4.6[c]	Regular users for whom the cap (with spermicide) was the sole method used "during the fertile portion of the cycle"

Notes:

[a] Updated from Trussell and Kost (1987), Table 4.

[b] 6-month net probability; 12-month probability not available.

[c] Calculated by James Trussell from data in the article.

[g] Most of these studies incorrectly report the loss to follow-up (LFU) probability as the number of women lost at any time during the study divided by the total number of women entering the study. Thus, these are the probabilities presented in the table. However, the correct measure of LFU would be a gross life-table probability. When available, gross 12-month probabilities are denoted by the letter "g."

[n] Only net probabilities available for this study.

For table references, see reference section.

Table 27–7 Summary of studies of contraceptive failure: sponge[a]

Reference	N for Analysis	Life-Table 12-Month % Pregnant	Characteristics of the Sample	LFU (%)[g]	Comments
Jones and Forrest, 1992	227	14.5	Aged 15–44[t]	21[r]	NSFG 1988
Edelman et al., 1984	722	17.0	89% aged 20–34, 28% married; 77% ≥13 years education; 94% white, 49% never-married; 38% used oral contraceptives prior to entering study	33.2[c-g]	Random assignment to the diaphragm or sponge
McIntyre and Higgins, 1986	723	17.4	89% aged 20–34, 28% married; 77% ≥13 years education; 94% white, 49% never-married; 38% used oral contraceptives prior to entering the study	33.2[c-g]	A reanalysis of data used by Edelman et al. (1984); random assignment to the diaphragm or sponge; much higher probability for parous women
Trussell and Vaughan, 1999	111	18.4	Aged 15–44[t]	21[r]	NSFG 1995
Bounds and Guillebaud, 1984	126	24.5	92% aged 20–34; all married/consensual union; "most" ≥13 years education; 99% white	1.7[g]	Britain; random assignment to the diaphragm or sponge

Notes:

[a] Updated from Trussell and Kost (1987), Table 4.

[c] Calculated by James Trussell from data in the article.

[g] Most of these studies incorrectly report the loss to follow-up (LFU) probability as the number of women lost at any time during the study divided by the total number of women entering the study. Thus, these are the probabilities presented in the table. However, the correct measure of LFU would be a gross life-table probability. When available, gross 12-month probabilities are denoted by the letter "g."

[r] Nonresponse rate for entire survey.

[t] Total for all methods in the study.

For table references, see reference section.

Table 27-8 Summary of studies of contraceptive failure: diaphragm with spermicide[a]

		Risk of Pregnancy					
		Life-Table 12-Month	Pearl Index Pregnancy Rate				
Reference	**N for Analysis**	**% Pregnant**	**Index**	**Total Exposure**	**Maximum Exposure**	**Characteristics of the Sample**	**LFU (%)[g]** **Comments**
Stim, 1980	1,238		1.1[c]	911 Yr.	4 Yr.	Median age = 24	19.5 Fit-free diaphragm without spermicides; continuous wearing with brief daily removal for cleaning but not within 6 hours after intercourse; 1,238 women given device, with follow-up of 997
Lane et al., 1976	2,168	2.1[c]				61% aged 21–34; 71% unmarried; 92% white	1.2[c-g] Probability downward biased due to improper exposure allocated to women LFU
Vessey and Wiggins, 1974	4,052		2.4	5,909 Mo.	>60 Mo.	All white; at recruitment aged 25–39 and married; all had been using the diaphragm for at least 5 months at enrollment; no previous pill use	1.0[v] Britain; Oxford/FPA study
Vessey et al., 1982	?		5.5	2,582 Yr.	24 Mo.	All white and aged 25–34; all married at recruitment; at enrollment, all women had been using the diaphragm, IUD, or pill successfully for at least 5 months	0.3[l,v] Britain; Oxford/FPA study
Mauck et al., 1999	403	7.9[d]				Mean age = 28.8; 25% null gravid	4.2[c] Ortho All-Flex diaphragm; random assignment to Ortho All-Flex diaphragm or FemCap

(continued)

Table 27–8 Summary of studies of contraceptive failure: diaphragm with spermicide[a]—(cont'd)

		Life-Table 12-Month % Pregnant	Pearl Index Pregnancy Rate					
Reference	N for Analysis		Index	Total Exposure	Maximum Exposure	Characteristics of the Sample	LFU (%)[g]	Comments
Trussell and Vaughan, 1999	166	8.1				Aged 15–44[t]	21[r]	NSFG 1995
Loudon et al., 1991	269		8.7	2,350 Mo.	12 Mo.	Mean age = 28.6; 57% gravidity 0; 68% married or cohabiting; 54% already using the diaphragm at start of trial	>3.7	Britain; random assignment of spermicide: either C-Film or jelly
Fu et al., 1999	?	9.2					21[r]	NSFG 1995; probability when standardized and corrected for estimated underreporting of abortion = 15.9s
Dubrow and Kuder, 1958	873		9.3	5,814 Mo.	48 Mo.	Mean age = 25; 39% black; 45% Puerto Rican; 93% ≤12 years education[t]	38.0[c]	
Jones and Forrest, 1992	472	10.4				Aged 15–44[t]	21[r]	NSFG 1988; probability when standardized and corrected for estimated underreporting of abortion = 22.0s
Hall, 1973	347	10.6				Approximately 75% aged 20–24; 47% black; 38% Hispanic; all postpartum	16.0	
Bounds and Guillebaud, 1984	123	10.9				90% aged 20–34; all married/consensual union; "most" ≥13 years education; 96% white	0.0	Britain; random assignment to the diaphragm or sponge

(continued)

Table 27–8 Summary of studies of contraceptive failure: diaphragm with spermicide[a]—(cont'd)

Reference	N for Analysis	Life-Table 12-Month % Pregnant	Pearl Index Pregnancy Rate — Index	Pearl Index Pregnancy Rate — Total Exposure	Maximum Exposure	Characteristics of the Sample	LFU (%)[g]	Comments
Edelman et al., 1984	717	12.5				88% aged 20–34; 55% never married; 76% ≥13 years education; 94% white; 35% used oral contraceptives prior to entering study	37.8[c,g]	Random assignment to the diaphragm or sponge
McIntyre and Higgins, 1986	717	12.9				88% aged 20–34; 55% never married; 76% ≥13 years education; 94% white; 35% used oral contraceptives prior to entering study	37.8[c,g]	A reanalysis of data used by Edelman et al. (1984); random assignment to the diaphragm or sponge
Vaughan et al., 1977	166	13.1[s]				Aged 15–44; all married[t]	19.0[r]	NSFG 1973
Dingle and Tietze, 1963	189		14.3	2,012 Mo.	36 Mo.	Median age = 22.8	3.2[t]	
Grady et al., 1983	349	14.3[c,s]				Aged 15–44; all married[t]	18.2[r]	NSFG 1973 and 1976
Bernstein et al., 1986	707[c]	16.7				96% aged ≤35; 17% married; 97% ≥ high school completion	33.5[c,g]	Random assignment to the diaphragm or cervical cap
Grady et al., 1986	257	17.0[s]				Aged 15–44; all married[t]	20.6[r]	NSFG 1982
Tietze and Lewit, 1967	1,197	17.9				86% aged <30; all married; 60% ≥ high school completion; 50% white	7.2[g]	

(continued)

Table 27–8 Summary of studies of contraceptive failure: diaphragm with spermicide[a]—(cont'd)

Reference	N for Analysis	Life-Table 12-Month % Pregnant	Pearl Index Pregnancy Rate Index	Risk of Pregnancy — Pearl Index Pregnancy Rate Total Exposure	Risk of Pregnancy — Pearl Index Pregnancy Rate Maximum Exposure	Characteristics of the Sample	LFU (%)[g]	Comments
Schirm et al., 1982	349	18.6[s]				Aged 15–44; all married[t]	18.2[r]	NSFG 1973 and 1976
Kovacs et al., 1986	324	20.9[t]				28% aged 24–26	52.2	Australia
Bracher and Santow, 1992	219	21.0				12% aged <20; 77% aged 20–29, 11% aged 30+; 56% parity 0; 87% married or cohabiting	25[r]	Australian Family Survey; first use of method
Bounds et al., 1995	80	21.2				Mean age = 29.6; 60% nulliparous	1.3	Britain; probability during consistent use = 12.3; random assignment to diaphragm with spermicide or diaphragm only
Smith et al., 1995	110	24.1				Mean age = 28.8	26.0	Britain; fit-free diaphragm without spermicide; continuous wearing with brief daily removal for cleaning but not within 6 hours after intercourse

(continued)

Table 27-8 Summary of studies of contraceptive failure: diaphragm with spermicide[a]—(cont'd)

| Reference | N for Analysis | Life-Table 12-Month % Pregnant | Pearl Index Pregnancy Rate | | | Characteristics of the Sample | LFU (%)[g] | Comments |
			Index	Total Exposure	Maximum Exposure			
Bounds et al., 1995	84	28.6				Mean age = 29.5; 55% nulliparous	0.0[g]	Britain; diaphragm without spermicide; probability during consistent use = 19.3; random assignment to diaphragm only or diaphragm with spermicide

Notes:

[a] Updated from Trussell and Kost (1987), Table 3.

[c] Calculated by James Trussell from data in the article.

[d] 6-month probability; 12-month probability not available.

[g] Most of these studies incorrectly report the loss to follow-up (LFU) probability as the number of women lost at any time during the study divided by the total number of women entering the study. Thus, these are the probabilities presented in the table. However, the correct measure of LFU would be a gross life-table probability. When available, gross 12-month probabilities are denoted by the letter "g."

[r] Nonresponse rate for entire survey.

[s] Standardized: Vaughan et al., (1977) (1973 NSFG)—intention (the average of probabilities for preventers and delayers); Grady et al., (1983) (1973 and 1976 NSFG)—intention. Our calculation (the average of probabilities for preventers and delayers); Schirm et al., (1982) (1973 and 1976 NSFG)—intention, age, and income; Grady et al., (1986) (1982 NSFG)—intention, age, poverty status, and parity; Jones and Forrest, (1992) (1988 NSFG)—age, marital status, and poverty status; Fu et al., (1999) (1995 NSFG)—age, union status, poverty status.

[t] Total for all methods in the study.

[v] The authors report that LFU "or "relevant reasons (withdrawal of cooperation or loss of contact)" was 0.3% per year in the 1982 study and "about 10 per 1,000" per year in the 1974 study. In the 1982 study, women had been followed for 9.5 years or average; if 0.3% are LFU per year, then 2.8% would be LFU in 9.5 years. LFU including death and emigration is about twice as high as LFU for "relevant reasons."

For table references, see reference section.

Table 27–9 Summary of studies of contraceptive failure: male condom[a]

			Risk of Pregnancy					
		Life-Table	Pearl Index Pregnancy Rate					
Reference	N for Analysis	12-Month % Pregnant	Index	Total Exposure	Maximum Exposure	Characteristics of the Sample[w]	LFU (%)[g]	Comments
Potts and McDevitt, 1975	397	2.1[b]				77% males ≥ age 40; all married	4.8[c]	Britain; postal trial of spermicidally lubricated condom
Steiner et al., 2003	436	3.3[d]				72% living with partner	5.8	Kimono Select latex condom; random assignment to Kimono Select latex or eZ-on plastic condom
Peel, 1972	96		3.9	3,689 Mo.	60 Mo.	All married	2.9[t]	Britain; Hull Family Survey
Frezieres et al., 1999	383	4.1[d]				Mean age of male and female subjects = 27	3.9[c]	Avanti plastic condom; random assignment to Avanti plastic or Ramses latex condom
Glass et al., 1974	2,057	4.2	4.4	10,000c Yr.	24 Mo.	All white; at recruitment aged 25–39 and married; at enrollment, all women had been using the diaphragm, IUD, or pill successfully for at least 5 months	<1.0[v]	Britain; Oxford/FPA study
Vessey et al., 1988	?					All white; at recruitment aged 25–39 and married; at enrollment, all women had been using the diaphragm, IUD, or pill successfully for at least 5 months	?	Britain; Oxford/FPA study
John, 1973	85		5.7[c]	261 Yr.	>7 Yr.	?	?	Britain; retrospective study

(continued)

Table 27-9 Summary of studies of contraceptive failure: male condom[a]—(cont'd)

Reference	N for Analysis	Life-Table 12-Month % Pregnant	Pearl Index Pregnancy Rate			Characteristics of the Sample[w]	LFU (%)[g]	Comments
			Index	Total Exposure	Maximum Exposure			
Vessey et al., 1982	?		6.0	4,317 Yr.	24 Mo.	All white and aged 25–34; all married at recruitment; at enrollment all women were using the diaphragm, IUD, or pill successfully for at least 5 months	0.3[t,v]	Britain; Oxford/FPA study
Frezieres et al., 1999	384	6.2[d]				Mean age of male and female subjects = 27	2.9[c]	Ramses latex condom; random assignment to Ramses latex or Avanti plastic condom
Jones and Forrest, 1992	1,728	7.2				Aged 15–44[t]	21[r]	NSFG 1988; probability when standardized and corrected for estimated underreporting of abortion = 15.8s
Walsh et al., 2003	415	7.9[d]				74% > high school education[t]	0.7	Trojan-Enz or LifeStyles latex condom; random assignment to Trojan-Enz latex or LifeStyles latex condom or Tacylon plastic condom
Bracher and Santow, 1992	262	8.1				16% aged <20, 65% aged 20–29, 19% aged 30+; 48% parity 0; 83% married or cohabiting	25[r]	Australian Family Survey; first use of method
Trussell and Vaughan, 1999	2,925	8.7				Aged 15–44[t]	21[r]	NSFG 1995
Steiner et al., 2003	442	9.2[d]				73% living with partner	5.1	eZ-on plastic condom; random assignment to eZ-on plastic or Kimono Select latex condom

(continued)

Table 27–9 Summary of studies of contraceptive failure: male condom[a]—*(cont'd)*

		Risk of Pregnancy					
		Life-Table	Pearl Index Pregnancy Rate				
Reference	N for Analysis	12-Month % Pregnant	Index	Total Exposure	Maximum Exposure	Characteristics of the Sample[w]	LFU (%)[g] Comments
Schirm et al., 1982	1,223	9.6[s]				Aged 15–44; all married[t]	18.2[r] NSFG 1973 and 1976
Grady et al., 1983	1,223	9.7[s,c]				Aged 15–44; all married[t]	18.2[r] NSFG 1973 and 1976
Fu et al., 1999	?	9.7					21[r] NSFG 1995; probability when standardized and corrected for estimated underreporting of abortion = 14.[s]
Vaughan et al., 1977	696	10.1[s]				Aged 15–44; all married[t]	19.0[r] NSFG 1973
Walsh et al., 2003	415	10.8[d]				74% > high school education[t]	0.7 Tactylon plastic condom; random assignment to Tactylon plastic or Trojan-Enz latex or LifeStyles latex condom
Grady et al., 1986	526	13.8[s]				Aged 15–44; all married[t]	20.6[r] NSFG 1982
Westoff et al., 1961	~212		13.8[c]	10,062 Mo.	?	All married	5.7[r] FGMA study

(continued)

CONTRACEPTIVE TECHNOLOGY

Table 27–9 Summary of studies of contraceptive failure: male condom—*(cont'd)*

Notes:

a Updated from Trussell and Kost (1987), Table 6.

b 24-month probability; 12-month probability not published.

c Calculated by James Trussell from data in the article.

d 6-month probability; 12-month probability not available.

g Most of these studies incorrectly report the loss to follow-up probability (LFU) as the number of women lost at any time during the study divided by the total number of women entering the study. Thus, these are the probabilities presented in the table. However, the correct measure of LFU would be a gross life-table probability. When available, gross 12-month probabilities are denoted by the letter "g."

r Nonresponse rate for entire survey.

s Standardized: Vaughan et al., (1977) (1973 NSFG)—intention (the average of probabilities for preventers and delayers); Grady et al., (1983) (1973 and 1976 NSFG)—intention. Our calculation (the average of probabilities for preventers and delayers); Schirm et al., (1982) (1973 and 1976 NSFG)—intention, age, and income; Grady et al., (1986) (1982 NSFG)—intention, age, poverty status, and parity; Jones and Forrest, (1992) (1988 NSFG)—age, marital status, and poverty status; Fu et al., (1999) (1995 NSFG)—age, union status, poverty status.

t Total for all methods in the study.

v The authors report that LFU for "relevant reasons (withdrawal of cooperation or loss of contact)" was 0.3% per year in 1982 study. In the 1982 study, women had been followed for 9.5 years on average; if 0.3% are LFU per year, then 2.8% would be LFU in 9.5 years. LFU including death and emigration is about twice as high as LFU for "relevant reasons."

w Unless otherwise noted, characteristics refer to female.

For table references, see reference section.

Table 27–10 Summary of studies of contraceptive failure: progestin-only pill[a]

Reference	Method Brand	N for Analysis	Risk of Pregnancy						Characteristics of the Sample	LFU (%)[g]	Comments
			Life-Table 12-Month % Pregnant	Pearl Index Pregnancy Rate							
				Index	Total Exposure	Maximum Exposure					
Broome and Fetherby, 1990	Femulen, Micronor, Microval, Neogest	358		0.2	18,125 Mo.	150 Mo.				?	At a minimum, 14,103 months (78% of the total exposure) capture use beyond the first year; 46% of women used for >4 years and 13% used for >8 years. Retrospective chart review; England
Postlethwaite, 1979	Femulen (Ethynodiol diacetate 0.5 mg)	309	1.1[c]						Aged 17–48	21.0[c]	Britain
Shroff et al., 1987	Femulen (Ethynodiol diacetate 0.5 mg)	425	1.1[n]						72% aged 16–34; 25% nulligravid	12.7[c]	Britain; authors employed by manufacturer
Board, 1971	Micronor (Norethindrone 0.35 mg)	154		1.3	1,882 Mo.	19 Mo.				?	
Keifer, 1973	Micronor (Norethindrone 0.35 mg)	151		1.68	2,141 Mo.	26 Mo.			Aged 18–45; 84% aged 21–35; 74% previous oral contraceptive users; at least 32% current users at start	4.6[c]	

(continued)

Table 27-10 Summary of studies of contraceptive failure: progestin-only pill[a]—(cont'd)

Reference	Method Brand	N for Analysis	Risk of Pregnancy — Life-Table 12-Month % Pregnant	Risk of Pregnancy — Pearl Index Pregnancy Rate Index	Risk of Pregnancy — Pearl Index Pregnancy Rate Total Exposure	Risk of Pregnancy — Pearl Index Pregnancy Rate Maximum Exposure	Characteristics of the Sample	LFU (%)[g]	Comments
Vessey et al., 1985		?		1.98[c]	404 Yr.	12 Mo.	All white and aged 25–34; all married at recruitment; at enrollment, all women had been using the diaphragm, IUD, or pill successfully for at least 5 months	0.3[t,v]	Britain; Oxford/FPA study
Korba and Paulson, 1974	Ovrette (Norgestrel 0.075 mg)	2,202		2.13[c]	29,306 Mo.	67 Mo.		?	Authors employed by manufacturer
McQuarrie et al., 1972	Micronor (Norethindrone 0.35 mg)	318		2.64[c]	3,453 Cy.	27 Mo.	Aged 16–42; mean age = 26; all white	2.2[c]	
Nelson, 1973	Megestrol acetate (0.5 mg)	342		2.7	3,552 Mo.	41 Mo.		14.6[c]	
Jubhari et al., 1974	Quingestanol acetate (0.3 mg)	382	2.9[r]				Mean age = 23; "predominantly white, single anc nulliparous"	14.0	
Hawkins and Benster, 1977	Norethisterone (0.35 mg)	200	6.8				Mean age = 25; postpartum women, 71% within 3 months cf delivery[t]	5.2[c]	Britain
Hawkins and Benster, 1977	Megestrol acetate (0.5 mg)	174	8.7				Mean age = 25; postpartum women, 71% within 3 months cf delivery[t]	8.4[c]	Britain
Sheth et al., 1982	Levonorgestrel (0.30 mg)	128	9.5[s]				Mean age = 25.7	2.1[t]	Yugoslavia, India
Hawkins and Benster, 1977	Chlormadinone acetate (0.5 mg)	182	9.6				Mean age = 26; postpartum women, 71% within 3 months of delivery[t]	3.3[c]	Britain

(continued)

Table 27–10 Summary of studies of contraceptive failure: progestin-only pill[a]—(cont'd)

Reference	Method Brand	N for Analysis	Risk of Pregnancy					Characteristics of the Sample	LFU (%)[g]	Comments
			Life-Table 12-Month % Pregnant	Pearl Index Pregnancy Rate						
				Index	Total Exposure	Maximum Exposure				
Sheth et al., 1982	Norethisterone (0.35 mg)	130	13.2[n]					Mean age = 25.6	2.1[t]	Yugoslavia, India

Notes:

[a] Updated from Trussell and Kost (1987), Table 8.

[c] Calculated by James Trussell from data in the article.

[g] Most of these studies incorrectly report the loss to follow-up (LFU) probability as the number of women lost at any time during the study divided by the total number of women entering the study. Thus, these are the probabilities presented in the table. However, the correct measure of LFU would be a gross life-table probability. When available, gross 12-month probabilities are denoted by the letter "g."

[n] Only net probabilities available for this study.

[t] Total for all methods in the study.

[v] The authors report that LFU for "relevant reasons (withdrawal of cooperation or loss of contact)" was 0.3% per year in the 1982 study. In the 1985 study, women had probably been followed for 12.5 years on average; if 0.3% are LFU per year, then 3.7% would be LFU in 12.5 years. LFU including death and emigration is about twice as high as LFU for "relevant reasons."

For table references, see reference section.

Table 27–11 Summary of studies of contraceptive failure: combined oral contraceptives, vaginal rings, and patches[a]

Reference	Method Brand	N for Analysis	Life-Table 12-Month % Pregnant	Pearl Index Pregnancy Rate — Index	Pearl Index Pregnancy Rate — Total Exposure	Pearl Index Pregnancy Rate — Maximum Exposure	Characteristics of the Sample	LFU (%)[g]	Comments
Preston, 1972	Norlestrin 2.5 (80%)	378	0.0[c]				Aged 15–46; 46% aged 25–34; 36% white; 64% on pill at start	9.5	Author employed by manufacturer; pill not marketed
Ledger, 1970	Ortho-Novum 1/80	144	0.0[c]				All aged 14–43; mean age = 24; mostly graduate students or wives of students	14.0[c]	
Woutersz, 1981	Lo/Ovral	1,700		0.12	22,489 Cy.	53 Cy.	65% aged 20–29; 55% on pill at start	23.8	Author employed by manufacturer
Korba and Heil, 1975	Ovral	6,806		0.19	127,872 Cy.	110 Cy.	Mean age = 25; 26% white; approximately 80% had not used other oral contraceptives within 3 months	?	Mexico, Puerto Rico, United States; author employed by manufacturer
Lammers and Oop ten Berg, 1991	Mercilon	1,684		0.20	25,970 Cy.	36 Cy.	23% aged <20, 51% aged 20–29, 14% aged 30–34; 12% aged 35+	?	Authors employed by manufacturer; Belgium, Denmark, Finland, France, Hungary, Netherlands, Norway, Poland, Sweden, Switzerland, West Germany, Yugoslavia
Ellis, 1987	Ortho-Novum 7/7/7	619		0.22	909[c] Yr.	?	Mean age = 24.5; 40.5% nulligravid	?	United States, Canada, France

(continued)

Table 27-11 Summary of studies of contraceptive failure: combined oral contraceptives, vaginal rings, and patches[a]—*(cont'd)*

Reference	Method Brand	N for Analysis	Life-Table 12-Month % Pregnant	Pearl Index Pregnancy Rate — Index	Pearl Index Pregnancy Rate — Total Exposure	Pearl Index Pregnancy Rate — Maximum Exposure	Characteristics of the Sample	LFU (%)[g]	Comments
Morigi and Pasquale, 1978	Modicon	1,168		0.24[c]	16,345 Cy.	53 Cy.	Aged 13–54; 85% aged 19–36; 61% previous use of oral contraceptives	?	Mexico, Puerto Rico, Canada, United States; author employed by manufacturer
Hughes, 1978	Ovamin	453	0.24[c]				Aged 16–40; % new users not stated	11.9[c]	Britain
Vessey et al., 1982	50 µg estrogen	?		0.25	10,400 Yr.	24 Mo.	All white and aged 25–34; all married at recruitment; at enrollment, all women had been using the diaphragm, IUD, or pill successfully for at least 5 months	0.3[t,v]	Britain; Oxford/FPA study
Runnebaum et al., 1992	Ortho-Cyclen	59,701		0.27[c]	342,348 Cy.	6 Cy.	Mean age = 24.0; 32% parous	?	Germany
Kaunitz et al., 1999	Ortho-Novum 7/7/7	321	0.30				Mean age = 27.8; 65% used hormonal contraception in prior month	6.9[c]	Trial design discontinued subjects who did not adhere to dosing schedule
Bannemerschult et al., 1997	Alesse	805		0.30	4,400 Cy.	6 Cy.	Mean age = 25.6	0.6[c]	Germany; some women who did not return for follow-up visits were excluded

(continued)

Table 27–11 Summary of studies of contraceptive failure: combined oral contraceptives, vaginal rings, and patches[a]—*(cont'd)*

				Risk of Pregnancy					
			Life-Table	Pearl Index Pregnancy Rate					
		N for	12-Month		Total	Maximum		LFU	
Reference	Method Brand	Analysis	% Pregnant	Index	Exposure	Exposure	Characteristics of the Sample	(%)[g]	Comments
Royal College, 1974		23,611		0.34	?	48 Mo.	75% aged 20–34; all married/living as married; 62% on pill at start (20% new users)	32.0[c]	Britain
Woutersz, 1983	Nordette	1,130		0.35	11,064 Cy.	31 Cy.	71% aged 20–30; 48% no use of hormones and not pregnant within 60 days of start	8.1[c]	Author employed by manufacturer
Vessey et al., 1982	<50 µg estrogen	?		0.38	5,158 Yr.	24 Mo.	All white and aged 25–34; all married at recruitment; at enrollment, all women had been using the diaphragm, IUD, or pill successfully for at least 5 months	0.3[v]	Britain; Oxford/FPA study
Kaunitz, 2000	Ortho-Novum 7/7/7	2,675	0.39[d]				Mean age = 28.5[t]	6.0[c]	Random assignment to Ortho-Novum 7/7/7 or Cyclessa; 2.5% of subjects discontinued for noncompliance
Parsey and Pong, 2000	Yasmin	326		0.41	3,201 Cy.	13 Cy.	Mean age = 26.4	?	
Kaunitz, 2000	Cyclessa	2,643	0.51[d]				Mean age = 28.5[t]	5.8[c]	Random assignment to Cyclessa or Ortho-Novum 7/7/7; 2.4% of subjects discontinued for non-compliance

(continued)

Table 27–11 Summary of studies of contraceptive failure: combined oral contraceptives, vaginal rings, and patches[a]—(cont'd)

Reference	Method Brand	N for Analysis	Risk of Pregnancy				Characteristics of the Sample	LFU (%)[g]	Comments
			Life-Table 12-Month % Pregnant	Pearl Index Pregnancy Rate					
				Index	Total Exposure	Maximum Exposure			
Anderson et al., 2003	Seasonale	456	0.055					8.6	Random assignment to Seasonale or Nordette; noncompliant patients excluded
Gauthier et al., 1992	Ortho Tri-Cyclen	661	0.57[b]				Mean age = 27.9; 24% nulligravid	?	France; 2 authors employed by manufacturer
Åkerlund et al., 1993	Mercilon	485		0.57[c]	4,543 Cy.	12 Mo.	Mean age = 23.8	?	Denmark, Norway, Sweden; random assignment to Mercilon or Marvelon; cycles excluded if the pill-taking period was less than 18 or more than 33 days or if the pill-free period was less than 5 or more than 9 days
Anderson et al., 2006	Seasonique	1,006	0.6				Mean age = 27.4	14.8	
Preston, 1974 and 1972	Norlestrin 2.5 (60%)	1,192		3[c]	14,536 Cy.	>18 Cy.	Aged 14-47; 35% aged 25-34; 47% white; 56% on pill at start	13.7	Author employed by manufacturer; pill not marketed

(continued)

Table 27-11 Summary of studies of contraceptive failure: combined oral contraceptives, vaginal rings, and patches[a]—*(cont'd)*

Reference	Method Brand	N for Analysis	Life-Table 12-Month % Pregnant	Risk of Pregnancy — Pearl Index Pregnancy Rate			Characteristics of the Sample	LFU (%)[g]	Comments
				Index	Total Exposure	Maximum Exposure			
Roumen et al., 2001	NuvaRing	1,145		0.64[c]	12,109 Cy.	13 Cy.	Mean age = 28.2	?	Austria, Belgium, Denmark, Finland, France, Germany, Israel, Netherlands, Norway, Spain, Sweden, United Kingdom
Archer et al., 1999	Alesse	1,708	0.69[b]				Mean age = 27.2	12.1	Cycles in which 3 or more consecutive active pills were missed and all subsequent cycles from that subject were excluded from the analysis
Smallwood et al., 2001	Evra patch	1,664	0.7				Mean age = 28.7	?	Australia, Austria, Belgium, France, Israel, Netherlands, Sweden, Switzerland, United Kingdom, United States
London et al., 1992	Triphasil (Tri-Levlen)	2,124		0.80	11,306 Cy.	6 Cy.	Mean age = 25.5	?	Random assignment to Triphasil or Ortho Tri-Cyclen

(continued)

| | | Life-Table 12-Month | Risk of Pregnancy | | | | | |
| | | | Pearl Index Pregnancy Rate | | | | | |
Reference	Method Brand	N for Analysis	% Pregnant	Index	Total Exposure	Maximum Exposure	Characteristics of the Sample	LFU (%)[g]	Comments
Åkerlund et al., 1993	Marvelon (Ortho-Cept, Desogen)	497		0.83[c]	4,688 Cy.	12 Mo.	Mean age = 23.1	?	Denmark, Norway, Sweden; random assignment to Marvelon or Mercilon; cycles excluded if the pill-taking period was less than 18 or more than 33 days or if the pill-free period was less than 5 or more than 9 days
Corson, 1990	Lo/Ovral	737		0.94[c]	9,727 Cy.	24 Cy.	Mean age = 24.3	?	Random assignment to Lo/Ovral or Ortho-Cyclen
London et al., 1992	Ortho Tri-Cyclen	2,110		0.94	11,006 Cy.	6 Cy.	Mean age = 25.6	?	Random assignment to Ortho Tri-Cyclen or Triphasil
Preston, 1974 and 1972	Norlestrin 2.5 (40%)	1,393		0.94[c]	15,265 Cy.	>18 Cy.	Aged 13–42; 27% aged 25–34; 39% white; 49% on pill at start	16.3	Author employed by manufacturer; pill not marketed
The Mircette Study Group, 1998	Mircette	1,226		1.02	14,050 Cy.	13 Cy.	Mean age = 28.3	6.8[c]	

(continued)

Table 27–11 Summary of studies of contraceptive failure: combined oral contraceptives, vaginal rings, and patches[a]—(cont'd)

Reference	Method Brand	N for Analysis	Life-Table 12-Month % Pregnant	Pearl Index Pregnancy Rate			Characteristics of the Sample	LFU (%)[g]	Comments
				Index	Total Exposure	Maximum Exposure			
Endrikat et al., 1995	Mercilon	219		1.04[c]	2,496 Cy.	12 Cy.	Mean age = 25.0	?	Austria, France; random assignment to Mercilon or Meliane; cycles excluded if more than two pills were missed or pill-taking was irregular
Oddsson et al., 2005	Microgynon	518	1.07				Mean age = 27.2; 53% nulligravid	6.4[c]	Random assignment to Microgynon or NuvaRing; Belgium, Brazil, Chile, Denmark, Finland, France, Germany, Italy, Norway, Spain, Sweden
Ellsworth, 1986	Triphasil	1,264		1.09	8,349 Cy.	34 Cy.	All < age 38	?	17 U.S. centers
Carson, 1990	Ortho-Cyclen	735		1.11[c]	9,351 Cy.	24 Cy.	Mean age = 24.6	?	Random assignment to Ortho-Cyclen or Lo/Ovral
Dieben et al., 2002	NuvaRing	2,322	1.18				Mean age = 28.2	?	United States, Canada, Europe; Pearl index for United States = 1.75; European results published separately by Roumen et al. (2001)

(continued)

Table 27–11 Summary of studies of contraceptive failure: combined oral contraceptives, vaginal rings, and patches[a]—(cont'd)

Reference	Method Brand	N for Analysis	Risk of Pregnancy					Characteristics of the Sample	LFU (%)[g]	Comments
			Life-Table 12-Month % Pregnant	Pearl Index Pregnancy Rate						
				Index	Total Exposure	Maximum Exposure				
Oddsson et al., 2005	NuvaRing	512	1.2					Mean age = 27.0; 57% nulligravid	6.4[c]	Random assignment to NuvaRing or Microgynon; Belgium, Brazil, Chile, Denmark, Finland, France, Germany, Italy, Norway, Spain, Sweden
Bachmann et al., 2004	Yaz	1,018	1.26					Mean age = 24.7	4.6	Argentina, Austria, Brazil, Poland, United States
Audet et al., 2001	Evra patch	811	1.3					Mean age = 28.0	3.9[c]	Random assignment to Evra patch or Triphasil
Anderson et al., 2003	Nordette	226	1.45						9.3	Random assignment to Nordette or Seasonale; noncompliant patients excluded
Preston, 1974 and 1972	Norlestrin 1.0 (60%)	1,872		1.47[c]	20,341 Cy.	>18 Cy.		Aged 14–44; 30% aged 25–34; 42% white; 55% on pill at start	13.1	Author employed by manufacturer; pill not marketed
Preston, 1974	Norlestrin 1.0 (20%)	276		1.59[c]	2,449 Cy.	?			?	Author employed by manufacturer; pill not marketed
Audet et al., 2001	Triphasil	605	1.8					Mean age = 27.8	7.9[c]	Random assignment to Triphasil or Evra patch

(continued)

Reference	Method Brand	N for Analysis	Risk of Pregnancy				Characteristics of the Sample	LFU (%)[g]	Comments
			Life-Table 12-Month % Pregnant	Pearl Index Pregnancy Rate					
				Index	Total Exposure	Maximum Exposure			
Vaughan et al., 1977		2,434	2.0[s]				Aged 15–44; all married[t]	19.0[r]	NSFG 1973
Bracher and Santow, 1992		1,830	2.2				42% aged <20, 49% aged 20–29, 9% aged 30+; 67% parity 0; 45% married or cohabiting	25[r]	Australian Family Survey, first use of method
Schirm et al., 1982		4,487	2.4[s]				Aged 15–44; all married[t]	18.2[r]	NSFG 1973 and 1976
Grady et al., 1983		4,487	2.5[c,s]				Aged 15–44; all married[t]	18.2[r]	NSFG 1973 and 1976
Bounds et al., 1979	Microgynon-30	55	2.6[c]				Aged 16–39; mean age = 26; 62% used oral contraceptives as last contraceptive before study	5.5[c]	Britain; probability based on only 12 cycles
Grady et al., 1986		856	2.9[s]				Aged 15–44; all married[t]	20.6[r]	NSFG 1982
Jones and Forrest, 1992		3,041	5.1				Aged 15–44; all married[t]	21[r]	NSFG 1988; probability when standardized and corrected for estimated under-reporting of abortion = 7.3s
Preston, 1974	Norlestrin 1.0 (40%)	313		5.80[c]	1.570 Cy.	?		?	Author employed by manufacturer; pill not marketed
Bounds et al., 1979	Loestrin-2C	55	5.3[c]				Aged 16–39; mean age = 26; 65% used oral contraceptives as last contraceptive before study	5.5[c]	Britain; probability based on only 12 cycles

(continued)

Table 27–11 Summary of studies of contraceptive failure: combined oral contraceptives, vaginal rings, and patches[a]—(cont'd)

Reference	Method Brand	N for Analysis	Life-Table 12-Month % Pregnant	Risk of Pregnancy Pearl Index Pregnancy Rate Index	Total Exposure	Maximum Exposure	Characteristics of the Sample	LFU (%)[g]	Comments
Trussell and Vaughan, 1999		2,130	6.9				Aged 15–44[t]	21[r]	NSFG 1995
Fu et al., 1999		?	7.3					21[r]	NSFG 1995; probability when standardized and corrected for estimated underreporting of abortion = 8.1[s]
Preston, 1974	Norlestrin 2.5 (20%)	178		10.45[c]	871 Cy.	?		?	Author employed by manufacturer; pill not marketed

Notes:

[a] Updated from Trussell and Kost (1987), Table 8.

[b] 12-cycle probability; 12-month probability not available.

[c] Calculated by James Trussell from data in the article.

[d] 6-cycle probability.

[g] Most of these studies incorrectly report the loss to follow-up (LFU) probability as the number of women lost at any time during the study divided by the total number of women entering the study. Thus, these are the probabilities presented in the table. However, the correct measure of LFU would be a gross life-table probability. When available, gross 12-month probabilities are denoted by the letter "g."

[r] Nonresponse rate for entire survey.

[s] Standardized: Vaughan et al., (1977) (1973 NSFG)—intention (the average of probabilities for preventers and delayers); Grady et al., (1983) (1973 and 1976 NSFG)—intention. Our calculation (the average of probabilities for preventers and delayers); Schirm et al., (1982) (1973 and 1976 NSFG)—intention, age, and income; Grady et al., (1986) (1982 NSFG)—intention, age, poverty status, and parity; Jones and Forrest, (1992) (1988 NSFG)—age, marital status, and poverty status; Fu et al., (1999) (1995 NSFG)—age, union status, poverty status.

[t] Total for all methods in the study.

[v] The authors report that LFU for "relevant reasons (withdrawal of cooperation or loss of contact)" was 0.3% per year in the 1982 study. In the 1982 study, women had probably been followed for 9.5 years on average; if 0.3% are LFU per year, then 2.8% would be LFU in 9.5 years. LFU including death and emigration is about twice as high as LFU for "relevant reasons."

For table references, see reference section.

Table 27–12 Summary of studies of contraceptive failure: injectables[a]

Reference	Method Brand	N for Analysis	Life-Table 12-Month % Pregnant	Characteristics of the Sample	LFU (%)[s]	Comments
Jain et al., 2004	Depo-Provera SC	1,779	0.0	Mean age = 30.6		Brazil, Bulgaria, Canada, Chile, Estonia, Indonesia, Latvia, Lithuania, Mexico, Norway, Pakistan, Peru, Poland, Romania, Russia, United Kingdom, United States
W.H.O., 1988	Depo-Provera 25 mg + Estradiol Cypionate 5 mg (30-Day)	1,168	0.0	Aged 18–35; mean age = 26; proven fertility	11.4[8]	Egypt, Thailand, Mexico, Guatemala, Cuba, Indonesia, Pakistan, U.S.S.R., Philippines, Italy, Hungary, Chile
W.H.O., 1986	Depo-Provera 150 mg (90-Day)	607	0.0	Mean age = 27.7[t]	8.6[8]	7 developing countries
Mishell et al., 1968	Depo-Provera 150 mg (90-Day)	100	0.0[c]	59% aged 21–30	24.0[c]	Injection immediately postpartum
Howard et al., 1982	Norigest 200 mg (56-Day)	383	0.0[c]		6.5[t]	Britain
Kaunitz et al., 1999	Lunelle	782	0.0	Mean age = 27.3; 44% used hormonal contraception in prior month	8.6[c]	Trial design discontinued subjects who did not adhere to dosing schedule
Hall et al., 1997	Cyclofem (Lunelle)	3,183	0.0		12.9[c]	Brazil, Chile, Colombia, Peru. Perfect use analysis since trial design discontinued women who were late for injections
W.H.O., 1983	Depo-Provera 150 mg (90-Day)	1,587	0.1	Mean age = 27.4[t]	8.1	87% of women from 9 developing countries

(continued)

Table 27–12 Summary of studies of contraceptive failure: injectables[a]—(cont'd)

Reference	Method Brand	N for Analysis	Life-Table 12-Month % Pregnant	Characteristics of the Sample	LFU (%)[g]	Comments
W.H.O., 1988	Norigest 50 mg + Estradiol Valerate 5 mg (30-Day)	1,152	0.18	Aged 18–35; mean age = 26.7; proven fertility	10.5[g]	Egypt, Thailand, Mexico, Guatemala, Cuba, Indonesia, Pakistan, U.S.S.R., Philippines, Italy, Hungary, Chile
Sangi-Haghpeykar et al., 1996	Depo-Provera 150 mg (3-Month)	536	0.2	25% nulligravid; mean age = 24.4; primarily low income	5.4[c]	
Scutchfield et al., 1971	Depo-Provera 150 mg (90-Day)	650	0.2[c]	66% aged 20–34; 50% married	6.8[n]	
Schwallie and Assenzo, 1973	Depo-Provera 150 mg (90-Day)	3,857	0.3	86% aged 20–39	18.6	Primarily United States; also Chile, Jamaica, Mexico; authors employed by manufacturer
W.H.O., 1983	Norigest 200 mg (60-Day)	789	0.4	Mean age = 27.4[t]	7.1	87% of women from 9 developing countries
W.H.O., 1986	Depo-Provera 100 mg (90-Day)	609	0.4	Mean age = 27.7[t]	8.2[g]	7 developing countries
W.H.O., 1983	Norigest 200 mg (84-Day)	796	0.6	Mean age = 27.4[t]	7.4	87% of women from 9 developing countries
W.H.O., 1977	Depo-Provera 150 mg (84-Day)	846	0.7	87% aged 20–34	6.2	10 developing countries
Schwallie and Assenzo, 1972	Depo-Provera 300 mg (180-Day)	991	2.3[n]	88% aged 20–39	28.9	United States, Chile; authors employed by manufacturer
Fu et al., 1999	Depo-Provera 150 mg	?	2.8		21[r]	NSFG 1995; probability when standardized and corrected for estimated underreporting of abortion = 2.6[s]

(continued)

Table 27–12 Summary of studies of contraceptive failure: injectables[a]—*(cont'd)*

Reference	Method Brand	N for Analysis	Life-Table 12-Month % Pregnant	Characteristics of the Sample	LFU (%)[z]	Comments
Trussell and Vaughan, 1999	Depo-Provera 150 mg	209	3.2	Aged 15–44[t]	21[r]	NSFG 1995
W.H.O., 1977	Norigest 200 mg (84-832 Day)		3.6	84% aged 20–34	5.8	10 developing countries

Notes:

[a] Updated from Trussell and Kost (1987), Table 9.

[c] Calculated by James Trussell from data in the article.

[g] Most of these studies incorrectly report the loss to follow-up (LFU) probability as the number of women lost at any time during the study divided by the total number of women entering the study. Thus, these are the probabilities presented in the table. However, the correct measure of LFU would be a gross life-table probability. When available, gross 12-month probabilities are denoted by the letter "g."

[n] Only net probabilities available for this study.

[r] Nonresponse rate for entire survey.

[s] Fu et al., (1995 NSFG)—age, union status, poverty status.

[t] Total for all methods in the study.

For table references, see reference section.

Table 27–13 Summary of studies of contraceptive failure: IUD[a]

Reference	Method Brand	N for Analysis	Life-Table 12-Month % Pregnant	Characteristics of the Sample	LFU (%)[g]	Comments
Luukkainen et al., 1987	LNG20	1,821	0.1	15% aged 17–25, 60% aged 26–35, 25% aged 36–40; 7% parity 0, 27% parity 1, 50% parity 2, 16% parity 3+	5.7[c]	Denmark, Finland, Hungary, Norway, Sweden
Sivin et al., 1990 Singapore, United States	LNG20	1,124	0.2	Mean age = 26.6; mean parity = 2.4	5.7[g,x]	Brazil, Chile, Dominican Republic, Egypt,
Sivin et al., 1990	TCu380A Slimline	698	0.3	Mean age = 28.5; mean parity = 2.7; 47.4% prior IUD use	6.0	Randomized trial of TCu380A and TCu380A Slimline. Egypt, Chile, Sweden, Dominican Republic, Brazil
Sivin et al., 1990	TCu380A	298	0.4	Mean age = 28.1; mean parity = 2.6; 49.0% prior IUD use	9.7	Randomized trial of TCu380A and TCu380A Slimline. Egypt, Chile, Sweden, Dominican Republic, Brazil
Cox and Blacksell, 2000	LNG20	692	0.6	All parous	?	United Kingdom
Sivin and Stern, 1979	TCu380A	3,536	0.8	72% aged 20–29; 64% nulliparous	18.3[n]	
Gibor and Mitchell, 1980	Progestasert	6,261	2.0[n]		?	Authors employed by manufacturer; United States (51%), Canada (5%), and at least 11 other countries
Trussell and Vaughan, 1999		59	3.7	Aged 15–44[t]	21[r]	NSFG 1995
Bracher and Santow, 1992		408	3.9	10% aged <20, 68% aged 20–29, 22% aged 30+; 25% parity 0; 87% married or cohabiting	25[r]	Australian Family Survey, first use of method

(continued)

Table 27–13 Summary of studies of contraceptive failure: IUD[a]—*(cont'd)*

Reference	Method Brand	N for Analysis	Life-Table 12-Month % Pregnant	Characteristics of the Sample	LFU (%)[g]	Comments
Vaughan et al., 1977		576	4.2[s]	Aged 15–44; all married[t]	19.0[r]	NSFG 1973
Schirm et al., 1982		1,070	4.5[s]	Aged 15–44; all married[t]	18.2[r]	NSFG 1973 and 1976
Grady et al., 1983		1,070	4.8[c,s]	Aged 15–44; all married[t]	18.2[r]	NSFG 1973 and 1976
Grady et al., 1985		235	5.3[s]	Aged 15–44; all married[t]	20.6[r]	NSFG 1982

Notes:

[a] Updated from Trussell and Kost (1987), Table 7.

[c] Calculated by James Trussell from data in the article.

[g] Most of these studies incorrectly report the loss to follow-up (LFU) probability as the number of women lost at any time during the study divided by the total number of women entering the study. Thus, these are the probabilities presented in the table. However, the correct measure of LFU would be a gross life-table probability. When available, gross 12-month probabilities are denoted by the letter "g."

[n] Only net probabilities available for this study.

[r] Nonresponse rate for entire survey.

[s] Standardized: Vaughan et al. (1977) (1973 NSFG)—intention (the average of probabilities for preventers and delayers); Grady et al. (1983) (1973 and 1976 NSFG)—intention. Our calculation (the average of probabilities for preventers and delayers); Schirm et al. (1982) (1973 and 1976 NSFG)—intention, age, and income; Grady et al. (1985) (1982 NSFG)—intention, age, poverty status, and parity.

[t] Total for all methods in the study.

[x] Irving Sivin, personal communication to James Trussell, August 13, 1992.

For table references, see reference section.

Table 27–14 Summary of studies of contraceptive failure: Implants[a]

Reference	Method Brand	N for Analysis	Life-Table 12-Month % Pregnant	Characteristics of the Sample	LFU (%)[g]	Comments
Croxotto et al., 1999	Implanon	635	0.0	Mean age = 29.1; 17% nulligravid	0.5	Canada, Chile, Finland, Hungary, Indonesia, Singapore, Sweden, Thailand, United Kingdom
Croxotto and Mäkäräinen, 1998	Implanon	1,716	0.0		?	
Funk et al., 2005	Implanon	330	0.0	13% aged 18–20, 39% aged 21–25, 26% aged 26–30, 17% aged 31–35, 5% aged 36–40; 37% nulligravid	?	
Sivin et al., 1997	Norplant-2 (2 Rods)	199	0.0		2.0	Chile, Dominican Republic, Singapore, Thailand, United States; current version with core of rods made of new elastomer; random assignment to new or old version of Norplant-2
Sivin et al., 2000	Norplant (6 capsules)	1,210	0.0	Mean age = 27.4; 13% nulliparous	1.2	Chile, Dominican Republic, Egypt, Finland, Singapore, Thailand, United States; current version with capsules made of new elastomer
Sivin et al., 1998[b]	Norplant (2 Rods)	600	0.0	Mean age = 28.3; 2% nulliparous	0.3[c]	Chile, Egypt, Finland, Singapore, Thailand, United States; current version with core of rods made of new elastomer
Sivin et al., 1998[a]	Norplant (2 Rods)	594	0.2	Mean age = 25.5; 17% nulliparous	2.2	Dominican Republic, United States; current version with core of rods made of new elastomer
Fu et al., 1999		?	1.8		21[r]	NSFG 1995; probability when standardized and corrected for estimated under-reporting of abortion = 1.4[s]

(continued)

Table 27–14 Summary of studies of contraceptive failure: Implants[a]—*(cont'd)*

Reference	Method Brand	N for Analysis	Life-Table 12-Month % Pregnant	Characteristics of the Sample	LFU (%)[g]	Comments
Trussell and Vaughan, 1999		146	2.3	Aged 15–44[t]	21[r]	NSFG 1995

Notes:

[a] Updated from Trussell and Kost (1987), Table 9.

[c] Calculated by James Trussell from data provided by Sivin (1992).

[g] Proportion LFU in the first year (number of women LFU in the first year divided by the number entering the study); gross 12-month life-table probabilities denoted by the letter "g."

[r] Nonresponse rate for entire survey.

[s] Fu et al., (1999) (1995 NSFG)—age, union status, poverty status.

[t] Total for all methods in the study.

For table references, see reference section.

Table 27–15 Summary of studies of contraceptive failure: female sterilization[a]

Reference	Procedure	N for Analysis	Risk of Pregnancy Life-Table 12-Month % Pregnant	Pearl Index Pregnancy Rate Index	Pearl Index Pregnancy Rate Total Exposure	Pearl Index Pregnancy Rate Maximum Exposure	Characteristics of the Sample	LFU (%)[g]	Comments
Engel, 1978	Laparoscopy	182	0.0[c]				"No failures" presumably some women followed for at least 12 months	?	
Valle and Battifora, 1978	Laparoscopy	165	0.0[c]				"Failure rate after 2 years follow-up is zero" all aged 22–38; 80% had at least 12 months follow-up	?	
Vessey et al., 1983	Procedures other than laparotomy and laparoscopy	345		0.0	331 Yr.	12 Mo.	All white; at recruitment aged 25–39 and married; at enrollment, all women had been using the diaphragm, IUD, or pill successfully for at least 5 months	0.3[v]	Britain; Oxford/FPA study
Chi et al., 1980	Culdoscopy: Pomeroy	392	0.0				Mean age = 32[t]	?	IFRP (19 countries)
Loffer and Pent, 1977	Laparoscopy	1,717		0.0[c]		>6 Mo.	Duration of follow-up not reported	?	
Chi et al., 1987	Minilaparotomy: Pomeroy	445	0.0[c]				Median age = 32	31.6	IFRP (19 countries)
Peterson et al., 1996	Postpartum partial salpingectomy	1,637	0.06				43% aged 18–27, 38% aged 28–33, 18% aged 34+	8.8	U.S. Collaborative Review of Sterilization

(continued)

Table 27-15 Summary of studies of contraceptive failure: female sterilization[a]—(cont'd)

Reference	Procedure	N for Analysis	Risk of Pregnancy				Characteristics of the Sample	LFU (%)[g]	Comments
			Life-Table 12-Month % Pregnant	Pearl Index Pregnancy Rate					
				Index	Total Exposure	Maximum Exposure			
Peterson et al., 1996	Unipolar coagulation	1,432	0.07				20% aged 18–27, 39% aged 28–33, 42% aged 34+	5.0	U.S. Collaborative Review of Sterilization
Dominik et al., 2000	Filshie Clip	1,063	0.11					31.3[c]	Dominican Republic, Guatemala, Haiti, Malaysia, Mexico, Panama, Venezuela
Sokal et al., 2000	Filshie Clip	1,378	0.17				Mean age = 31	18.1[c]	Brazil, Dominican Republic, Indonesia, Kenya, Mexico, Panama, Peru, Thailand
Sokal et al., 2000	Tubal Ring	1,355	0.17				Mean age = 31	17.6[c]	Brazil, Dominican Republic, Indonesia, Kenya, Mexico, Panama, Peru, Thailand
Bhiwandiwala et al., 1982	Rocket Clip	630	0.18[u]					42.1[ct]	IFRP (27 countries)
Peterson et al., 1996	Bipolar coagulation	2,267	0.23				31% aged 18–27, 35% aged 28–33, 35% aged 34+	10.5	U.S. Collaborative Review of Sterilization
Chi et al., 1980	Minilaparotomy	3,988	0.24				Mean age = 32[t]	?	IFRP (19 countries)

(continued)

Table 27–15 Summary of studies of contraceptive failure: female sterilization[a]—(cont'd)

Reference	Procedure	N for Analysis	Life-Table 12-Month % Pregnant	Risk of Pregnancy — Pearl Index Pregnancy Rate — Index	Total Exposure	Maximum Exposure	Characteristics of the Sample	LFU (%)[g]	Comments
Bhiwandiwala et al., 1982	Electro-coagulation	6,542	0.26[u]					42.1[c,t]	IFRP (27 countries)
Vessey et al., 1983	Laparotomy: all procedures	743		0.28	716 Yr.	12 Mo.	All white; at recruitment aged 25–39 and married; at enrollment, all women had been using the diaphragm, IUD, or pill successfully for at least 5 months	0.3[v]	Britain; Oxford/FPA study
Mumford et al., 1980	Minilaparoscopy: Pomeroy	2,022	0.3[u]					?	IFRP (23 countries)
Chi et al., 1980	Electro-coagulation	3,594	0.32[c]					?	IFRP (19 countries)
Bhiwandiwala et al., 1982	Tubal Ring	5,046	0.47[u]					42.1[c,t]	IFRP (27 countries)
Mumford et al., 1980	Minilaparoscopy: Ring	1,324	0.51[u]					?	IFRP (23 countries)
Vessey et al., 1983	Laparoscopy: Tubal Diathermy	776		0.53	755 Yr.	12 Mo.	All white; at recruitment aged 25–39 and married; at enrollment, all women had been using the diaphragm, IUD, or pill successfully for at least 5 months	.3[v]	Britain: Oxford/FPA study

(continued)

Table 27-15 Summary of studies of contraceptive failure: female sterilization[a]—*(cont'd)*

				Risk of Pregnancy					
			Life-Table	Pearl Index Pregnancy Rate					
Reference	Procedure	N for Analysis	12-Month % Pregnant	Index	Total Exposure	Maximum Exposure	Characteristics of the Sample	LFU (%)[g]	Comments
Chi et al., 1981	Tubal Ring	4,106	0.54[c]					?	IFRP (19 countries)
Peterson et al., 1996	All methods combined	10,685	0.55				33% aged 18–27, 35% aged 28–33, 32% aged 34+	10.8	U.S. Collaborative Review of Sterilization
Chi et al., 1980	Laparoscopy: Rocket Clip	457	0.59				Mean age = 32[t]	?	IFRP (19 countries)
Peterson et al., 1996	Rubber band	3,329	0.59				30% aged 18–27, 36% aged 28–33, 34% aged 34+	12.1	U.S. Collaborative Review of Sterilization
Mumford et al., 1980	Laparoscopy: Rings	4,262	0.60[u]					?	IFRP (23 countries)
Vessey et al., 1983	Laparoscopy: Rings, Clips, etc.	379		3.60	334 Yr.	12 Mo.	All white; at recruitment aged 25–39 and married; at enrollment, all women had been using the diaphragm, IUD, or pill successfully for at least 5 months	0.3[v]	Britain; Oxford/FPA study
Dominik et al., 2000	Hulka Clip	1,062	0.69					33.1[c]	Dominican Republic, Guatemala, Haiti, Malaysia, Mexico, Panama, Venezuela
Peterson et al., 1996	Interval partial salpingectomy	425	0.73				28% aged 18–27, 32% aged 28–33, 40% aged 34+	7.3	U.S. Collaborative Review of Sterilization

(continued)

Table 27–15 Summary of studies of contraceptive failure: female sterilization[a]—(cont'd)

Reference	Procedure	N for Analysis	Life-Table 12-Month % Pregnant	Pearl Index Pregnancy Rate — Index	Pearl Index Pregnancy Rate — Total Exposure	Pearl Index Pregnancy Rate — Maximum Exposure	Characteristics of the Sample	LFU (%)[g]	Comments
Chi et al., 1987	Minilaparotomy; Rings and Clips	1,146		0.79	1,143 Yr.	12 Mo.	Median age = 32 years	13.5	IFRP (19 countries)
Yoon et al., 1977	Falope Ring	902		1.33[c]	3,617[c] Mo.	12 Mo.		21.0[c]	
Peterson et al., 1996	Spring Clip	1,595	1.82				44% aged 18–27, 30% aged 28–33, 26% aged 34+	16.4	U.S. Collaborative Review of Sterilization
Hulka et al., 1976	Spring Clip	1,079	2.3[z]					9.5[c]	United States, UK, Jamaica, Thailand, Singapore, El Salvador (defective clips)
Chi et al., 1981	Spring Clip	1,699	4.19[c]					?	IFRP (19 countries) (defective clips)
Chi et al., 1980	Culdoscopy; Tantalum Clip	498	8.19				Mean age = 32[t]	?	IFRP (19 countries)

Notes:

[a] Updated from Trussell and Kost (1987), Table 10.

[c] Calculated by James Trussell from data in the article.

[g] Most of these studies incorrectly report the loss to follow-up (LFU) probability as the number of women lost at any time during the study divided by the total number of women entering the study. Thus, these are the probabilities presented in the table. However, the correct measure of LFU would be a gross life-table probability. When available, gross 12-month probabilities are denoted by the letter "g."

[t] Total for all methods in the study.

[u] Study did not report whether the cumulative life-table probability was net or gross.

[v] The authors report that LFU for "relevant reasons" (withdrawal of cooperation or loss of contact)[v] was 0.3% per year in the 1983 study. In the 1983 study, women had probably been followed for 10 years on average; if 0.3% are LFU per year, then 3.0% would be LFU in 10 years. LFU including death and emigration is about twice as high as LFU for "relevant reasons."

For table references, see reference section.

Table 27-16 Summary of studies of contraceptive failure: vasectomy[a]

		Risk of Pregnancy				
		Life-Table	Pearl Index Pregnancy Rate			
Moss, 1992	6,220	0.0c			?	1 pregnancy 10 years after vasectomy
Schmidt, 1988	5,000	0.0c			?	Presumably 0 pregnancies
Alderman, 1988	5,331	0.0c		5,331 of 8,879 had at least 2 post-op semen tests	?	Canada; 4 pregnancies, 4.5–8.6 years after vasectomy
Philip et al., 1984	16,039	0.0c		16,039 of 16,796 provided requested post-op semen samples	?	Britain; 6 pregnancies, 1.3–3 years after vasectomy; 3 pregnancies in first year among 757 men who did not supply post-op semen samples
Kase and Goldfarb, 1973	500	0.0c		2% ≥ aged 41	?	1 pregnancy 15 months after vasectomy
Vessey et al., 1982	?		0.08 2,500 Yr. 24 Mo.	Females all white; females at recruitment aged 25–39 and married; at enrollment, all women had been using the diaphragm, IUD, or pill successfully for at least 5 months	0.3t,v	Britain; Oxford/FPA study
Margaret Pyke Center, 1973	1,000	0.1c		24% ≥ age 41	?	Britain; 1 pregnancy in first year
Klapproth and Young, 1973	1,000	0.2c		35% ≥ age 41	10.0?	2 pregnancies, 3 and 4 months after vasectomy

(continued)

Table 27–16 Summary of studies of contraceptive failure: vasectomy[a]—(cont'd)

| | | Risk of Pregnancy | | | | | | |
| | | Life-Table | Pearl Index Pregnancy Rate | | | | | |
Reference	N for Analysis	12-Month % Pregnant	Index	Total Exposure	Maximum Exposure	Characteristics of the Sample	LFU (%)[g]	Comments
Marshall and Lyon, 1972	200	0.5[c]				Age 25–60; "majority" aged 35–39	?	1 pregnancy 3 months after vasectomy
Jamieson et al., 2004	544	0.74					6.1	U.S. Collaborative Review of Sterilization; women interviewed after husbands' vasectomy

Notes:

[a] Updated from Trussell and Kost (1987), Table 10.

[c] Calculated by James Trussell from data in the article.

[g] Most of these studies incorrectly report the loss to follow-up (LFU) probability as the number of women lost at any time during the study divided by the total number of women entering the study. Thus, these are the probabilities presented in the table. However, the correct measure of LFU would be a gross life-table probability. When available, gross 12-month probabilities are denoted by the letter "g."

[t] Total for all methods in the study.

[v] The authors report that LFU for "relevant reasons (withdrawal of cooperation or loss of contact)" was 0.3% per year in the 1982 study. In the 1982 study, women had probably been followed for 9.5 years on average; if 0.3% are LFU per year, then 2.8% would be LFU in 9.5 years. LFU including death and emigration is about twice as high as LFU for "relevant reasons."

For table references, see reference section.

TABLE REFERENCES

Åkerlund M, Røde A, Westergaard J. Comparative profiles of reliability, cycle control and side effects of two oral contraceptive formulations containing 150 μg desogestrel and either 30 μg or 20 μg ethinyl oestradiol. Brit J Obstet Gynaecol 1993;100:832–838.

Alderman PM. The lurking sperm: a review of failures in 8879 vasectomies performed by one physician. JAMA 1988;259:3142–3144.

Anderson FD, Hait H, the Seasonale-301 Study Group. A multicenter, randomized study of an extended cycle oral contraceptive. Contraception 2003;68:89–96.

Anderson FD, Gibbons W, Portman D, the Seasonique® Study Group. Safety and efficacy of an extended-regimen oral contraceptive utilizing continuous low-dose ethinyl estradiol. Contraception 2006;73:229–234.

Apothecus Pharmaceutical Corporation. VCF®: Vaginal Contraceptive Film®. East Norwich NY: Apothecus Inc, 1992.

Archer DF, Maheux R, DelConte A, O'Brien FB. North American levonorgestrel study group (NALSG). Efficacy and safety of a low-dose monophasic combination oral contraceptive containing 100 μg levonorgestrel and 20 μg ethinyl estradiol (Alesse). Am J Obstet Gynecol 1999;181:S39-S44.

Aérvalo M, Jennings V, Nikula M, Sinai I. Efficacy of the new TwoDay Method of family planning. Fertil Steril 2004;82:885–892.

Arévalo M, Jennings V, Sinai I. Efficacy of a new method of family planning: the Standard Days Method. Contraception 2002;65:333–338.

Audet MC, Moreau M, Koltun WD, Waldbaum AS, Shangold G, Fisher AC, Creasy GW. Evaluation of contraceptive efficacy and cycle control of a transdermal contraceptive patch vs an oral contraceptive. JAMA 2001;285:2347–2354.

Bachmann G, Sulak PJ, Sampson-Landers C, Benda N, Marr J. Efficacy and safety of a low-dose 24-day combined oral contraceptive containing 20 micrograms ethinylestradiol and 3 mg drospirenone. Contraception 2004;70:191–198.

Ball M. A prospective field trial of the ovulation method of avoiding conception. Eur J Obstet Gynecol Reprod Biol 1976;6:63–66.

Bannemerschult R, Hanker JP, Wunsch C, Fox P, Albring M, Brill K. A multicenter, uncontrolled clinical investigation of the contraceptive efficacy, cycle control, and safety of a new low dose oral contraceptive containing 20 μg ethinyl estradiol and 100 μg levonorgestrel over six treatment cycles. Contraception 1997;56:285–290.

Bartzen PJ. Effectiveness of the temperature rhythm system of contraception. Fertil Steril 1967;18:694–706.

Belhadj H, Sivin I, Diaz S, Pavez M, Tejada AS, Brache V, Alvarez F, Shoupe D, Breaux II, Mishell DR, McCarthy T, Yo V. Recovery of fertility after use of the levonorgestrel 20 mcg/d or copper T 380 Ag intrauterine device. Contraception 1986;34.261–267.

Bernstein GS. Clinical effectiveness of an aerosol contraceptive foam. Contraception 1971;3:37–43.

Bernstein GS, Clark V, Coulson AH, Frezieres RG, Kilzer L, Moyer D, Nakamura RM, Walsh T. Use effectiveness study of cervical caps. Final report. Washington DC: National Institute of Child Health and Human Development, Contract No. 1-HD-1-2804, July, 1986.

Bhiwandiwala PP, Mumford SD, Feldblum PJ. A comparison of different laparoscopic sterilization occlusion techniques in 24,439 procedures. Am J Obstet Gynecol 1982;144:319–331.

Board JA. Continuous norethindrone, 0.35 mg, as an oral contraceptive agent. Am J Obstet Gynecol 1971;109:531–535.

Boehm D. The cervical cap: effectiveness as a contraceptive. J Nurse Midwifery 1983;28:3–6.

Bounds W, Guillebaud J. Randomised comparison of the use-effectiveness and patient acceptability of the Collatex (Today) contraceptive sponge and the diaphragm. Br J Fam Plann 1984;10:69–75.

Bounds W, Guillebaud J, Dominik R, Dalberth BT. The diaphragm with and without spermicide: a randomized, comparative efficacy trial. J Reprod Med 1995;40:764–774.

Bounds W, Vessey M, Wiggins P. A randomized double-blind trial of two low dose combined oral contraceptives. Brit J Obstet Gynaecol 1979;86:325–329.

Bracher M, Santow G. Premature discontinuation of contraception in Australia. Fam Plann Perspect 1992;24:58–65.

Brehm H, Haase W. Die alternative zur hormonalen kontrazeption? Med Welt 1975;26:1610–1617.

Brigato G, Pisano G, Bergamasco A, Pasqualini M, Cutugno G, Luppari T. Vaginal topical chemical contraception with C-Film. Ginecol Clinica 1982;3:77–80. (In Italian; translation supplied by Apothecus Inc.)

Broome M, Fotherby K. Clinical experience with the progestogen-only pill. Contraception 1990;42:489–495.

Bushnell LF. Aerosol foam: a practical and effective method of contraception. Pac Med Surg 1965;73:353–355.

Cagen R. The cervical cap as a barrier contraceptive. Contraception 1986;33:487–496.

Carpenter G, Martin JB. Clinical evaluation of a vaginal contraceptive foam. Adv Plann Parent 1970;5:170–175.

Chi IC, Laufe LE, Gardner SD, Tolbert MA. An epidemiologic study of risk factors associated with pregnancy following female sterilization. Am J Obstet Gynecol 1980;136:768–773.

Chi IC, Mumford SD, Gardner SD. Pregnancy risks following laparoscopic sterilization in nongravid and gravid women. J Reprod Med 1981;26:289–294.

Chi IC, Siemens AJ, Champion CB, Gates D, Cilenti D. Pregnancy following minilaparotomy tubal sterilization: an update of an international data set. Contraception 1987;35:171–178.

Cliquet RL, Schoenmaeckers R, Klinkenborg L. Effectiveness of contraception in Belgium: results of the second national fertility survey, 1971 (NEGO II). J Biosoc Sci 1977;9:403–416.

Cox M, Blacksell S. Clinical performance of the levonorgestrel intra-uterine system in routine use by the UK Family Planning and Reproductive Health Research Network: 12-month report. Br J Fam Plann 2000;26:143–147.

Croxatto HB, Mäkäräinen L. The pharmacodynamics and efficacy of Implanon. An overview of the data. Contraception. 1998;58:91S-97S. Retraction in: Rekers H, Affandi B. Contraception. 2004;70:433.

Croxatto HB, Urbancsek J, Massai R, Coelingh Bennink H, van Beek A. A multicentre efficacy and safety study of the single contraceptive implant Implanon. Implanon Study Group. Hum Reprod 1999;14:976–981.

Debusschere R. Effectiviteit van de anticonceptie in Vlaanderen: resultaten van het NEGO-III-onderzoek 1975–1976. Bevolking en Gezin 1980;1:5–28.

Denniston GC, Putney D. The cavity rim cervical cap. Adv Plann Parent 1981;16:77–80.

Dieben TOM, Roumen JME, Apter D. Efficacy, cycle control and user acceptability of a novel combined contraceptive vaginal ring. Obstet Gynecol 2002;100:585–593.

Dimpfl J, Salomon W, Schicketanz KH. Die spermizide barriere. Sexualmedizin 1984;13:95–98.

Dingle JT, Tietze C. Comparative study of three contraceptive methods: vaginal foam tablets, jelly alone, and diaphragm with jelly or cream. Am J Obstet Gynecol 1963;85:1012–1022.

Dolack L. Study confirms values of ovulation method. Hospital Progress 1978;59:64–66,72–73.

Dominik R, Gates D, Sokal D, Cordero M, Lasso de la Vega J, Remes Ruiz A, Thambu J, Lim D, Louissaint S, Galvez RS, Uribe L, Zighelboim I. Two randomized controlled trials comparing the Hulka and Filshie Clips for tubal sterilization. Contraception 2000;62:169–175.

Dubrow H, Kuder K. Combined postpartum and family-planning clinic. Obstet Gynecol 1958;11:586–590.

Edelman DA. Nonprescription vaginal contraception. Int J Gynecol Obstet 1980;18:340–344.

Edelman DA, McIntyre SL, Harper J. A comparative trial of the Today contraceptive sponge and diaphragm. Am J Obstet Gynecol 1984;150:869–876.

Ellis JW. Multiphasic oral contraceptives: efficacy and metabolic impact. J Reprod Med 1987;32:28–36.

Ellsworth HS. Focus on triphasil. J Reprod Med 1986;31:559–564.

Endrikat J, Jaques MA, Mayerhofer M, Pelissier C, Müller U, Düsterberg B. A twelve-month comparative clinical investigation of two low-dose oral contraceptives containing 20 μg ethinylestradiol/75 μg gestodene and 20 μg ethinylestradiol/150 μg desogestrel, with respect to efficacy, cycle control and tolerance. Contraception 1995;52:229–235.

Engel T. Laparoscopic sterilization: electrosurgery or clip application? J Reprod Med 1978;21:107–110.

Florence N. Das kontrazeptive vaginal-suppositorium: ergebnisse einer klinischen fünfjahresstudie. Sexualmedizin 1977;6:385–386.

Frank R. Clinical evaluation of a simple jelly-alone method of contraception. Fertil Steril 1962;13:458–464.

Frankman O, Raabe N, Ingemansson CA. Clinical evaluation of C-Film, a vaginal contraceptive. J Int Med Res 1975;3:292–296.

Frezieres RG, Walsh TL, Nelson AL, Clark VA, Coulson AH. Evaluation of the efficacy of a polyurethane condom: results from a randomized controlled clinical trial. Fam Plann Perspect 1999;31:81–87.

Fu H, Darroch JE, Haas T, Ranjit N. Contraceptive failure rates: new estimates from the 1995 National Survey of Family Growth. Fam Plann Perspect 1999; 31:56–63.

Funk S, Miller MM, Mishell DR, Archer DF, Poindexter A, Schmidt J, Zampaglione E and for the Implanon® US Study Group. Safety and efficacy of Implanon®, a single-rod implantable contraceptive containing etonogestrel. Contraception 2005;71:319–326.

Gibor Y, Mitchell C. Selected events following insertion of the Progestasert system. Contraception 1980;21:491–503.

Glass R, Vessey M, Wiggins P. Use-effectiveness of the condom in a selected family planning clinic population in the United Kingdom. Contraception 1974;10:591–598.

Godts P. Klinische prüfung eines vaginalem antikonzipiens. Ars Medici 1973;28:584–593.

Grady WR, Hayward MD, Yagi J. Contraceptive failure in the United States: estimates from the 1982 National Survey of Family Growth. Fam Plann Perspect 1986;18:200–209.

Grady WR, Hirsch MB, Keen N, Vaughan B. Contraceptive failure and continuation among married women in the United States, 1970–75. Stud Fam Plann 1983;14:9–19.

Hall P, Bahamondes L, Diaz J, Petta C. Introductory study of the once-a-month, injectable contraceptive Cyclofem in Brazil, Chile, Colombia, and Peru. Contraception 1997;56:353–359.

Hall RE. Continuation and pregnancy rates with four contraceptive methods. Am J Obstet Gynecol 1973;116:671–681.

Hawkins DF, Benster B. A comparative study of three low dose progestogens, chlormadinone acetate, megestrol acetate and norethisterone, as oral contraceptives. Br J Obstet Gynaecol 1977;84:708–713.

Howard G, Blair M, Chen JK, Fotherby K, Muggeridge J, Elder MG, Bye PG. A clinical trial of norethisterone oenanthate (Norigest) injected every two months. Contraception 1982;25:333–343.

Hughes I. An open assessment of a new low dose estrogen combined oral contraceptive. J Int Med Res 1978;6:41–45.

Hulka JF, Mercer JP, Fishburne JI, Kumarasamy T, Omran KF, Phillips JM, Lefler HT, Lieberman B, Lean TH, Pai DN, Koetsawang S, Castro VM. Spring clip sterilization: one-year follow-up of 1,079 cases. Am J Obstet Gynecol 1976;125:1039–1043.

Iizuka R, Kobayashi T, Kawakami S, Nakamura Y, Ikeuchi M, Chin B, Mochimaru F, Sumi K, Sato H, Yamaguchi J, Ohno T, Shiina M, Maeda N, Tokoro H, Suzuki T, Hayashi K, Takahashi T, Akatsuka M, Kasuga Y, Kurokawa H. Clinical experience with the Vaginal Contraceptive Film containing the spermicide polyoxyethylene nonylphenyl ether (C-Film study group). Jpn J Fertil Steril 1980;25:64–68. (In Japanese; translation supplied by Apothecus Inc.)

Jain J, Jakimiuk AJ, Bode FR, Ross D, Kaunitz AM.Contraceptive efficacy and safety of DMPA-SC. Contraception 2004;70:269–275.

Jamieson DJ, Costello C, Trussell J, Hillis SD, Marchbanks PA, Peterson HB; US Collaborative Review of Sterilization Working Group. The risk of pregnancy after vasectomy. Obstet Gynecol. 2004;103:848–850. Erratum in: Obstet Gynecol 2004;104:200.

John APK. Contraception in a practice community. J R Coll Gen Pract 1973;23:665–675.

Johnston JA, Roberts DB, Spencer RB. A survey evaluation of the efficacy and efficiency of natural family planning services and methods in Australia: report of a research project. Sydney, Australia: St. Vincent's Hospital, 1978.

Jones EF, Forrest JD. Contraceptive failure rates based on the 1988 NSFG. Fam Plann Perspect 1992;24:12–19.

Jubhari S, Lane ME, Sobrero AJ. Continuous microdose (0.3 mg) quingestanol acetate as an oral contraceptive agent. Contraception 1974;9:213–219.

Kambic R, Kambic M, Brixius AM, Miller S. A thirty-month clinical experience in natural family planning. Am J Public Health 1981;71:1255–1258. Erratum. Am J Public Health 1982;72:538.

Kasabach HY. Clinical evaluation of vaginal jelly alone in the management of fertility. Clin Med 1962;69:894–897.

Kase S, Goldfarb M. Office vasectomy review of 500 cases. Urology 1973;1:60–62.

Kassell NC, McElroy MP. Emma Goldman Clinic for Women study. In: King L (ed). The cervical cap handbook for users and fitters. Iowa City IA: Emma Goldman Clinic for Women, 1981:11–19.

Kaunitz AM. Efficacy, cycle control, and safety of two triphasic oral contraceptives: Cyclessa (desogestrel/ethinyl estradiol) and Ortho-Novum 7/7/7 (norethindrone/ethinyl estradiol): a randomized clinical trial. Contraception 2000;61:295–302.

Kaunitz AM, Garceau RJ, Cromie MA, Lunelle Study Group. Comparative safety, efficacy, and cycle control of Lunelle monthly contraceptive injection (medroxyprogesterone acetate and estradiol cypionate injectable suspension) and Ortho-Novum 7/7/7 oral contraceptive (norethindrone/eithinyl estradiol triphasic). Contraception 1999;60:179–187.

Keifer W. A clinical evaluation of continuous Norethindrone (0.35 mg). In: Ortho Pharmaceutical Corporation. A clinical symposium on 0.35 mg. Norethindrone: continuous regimen low-dose oral contraceptive. Proceedings of a symposium, New York City, February 22, 1971. Raritan NJ: Ortho Pharmaceutical Corporation, 1973:9–14.

Klapproth HJ, Young IS. Vasectomy, vas ligation and vas occlusion. Urology 1973;1:292–300.

Klaus H, Goebel JM, Muraski B, Egizio MT, Weitzel D, Taylor, RS, Fagan MU, Ek K, Hobday K. Use-effectiveness and client satisfaction in six centers teaching the Billings ovulation method. Contraception 1979;19:613–629.

Kleppinger RK. A vaginal contraceptive foam. Penn Med J 1965;68:31–34.

Koch JP. The Prentif contraceptive cervical cap: a contemporary study of its clinical safety and effectiveness. Contraception 1982;25:135–159.

Korba VD, Heil CG. Eight years of fertility control with norgestrel-ethinyl estradiol (Ovral): an updated clinical review. Fertil Steril 1975;26:973–981.

Korba VD, Paulson SR. Five years of fertility control with microdose norgestrel: an updated clinical review. J Reprod Med 1974;13:71–75.

Kovacs GT, Jarman H, Dunn K, Westcott M, Baker HWG. The contraceptive diaphragm: is it an acceptable method in the 1980s? Aust NZ J Obstet Gynaecol 1986;26:76–79.

Lane ME, Arceo R, Sobrero AJ. Successful use of the diaphragm and jelly by a young population: report of a clinical study. Fam Plann Perspect 1976;8:81–86.

Ledger WJ. Ortho 1557-O: a new oral contraceptive. Int J Fertil 1970;15:88–92.

Lehfeldt H, Sivin I. Use effectiveness of the Prentif cervical cap in private practice: a prospective study. Contraception 1984;30:331–338.

Loffer FD, Pent D. Risks of laparoscopic fulguration and transection of the fallopian tube. Obstet Gynecol 1977;49:218–222.

Loudon NB, Barden ME, Hepburn WB, Prescott RJ. A comparative study of the effectiveness and acceptability of the diaphragm used with spermicide in the form of C-film or a cream or jelly. Br J Fam Plann 1991;17:41–44.

Luukkainen T, Allonen H, Haukkamaa M, Holma P, Pyörälä T, Terho J, Toivonen J, Batar I, Lampe L, Andersson K, Atterfeldt P, Johansson EDB, Nilsson S, Nygren KG, Odlind V, Olsson SE, Rybo G, Sikström B, Nielsen NC, Buch A, Osler M, Steier A, Ulstein M. Effective contraception with the levonorgestrel-releasing intrauterine device: 12-month report of a European multicenter study. Contraception 1987;36:169–179.

Margaret Pyke Centre. One thousand vasectomies. Br Med J 1973;4:216–221.

Marshall J. Cervical-mucus and basal body-temperature method of regulating births: field trial. Lancet 1976;2:282–283.

Marshall S, Lyon RP. Variability of sperm disappearance from the ejaculate after vasectomy. J Urol 1972;107:815–817.

Mauck C, Callahan M, Weiner DH, Dominik R, FemCap investigators' group. A comparative study of the safety and efficacy of FemCap, a new vaginal barrier contraceptive, and the Ortho All-Flex diaphragm. Contraception 1999;60:71–80.

Mauck C, Glover LH, Miller E, Allen S, Archer DF, Blumenthal P, Rosenzweig BA, Dominik R, Sturgen K, Cooper J, Fingerhut F, Peacock L, Gabelnick HL. Lea's Shield®: a study of the safety and efficacy of a new vaginal barrier contraceptive used with and without spermicide. Contraception 1996;53:329–335.

McIntyre SL, Higgins JE. Parity and use-effectiveness with the contraceptive sponge. Am J Obstet Gynecol 1986;155:796–801.

McQuarrie HG, Harris JW, Ellsworth HS, Stone RA, Anderson AE. The clinical evaluation of norethindrone in cyclic and continuous regimens. Adv Plann Parent 1972;7:124–130.

Mears E. Chemical contraceptive trial: II. J Reprod Fertil 1962;4:337–343.

Mears E, Please NW. Chemical contraceptive trial. J Reprod Fertil 1962;3:138–147.

The Mircette Study Group. An open-label, multicenter, noncomparative safety and efficacy study of Mircette, a low-dose estrogen-progestin oral contraceptive. Am J Obstet Gynecol 1998;179:S2-S8.

Mishell DR, El-Habashy MA, Good RG, Moyer DL. Contraception with an injectable progestin. Am J Obstet Gynecol 1968;101:1046–1053.

Morigi EM, Pasquale SA. Clinical experience with a low dose oral contraceptive containing norethisterone and ethinyl oestradiol. Curr Med Res Opin 1978;5:655–662.

Moss WM. A comparison of open-end versus closed-end vasectomies: a report on 6220 cases. Contraception 1992;46:521–525.

Mumford SD, Bhiwandiwala PP, Chi IC. Laparoscopic and minilaparotomy female sterilisation compared in 15,167 cases. Lancet 1980;2:1066–1070.

Nelson JH. The use of the mini pill in private practice. J Reprod Med 1973;10:139–143.

Oddsson K, Leifels-Fischer B, de Melo NR, Wiel-Masson D, Benedetto C, Verhoeven CH, Dieben TO. Efficacy and safety of a contraceptive vaginal ring (NuvaRing) compared with a combined oral contraceptive: a 1-year randomized trial. Contraception 2005;71:176–182.

Parsey KS, Pong A. An open-label, multicenter study to evaluate Yasmin, a low-dose combination oral contraceptive containing drospirenone, a new progestogen. Contraception 2000;61:105–111.

Peel J. The Hull family survey: II. Family planning in the first five years of marriage. J Biosoc Sci 1972;4:333–346.

Peterson HB, Xia Z, Hughes JM, Wilcox LS, Tylor LR, Trussell J. The risk of pregnancy after tubal sterilization: findings from the U.S. Collaborative Review of Sterilization. Am J Obstet Gynecol 1996;174:1161–1170.

Philp T, Guillebaud J, Budd D. Complications of vasectomy: review of 16,000 patients. Br J Urol 1984;56;745–748.

Postlethwaite DL. Pregnancy rate of a progestogen oral contraceptive. Practitioner 1979;222:272–275.

Potts M, McDevitt J. A use-effectiveness trial of spermicidally lubricated condoms. Contraception 1975;11:701–710.

Powell MG, Mears BJ, Deber RB, Ferguson D. Contraception with the cervical cap: effectiveness, safety, continuity of use, and user satisfaction. Contraception 1986;33:215–232.

Preston SN. A report of a collaborative dose-response clinical study using decreasing doses of combination oral contraceptives. Contraception 1972;6:17–35.

Preston SN. A report of the correlation between the pregnancy rates of low estrogen formulations and pill-taking habits of females studied. J Reprod Med 1974;13:75–77.

Raymond EG, Chen PL, Luoto J. Contraceptive effectiveness and safety of five nonoxynol-9 spermicides: a randomized trial. Obstet Gynecol 2004;103:430–439.

Raymond E, Dominik R, the spermicide trial group. Contraceptive effectiveness of two spermicides: a randomized trial. Obstet Gynecol 1999;93:896–903.

Rice FJ, Lanctôt CA, Garcia-Devesa C. Effectiveness of the sympto-thermal method of natural family planning: an international study. Int J Fertil 1981;26:222–230.

Richwald GA, Greenland S, Gerber MM, Potik R, Kersey L, Comas MA. Effectiveness of the cavity-rim cervical cap: results of a large clinical study. Obstet Gynecol 1989;74:143–148.

Roumen FJME, Apter D, Mulders TMT, Dieben TOM. Efficacy, tolerability and acceptability of a novel contraceptive vaginal ring releasing etonogestrel and ethinyl oestradiol. Hum Reprod 2001;16:469–475.

Rovinsky JJ. Clinical effectiveness of a contraceptive cream. Obstet Gynecol 1964;23:125–131.

Royal College of General Practitioners. Oral contraceptives and health. New York NY: Pitman Publishing Corp., 1974.

Salomon W, Haase W. Intravaginale kontrazeption. Sexualmedizin 1977;6:198–202.

Sangi-Haghpeykar H, Poindexter AN, Bateman L, Ditmore JR. Experiences of injectable contraceptive users in an urban setting. Obstet Gynecol 1996;88:227–233.

Schirm AL, Trussell J, Menken J, Grady WR. Contraceptive failure in the United States: the impact of social, economic, and demographic factors. Fam Plann Perspect 1982;14:68–75.

Schmidt SS. Vasectomy. JAMA 1988;259:3176.

Schwallie PC, Assenzo JR. Contraceptive use-efficacy study utilizing Depo-Provera administered as an injection once every six months. Contraception 1972;6:315–327.

Schwallie PC, Assenzo JR. Contraceptive use-efficacy study utilizing medroxyprogesterone acetate administered as an intramuscular injection once every 90 days. Fertil Steril 1973;24:331–339.

Scutchfield FD, Long WN, Corey B, Tyler CW. Medroxyprogesterone acetate as an injectable female contraceptive. Contraception 1971;3:21–35.

Sheps MC. An analysis of reproductive patterns in an American isolate. Popul Stud 1965;19:65–80.

Sheth A, Jain U, Sharma S, Adatia A, Patankar S, Andolsek L, Pretnar-Darovec A, Belsey MA, Hall PE, Parker RA, Ayeni S, Pinol A, Foo CLH. A randomized, double-blind study of two combined and two progestogen-only oral contraceptives. Contraception 1982;25:243–252.

Shihata AA, Trussell J. New female intravaginal barrier contraceptive device: preliminary clinical trial. Contraception 1991;44:11–19.

Shroff NE, Pearce MY, Stratford ME, Wilkinson PD. Clinical experience with ethynodiol diacetate 0.5 mg daily as an oral contraceptive. Contraception 1987;35:121–134.

Sivin I, Alvarez F, Mishell DR Jr, Darney P, Wan L, Brache V, Lacarra M, Klaisle C, Stern J. Contraception with two levonorgestrel rod implants: a 5-year study in the United States and Dominican Republic. Contraception 1998a;58:275–282.

Sivin I, Campodonico I, Kiriwat O, Holma P, Diaz S, Wan L, Biswas A, Viegas O, el din Abdalla K, Anant MP, Pavez M, Stern J. The performance of levonorgestrel rod and Norplant contraceptive implants: a 5 year randomized study. Hum Reprod 1998b;13:3371–3378.

Sivin I, El Mahgoub S, McCarthy T, Mishell DR, Shoupe D, Alvarez F, Brache V, Jimenez E, Diaz J, Faundes A, Diaz MM, Coutinho E, Mattos CER, Diaz S, Pavez M, Stern J. Long-term contraception with the Levonorgestrel 20 mcg/day (LNG-IUS) and the Copper T 380Ag intrauterine devices: a five-year randomized study. Contraception 1990;42:361–378.

Sivin I, Lähteenmäki P, Ranta S, Darney P, Klaisle C, Wan L, Mishell DR, Lacarra M, Viegas OAC, Bilhareus P, Koetsawang S, Piya-Anant M, Diaz S, Pavez M, Alvarez F, Brache V, LaGuardia K, Nash H, Stern J. Levonorgestrel concentrations during use of levonorgestrel rod (LNG ROD) implants. Contraception 1997;55:81–85.

Sivin I, Mishell DR Jr, Diaz S, Biswas A, Alvarez F, Darney P, Holma P, Wan L, Brache V, Kiriwat O, Abdalla K, Campodonico I, Pasquale S, Pavez M, Schechter J. Prolonged effectiveness of Norplant capsule implants: a 7-year study. Contraception 2000;61:187–194.

Sivin I, Shaaban M, Odlind V, Olsson SE, Diaz S, Pavez M, Alvarez F, Brache V, Diaz J. A randomized trial of the Gyne T 380 and Gyne T 380 Slimline intrauterine copper devices. Contraception 1990;42:379–389.

Sivin I, Stern J. Long-acting, more effective copper T IUDs: a summary of U.S. experience, 1970–1975. Stud Fam Plann 1979;10:263–281.

Smallwood GH, Meador ML, Lenihan JP, Shangold GA, Fisher AC, Creasy GW, ORTHO EVRA/EVRA 002 Study Group. Efficacy and safety of a transdermal contraceptive system. Obstet Gynecol 2001;98:799–805.

Smith C, Farr G, Feldblum PJ, Spence A. Effectiveness of the non-spermicidal fit-free diaphragm. Contraception 1995;51:289–291.

Smith GG, Lee RJ. The use of cervical caps at the University of California, Berkeley: a survey. Contraception 1984;30:115–123.

Smith M, Vessey MP, Bounds W, Warren J. C-Film as a contraceptive. Br Med J 1974;4:291.

Sokal D, Gates D, Amatya R, Dominik R, Clinical investigator team. Two randomized controlled trials comparing the tubal ring and Filshie Clip for tubal sterilization. Fertil Steril. 2000;74:525–533.

Steiner MJ, Dominik R, Rountree RW, Nanda K, Dorflinger LJ. Contraceptive effectiveness of a polyurethane condom and a latex condom: a randomized controlled trial. Obstet Gynecol 2003;101:539–547.

Stim EM. The nonspermicidal fit-free diaphragm: a new contraceptive method. Adv Plann Parenthood 1980;15:88–98.

Squire JJ, Berger GS, Keith L. A retrospective clinical study of a vaginal contraceptive suppository. J Reprod Med 1979;22:319–323.

Tatum HJ. Comparative experience with newer models of the copper T in the United States. In: Hefnawi F, Segal SJ (eds). Analysis of intrauterine contraception. Amsterdam, Netherlands: North Holland, 1975:155–163.

Tietze C, Lewit S. Comparison of three contraceptive methods: diaphragm with jelly or cream, vaginal foam, and jelly/cream alone. J Sex Res 1967;3:295–311.

Tietze C, Lewit S. Evaluation of intrauterine devices: ninth progress report of the cooperative statistical program. Stud Fam Plann 1970;1:1–40.

Tietze C, Poliakoff SR, Rock J. The clinical effectiveness of the rhythm method of contraception. Fertil Steril 1951;2:444–450.

Trussell J, Grummer-Strawn L. Contraceptive failure of the ovulation method of periodic abstinence. Fam Plann Perspect 1990;22:65–75.

Trussell J, Hatcher RA, Cates W, Stewart FH, Kost K. Contraceptive failure in the United States: an update. Stud Fam Plann 1990;21:51–54.

Trussell J, Kost K. Contraceptive failure in the United States: a critical review of the literature. Stud Fam Plann 1987;18:237–283.

Trussell J, Vaughan B. Contraceptive Failure, method-related discontinuation and resumption of use: results from the 1995 National Survey of Family Growth. Fam Plann Perspect 1999;31:64–72 & 93.

Tyler ET. Current developments in systemic contraception. Pac Med Surg 1965;93:79–85.

Valle RF, Battifora HA. A new approach to tubal sterilization by laparoscopy. Fertil Steril 1978;30:415–422.

Vaughan B, Trussell J, Menken J, Jones EF. Contraceptive failure among married women in the United States, 1970–1973. Fam Plann Perspect 1977;9:251–258.

Vessey M, Huggins G, Lawless M, McPherson K, Yeates D. Tubal sterilization: findings in a large prospective study. Br J Obstet Gynaecol 1983;90:203–209.

Vessey M, Lawless M, Yeates D. Efficacy of different contraceptive methods. Lancet 1982;1:841–842.

Vessey MP, Lawless M, Yeates D, McPherson K. Progestogen-only oral contraception. Findings in a large prospective study with special reference to effectiveness. Br J Fam Plann 1985;10:117–121.

Vessey MP, Villard-Mackintosh L, McPherson K, Yeates D. Factors influencing use-effectiveness of the condom. Br J Fam Plann 1988;14:40 43.

Vessey M, Wiggins P. Use-effectiveness of the diaphragm in a selected family planning clinic population in the United Kingdom. Contraception 1974;9:15–21.

Vessey MP, Wright NH, McPherson K, Wiggins P. Fertility after stopping different methods of contraception. Br Med J 1978;1:265–267.

Wade ME, McCarthy P, Braunstein GD, Abernathy JR, Suchindran CM, Harris GS, Danzer HC, Uricchio WA. A randomized prospective study of the use-effectiveness of two methods of natural family planning. Am J Obstet Gynecol 1981;141:368–376.

Walsh TL, Frezieres RG, Peacock K, Nelson AL, Clark VA, Bernstein L. Evaluation of the efficacy of a nonlatex condom: results from a randomized, controlled clinical trial. Perspect Sex Reprod Health 2003;35:79–86.

Westoff CF, Potter RG, Sagi PC, Mishler FG. Family growth in metropolitan America. Princeton NJ: Princeton University Press, 1961.

Wolf L, Olson HJ, Tyler ET. Observations on the clinical use of cream-alone and gel-alone methods of contraception. Obstet Gynecol 1957;10:316–321.

World Health Organization. A multicentered phase III comparative clinical trial of depot-medroxyprogesterone acetate given three-monthly at doses of 100 mg or 150 mg: I. Contraceptive efficacy and side effects. Contraception 1986;34:223–235.

World Health Organization. A multicentered phase III comparative study of two hormonal contraceptive preparations given once-a-month by intramuscular injection: I. Contraceptive efficacy and side effects. Contraception 1988;37:1–20.

World Health Organization. A prospective multicentre trial of the ovulation method of natural family planning. II. The effectiveness phase. Fertil Steril 1981;36:591–598.

World Health Organization. Multinational comparative clinical evaluation of two long-acting injectable contraceptive steroids: norethisterone oenanthate and medroxyprogesterone acetate. Contraception 1977;15:513–533.

World Health Organization. Multinational comparative clinical trial of long-acting injectable contraceptives: norethisterone enanthate given in two dosage regimens and depot-medroxyprogesterone acetate. Final report. Contraception 1983;28:1–20.

Woutersz TB. A low-dose combination oral contraceptive: experience with 1,700 women treated for 22,489 cycles. J Reprod Med 1981;26:615–620.

Woutersz TB. A new ultra-low-dose combination oral contraceptive. J Reprod Med 1983;28:81–84.

Wyeth Laboratories. NORPLANT® SYSTEM Prescribing Information. Philadelphia PA: Wyeth Laboratories, December 10, 1990.

Yoon IB, King TM, Parmley TH. A two-year experience with the Falope ring sterilization procedure. Am J Obstet Gynecol 1977;127:109–112.

Appendix 1

Webpages with Active Links to Many Other Websites

CDC National Prevention Network . . . . .http://cdcnpin.org

Contraceptive Technology . . . . www.contraceptivetechnology.com

Department of Health and Human Services . . . . www.healthfinder.gov

MedWeb at Emory University . . . . www.medweb.emory.edu/MedWeb

Princeton University . . . . http://ec.princeton.edu/info/contrac.html

Appendix 2

Network of Professional Organizations

Advocates for Youth
www.advocatesforyouth.org

AIDS Clinical Trials Information
Service (ACTIS)
www.aidsinfo.nih.gov

Alan Guttmacher Institute (AGI)
www.guttmacher.org

Alliance for Microbicide Development
www.microbicide.com

American Association of Sex Educators,
Counselors, and Therapists
www.aasect.org

American College Health Association
www.acha.org

American College of Obstetricians and
Gynecologists (ACOG)
www.acog.org

American Public Health Association
(APHA)
www.apha.org

American Social Health Association
(ASHA)
www.ashastd.org

American Society for Reproductive
Medicine (ASRM)
www.asrm.org

Association of Reproductive Health
Professionals (ARHP)
www.arhp.org

California Family Health Council
www.cfhc.org

Catholics for a Free Choice
www.cath4choice.org

Centre for Development and
Population Activities (CEDPA)
www.cedpa.org

Centers for Disease Control and
Prevention (CDC)
www.cdc.gov/netinfo.htm

CDC Division of HIV/AIDS Prevention
www.cdc.gov/hiv/contactus.htm

Columbia University
www.mailman.columbia.edu/popfam

Committee on Population, National
Research Council
www7.nationalacademies.org/cpop

Contraceptive Research and
Development Program (CONRAD)
www.conrad.org

Contraceptive Technology
Communications, Inc.
P.O. Box 49007
Atlanta, GA 30359
www.contraceptivetechnology.org

East-West Center Program on
Population
www.eastwestcenter.org/res-ph.asp

Education and Training Resource
Associates (ETR)
www.etr.org

Engender Health
www.engenderhealth.org

Family Health International (FHI)
www.fhi.org

Family Violence Prevention Fund
www.endabuse.org

Ford Foundation
www.fordfound.org

Hewlett Foundation
www.hewlett.org

Ibis Reproductive Health
www.ibisreproductivehealth.org

Institute for Reproductive Health
www.irh.org

International Partnership for
Microbicides
www.ipm-microbicides.org

International Planned Parenthood
Federation (IPPF)
www.ippfwhr.org

International Union for the Scientific
Study of Population (IUSSP)
www.iussp.org

IPAS
www.ipas.org

John Snow, Inc.
www.jsi.com

Johns Hopkins University
www.jhuccp.org

Kaiser Family Foundation
www.kff.org

National Abortion Federation (NAF)
www.prochoice.org

National Abortion and Reproductive
Rights Action League (NARAL)
www.prochoiceamerica.org

National Association of Nurse
Practitioners Women's Health
(NPWH)
www.npwh.org

National Family Planning and
Reproductive Health Association
(NFPRHA)
www.nfprha.org

National Institute of Child Health and
Human Development (NICHD)
www.nichd.nih.gov/about/cpr/cpr.htm

Office on Women's Health
www.4woman.gov/healthpro.index.htm

Pathfinder International
www.pathfind.org

Planned Parenthood Federation of
America (PPFA)
www.plannedparenthood.org

Population Action International (PAI)
www.populationaction.org

Population Association of America
(PAA)
www.popassoc.org

Population Council
www.popcouncil.org

Population Institute
www.populationinstitute.org

Population Reference Bureau (PRB)
www.prb.org

Princeton University
http://opr.princeton.edu

Program for Appropriate Technology in
Health (PATH)
www.path.org

Program for International Training and
Health (INTRAH)
www.intrahealth.org

Religious Institute on Sexual Morality,
Justice, and Healing
www.religiousinstitute.org

Reproductive Health Technologies
Project (RHTP)
www.rhtp.org

Rockefeller Foundation
www.rockfound.org

Sexuality Information and Education Council of the United States (SIECUS)
www.siecus.org

United Nations Population Division
www.un.org/popin

United Nations Population Fund (UNFPA)
www.unfpa.org/

University of Michigan
www.psc.lsa.umich.edu/

University of North Carolina
www.cpc.unc.edu

U.S. Agency for International Development (USAID)
www.maqweb.org

World Bank
www.worldbank.org

World Health Organization
www.who.int

Appendix 3

Pharmaceutical Company Websites and Toll-free Phone Numbers

Allendale Pharmaceuticals: sponge	1-888-343-4499	www.todaysponge.com
Ansell Healthcare: condoms		www.ansell.com
Apothecus: VCF	1-800-227-2393	www.apothecus.com
Barr Pharmaceuticals: Plan B ECP	1-800-330-1271	www.go2planb.com
Berlex Laboratories: OCs, progestin IUD	1-888-237-5394	www.berlex.com
Bristol-Myers Squibb Company: OCs, ERT	1 800 321 1335	www.bms.com
Church & Dwight: condoms	1-800-833-9532	www.churchdwight.com
Danco Laboratories: mifepristone	1-877-432-7596	www.earlyoptionpill.com
GlaxoSmithKline: antivirals, antibiotics	1-888-825-5249	www.gsk.com
Mayer Laboratories: condoms, female condoms	1-800-426-6366	www.mayerlabs.com
Okamoto: condoms	1-800-283-7546	www.okamotousa.com
Organon: OCs, vaginal ring	1-800-631-1253	www.organon.com
Ortho-McNeil Pharmaceutical: OCs, patch, diaphragm, IUD	1-800-682-6532	www.ortho-mcneil.com
Parke Davis (Pfizer): OCs	1-800-223-0432	www.pfizer.com

Pharmacia (Pfizer): injectables, ERT	1-800-323-4204	www.pfizer.com
Smart Practice: non-allergenic gloves	1-800-522-0800	www.smartpractice.com
3M Pharmaceuticals: wart treatment, BV treatment	1-800-328-0255	www.3m.com/us/healthcare
Watson Pharmaceuticals: OCs	1-800-272-5525	www.watsonpharm.com
Wyeth Ayerst: OCs	1-800-934-5556	www.wyeth.com

Appendix 4

Hotlines and Websites

Topic	Organization	Hotline	Website
Abortion	Abortion Clinics OnLine		www.gynpages.com
	NARAL Pro-Choice America		www.naral.org
	National Abortion Federation	1-800-772-9100	www.prochoice.org
	Ibis Reproductive Health		www.medicationabortion.org
Adoption	Adopt a Special Kid-America	1-888-680-7349	www.adoptaspecialkid.org
	Adoptive Families	1-800-372-3300	www.adoptivefamilies.com
AIDS (see HIV/AIDS)			
AIDS Advocacy	Gay Men's Health Crisis	1-800-AIDS-NYC	www.gmhc.org
	Project Inform	1-800-822-7422	www.projinf.org
Alcoholism	Alcoholics Anonymous		www.aa.org
	Al-Anon & Alateen Family Groups	1-888-4AL-ANON	www.al-anon.org
	American Council on Alcoholism	1-800-527-5344	www.aca-usa.org
	Children of Alcoholics Foundation		www.coaf.org
	Co-Dependents Anonymous		www.codependents.org
	National Organization on Fetal Alcohol Syndrome	1-800-66-NOFAS	www.nofas.org
Anxiety (see also Depression)	Anxiety Disorders Association of America		www.adaa.org
	Freedom from Fear		www.freedomfromfear.org
	NIMH Panic Disorder Information Line	1-866-615-6464	www.nimh.nih.gov/healthinformation/panicmenu.cfm
Breast Cancer (see also Cancer)	National Alliance of Breast Cancer Organizations		www.nabco.org
	Reach to Recovery (mastectomy patients)	1-800-ACS-2345	www.cancer.org
	Y-Me National Breast Cancer Organization	1-800-221-2141	www.y-me.org
Breastfeeding	International Lactation Consultant Association		www.ilca.org
	La Leche League International		www.lalecheleague.org
	The Linkages Project		www.linkagesproject.org

(continued)

Topic	Organization	Hotline	Website
Cancer (see also specific cancers)	American Cancer Society	1-800-ACS-2345	www.cancer.org
	Candlelighters Childhood Cancer Foundation	1-800-366-2223	www.candlelighters.org
	National Cancer Institute's Cancer Information	1-800-4-CANCER	http://cancer.gov
Child Abuse	Childhelp USA National Child Abuse Hotline	1-800-4-A-CHILD	www.childhelpusa.org
	KidsPeace National Center for Kids Overcoming Crisis	1-800-8KID-123	www.kidspeace.org
	National Center for Missing & Exploited Children	1-800-THE-LOST	www.ncmec.org
	Prevent Child Abuse America	1-312-663-3520	www.preventchildabuse.org
Contraception	Association of Reproductive Health Professionals	1-202-466-3825	www.arhp.org/patienteducation
	EngenderHealth	1-212-561-8000	www.engenderhealth.org
	Planned Parenthood Federation of America	1-800-230-PLAN	www.ppfa.org
	World Health Organization		www.who.int/health_topics/contraception/en/
Depression	Depression and Bipolar Support Alliance	1-800-826-3632	www.dbsalliance.org
	National Foundation for Depressive Illness	1-800-784-2433	www.depression.org
Domestic Violence	Family Violence Prevention Fund (for clinicians)	1-415-252-8900	http://endabuse.org/programs/healthcare
	Family Violence Prevention Fund (for women)	1-415-252-8900	http://endabuse.org
	National Domestic Violence Hotline	1-800-799-SAFE	www.ndvh.org
	National Resource Center on Domestic Violence	1-800-537-2238	www.pcadv.org
Drug Abuse	Alcohol & Drug Helpline	1-800-821-4357	www.wellplace.com
	Narcotics Anonymous World Services	1-818-773-9999	www.na.org
Eating Disorders	National Association of Anorexia Nervosa and Associated Disorders (ANAD)	1-847-831-3438	www.anad.org
	National Eating Disorders Association	1-800-931-2237	www.nationaleatingdisorders.org
Emergency Contraception	Emergency Contraception Website & Hotline	1-888-NOT-2-LATE	http://not-2-late.com
	Planned Parenthood Federation of America	1-800-230-PLAN	www.ppfa.org/ec

(continued)

Topic	Organization	Hotline	Website
Endometriosis	Endometriosis Association	1-800-992-ENDO	www.EndometriosisAssn.org
Family/parenting	American Academy of Family Physicians	1-800-274-AAFP	www.aafp.org
	American Academy of Pediatrics	1-800-433-9016	www.aap.org
Fitness	Aerobics and Fitness Association of America	1-800-YOUR-BODY	www.afaa.com
Headaches	National Headache Foundation	1-888-NHF-5552	www.headaches.org
Hepatitis	Hepatitis B Coalition	1-651-647-9009	www.immunize.org
Herpes	National Herpes Hotline (ASHA)	1-919-361-8488	www.ashastd.org
HIV/AIDS	AIDSinfo	1-800-HIV-0440	www.aidsinfo.nih.gov/
	American Red Cross	1-202-303-4498	www.redcross.org/services/hss/hivaids
	CDC National HIV/AIDS Hotline		www.cdc.gov/hiv/pubs/facts.htm
	International AIDS Society-USA	1-415-544-9400	www.iasusa.org
	UNAIDS		www.unaids.org
Hospice	National Hospice and Palliative Care Organization	1-800-658-8898	www.nhpco.org
HPV	National HPV and Cervical Cancer Prevention Hotline	1-919-361-4848	www.ashastd.org
Hypertension	American Heart Association	1-800-AHA-USA-1	www.americanheart.org
Infertility	Resolve National Infertility Helpline	1-888-623-0744	www.resolve.org
Interstitial Cystitis	Interstitial Cystitis Association	1-800-HELP-ICA	www.ichelp.org
Lactational Amenorrhea Method	The Linkages Project	1-202-884-8221	www.linkagesproject.org
Menopause	North American Menopause Society	1-440-442-7550	www.menopause.org
Natural Family Planning	FertilityUK		www.fertilityUK.org

(continued)

Topic	Organization	Hotline	Website
Osteoporosis	National Osteoporosis Foundation	1-800-223-9994	www.nof.org
Ovarian Cancer (see also Cancer)	National Ovarian Cancer Coalition	1-888-OVARIAN	www.ovarian.org
Pregnancy, crisis (see also Adoption)	America's Pregnancy Helpline	1-888-672-2296	www.thehelpline.org
Pregnancy, delivery and postpartum	Bradley Method	1-800-4-A-BIRTH	www.bradleybirth.com
	Depression After Delivery, Inc.		www.depressionafterdelivery.com
	Lamaze International	1-800-368-4404	www.lamaze.org
	Postpartum Support International	1-805-967-7636	www.chss.iup.edu/postpartum
Q & A	Go Ask Alice		www.goaskalice.columbia.edu
Sexual Assault	Rape Abuse & Incest National Network	1-800-656-HOPE	www.rainn.org
Sexually Transmitted infections	American Social Health Association	1-800-227-8922	www.ashastd.org
	CDC Sexually Transmitted Disease Hotline	1-800-344-7432	www.cdc.gov/std.html
Smoking	American Cancer Society	1-800-ACS-2345	www.cancer.org
	American Lung Association	1-800-LUNGUSA	www.lungusa.org
Teens	Teenwire		www.teenwire.com
Urinary Incontinence	National Association for Continence	1-800-BLADDER	www.nafc.org
Women's Health	Office of Women's Health (DHHS)	1-800-994-9662	www.4women.gov

Index

Asthma, 208
Atrophy, cervical, 575
Attributable risk, 212
Atypical glandular cells (AGC), 576, 578(t), 579(t)
Atypical squamous cell (ASC), 575–576
Atypical squamous cell of undetermined significance (ASC-US), 565, 571, 575, 576, 577(t)
Auras, migraine, 478
Avanti, 442–443
Azoospermia, 686

B

Bacterial vaginosis (BV), 249, **533–534,** 573–574
Barrier methods. *See also* Diaphragms; Female condoms; Male condoms; Sponges, contraceptive
· advantages, 324–325
· breastfeeding and, 403, 415
· cervical cap, 442
· clinician's role, 329
· disadvantages/cautions, 326–327
· effectiveness, 323
· efficacy, 323
· failure rates, 777(t)–779(t)
· guidelines for use, 328(t), 333–334
· lubricants with, 330
· mechanism of action, 318–321
· medical eligibility criteria for, 58–71
· perimenopause and, 704
· postpartum use, 411–412
· pregnancy, first-year probability of, 322(t)
· problems, managing, 332
· providing, 327–331
· research on, 441–443
· spermicide with, 324
Basal body temperature (BBT), 683
· breastfeeding and, 415
· menstrual cycle and, 13

Bellergal-S, 711–712
Benign breast conditions, 205
Benzalkonium chloride, 318, 442
Beta hCG
· after pregnancy, 600–602, 601(f)
· in pregnancy, 599–600, 599(t)
· serum quantitative assay of, 605–606
· ultrasound and, 609–611
Beta hCG assay, 620–622
Bethesda System classification, 571, 572(t)
"Bi-cycling,", 230
Billings Ovulation Method, 344, 345, 353–354
Binding affinity, 197
Bioavailability, 196
Bioidentical hormones, 713
Biphasic formulations, 200
BI-RADS. *See* Breast Imaging Reporting and Data System
Birth defects, 692–693
Bisphosphonates, 723
Black cohosh, 710–711
Bleeding problems
· abortion and, 661
· IUDs and, 123
Blood clots, 662
Blood loss, 456(t)
· with abortion, 655
· COCs and decreased, 202–203
· levonorgestrel system and, 41, 122
· and menorrhagia, 456–457, 459
· menstrual cycle and, 14
BMD. *See* Bone mineral density
Bone density. *See also* Osteopenia/osteoporosis
· COCs and, 207–208
· DMPA and, 163, 165–167
Bone mass, 721(t)
Bone mineral density (BMD), 207–208, 721
BRCA1, 204–205
· and ovarian cancer, 581
· tubal sterilization and, 366

BRCA2, 205
· and ovarian cancer, 581
· tubal sterilization and, 366
Breast cancer
· abortion and, 665–666
· COCs and, 35–37, 223–224, 257
· DMPA and, 164–165
· menopause and, 707
· postmenopausal hormone therapy and, 729–731
· risk characteristics of, 584(t)
Breast cancer screening, **583–587**
· mammography, 585–587, 586(t)
· techniques, 583–585
Breast conditions
· COCs and, 205, 248
· postmenopausal hormone therapy and, 732
Breastfeeding
· COCs and, 234
· contraception and, 414–420
· DMPA and, 164
· ECPs and, 101
· emergency contraception and, 420
· full/partial/token, 408(f)
· guidelines for, 405(f)
· HIV and, 421–422
· hormonal contraception and, 415–420
· infant, advantages to, 420–421
· instructions/information, 422–424
· lactational infertility and, 404, 406
· LAM contraception and, 407–408
· Medical Eligibility Criteria and, 57-58, 79
· mother, effects on, 422
· nonhormonal contraception and, 414–415
· POPs and, 186
· resource materials for, 424
Breast Imaging Reporting and Data System (BI-RADS), 586, 586(t)
Breastmilk, 403, 404
Breast self-examination (BSE), 583, 584

Breast symptoms, patches and, 275
Broad-spectrum antibiotics, 237
BSE. *See* Breast self-examination
Buccal dose, 647
BufferGel Duet, 442
Bulimia, 465–466
Bupivacaine, 124
BV. *See* Bacterial vaginosis

C

CAD (coronary artery disease), 707
CAH (congenital adrenal hyperplasia), 467
Calcium, 718, 719(t)
· dietary sources of, 719(t)
· PMS and, 473–474
Calendar Rhythm Method, 20, 344, 345, 351–352
Calendars
· migraines charted on, 477
· PMS charted on, 472
Cancer(s). *See also* Breast cancer *and* Cervical cancer
· COCs and, 223(t)
· DMPA and, 164–165
· quinacrine and, 446
· risk of, 35–37
Cancer prevention/protection
· COCs and, 204–207
· IUDs and, 121–122
· tubal sterilization and, 366–367
Candida spp., 573
Candidiasis, **534–535**
Cardiovascular disease (CVD)
· female surgical sterilization procedures, 73–74
· medical eligibility criteria, 60–63
· menopause and, 707
· postmenopausal hormone therapy and, 728
· risk of, 35
Caruncles, 716
Catamenial seizures, 208, **478**
Cautery, 387, 389

Depo-Provera (DMPA)—*continued*
· PMS and, 475
· postpartum use, 410, 411, 414
· precautions, 164
· pregnancy rate with, 24(t)
· primary dysmenorrhea and,
    453–454
· problems, managing, 169–170
· providing, 168–169
· reported use, 20
· reproductive tract
    infections/disorders, 64–67
· schistosomiasis, 68
· STIs and, 167–168
· TSS, history of, 68
· tuberculosis, 68
· user instructions, 170–174
· UTIs, 68
Depo-subQ provera 104 (DMPA-SC
104), 157, 158, 161
Depression
· COCs and, 245–247
· DMPA and, 162–163
· female surgical sterilization
    procedures, 74
· male surgical sterilization
    procedures, 78
· medical eligibility criteria, 64
· PCOS and, 468
DES (diethylstilbestrol), 90
Desogestrel, 145, 151, 182, 183, 185,
196
DEXA (dual-energy X-ray
absorptiometry), 721
Dextronorgestrel, 196
DHEA. *See* Dehydroepiandrosterone
DHEAS (dehydroepiandrosterone
sulfate), 469
Diabetes
· COCs and, 220
· IUDs and, 129
· medical eligibility criteria, 69, 76
· PCOS and, 468
· POPs and, 185

Diaphragms, 320(f)
· allergies, 71
· anemias, 71
· cardiovascular disease, 60–63
· dangers/side effects/benefits, 40(t)
· depressive disorders, 64
· drug interactions, 71
· endocrine conditions, 69
· failure rates, 781(t)–785(t)
· fitting, 330–331
· gastrointestinal conditions, 70
· HIV/AIDS, 68
· improving effectiveness of, 26(f)
· malaria, 68
· medical eligibility criteria for,
    58–71
· neurologic conditions, 64
· as ongoing contraception, 107(t)
· perfect use, 749
· personal characteristics and
    reproductive history, 58–60
· postpartum use, 411
· pregnancy, first-year probability of,
    322(t)
· pregnancy rate with, 24(t)
· reported use, 20
· reproductive tract
    infections/disorders, 64–67
· research on, 442
· schistosomiasis, 68
· with spermicides, 781(t)–785(t)
· TSS, history of, 68
· tuberculosis, 68
· UTIs, 68
Diarrhea, 248
Diazepam, 237
Diet
· osteoporosis and, 718, 719(t)
· PMS and, 473
Diethylstilbestrol (DES), 90
Dilapan, 658
Dilating devices, 658–659
Dilation and evacuation (D&E), 642,
643(f), 645, 657–658

Emergency contraception
(EC)—*continued*
· effectiveness, 86, 96–97
· future potential for, 90–94
· history, 88, 90
· impact of, 434
· initiating ongoing contraception
  after, 107(t)
· mechanism of action, 94–96
· pills (*See* Emergency contraception
  pills)
· and pregnancy probability by cycle
  day, 103(f)
· providing, 102–109
· research on, 443–444
· side effects, 99–100
· usage, 755
· user instructions, 109–110
Emergency contraception pills (ECPs),
87, 88, 89(t), 90–94, 322
· advantages/indications, 97–99
· cautions, 100–101
· counseling for, 102–106
· effectiveness, 96–97
· mechanism of action, 94–95
· providing, 102–108
· side effects, 99–100
· treatment regimen, 106, 107
· user instructions, 109–110
Emergency contraception services,
108–109
Emko, 751
Endocrine conditions
· amenorrhea and, 464–466
· female surgical sterilization
  procedures, 76
· medical eligibility criteria, 69
Endometrial cancer, 205
Endometrial cavity line, 615(f)
Endometrial cells, 575
Endometrial proliferation, 468
Endometriosis, **479–481**
· chronic pelvic pain and, 482
· clinical presentation, 479–480
· COCs and, 206–207

Endometriosis—*continued*
· DMPA and, 160–161
· hormonal therapies for, 487–488
· implants and, 148
· infertility treatment and, 691
· secondary dysmenorrhea and, 455
· treatment, 480–481
Endometrium
· implants and, 148
· menstrual cycle and, 9–10, 12(f)
· POPs and, 182
Enovid, 193–194
Epilepsy, 478
Epithelial cell abnormalities, 575–576
EPT. *See* Estrogen-progestin therapy
Erythromycin, 446–447
"Escape ovulation,", 198
Essure microinsert device, 362, 363,
369, 372, 373, 376, 378, 446
Estradiol, 733
· breastfeeding and, 419
· implants and, 148
· menstrual cycle and, 9, 13
· menstrual cycle and, 10
Estranes, 196
Estriol, 733
Estrogen
· breastfeeding and, 419
· in COCs, 194–195
· implants and, 149
· menopause and, 725
· menstrual cycle and, 8–10, 11(f), 14,
  15, 16
· menstrual migraines and, 476–478
· osteoporosis and, 721, 722
Estrogen dermatitis, 184
Estrogen-progestin therapy (EPT),
712, 714, 722, 727–734
Estrogen therapy (ET), 712, 713, 722
Estrone, 468
Estrostep, 205, 247
ET. *See* Estrogen therapy
Ethinyl estradiol (EE), 88, 92, 194–195,
271, 272, 282, 284, 419, 733
Ethyndiol diacetate, 195

Etonogestrel, 145, 147, 151, 152, 282
Evening primrose oil, 474, 714
Evra patch, 753–754
· dangers/side effects/benefits, 39(t)
· pregnancy rate with, 24(t)
· usage, 753–754
Exercise
· osteoporosis and, 718
· perimenopause and, 703
· PMS and, 473
· pregnancy and, 594, 595
Expectant management, 623
Expelled vaginal ring, 289–290
Expulsion, IUD, 124
Eye problems, 255(f)
EZ-on, 442–443

F

FAB methods. *See* Fertility
  awareness-based methods
FACE (Freedom of Access to Clinic
  Entrances Act), 639
Fallopian tubes, 14–15, 680
Falope Ring, 376
Family planning guidance, four
  cornerstones of, 50, 51
Fascial interposition (vasectomy), 389
FC2 Female Condom, 442
FC Female Condom, 442
Fecundity, 675(t)
Female condoms
· dangers/side effects/benefits, 39(t)
· mechanism of action, 318–320
· pregnancy, first-year probability of,
    322(t)
· pregnancy rate with, 24(t)
· research on, 442
· typical use, 750
Female fertility
· abortion and, 664–665
· evaluation of, 679–681, 681(t), 682(t)
· infertility treatment, 688–691
· requirements for, 676

Female genital tract cancer screening,
  559–587
· breast cancer, 583–587
· cervical cancer, 561–581
· ovarian cancer, 581–582
Female sterilization procedures,
  362–380
· advantages/indications, 364–365
· anesthesia/pain management, 378
· approaches to, 373–375
· counseling guidelines for, 370–372
· disadvantages/cautions, 365–370
· effectiveness, 362–364
· failure rates, 810(t)–814(t)
· follow-up, 378–380
· mechanism of action, 364, 364(f)
· medical eligibility criteria, 72–77
· occlusion method, 375–378
· pregnancy rate with, 24(t)
· problems, managing, 378–380
· providing, 370–378
· reported use, 20
· timing of, 372–373
· usage, 754–755
FemCap, 321, 442
Fertility
· breastfeeding and, 403–404
· COCs and, 255–256
· female (*See* Female fertility)
· male (*See* Male fertility)
· requirements of, 676–677
· secondary dysmenorrhea and, 455
Fertility awareness-based (FAB)
  methods, **343–359**
· advantages/indications, 346
· breastfeeding and, 415
· classification of conditions for, 54
· comparison of methods, 358(t)
· disadvantages/cautions, 347–348
· effectiveness, 344–346
· failure rates, 772(t)–776(t)
· home test kits, 358–359
· improving effectiveness of, 26(f)
· instructions for using, 349–358
· mechanism of action, 343–344

LNG/ETG implants—*continued*
· reproductive tract
infections/disorders, 64–67
· schistosomiasis, 68
· TSS, history of, 68
· tuberculosis, 68
· UTIs, 68
LNG IUD
· allergies, 71
· anemias, 71
· cardiovascular disease, 60–63
· depressive disorders, 64
· drug interactions, 71
endocrine conditions, 69
· gastrointestinal conditions, 70
· HIV/AIDS, 68
· malaria, 68
· medical eligibility criteria for,
58–71
· neurologic conditions, 64
· personal characteristics and
reproductive history, 58–60
· reproductive tract
infections/disorders, 64–67
· schistosomiasis, 68
· TSS, history of, 68
· tuberculosis, 68
· UTIs, 68
LNG-IUS. *See* Levonorgestrel-
releasing intrauterine system
Loestrin 24-Fe, 229
Longitudinal ultrasound, 611, 612(f),
615(f)
Lonidamine, 445
Loop electrosurgical excision (LEEP),
565
Lo-Ovral, 196
Loss-to-follow-up (LFU), 33
Lower genital tract, 463–464
Low-grade squamous intraepithelial
lesions (LSIL), 571, 577(t), 578(t)
Lubricants, oil-based, 330
Lubrication, 307, 307(t), 308, 440–441
LUNA (laparoscopic uterosacral
nerve ablation), 488

Lunelle, 157, 411, 443
Luteal phase, 12(f), 13
Luteinizing hormone (LH), 13
· anovulation and, 15
· breastfeeding and, 404, 406
· menstrual cycle and, 8, 9, 10, 11(f),
16
Lymphogranuloma venereum (LGV),
547–548
Lynestrenol, 195

M

Magnesium, 473
Magnetic field therapy, 489
Male condoms, **297–311**
· advantages/indications, 301
· anal intercourse, use during, 303
· characteristics, 299(t)
· dangers/side effects/benefits, 39(t)
· disadvantages/cautions, 301–302
· effectiveness, 299–301
· failure rates, 786(t)–789(t)
· follow-up, 308
· history, 298
· improving effectiveness of, 26(f),
306–308
· and lubricants, 307(t)
· mechanism of action, 298–299
· options, 298, 299
· oral intercourse, use during, 303
· perfect use, 752
· pregnancy, first-year probability of,
322(t)
· pregnancy probability, 300(t)
· pregnancy rate with, 24(t)
· problems, managing, 308
· promotion of, 304
· providing, 304–308
· reported use of, 20
· research on, 442–443
· special issues, 302–304
· STI protection, 302–303
· storage of, 310–311
· user instructions, 308–311

Menopause—*continued*
· postmenopause, symptoms of,
708–724
· vasomotor symptoms, 709–714
Menorrhagia, 451, **456–460**
· evaluation, 458
· treatment, 458–460
Menstrual calendars, 456, 682
Menstrual changes
· DPMA and, 169–170
· ECPs and, 100
· POPs and, 183
Menstrual cycle, **7–16**
· aging and, 15
· anovulation and, 15
· anterior pituitary and, 8
· cervical secretion variations chart,
355(f)
· cervix and, 10
· DMPA and, 161–162
· endometrium and, 9–10
· fertility and, 679–680
· fertilization and, 14
· follicular phase, 10, 11(f), 12(f), 13
· hormonal contraceptives and,
15–16
· hypothalamus and, 8
implantation and, 14–15
· integrated, 10–14
· luteal phase, 13
· menstrual phase, 13–14
· ovulatory phase, 13
· peptide hormones in ovaries, 9
· POPs and, 184
· pregnancy probability by day of,
103(t)
· regularity of, 31
· regulation of, 8–10, 11(f), 12(f)
· steroid production in ovaries, 8–9
· symptothermal variations during,
357(f)
Menstrual cycle regulation, 8–10,
11(f), 12(f)
· cervix and, 10
· COCs for, 203

Menstrual cycle regulation—*continued*
· endometrium and, 9–10
· peptide hormones in ovaries, 9
· steroid production in ovaries, 8–9
Menstrual migraines, 204, **476–478**
Menstrual phase, 12(f), 13–14
Menstrual problems, **451–489**
· amenorrhea, 461–466, 462(f), 464(f)
· DUB characteristics/treatments,
460(t)
· dysmenorrhea, 451–454
· endometriosis, 479–481
· IUDs and, 123
· medical problems and, 476–479
· menorrhagia, 456–460
· normal values, ranges, 456(t)
· NSAIDs, 459(t)
· oligomenorrhea, 466–469
· pelvic pain, chronic, 481–489
· PMS/PMDD, 469–476, 470(t)
· tubal sterilization and, 367
Menstrual-related migraines, 476
Mestranol, 194–195
Metformin, 690
Methergine, 659
Method failure rates, 32–33
Methotrexate, 643, 646, 648
Metrorrhagia, 456
MI. *See* Myocardial infarction
Microbicides, 439–441
Mifeprex, 90
Mifepristone, 90, 443–444, 642–649,
648(t), 651, 652, 655, 658
Migraine headaches, 204, 245, 476–478
Minerals, 473–474
Minilaparoscopy, 377(t), 379
Minilaparotomy, 373, 375(f), 413
Minipills. *See* Progestin-only pills
Mircette, 228
Mirena IUDs, 445
· blood loss and, 41
· insertion instructions, **135–138,**
135(f)–138(f)
· pregnancy rate with, 24(t)
· vaginal ring and, 288

No-scalpel vasectomy (NSV), 386, 387, 388(f)

NSAIDs. *See* Non-steroidal anti-inflammatory drugs

NSV. *See* No-scalpel vasectomy

Nulliparity, 128

NuvaRing®, 282, 283, 286–292, 753–754
· dangers/side effects/benefits, 39(t)
· pregnancy rate with, 24(t)
· usage, 754

O

Obesity
· DMPA and, 159
· patches and, 276
· perimenopause and, 702–703

Occlusion methods
· electrocoagulation, 376
· female, 375–378, 377(t)
· male, 387, 389
· mechanical, 376, 378

OCs. *See* Oral contraceptives

Oil-based lubricants, 330

Oligomenorrhea, **466–469**

Omega-3 polyunsaturated fatty acids, 454

OMI (oocyte maturation inhibitor), 9

Ongoing contraception, 107(t)

Oocyte maturation inhibitor (OMI), 9

Oocytes, 7, 13–15

Opioids, 487

Oral contraceptives (OCs)
· as emergency contraceptives, 89(t)
· first, 435
· perfect use, 753
· postpartum use, 411
· reported use, 20

Oral dose, 647

Oral intercourse, 303

Organic gynecologic disease, 457

Organon, 146

Organ trauma, 662–663

Orlistat, 238

Ortho Evra®, 271, 272, 275, 277, 278

Ortho TriCyclen, 196, 205, 247

Osmotic dilating devices, 658–659

Osteopenia/osteoporosis, 716–724
· drug therapies for, 721–724
· medical conditions with increased risk of, 720(t)
· prevention measures for, 718–719
· risk factors for, 720(t)
· screening for, 719–721

OTC drugs. *See* Over-the-counter drugs

Ovarian cancer, 731
· COCs and, 204–205
· screening, 581–582
· tubal sterilization and, 366–367

Ovarian cysts
· COCs and, 204
· implants and, 150
· POPs and, 185

Ovarian reserve, 683

Ovaries
· amenorrhea and, 464–466
· anovulation and, 15
· breastfeeding and, 404
· menstrual cycle and, 11(f), 12(f)
· peptide hormones in, 9
· steroid production in, 8–9
· tubal sterilization and, 367

Over-the-counter (OTC) drugs, 93–94

Oves cap, 442

Ovrette, 88, 90

Ovulation Method, 24(t)

Ovulation suppressants, 475, 476

Ovulatory dysfunction, 681–683

Ovulatory menorrhagia, 460(t)

Ovulatory phase, 13

Oxytocin, 422, 659

P

Pain
· IUDs and, 123–124
· tubal ligation and management of, 378

Spermicides—*continued*
· reproductive tract
infections/disorders, 64–67
· research on, 439–441
· schistosomiasis, 68
· TSS, history of, 68
· tuberculosis, 68
· UTIs, 68
· vaginal barriers with, 324
Spironolactone, 196, 475
Sponges, contraceptive, 321(f)
· dangers/side effects/benefits, 40(t)
· failure rates, 780(t)
· mechanism of action, 320
· as ongoing contraception, 107(t)
· perfect use, 749
· postpartum use, 411–412
· pregnancy, first-year probability of,
322(t)
· pregnancy rate with, 24(t)
· research on, 441–442
· typical use, 750
Spontaneous abortion, **624–625**
Spotting, 242–243, 732
Squamous epithelium, 562
Squamous intraepithelial lesions
(SILs), 565, 580–581
SSRIs. *See* Selective serotonin
reuptake inhibitors
Stages of reproductive life, 42(t),
700(f)
Standard Days Method, 24(t), 344,
345, 349–350, 350(f), 351(t)
Stein-Leventhal syndrome. *See*
Polycystic ovarian syndrome
(PCOS)
Sterilization procedures
· dangers/side effects/benefits, 40(t)
· as ongoing contraception, 107(t)
· perimenopause and, 704–705
· research on, 446–447
· surgical (*See* Surgical sterilization
procedures)
· usage, 754–755

Steroids
· breastfeeding and, 404, 415–416,
419
· epilepsy and, 478
· menstrual cycle and, 8–9
· production, 8–9, 404
STIs. *See* Sexually transmitted
infections
STRAW Regime recommendations,
700(f)
Strings, IUD, 125
Stroke
· COCs and, 214–216
· headaches and, 245
· postmenopausal hormone therapy
and, 728–729
Stromal tissue, 13
Subfertility, 674
Sublingual dose, 647
Sub Q 104 DMPA, 480
Substance abuse, 475
Subumbilical minilaparotomy, 377(t)
Sunday start, 227–228
Suppositories, spermicide, 321–322
Suppressed estrogen production, 466
Suppression of testicular cells,
444–445
Suprapubic minilaparoscopy, 377(t)
Supreme Court, U.S., 638
Surgery
· for chronic pelvic pain, 488
· as infertility treatment, 690–691
· for menorrhagia, 460
Surgical sterilization procedures,
361–394
· anemias, 77, 78
· cardiovascular disease, 73–74
· classification of conditions for,
53–54
· depressive disorders, 74, 78
· endocrine conditions, 76, 78
· female (*See* Female sterilization
procedures)
· gastrointestinal conditions, 76
· HIV/AIDS, 75

Surgical sterilization
procedures—*continued*
· malaria, 76
· male (*See* Vasectomy)
· medical eligibility criteria, 72–78
· neurologic conditions, 74
· personal characteristics and
reproductive history, 72–73, 78
· postpartum, 410, 412–413
· reproductive tract
infections/disorders, 74–75
· research on, 446–447
· schistosomiasis, 75
· tuberculosis, 75
Symptothermal Method, 345–346, 356,
357, 357(f), 415
Synthetic condoms, 298, 299, 299(t)
Synthetic hygroscopic dilators, 658
Syphilis, **551–552**
Systemic methods, 444–445

T

Tamoxifen, 730
TCu 380A. *See* Copper T 380A IUDs
Telangiectasias, 247
TENS (transcutaneous electrical nerve
stimulation), 454
Tension headaches, 244–245
Teratogens, 628–629, 643
Testosterone, 206, 444–445
Testosterone patches, 724
Testosterone undecanoate (TU), 445
Theophylline, 237
Thin layer preparation technique, 562
Third generation progestins, 196
Three-month injectable, 107(t)
Thromboembolic conditions
· implants and, 151
· patches and, 274–275
· POPs and, 185
· postpartum, 413–414
· vaginal ring and, 285–286
Thyroxine stimulating hormone
(TSH), 463, 465

Tibolone, 713, 723
Tissue evaluation, 622–623
Today contraceptive sponge, 441
Topical ET/EPT, 733
Toxic shock syndrome (TSS)
· diaphragm and, 319, 334
· history of, 68
· vaginal barriers and, 326, 328–329
· vaginal ring and, 286
Transabdominal tubal sterilization,
373, 379–380
Transcervical tubal sterilization, 373,
374, 375(f), 377(t), 378, 446
Transcutaneous electrical nerve
stimulation (TENS), 454
Transdermal contraceptive patch, 271
Transverse ultrasound, 611, 612(f)
Trichomonas, 573
Trichomoniasis, **552–553**
Tricyclic antidepressants, 237
"Tri-cycling," 230
Trimester framework, 638
Triphasic formulations, 200
TSH. *See* Thyroxine stimulating
hormone
TSS. *See* Toxic shock syndrome
TU (testosterone undecanoate), 445
Tubal damage
· fertility and, 684–685
· infertility treatment and, 691
Tubal ligation
· breastfeeding and, 414
· methods of, 378
· postpartum, 413
Tubal reversal surgery, 369 370
Tubal sterilization, 361
· failure rate, 120
· hysterectomy and, 368
· interval, 372
· postabortion, 373
· postpartum, 372
· safety, 365–366
· sexuality and, 368
Tuberculosis, 68, 75
Turner's syndrome, 464, 680

TwoDay Method, 24(t), 344, 345, 352, 352(f), 353, 415
Typical use, 23, 24(t)–25(t), 25

U

Uchida method, 378
Ultrasound, 609–618, 685
· beta hCG and, 609–611
· choriodecidual reaction, 614(f), 615(f)
· earliest visualization with, 611–618
· eccentric implantation, 615(f)
· ectopic pregnancy and, 623
· free fluid in cul-de-sac, 617(f)
· landmark timings and, 610(t)
· longitudinal/transverse view, 612(f)
· osteoporosis and, 721
· pseudosac, 616(f), 617(f)
· yolk sac, 618(f)
Unintended pregnancy(-ies), 434, 759(t)–760(t)
· contraceptive failure and, 20–22
· number of, 19
Unopposed estrogen, 466
Upper-genital-tract infection, 125–127
Urethritis, **553–554**
Urinary tract infection (UTI)
· medical eligibility criteria, 68
· menopause and, 715–716
· vaginal barriers and, 332, 333
Urine tests, pregnancy
· high-sensitivity, 602–604
· reduced-sensitivity, 604–605
User characteristics, 30–31
Uterine abnormalities, 685–686
Uterine bleeding, 149–150, 457–458
Uterine cancer, 729
Uterine fibroids, 207, 222, 455
Uterotonic agents, 659
Uterus
· abortion and trauma to, 662–663
· amenorrhea and, 463–464
· fertility and, 680

Uterus—*continued*
· menstrual cycle and, 11(f)
· pregnancy and size of, 599(t)
· ultrasound of, 611
UTI. *See* Urinary tract infection

V

VA feminine condom, 442
Vagina
· bleeding, 154
· irritation, 440–441
· lubrication, 422
· menopause and, 715
· vaginal ring and, 286, 290
Vaginal barriers. *See* Barrier methods
Vaginal cream, 733
Vaginal discharge, 249
Vaginal ring, **282–292**
· advantages, 283–285
· allergies, 71
· anemias, 71
· breastfeeding and, 417
· cardiovascular disease, 60–63
· depressive disorders, 64
· description, 282
· disadvantages/cautions, 285–287
· disconnected/broken, 290
· drug interactions, 71
· effectiveness, 282–283
· endocrine conditions, 69
· estradiol-releasing, 733
· expelled, 289–290
· failure rates, 793(t)–802(t)
· follow-up, 289–291
· gastrointestinal conditions, 70
· HIV/AIDS, 68
· improving effectiveness of, 26(f)
· inserting NuvaRing, 291(f)
· malaria, 68
· mechanism of action, 283
· medical eligibility criteria for, 58–71
· neurologic conditions, 64
· as ongoing contraception, 107(t)

WHO. *See* World Health
  Organization
Wide-seal diaphragms, 319, 320
Withdrawal. *See* Coitus interruptus
Women's Health Initiative (WHI),
  725(t)
Women's reproductive rights,
  638–639
World Health Organization (WHO),
  49–56

Y

Yaz, 228–229
Yolk sac, 618(f)
Yuzpe regimen, 88

Z

ZIFT (zygote intra-fallopian transfer),
  688(t)
Zona pellucida binding of sperm, 444
Zygote intra-fallopian transfer (ZIFT),
  688(t)

Notes

Notes

Notes

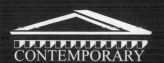

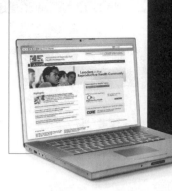
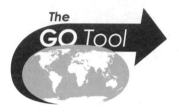
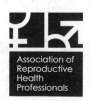

Contraceptive Technology

❏ CD-ROM
Registration is required to activate your CD-ROM.
If you have already purchased, please include your receipt or proof of purchase.
If purchasing, please include the order form in the back of this
book along with your payment.
(See other side of this form for address.)

or

❏ New Media Survey

ABOUT YOU

1. Educational degree: _____
   Note: *If you're a student, list degree you're studying for and expected date of graduation.*

2. Describe your current position: _____

3. Circle your most important site of work:

   Managed care organization   Private practice   Health department

   Family planning clinic   Hospital   Other _____

4. Circle the number of women you have provided personal contraceptive or STI services in the past year:

   None   1-10   11-100   101-500   501-5000   More than 5000

5. I use a ❏ PDA or ❏ laptop while counseling patients. *(please check one or both)*
   PDA device type: _____

6. Name and address:
   Name _____
   Organization/Institution _____
   Address _____
   _____
   City _____ State _____ Zip _____
   Fax _____
   Email _____
   Website URL _____
   ❏ I am interested in linking my health related website to yours.

   (Please complete the Form found on the back of this page.)

   Thank you for taking the time to help us serve you better!

   Please photocopy or clip out both pages of this form and mail to:

   Ardent Media Inc.
   Box 286 Cooper Station P.O.
   New York, New York 10276-0286
   Please mail it along with your order.

Contraceptive Technology

❏ CD-ROM

*If you have already purchased, please include your receipt or proof of purchase.
If purchasing, please include the order form in the back of this
book along with your payment.
(See other side of this form for address.)*

or

❏ New Media Survey

As our thank you for completing this form and the ABOUT YOU form on the adjoining page, you will receive a special prepublication discount on future new media published by us.

In addition, the most helpful surveys will receive a free copy of *Safety Sexual* upon publication.

1. Would you be interested in having access to an electronic version of *Safely Sexual* or *Contraceptive Technology* if it were offered on the Internet, PDA or on a CD-ROM?
   ❏ **CT**   ❏ **Safely Sexual**   ❏ **CD-ROM**   ❏ **PDA**   ❏ **Internet**

2. Would you be interested in receiving electronic updates of *Contraceptive Technology* and/or *Safely Sexual* with new developments in the field?
   ❏ **CT**   ❏ **Safely Sexual**   ❏ **Both**

3. How often would you like to receive electronic updates?
   ❏ Every 3 months   ❏ Every 6 months   ❏ Other _____

4. What would you consider a fair price for an update as often as you specified above of a chapter or the entire *CT* book?
   Chapter $_____   Book $ _____

5. Would you be interested primarily in receiving electronic updates of specific chapters of CT? If yes, please specify your top 5 choices in order of preference by chapter number.
   1 _____   2 _____   3 _____   4 _____   5 _____

6. Let us know if you are interested in a CT and Safely Sexual CD-ROM or PDA:
   ❏   I am interested in a CD-ROM of   ❏ *CT*   ❏ *Safely Sexual* to printout information for patients.
   ❏   I am interested in a CD-ROM of   ❏ *CT*   ❏ *Safely Sexual* with additional information.
   Such as: ❏ audio ❏ video ❏ color graphics
   ❏ selected readings or source material
   ❏   I am interested in approximately ___ copies of a ❏ **CD-ROM** ❏ **PDA** for ❏ *CT* ❏ *Safely Sexual*.
   ❏   I am part of a network of ___ users and would like information on a net work license or bulk purchase of ___ copies of a ❏ *CT* ❏ *SS* on ❏ **CD-ROM** ❏ **PDA**.
   ❏   I am interested in a ❏ CD-ROM ❏ PDA with high-end capabilities such as searching with Boolean logic, word proximity, and key words or phrases for ❏ *CT* ❏ *SS*.

7. What could we do to improve the book and electronic media to make it more useful to you?

8. What type of PDA do you have? _____

Please use additional sheet re: above questions 1-7 with your specific suggestions.

Please complete the other side of this form.

PLEASE PHOTOCOPY THIS FORM OR CUT OUT AND MAIL TO ARDENT MEDIA, INC. BOX 286, COOPER STATION P.O., NEW YORK. NY 10276-0286

ARDENT MEDIA INC
is pleased to announce the birth of:
CONTRACEPTIVE TECHNOLOGY

in PDF format on CD-ROM
Included with purchase of book and sold separately

For the first time, *Contraceptive Technology* (CT) books also include a CD-ROM with the complete text of CT in direct electronic conversion. Jump links are included so that you can go directly from the table of contents to any chapter or any topic listed in the subheads in the contents. Electronic links are included to the 300 Web sites recommended by the authors so that you can go online with your electronic version of CT and access instantly a wealth of helpful information to complement CT. This electronic format also enables you to quickly perform a keyword search of the entire book, including tables and footnotes, to help speed up the process of finding the information you need. As well, you will be able to quickly print out patient instructions for those you counsel, or other content for your own use.

Please read this overview BEFORE opening your CD-ROM.

Please save your receipt if you have purchased or when you do purchase the CD-ROM or book/CD combo. Your purchase information will be needed to register your product.

Each CD-ROM is for a single-user only unless you purchase a network license. The CD-ROM is protected and you must register it to receive a password to unlock and view the electronic document. In addition, you must have the CD-ROM in your drive to view the electronic document. You may register your CD-ROM at www.contraceptivemedia.com.

If you are considering the purchase of additional CD-ROMs, but are not sure if it is right for the needs of your organization, we ask that you fill out and send in the New Media Survey in the back of this book. Please include your specific needs and we will help you meet those needs.

For organizations with multiple computer users, we can provide either bulk quantity CD-ROMs at a discount, or you can purchase a network license if your computers are networked. Please fill out the New Media Survey in the back of this book, describe your needs and send it to us so that we can provide a solution. If your organization desires the ability to cut and paste for use within the network, a network license must be purchased as this function is not supported on single-user CD-ROMs.

You may use the CD-ROM on your computer or workstation but may not copy it or reproduce it through a LAN or other network.

If you or your organization wish to print out, reproduce or distribute any of the content on the CD for a purpose other than individual counseling or use (for example, for a class, workshop or seminar with multiple participants) please send us the New Media Survey near the back of this book or fill out the Survey on either of our websites describing your permissions request and we will contact you with a solution to obtain the written permission you need for a network license, other license, or provide you bulk CDs at a discount.

Hardware requirements:
PC or Mac with CD-ROM Drive

Software requirements:
PC; Win 95 or greater
Mac; OS 7 or greater

IMPORTANT: Access to the internet is required to register online. If you do not have internet access, please fill out the Registration Form in the back of this book.

Please carefully read the complete Single-User Purchaser Agreement for the CD-ROM at http://www.contraceptivemedia.com/terms before opening the CD-ROM package. CD-ROMs are returnable only if defective, and will be replaced in that event. By clicking on "I Agree" when you register, you are agreeing to be bound by the terms of the Purchaser Agreement.

ACCESSING THE CD ON A PC:
Place the CD in the CD Drive. A menu with instructions should automatically start. If you do not see a menu come up, navigate to your CD drive and click on CDRUN.EXE. Follow the on screen instructions to register and activate the CD-ROM.

ACCESSING THE CD ON A MAC:
Place the CD in the CD Drive. A menu with instructions should automatically start. If you do not see a menu come up, navigate to your CD drive and click on MACRUN.APP. Follow the on screen instructions to register and activate the CD-ROM.

Please visit our new web site to order or for more information:
contraceptivemedia.com

Thank you for helping *Contraceptive Technology* enter the electronic era.

ARDENT MEDIA INC.
Box 286 Cooper Station P.O.
New York, New York 10276-0286

Please Print Clearly

Name _____

Address _____

City _____

State _____ Zip _____

Telephone _____

Fax _____

Email _____

Method of Payment: ☐ Purchase Order enclosed (Institutions only)
☐ Check ☐ Money Order ☐ MasterCard ☐ Visa

Credit Card #: _____

Expiration Date _____

Name on Card _____
(Please Print Above)

Signature _____

Contact Ardent Media for discount information on bulk orders (*Managing Contraception*: 100 copies or more) at our fax 212-861-0998, phone 212-861-1501 or write to our New York address listed on this page. Please see reverse side for more information on bulk discounts.

Prices are subject to change without notice. All sales final. No returns. Our standard returns policy applies for bookstores.

Subtotal

10% Postage and handling (minimum $2.50)
International shipping additional (minimum $10.00)

NY residents add sales tax (NYC 8.875%)

TOTAL DUE (US funds only)

ORDER FORM

Ardent Media Inc Federal ID # 13-3984679

Managing Contraception
For Your Pocket
2007-2009 Edition
by Mimi Zieman, MD et al.

Description	Unit Price	Quantity	Total
3.5"x5.5" Paperback - 196 pages	$10.00		
ISBN 978-0-9794395-0-6			
ISBN 0-9794395-0-6			

- Most recent WHO Medical Eligibility Criteria
- Implanor — Now Available! Find out how to be trained and much, much more!
- New info on HPV vaccine
- How to order and stock IUDs and Implanon
- Updated NEW medical evidence
- Screening & Risk Assessment by Age
- Counseling, Sexual HX/Dysfunction, Adolescent Issues
- Perimenopause, Menopause, HRT
- Pregnancy Preplanning/Tests, PF, Termination
- Timing Issues, Choosing a Method, Failure Rates
- Abstinence, Breast-Feeding, FAM
- Barriers: Cap, Diaphragm, Spermicides, Withdrawal
- Emergency Contraception: COCS, POPS, IUD, RU-486
- Updated CDC STI Guidelines
- Combined Contraceptives: Pills, Patches, Injections, Rings

ARDENT MEDIA INC
Ordering Information
1-800-218-1535

Credit card orders (VISA or Mastercard) or institutional purchase orders may be placed toll-free 9AM-5PM EST weekdays at the above telephone number.

Credit card orders (VISA or Mastercard) or institutional purchase orders may be faxed toll free 24 hours to 1-800-711-3724.

or

Please photocopy or clip the Order Form on the opposite side and mail with your check, money order, credit card information, or purchase order to: ARDENT MEDIA INC Box 286, Cooper Station P.O., New York, NY 10276-0286

or

Visit the website of ARDENT MEDIA INC
www.ardentmediainc.com

The 2007-2009 edition of *Managing Contraception* is current until publication of the next edition, scheduled for release in early 2010. Please write or fax ARDENT MEDIA to be notified of the publication of the next edition and receive a prepublication discount offer. Please state if you are a nonprofit organization and the number of copies you are interested in purchasing. Also check our website listed above for further information, sign up for email notification and prepublication discount offer.

Bulk Purchase Discounts: Managing Contraception. Minimum quantity for bulk discount is 100 copies. Please state if you are a nonprofit organization and the number of copies you are interested in purchasing. Bulk discount orders are nonreturnable. Please contact Special Sales Department at 212-861-1501, fax 212-861-0998 or write the address above.

Note to Book sellers:
All returns require written permission from the publisher.
Please fax to 1-800-711-3124 for permission.

ARDENT MEDIA INC
is pleased to announce that it's expecting
the birth in Fall 2009 of

SAFELY SEXUAL
Formatted for CD-ROM
and other electronic formats

This single-user version now being completed will be a direct electronic conversion on CD-ROM, including word searching capability and the ability to print out patient instructions. Visit our web site in early Fall 2009 to see information about accessing *Safely Sexual* in electronic format. For information on other direct electronic conversions of *Safely Sexual*, such as media for PDAs, eBooks, Kindle or online access, please visit ardentmediainc.com or email info@ardentmediainc.com.

Some of the exciting features that will be available with many electronic formats are:

- •Keyword Search
- •Notes
- •Bookmarks
- •Tables and Figures

If you have special requests, please call us, email us at info@ardentmediainc.com, or mail the New Media Survey near the back of this book. Please include your email address so we can notify you of pre-publication offers, such as a sample chapter in various electronic formats that we will make available for download. Please specify your preferred format.

For organizations with multiple computer users, we can provide either bulk quantity CD-ROMs at a discount, or you can purchase a network license if your computers are networked. Please fill out the New Media Survey in the back of this book, describe your needs and send it to us so that we can provide a solution. If your organization desires the ability to cut and paste for use within the network, a network license must be purchased as this function is not supported on single-user CD-ROMs.

Please visit our web site to order or for more information:
ardentmediainc.com

Please call Ardent Media at 1-800-218-1535 or
email info@ardentmediainc.com for more information.

Thank you for your interest in this exciting new way to access *Safely Sexual*.

Ardent Media invites you to link your health related web site to www.ardentmediainc.com and/or www.contraceptivemedia.com. Please email info@ardentmediainc.com for inquiries.

ARDENT MEDIA INC.
Box 286 Cooper Station P.O.
New York, New York 10276-0286

Please Print Clearly

Name _____
Address _____
City _____
State _____ Zip _____
Telephone _____
Fax _____
Email _____
Method of Payment: ❑ Purchase Order enclosed (Institutions only)
❑ Check ❑ Money Order ❑ MasterCard ❑ Visa
Credit Card #: _____
Expiration Date _____
Name on Card _____
(Please Print Above)
Signature _____

Contact Ardent Media for discount information on bulk orders (*Contraceptive Technology*: 25 copies or more) at our fax 212-861-0998, phone 212-861-1501 or write to our New York address listed on this page. Please see reverse side for more information on bulk discounts.

Prices are subject to change without notice. All sales final. No returns. Our standard returns policy applies for bookstores.

Subtotal
10% Postage and handling (minimum $8.00)
International shipping additional (minimum $12.00)
NY residents add sales tax (NYC 8.875%)
TOTAL DUE (US funds only)

ORDER FORM
Ardent Media Inc Federal ID # 13-3984679

NOW AVAILABLE
Contraceptive Technology- New 19th Edition
New STD Treatment Guidelines • Medical Eligibility Criteria for Contraceptive Use

Description	Unit Price	Quantity	Total
Hardback with Single-User CD-ROM ISBN 978-1-59708-002-6 ISBN 1-59708-002-0	$99.95		
Paperback with Single-User CD-ROM ISBN 978-1-59708-001-9 ISBN 1-59708-001-2	$79.95		
Single-User CD-ROM (PC or MAC Compatible Electronic Edition) ISBN 978-1-59708-003-3 ISBN 1-59708-003-9	$59.95		

Note: Please send the New Media Form along with your order.

You may also order online at contraceptivemedia.com

ARDENT MEDIA INC
Ordering Information
1-877-CT2-3360

Credit card orders (VISA or Mastercard) or institutional purchase orders may be placed toll-free 9AM-5PM EST weekdays at the above telephone number.

Credit card orders (VISA or Mastercard) or institutional purchase orders may be faxed toll free 24 hours to 1-800-711-3724.

or

Please photocopy or clip the Order Form on the opposite side and mail with your check, money order, credit card information, or purchase order to:
ARDENT MEDIA INC Box 286, Cooper Station P.O., New York, NY 10276-0286

or

Visit our new website
www.contraceptivemedia.com

This 19th edition of *Contraceptive Technology* is current until publication of the 20th edition, scheduled for release in Spring 2011. Please write or fax ARDENT MEDIA to be notified of the publication of the 20th edition and receive a prepublication discount offer. Please state if you are a nonprofit organization and the number of copies you are interested in purchasing. Also check our website listed above for further information, sign up for email notification and prepublication discount offer.

Bulk Purchase Discounts: Contraceptive Technology. For discounts on orders of 25 copies or more please call 212-861-1501, fax 212-861-0998 or write the address above. Please state if you are a nonprofit organization and the number of copies you are interested in purchasing. Bulk discount orders are nonreturnable. *Note:* Any of the ISBNs listed for *Contraceptive Technology,* including the electronic formats, may be combined to qualify for the 25 copy minimum: for example, 10 paperbacks, 10 hardbacks, and 5 CD-ROMs.

Note to Book sellers:
All returns require written permission and label from the publisher. Write to the address above or fax to the number above for permission.

ARDENT MEDIA INC.
Box 286 Cooper Station P.O.
New York, New York 10276-0286

ORDER FORM
Ardent Media Inc Federal ID # 13-3984679

NOW AVAILABLE
Contraceptive Technology • **New 19th Edition**
New STD Treatment Guidelines • Medical Eligibility Criteria for Contraceptive Use

Description	Unit Price	Quantity	Total
Hardback with Single-User CD-ROM SBN 978-1-59708-002-6 SBN 1-59708-002-0	$99.95		
Paperback with Single-User CD-ROM ISBN 978-1-59708-001-9 ISBN 1-59708-001-2	$79.95		
Single-User CD-ROM (PC or MAC Compatible Electronic Edition) ISBN 978-1-59708-003-3 ISBN 1-59708-003-9	$59.95		

Note: Please send the New Media Form along with your order.
You may also order online at contraceptivemedia.com

Please Print Clearly

Name _____
Address _____
City _____ Zip _____
State _____
Telephone _____
Fax _____
Email _____
Method of Payment: ❑ Purchase Order enclosed (Institutions only)
❑ Check ❑ Money Order ❑ MasterCard ❑ Visa
Credit Card #: _____
Expiration Date _____
Name on Card _____
(Please Print Above)
Signature _____

Contact Ardent Media for discount information on bulk orders (*Contraceptive Technology* 25 copies or more) at our fax 212-861-0998, phone 212-861-1501 or write to our New York address listed on this page. Please see reverse side for more information on bulk discounts.

Prices are subject to change without notice. All sales final. No returns. Our standard returns policy applies for bookstores.

Subtotal
10% Postage and handling (minimum $8.00)
International shipping additional (minimum $12.00)
NY residents add sales tax (NYC 8.875%)
TOTAL DUE (US funds only)

ARDENT MEDIA INC
Ordering Information
1-877-CT2-3360

Credit card orders (VISA or Mastercard) or institutional purchase orders may be placed toll-free 9AM-5PM EST weekdays at the above telephone number.

Credit card orders (VISA or Mastercard) or institutional purchase orders may be faxed toll free 24 hours to 1-800-711-3724.

or

Please photocopy or clip the Order Form on the opposite side and mail with your check, money order, credit card information, or purchase order to: ARDENT MEDIA INC Box 286, Cooper Station P.O., New York, NY 10276-0286

or

Visit our new website
www.contraceptivemedia.com

This 19th edition of *Contraceptive Technology* is current until publication of the 20th edition, scheduled for release in Spring 2011. Please write or fax ARDENT MEDIA to be notified of the publication of the 20th edition and receive a prepublication discount offer. Please state if you are a nonprofit organization and the number of copies you are interested in purchasing. Also check our website listed above for further information, sign up for email notification and prepublication discount offer.

Bulk Purchase Discounts: Contraceptive Technology. For discounts on orders of 25 copies or more please call 212-861-1501, fax 212-861-0998 or write the address above. Please state if you are a nonprofit organization and the number of copies you are interested in purchasing. Bulk discount orders are nonreturnable. *Note:* Any of the ISBNs listed for *Contraceptive Technology,* including the electronic formats, may be combined to qualify for the 25 copy minimum: for example, 10 paperbacks, 10 hardbacks, and 5 CD-ROMs.

Note to Book sellers:
All returns require written permission and label from the publisher. Write to the address above or fax to the number above for permission.